Study Guide

Today's Medical Assistant

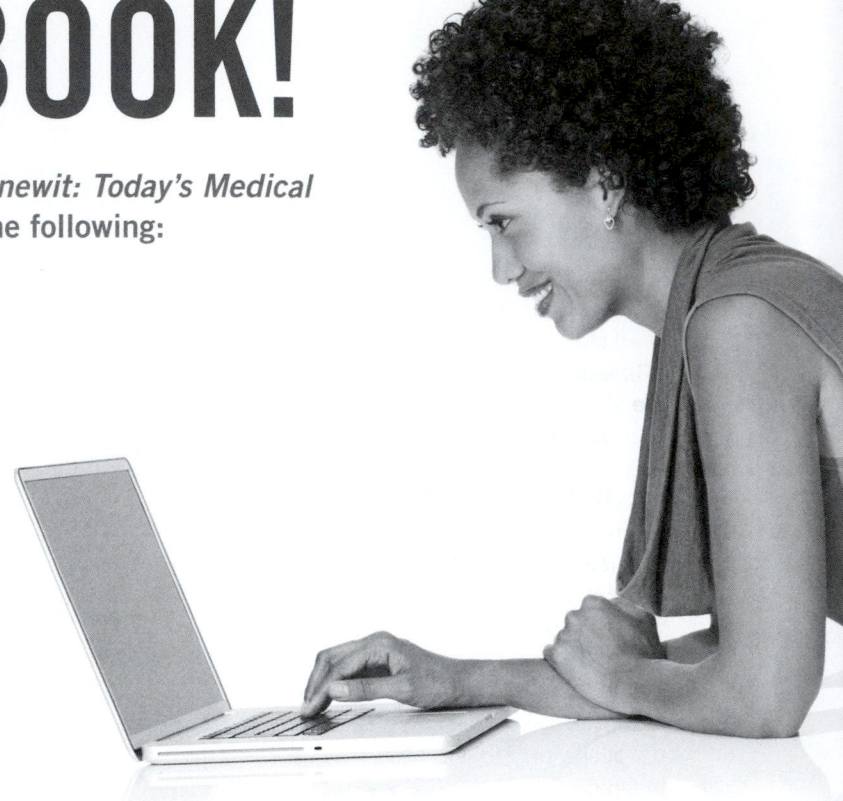

Study Guide

Today's Medical Assistant: Clinical and Administrative Procedures

Third Edition

Kathy Bonewit-West, BS, MEd
Coordinator and Instructor
Medical Assistant Program
Hocking College
Nelsonville, Ohio
Former Member, Curriculum Review Board of the American Association of Medical Assistants

Sue A. Hunt, MA, RN, CMA (AAMA)
Professor Emeritus
Medical Assisting Program
Middlesex Community College
Lowell, Massachusetts

Edith Applegate, MS
Professor of Biological Sciences
Kettering College of Medical Arts
Kettering, Ohio

ELSEVIER

ELSEVIER

3251 Riverport Lane
St. Louis, Missouri 63043

STUDY GUIDE FOR TODAY'S MEDICAL ASSISTANT: CLINICAL AND ADMINISTRATIVE PROCEDURES, THIRD EDITION ISBN: 978-0-323-31128-1

This book and the individual contributions contained in it are protected under copyright by the Publisher (other than as may be noted herein).

Previous editions copyrighted 2013 and 2009.

International Standard Book Number: 978-0-323-31128-1

Executive Content Strategist: Jennifer Janson
Content Development Manager: Luke Held
Senior Content Development Specialist: Jennifer Bertucci
Publishing Services Manager: Julie Eddy
Book Production Specialist: Celeste Clingan
Design Direction: Maggie Reid

Printed in the United States of America

Last digit is the print number: 9 8 7 6

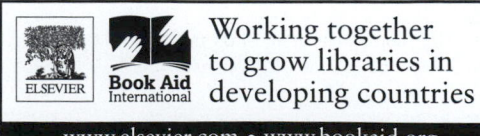

Preface

Outcome-based education prepares individuals to perform the prespecified tasks of an occupation under real-world conditions at a level of accuracy and speed required of the entry-level practitioner of that profession. Outcome-based education plays an important role in medical assisting programs in preparing qualified individuals for careers in medical offices, clinics, and related health care facilities. The *Study Guide for Today's Medical Assistant* has been developed using a thorough outcome-based approach. It meets the criteria stipulated by the Commission on Accreditation of Allied Health Education (CAAHEP)* Standards and Guidelines for the Medical Assisting Educational Programs and the Accrediting Bureau of Health Education Schools (ABHES)** Programmatic Evaluation Standards for Medical Assisting. Instructors should find this Study Guide a valuable teaching aid for training students who are able to think critically and to perform competently in the clinical setting.

Each study guide chapter is organized into the following sections:

1. **ASSIGNMENT SHEETS:** The Study Guide Assignment Sheets indicate the assignments required for each chapter, along with a space provided for the student to document the following: the date each assignment is due, completion of the assignment, and points earned for each assignment. The Laboratory Assignment Sheet indicates the procedures required for each chapter, along with the textbook and Study Guide reference pages, the number of practices required to attain competency, and a space for documenting the score earned on the Performance Evaluation Checklist.
2. **PRETEST AND POSTTEST:** These tests have been included for each chapter using true/false questions that allow the student to test his or her acquisition of knowledge for each chapter before and after completing the chapter. These tests can be used as a study guide to prepare for chapter tests.
3. **KEY TERM ASSESSMENT:** This section provides the student with an assessment of his or her knowledge of the medical terms covered in each chapter. This section also includes an assessment of the word parts of the medical terms (prefixes, suffixes, and combining forms) to evaluate the student's knowledge of the meaning of the medical term through its word parts.
4. **EVALUATION OF LEARNING:** These questions help the student evaluate his or her progress throughout each chapter. After the student has completed these questions and checked them for accuracy, they provide an ongoing review of the textbook material. Individuals preparing for a certification examination will find the completed Evaluation of Learning sections a useful study aid for the clinical aspect of the examination.
5. **CRITICAL THINKING ACTIVITIES:** In this section, the student performs activities that enhance his or her ability to think critically. Some situations require the student to become involved in a game or play a role; others require the student to use independent study to answer questions posed by a patient. Independent study helps the student become familiar with resources available to acquire additional knowledge and skills outside the classroom. By learning techniques of self-development, the medical assisting student may become aware of the necessity for continuing education after graduation and entrance into the medical assisting profession.
6. **PRACTICE FOR COMPETENCY:** This section consists of worksheets that provide the student with a guide for the practice of each clinical skill presented in the textbook.
7. **EVALUATION OF COMPETENCY:** This section has two parts. The first part is the Performance Objective, which provides an exact description of what the learner must be able to demonstrate to attain competency and has been developed to correspond with the procedures presented in the textbook. A performance objective consists of the (1) outcome, (2) conditions, and (3) standards. The second part is the Performance Evaluation Checklist, which provides quality control by comparing the student's performance against an established set of performance standards.
8. **SUPPLEMENTAL EDUCATION:** Several medical assisting content areas are more difficult than others for the student to comprehend and perform. Because students have special difficulty in taking patients' symptoms and in calculating drug dosage, two supplemental education sections have been incorporated into this manual. The section "Taking Patients' Symptoms" provides supplemental education for Chapter 38 (The Medical Record) in the textbook;

---

*CAAHEP competencies used on the "Evaluation of Competency" checklists are from the American Association of Medical Assistants, Chicago, Illinois, and the Commission on Accreditation of Allied Health Education Programs, Clearwater, Florida. Both 2008 and 2015 competencies are mapped in this book.

**ABHES competencies used on the "Evaluation of Competency" checklists are from the Accrediting Bureau of Health Education Schools, Falls Church, Virginia.

the section "Drug Dosage Calculation" provides supplemental education for Chapter 26 (Administration of Medication and Intravenous Therapy). In these two sections, a step-by-step, self-directed approach has been used, beginning with basic concepts and advancing to more difficult ones. The student should find that this type of approach facilitates the process of becoming proficient in these areas.

9. **EVOLVE SITE:** The Evolve site (http://evolve.elsevier.com/Bonewit/today/) offers many opportunities for students to apply the theory and skills learned throughout the textbook. Organized by chapter, the Evolve site includes all procedural videos, several games (e.g., Quiz Show, Road to Recovery) and question sets (e.g., Apply Your Knowledge) to provide entertainment while learning important concepts related to selected chapters, matching exercises, labeling exercises, identification exercises, multiple-choice and drag-and-drop questions, and other helpful activities for the student. Also, there are helpful supplemental resources like Practicum Activities (which assist the student in relating classroom knowledge to the real-world setting of the medical office) and Video Evaluations (which assess the student's knowledge of key points in the procedural videos that accompany the textbook).

We would like to thank the staff at Elsevier for their assistance and support in preparing this Study Guide, especially Jennifer Bertucci, Senior Content Development Specialist, and Celeste Clingan, Book Production Specialist.

Kathy Bonewit-West, BS, MEd
Sue A. Hunt, MA, RN, CMA (AAMA)
Edith Applegate, MS

Message to the Student

This Study Guide has been designed to facilitate the attainment of competency in the clinical theory and procedures in your textbook. Each chapter of the manual has been organized into the ten components outlined below. By completing each component, it is hoped that your ability to assimilate the theory and perform the clinical skills will be greatly enhanced.

1. **STUDY GUIDE ASSIGNMENT SHEETS**
   A. Each time your instructor makes an assignment from the Study Guide or Evolve site, document the date due in the appropriate space on the Assignment Sheet.
   B. Complete each assignment by the due date. Place a checkmark in the appropriate space on the Assignment Sheet after completing each assignment.
   C. Grade the assignment according to the directions stipulated by your instructor.
   D. Record your points earned in the appropriate space on the Assignment Sheet.
2. **LABORATORY ASSIGNMENT SHEET**
   A. Your instructor will assign the procedures to be completed for each laboratory practice session. Check the assigned procedures in the appropriate space on the Laboratory Assignment Sheet.
   B. Refer to the page numbers on the Laboratory Assignment Sheet for the Practice for Competency and Evaluation of Competency worksheets required for each procedure your instructor assigned.
   C. Locate and tear out the worksheets required for each procedure to be performed and bring them to your laboratory practice session.
   D. Record the score you earned on the Evaluation of Competency Performance Evaluation Checklist in the appropriate space on the Laboratory Assignment Sheet. This will provide you with a record of your progress on clinical procedures.
3. **PRETEST AND POSTTEST**
   A. Complete the Pretest before beginning a study of each chapter. Complete the Posttest after completing the study of the chapter. Place a checkmark in the appropriate space on the Study Guide Assignment Sheet after completing each test.
   B. Check your work for accuracy against the textbook and correct any errors.
   C. Grade the tests according to the directions stipulated by your instructor.
   D. Record the points you earned in the appropriate space on the Study Guide Assignment Sheet.
   E. Review the Pretest and Posttest before taking your chapter test.
4. **KEY TERM ASSESSMENT**
   A. Study the Terminology Review section located at the end of each chapter in the textbook.
   B. Match the medical terms with the definitions and complete the word parts table. Place a checkmark in the appropriate space on the Study Guide Assignment Sheet after completing the exercise.
   C. Check your work for accuracy against the textbook and correct any errors.
   D. Grade the exercise according to the directions stipulated by your instructor.
   E. Record the points you earned in the appropriate space on the Study Guide Assignment Sheet.
   F. Review the Key Term Assessment before taking your chapter test.
5. **EVALUATION OF LEARNING QUESTIONS**
   A. Read the textbook chapter.
   B. Complete the Evaluation of Learning questions. Place a checkmark in the appropriate space on the Study Guide Assignment Sheet after completing the questions.
   C. Check your work for accuracy against the textbook and correct any errors.
   D. Grade the questions according to the directions stipulated by your instructor.
   E. Record the points you earned in the appropriate space on the Textbook Assignment Sheet.
   F. Review the Evaluation of Learning questions before taking your chapter test.

6. **CRITICAL THINKING ACTIVITIES**
   A. Review the information required to complete the Critical Thinking Activities.
   B. Obtain any additional materials or resources required.
   C. Complete each Critical Thinking Activity. Place a checkmark in the appropriate space on the Study Guide Assignment Sheet after completing each assigned activity.
   D. Grade each Critical Thinking Activity according to the directions stipulated by your instructor.
   E. Record the points you earned in the appropriate space on the Textbook Assignment Sheet.
7. **EVOLVE SITE ACTIVITIES**
   A. Review the information required to complete the Evolve site activities.
   B. Using the Evolve site, complete the activities.
   C. Place a checkmark in the appropriate section on the Study Guide Assignment Sheet after completing each Evolve site activity.
   D. Record the points you earned in the appropriate space on the Study Guide Assignment Sheet.
8. **VIDEO EVALUATION**
   A. If applicable to the chapter, view the videos (located on the Evolve site) assigned by your instructor.
   B. Complete the video evaluation questions and place a checkmark in the appropriate space on the Study Guide Assignment Sheet.
   C. Check your work for accuracy, and correct any errors.
   D. Grade the questions according to the directions stipulated by your instructor.
   E. Record the points you earned in the appropriate space on the Study Guide Assignment Sheet.
   F. Review the Video Evaluation questions before being evaluated on each clinical skill by your instructor.
9. **PRACTICE FOR COMPETENCY**
   A. Your instructor will assign the procedure(s) to be completed for each laboratory practice session. For each procedure assigned, place a checkmark in the appropriate space on the Laboratory Assignment Sheet.
   B. Refer to the page numbers on the Laboratory Assignment Sheet for the Practice for Competency and Evaluation of Competency sheets required for each procedure your instructor assigned. Locate and tear out the sheets required for each procedure to be performed and bring them to your laboratory practice session.
   C. Practice each assigned procedure the required number of times indicated on the Laboratory Assignment Sheet or as designated by your instructor. Use the following guidelines when practicing the procedure to attain competency over each procedure:
      1. Information indicated on the Practice for Competency sheet
         - Record your practices in the chart provided.
      2. Procedure as presented in your textbook
      3. Video of the procedure (on the Evolve site)
         - View each procedure several times to make sure you understand the correct technique and theory.
      4. Evaluation of Competency Performance Checklist
         - Make sure that you can perform each procedure according to the criteria stipulated under conditions and standards.
      5. Peer evaluation
         - If directed by your instructor, obtain a peer evaluation using the Evaluation of Competency Performance Evaluation Checklist.
   D. Bring the completed Practice for Competency sheet to your laboratory testing session and present it to your instructor for his or her review before testing on the procedure.
10. **EVALUATION OF COMPETENCY PERFORMANCE CHECKLIST**
    A. Write your name and date in the space indicated on the Evaluation of Competency Performance Evaluation Checklist.
       1. Do not chart the procedure (in advance) on the Evaluation of Competency sheet. You do this after you have been tested on the procedure.

B. For each procedure being evaluated, bring the following to your laboratory testing session, and present them to your instructor:
    1. Completed Practice for Competency sheet
    2. Evaluation of Competency Performance Checklist
    3. Outcome Assessment Record
C. Demonstrate the proper procedure for performing the clinical skill for your instructor.
D. Record results (if required) in the chart provided on the Evaluation of Competency Checklist.
E. Obtain your instructor's initials on your Outcome Assessment Record indicating you have performed the procedure with competency.
F. Record the score you earned in the appropriate space on your Laboratory Assignment Sheet.

After you have completed each chapter in this Study Guide, it is suggested that you place the perforated sheet into a three-ring notebook. This will provide an ongoing record of your academic progress. In addition, the notebook will be useful both as a classroom reference and as a certification examination review resource.

We hope that this Study Guide will assist your attainment of competency in medical assisting procedures and will facilitate your transition from the classroom to the workplace.

Kathy Bonewit-West, BS, MEd
Sue A. Hunt, MA, RN, CMA (AAMA)
Edith Applegate, MS

Outcome Assessment Record

This list of outcomes is used to maintain an ongoing record of classroom and practicum outcome assessment. Your instructor should initial each outcome when you have performed it with competency in the classroom. When you have performed the outcome with competency at your practicum facility, it should be initialed by your practicum supervisor. Space is provided for three practicum experiences in the event that you extern at more than one practicum site.

Name________	Classroom Performance	Practicum	Practicum	Practicum
MEDICAL ASEPSIS AND THE OSHA STANDARD				
Perform handwashing.				
Apply an alcohol-based hand rub.				
Apply and remove clean disposable gloves.				
Demonstrate the proper use of a sharps container.				
Prepare regulated waste for pickup by a medical waste service.				
STERILIZATION AND DISINFECTION				
Sanitize instruments.				
Wrap an instrument for autoclaving.				
Sterilize articles in the autoclave.				
VITAL SIGNS				
Measure and record oral body temperature.				
Measure and record axillary body temperature.				
Measure and record rectal body temperature.				
Measure and record aural body temperature.				
Measure and record temporal body temperature.				
Measure and record (radial) pulse and respiration.				
Measure and record apical pulse.				
Perform and record pulse oximetry.				
Measure and record blood pressure.				

Name______________	Classroom Performance	Practicum	Practicum	Practicum
THE PHYSICAL EXAMINATION				
Measure weight and height.				
Demonstrate proper body mechanics.				
Position and drape an individual.				
Transfer a patient from and to a wheelchair.				
Prepare a patient for a physical examiniation.				
Assist the physician with the physical examination.				
EYE AND EAR PROCEDURES				
Assess distance visual acuity.				
Assess color vision.				
Perform an eye irrigation.				
Perform an eye instillation.				
Perform an ear irrigation.				
Perform an ear instillation.				
PHYSICAL AGENTS TO PROMOTE TISSUE HEALING				
Apply a heating pad.				
Apply a hot soak.				
Apply a hot compress.				
Apply an ice bag.				
Apply a cold compress.				
Apply a chemical pack.				
Measure a patient for axillary crutches.				
Instruct a patient in mastering crutch gaits.				
Instruct a patient in the use of a cane.				
Instruct a patient in the use of a walker.				
THE GYNECOLOGIC EXAMINATION AND PRENATAL CARE				
Provide instructions for a breast self-examination.				
Assist with a gynecologic examination.				
Assist with a return prenatal examination.				

Name________	Classroom Performance	Practicum	Practicum	Practicum
THE PEDIATRIC EXAMINATION				
Carry an infant in the following positions: cradle and upright.				
Measure the weight and length of an infant.				
Measure the head and chest circumference of an infant.				
Plot pediatric measurements on a growth chart.				
Apply a pediatric urine collector.				
MINOR OFFICE SURGERY				
Apply and remove sterile gloves.				
Open a sterile package.				
Add a sterile article to a sterile field from a peel-apart package.				
Pour a sterile solution into a container on a sterile field.				
Change a sterile dressing.				
Remove sutures.				
Remove staples.				
Apply and remove adhesive skin closures.				
Prepare a sterile field for minor office surgery.				
Assist with minor office surgery.				
Apply the following bandage turns: circular, spiral, spiral-reverse, figure-eight, and recurrent.				
ADMINISTRATION OF MEDICATION AND INTRAVENOUS THERAPY				
Prepare and administer oral medication.				
Prepare an injection from a vial.				
Prepare an injection from an ampule.				
Reconstitute a powdered drug.				
Administer a subcutaneous injection.				
Locate the following intramuscular injection sites: dorsogluteal, deltoid, vastus lateralis, and ventrogluteal.				
Administer an intramuscular injection.				
Administer an injection using the Z-track method.				
Administer an intradermal injection.				
Administer a tuberculin skin test and read the test results.				

Name________	Classroom Performance	Practicum	Practicum	Practicum
CARDIOPULMONARY PROCEDURES				
Record a 12-lead, three-channel electrocardiogram (ECG).				
Perform a spirometry test.				
Measure a peak flow rate.				
COLON PROCEDURES AND MALE REPRODUCTIVE HEALTH				
Instruct a patient for a fecal occult blood test.				
Develop a fecal occult blood test.				
Provide instructions for a testicular self-examination.				
RADIOLOGY AND DIAGNOSTIC IMAGING				
Instruct a patient in the proper preparation required for each of the following x-ray examinations: mammogram, bone density scan, upper GI, lower GI, and intravenous pyelogram.				
Instruct a patient in the proper preparation required for each of the following: ultrasonography, computed tomography, magnetic resonance imaging, and nuclear medicine.				
INTRODUCTION TO THE CLINICAL LABORATORY				
Operate an emergency eyewash station.				
Use a laboratory directory.				
Complete a laboratory request form.				
Prepare a laboratory report for review by the physician.				
Instruct the patient in advance preparation requirements for a laboratory test.				
Collect a specimen.				
Properly handle and store a specimen.				
Review a laboratory report.				
URINALYSIS				
Instruct a patient in clean-catch midstream urine specimen collection.				
Assess the color and appearance of a urine specimen.				
Perform a CLIA-waived chemical assessment of a urine specimen.				
Prepare a urine specimen for microscopic examination.				
Perform a CLIA-waived urine pregnancy test.				

Name____________	Classroom Performance	Practicum	Practicum	Practicum
PHLEBOTOMY				
Perform a venipuncture using the vacuum tube method.				
Perform a venipuncture using the butterfly method.				
Perform a skin puncture using a disposable semiautomatic lancet device.				
Perform a skin puncture using a reusable semiautomatic lancet device.				
HEMATOLOGY				
Perform a CLIA-waived hemoglobin determination.				
Perform a CLIA-waived hematocrit determination.				
Prepare a blood smear for a differential cell count.				
Perform a CLIA-waived PT/INR test.				
BLOOD CHEMISTRY AND IMMUNOLOGY				
Perform a CLIA-waived blood glucose test.				
Perform a CLIA-waived blood chemistry test.				
Perform a CLIA-waived rapid mononucleosis test.				
MEDICAL MICROBIOLOGY				
Use a microscope.				
Collect a throat specimen.				
Obtain a specimen using a collection and transport system.				
Perform a CLIA-waived rapid strep test.				
NUTRITION				
Instruct a patient according to patient's special dietary needs.				
EMERGENCY PREPAREDNESS AND PROTECTIVE PRACTICES				
Demonstrate proper use of a fire extinguisher.				
Participate in a mock exposure event.				

Name________	Classroom Performance	Practicum	Practicum	Practicum
THE MEDICAL RECORD				
Complete a procedure consent form.				
Assist a patient in the completion of a medical records release form.				
Release medical information according to a completed medical records release form.				
Obtain a patient history using reflection, restatement, and clarification techniques.				
Formulate and document the patient's chief complaint and/or patient symptoms.				
PATIENT RECEPTION				
Open the medical office.				
Close the medical office.				
Obtain information from a new patient, obtain consents, and validate insurance coverage.				
Respond to issues of confidentiality.				
Input patient data utilizing a practice management system.				
Coach a patient regarding office policies and procedures.				
TELEPHONE TECHNIQUES				
Screen incoming telephone calls.				
Take a telephone message.				
Take a message requesting medication or a prescription refill.				
Place an outgoing telephone call to a patient for follow-up.				
SCHEDULING APPOINTMENTS				
Set up the appointment schedule.				
Implement time management principles to maintain effective office functions.				
Make an appointment for a patient.				
Review the daily appointment schedule.				
Cancel a patient appointment.				
Change a patient appointment.				
Indicate a missed appointment.				
Document cancellations and missed appointments on the day of the appointment.				
Schedule an inpatient or outpatient diagnostic test or procedure.				
Schedule an inpatient or outpatient admission for a patient.				

Name________	Classroom Performance	Practicum	Practicum	Practicum
MEDICAL RECORDS MANAGEMENT				
Prepare a medical record.				
Organize a patient's medical record.				
File patient records correctly using an alphabetic filing system.				
Maintain organization by filing.				
File patient records correctly using a terminal digit filing system.				
Maintain organization by filing.				
File reports, correspondence, and other material in a patient record.				
Organize a patient's medical record.				
WRITTEN COMMUNICATIONS				
Compose a professional business letter.				
Send a fax.				
Apply HIPAA rules in regard to privacy/ release of information.				
Prepare copies of multiple-page documents.				
MAIL				
Process incoming mail.				
Implement time management principles to maintain effective office function.				
Use the internet to find the correct ZIP+4 code for a given address.				
Address an envelope, and process envelopes to be mailed.				
MANAGING PRACTICE FINANCES				
Complete an itemized charge slip or superbill for a patient using a fee schedule.				
Using the information from the completed charge slip, post patient charges to a patient account.				
Post payments and/or adjustments to a patient account.				
Write checks to pay bills for a medical office and record them in the checkbook or check register.				
Prepare a bank deposit.				

Name____________	Classroom Performance	Practicum	Practicum	Practicum
MEDICAL CODING				
Perform CPT coding for procedures.				
Perform HCPCS coding for services of equipment.				
Perform ICD coding for a patient's diagnosis.				
MEDICAL INSURANCE				
Interpret information on an insurance card.				
Verify insurance or managed care eligibility.				
Obtain insurance preauthorization (precertification).				
Complete or review an insurance claim form.				
Interact professionally with third party representatives.				
Display tactful behaviour when communicating with medical providers regarding third party requirements.				
Show sensitivity when communicating with patients regarding third party requirements.				
BILLING AND COLLECTIONS				
Prepare patient statements.				
Post a check returned for not sufficient funds (NSF).				
Process a credit balance and issue a refund.				
Create and examine an accounts receivable aging record.				
Write a collection letter.				
THE MEDICAL ASSISTANT AS OFFICE MANAGER				
Perform and document a safety inspection after creating an environment checklist.				
Comply with safety signs, symbols, and labels.				
Perform equipment maintenance and document on equipment maintenance log.				
Take a supply or equipment inventory.				
Develop a current list of community resources.				
Facilitate referrals to community resources.				
Complete an incident report.				

Name_______________	Classroom Performance	Practicum	Practicum	Practicum
ADDITIONAL OUTCOMES (List)				

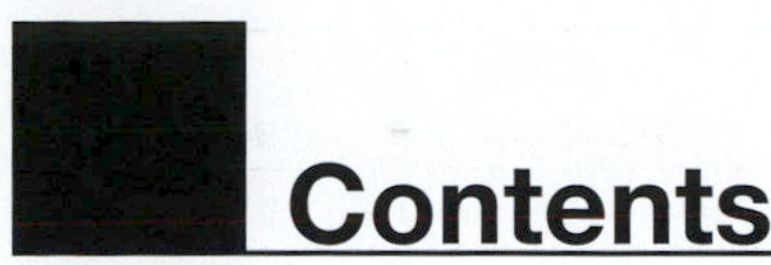

Contents

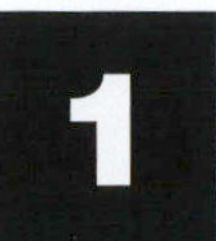

1 The Health Care System

CHAPTER ASSIGNMENTS

✓ After Completing	Date Due	Study Guide Page(s)	Study Guide Assignments (CTA: Critical Thinking Activity)	Possible Points	Points You Earned
		3	Pretest	10	
		4	Term Key Term Assessment A. Definitions B. Word Parts (Add 1 point for each key term)	 13 6	
		4-7	Evaluation of Learning questions	24	
		7	CTA A: Allied Health Professionals	10	
		8	CTA B: The Medical Office	10	
		8	CTA C: Medical Specialties	10	
			Evolve Site: Apply Your Knowledge questions	10	
		3	Posttest	10	
			ADDITIONAL ASSIGNMENTS		
			TOTAL POINTS		

Notes

Name ______________________________ Date ______________

PRETEST

True or False

_______ 1. Palliative treatment attempts to reduce the effects of a disease or condition but does not cure disease.

_______ 2. In the past 30 years there has been a trend to avoid admitting patients to the hospital if possible.

_______ 3. The first health insurance plans in the United States were provided by the federal government.

_______ 4. The managed care movement has put pressure on physicians to limit time spent with individual patients.

_______ 5. After graduating from medical school, a physician spends 2 to 5 years in postgraduate training called an internship.

_______ 6. If laboratory tests are done in the medical office, there is a specific room or area set aside for this.

_______ 7. Some medical offices use paper medical records, but it is becoming increasingly more common to store patient records electronically.

_______ 8. The physician who provides general medical care to an adult is usually an internist or a family practitioner.

_______ 9. A group practice often consists of three or four physicians in the same specialty.

_______ 10. Only a few patients, in addition to receiving standard medical treatment, also receive treatments that can be called complementary medicine.

POSTTEST

True or False

_______ 1. In order to be hospitalized, a patient's condition must be very unstable or require regulation of therapy.

_______ 2. Managed care insurance is another name for fee-for-service insurance.

_______ 3. A nurse practitioner manages routine patient care and can write prescriptions in most states.

_______ 4. When a patient enters the office, he or she is immediately taken to a treatment room.

_______ 5. The government agency that provides for health and safety in the workplace is CLIA.

_______ 6. The movement in primary care that emphasizes health care based on a personal relationship between a patient, physician, and the patient's care team is the patient-centered medical home (PCMH).

_______ 7. The medical office may have a special room just for treatments or procedures.

_______ 8. An osteopathic physician (DO) provides primary care and has the same legal status as a physician with an MD degree.

_______ 9. The physician who specializes in diseases of the nervous system is a neurologist.

_______ 10. Acupuncture is considered to be a standard medical treatment.

KEY TERM ASSESSMENT

Directions: Match each key term with its definition.

_______ 1. Ambulatory care
_______ 2. Capitation
_______ 3. Curative
_______ 4. Empirical
_______ 5. Fee-for-service
_______ 6. Formulary
_______ 7. Health insurance
_______ 8. Holistic
_______ 9. Managed care
_______ 10. Palliative treatment
_______ 11. Patient-centered medical home
_______ 12. Residency
_______ 13. Symptomatic treatment
_______ 14. Utilization review

A. A system that manages the delivery of health care with the intention of controlling costs
B. A set payment provided by managed care insurance per patient per month regardless of the amount of service the patient receives
C. Considering the whole; in medicine, considering the entire person when providing health care
D. Therapy that reduces the effects of disease or condition but does not remove the disease itself
E. A program to provide training in a medical specialty to a physician who has finished medical school
F. Medical care that is provided on an outpatient basis
G. Therapy for symptoms of a disease or condition
H. Purchase of protection for covered services related to health care
I. Assessing medical services to determine whether they are appropriate, necessary, and of high quality
J. A means of payment for health care in which each service provided is reimbursed in full or in part
K. Learned from observation or experiment
L. A list of prescription drugs covered or preferred by a managed care insurance company
M. Treatment that cures disease
N. A model of primary care that emphasizes care based on a personal relationship between a patient, physician, and the patient's health care team

B. Word Parts

Directions: Indicate the meaning of each word part in the space provided. List as many medical terms as possible that incorporate the word part in the space provided.

Word Part	Meaning of Word Part	Medical Terms That Incorporate Word Part
1. –al		
2. ambul/o		
3. empiric/o		
4. hol/o		
5. –ic		
6. –ory		

EVALUATION OF LEARNING

Directions: Fill in each blank with the correct answer.

1. What is the World Health Organization's definition of health?

____

____

____

2. What historical figure is considered to be the first to see illness as a result of physical and environmental factors? When did he live?

____

3. What three trends in modern medicine have a strong influence on health care in ambulatory settings?

4. What is fee-for-service health insurance?

5. List and give a short description of three government insurance plans that were introduced starting in the 1960s.

6. Briefly describe what managed care is.

7. If a managed care insurance plan uses capitation to pay for health care, what does this mean?

8. How do managed care plans attempt to reduce the cost of prescription medications?

9. List the six steps of an ordinary patient visit to a medical office.

10. Identify at least six other health professionals beside the physician and the medical assistant who may work in the medical office.

11. Describe briefly how physicians are educated.

12. What examination does a physician take to obtain a state license to practice medicine? How does a physician become "board certified?"

13. Describe the education and training of a physician assistant (PA) and a nurse practitioner (NP).

14. What is teamwork? Identify at least four components of effective teamwork.

15. Identify the major areas of a typical medical office and their functions.

16. Identify four other areas that can be found in larger offices.

17. Identify three types of primary care physicians.

18. Briefly describe the emphasis of the patient-centered medical home (PCMH).

19. Describe osteopathy. Are osteopaths licensed to practice medicine?

____

____

20. What is podiatry, and what kinds of patients might be referred to a podiatrist?

____

21. What is chiropractic, and what kinds of patients seek care from a chiropractor?

____

22. What is the difference between a solo practice and a group practice?

____

____

23. What type of medical facility was traditionally called a clinic?

____

____

24. What is acupuncture?

____

____

____

25. What is the role of complementary medicine in the United States today?

____

____

CRITICAL THINKING ACTIVITIES

A. Allied Health Professionals

Refer to Table 1-1 and select the allied health professionals, other than a medical assistant, who are most qualified to perform each of the following tasks.

1. Take an x-ray of the lower leg: _______________
2. Create a meal plan for a patient with a gastrointestinal disease: _______________
3. Supervise laboratory operations: _______________
4. Pass instruments during surgery to repair a hernia: _______________
5. Plan an exercise program for a patient after replacement of a hip: _______________
6. Help a patient learn how to get dressed after a stroke: _______________
7. Provide respiratory treatments to a patient with pneumonia: _______________
8. Perform an ultrasound of the gallbladder: _______________
9. Assign codes to office surgical procedures for billing: _______________
10. Set up a medical record filing system: _______________

B. The Medical Office

Where in the medical office shown in Figure 1-3 would the following activities probably take place?

1. Put a patient's paper medical record after use: ____________________
2. Physical examination by the physician: ____________________
3. Make an appointment for a patient during a telephone call: ____________________
4. Patient is weighed: ____________________
5. Test urine specimens: ____________________
6. Physician meeting with patient and family: ____________________
7. Prepare patient bills for mailing: ____________________
8. Suture a laceration: ____________________
9. Patient checks in: ____________________
10. Patient charges posted to patient accounts: ____________________

C. Medical Specialties

Look up each of the following conditions as needed and refer to Box 1-1 in the textbook to identify which medical specialist would treat an adult patient with the following problems:

1. Recurrent urinary tract infections: ____________________
2. Tumor of the colon: ____________________
3. Acne: ____________________
4. Brain tumor: ____________________
5. Ovarian cyst: ____________________
6. Cataract: ____________________
7. Hip fracture: ____________________
8. Growth on the vocal cords: ____________________
9. Stroke with paralysis: ____________________
10. Repair of fractured cheek bone: ____________________

2 The Professional Medical Assistant

CHAPTER ASSIGNMENTS

✓ After Completing	Date Due	Study Guide Page(s)	STUDY GUIDE ASSIGNMENTS (CTA: Critical Thinking Activity)	Possible Points	Points You Earned
		11	Pretest	10	
		12	Term Key Term Assessment	9	
		12-15	Evaluation of Learning questions	28	
		15	CTA A: Professional Appearance	20	
		15	CTA B: Professional Behavior for Physicians	6	
		16	CTA C: Professional Organizations	6	
		16-17	CTA D: Scope of Practice	7	
			Evolve Site: Apply Your Knowledge questions	10	
		11	Posttest	10	
			ADDITIONAL ASSIGNMENTS		
			TOTAL POINTS		

✓ When Assigned by Your Instructor	Study Guide Page(s)	Practices Required	LABORATORY ASSIGNMENTS (Procedure Number and Name)	Score*
	19	1	**Practice for Competency 2-1:** Locating and Defining a State's Legal Scope of Practice Textbook reference: p. 24	
	21-22		**Evaluation of Competency 2-1:** Locating and Defining a State's Legal Scope of Practice	*
			ADDITIONAL ASSIGNMENTS	

Name ______________________________ Date ______________

PRETEST

True or False

_______ 1. The American Medical Technologists was the first professional organization for medical assistants.

_______ 2. A medical assistant who accepts that patients often have different beliefs is displaying dependability.

_______ 3. Being well organized helps the medical assistant respond to sudden changes in schedule or plans.

_______ 4. A medical assistant should always wait for instructions before beginning a new task.

_______ 5. Professionalism is based on both scientific knowledge and a code of ethical behavior.

_______ 6. If a physician engages in unprofessional behavior, the state may suspend or revoke his or her license to practice medicine.

_______ 7. A registered medical assistant has passed a national examination given by the American Association of Medical Assistants (AAMA).

_______ 8. Continuing education is required if a medical assistant wants to maintain certification as a certified medical assistant (CMA [AAMA]) or registered medical assistant (RMA).

_______ 9. Professional organizations for medical assistants publish journals to help medical assistants stay current.

_______ 10. Billing is performed by a specialist in the medical office, not the medical assistant.

POSTTEST

True or False

_______ 1. Medical assisting programs seek accreditation from the American Association of Medical Assistants or the American Medical Technologists.

_______ 2. To be suited for the profession of medical assisting, an individual must be able to put the needs of a patient first.

_______ 3. In almost all offices, the medical assistant wears professional street clothes for both clinical and administrative tasks.

_______ 4. A medical assistant can demonstrate initiative by restocking examination rooms without having to be told to do so.

_______ 5. A professional medical assistant may have to report a colleague who breaks patient confidentiality.

_______ 6. If a medical assistant is certified, he or she has a state license to be a medical assistant.

_______ 7. To sit for a certification examination from any national agency, an individual must have graduated from a medical assisting program that has been accredited by CAAHEP (Commission on Accreditation of Health Education Programs).

_______ 8. Professional organizations provide programs that carry continuing education credit so that medical assistants can maintain certification.

_______ 9. State, local, and national meetings are held by professional organizations to help medical assistants meet their professional needs.

_______ 10. *Risk management* is a term used specifically for measures to prevent the spread of infection in a health care setting.

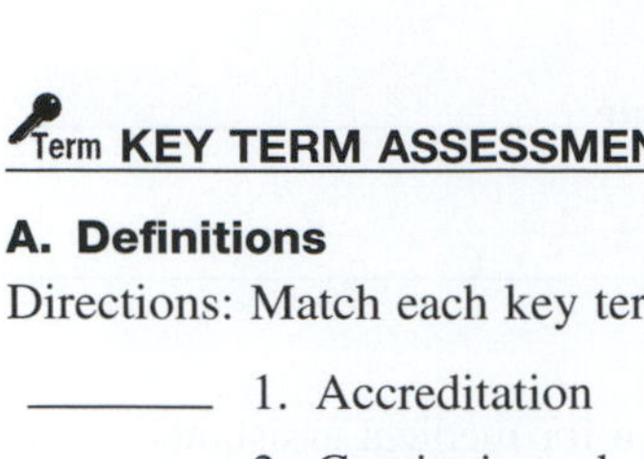

KEY TERM ASSESSMENT

A. Definitions

Directions: Match each key term with its definition.

_______ 1. Accreditation
_______ 2. Continuing education unit (CEU)
_______ 3. Fee splitting
_______ 4. Health coaching
_______ 5. Initiative
_______ 6. Patient navigator
_______ 7. Practicum
_______ 8. Risk management
_______ 9. Time management

A. A work supervised experience that is required in an educational program and usually unpaid
B. Processes to protect a health care facility from the risk of legal action
C. The ability to begin or carry through on a plan of action independently
D. Credit or recognition for maintaining certain standards by a regional or national organization
E. A process that helps patients identify their values related to health, set health goals, and take steps to meet their goals.
F. Skills and techniques used to accomplish tasks and meet goals in a timely manner
G. The unethical practice of sharing fees with colleagues, especially for making referrals
H. A standard unit of continuing education for professionals
I. A person whose role is to remove obstacles that patients face in accessing and receiving treatment.

EVALUATION OF LEARNING

Directions: Fill in each blank with the correct answer.

1. Identify five changes in medical care over the past 25 years that have affected the profession of medical assisting.

____

____

2. List two organizations that have worked to define professionalism for medical assistants.

____

3. What are three important character traits of a professional medical assistant?

____

4. How is caring expressed by a medical assistant?

____

5. Identify three reasons why neatness and good grooming are important for the medical assistant.

____

____

____

6. What does the medical assistant usually wear when performing clinical tasks? Administrative tasks?

____

7. Give two specific examples of how the medical assistant can demonstrate initiative.

____

8. List three general principles of effective time management.

9. List four tools that facilitate effective use of time.

10. Identify four sources of information about professional practice for physicians.

11. Who is thought to be the author of the oath that served as a guide for good conduct for ancient physicians?

12. What are five ethical responsibilities of a professional medical assistant?

13. Identify two written sets of standards that provide guidance for professional medical assistants.

14. What is the difference between certification and licensure?

15. Describe how an individual becomes a certified medical assistant through the American Association of Medical Assistants.

16. Describe how an individual becomes a registered medical assistant through the American Medical Technologists.

17. Identify three other organizations that provide certification for medical assistants.

18. What are three credentials other than certification that the medical assistant may be advised to obtain?

____

____

19. In general what continuing education requirements are required for recertification?

____

____

20. Describe the medical assistant's role related to making appointments and medical records.

____

____

____

21. Describe the medical assistant's role in billing, accepting payments, and recording payments.

____

____

22. Describe any six areas of clinical responsibility for the medical assistant.

____

____

____

23. Describe the medical assistant's responsibility if an emergency occurs in the medical office.

____

24. Explain the medical assistant's responsibility related to supplies and equipment.

____

____

25. Give examples of three different types of instruction that a medical assistant might give to patients.

____

____

26. Differentiate between patient education and health coaching.

____

____

27. Explain how a medical assistant might function as a patient navigator.

____

____

28. Discuss three common types of health care facilities where medical assistants often find employment.

____

____

CRITICAL THINKING ACTIVITIES

A. Professional Appearance

Create a poster with pictures and comments to show the proper clothing, hairstyle, and jewelry (if any) for a medical assistant assigned to various areas in the medical office. If you are female, illustrate female attire. If you are male, illustrate male attire. After your poster is completed, discuss your choices in class with a partner and/or the entire class.

1. Using items cut from a magazine (such as a uniform supply company) and items printed from the Internet, colored pencils, and markers, illustrate professional attire for the clinical or laboratory area on one half of your poster. Illustrate both short-sleeve and long-sleeve options. Write comments on the poster to describe appropriate hairstyle, jewelry, fingernail appearance, and footwear as needed.
2. Using items cut from a magazine and items printed from the Internet, colored pencils, and markers, illustrate professional attire for the administrative area of the medical office using business casual attire. Write comments on the poster to describe appropriate hairstyle, jewelry, fingernail appearance, and footwear as needed.

B. Professional Behavior For Physicians

Give reasons why each of the following behaviors by a physician would be considered professional or unprofessional.

1. Requiring a payment from any physician to whom a patient is referred

____

____

2. Sending prescriptions automatically to a pharmacy in which the physician owns stock without asking the patient if that is his or her preferred pharmacy

____

____

3. Meeting with pharmacy representatives during the lunch hour and accepting samples of new medications

____

____

4. Allowing the medical assistant to obtain blood specimens and perform blood tests

____

____

5. Dating a former patient who now obtains care from another primary care physician

____

____

6. Treating a patient outside the physician's specialty (e.g., a gynecologist treating a patient for diabetes mellitus)

____

____

C. Professional Organizations

Find information about local/state/regional chapters of the American Association of Medical Assistants (AAMA) and the American Medical Technologists (AMT). The websites of the national organizations have links to state associations.

1. What is the location of the nearest chapter of the AAMA to your school? ____________________

2. What is the location of the nearest chapter of the AMT to your school? ____________________

3. Is your medical assisting program accredited? ______________ If so, by whom? ______________

4. When is the next state meeting of the AAMA in your state? ______________ AMT? ______________

5. Are students and nonmembers welcome to attend state meetings? ____________________

6. From your research, identify five reasons to attend the state meeting of one or more of these organizations:

____

____

____

____

____

D. Scope of Practice

Based on the description of the medical assistant's role in Chapter 2, investigate and discuss whether each of the following is within the medical assistant's scope of practice in your state.

1. The medical assistant obtains and tests urine specimens.

____

____

2. The medical assistant performs routine physical examinations on children and adults.

____

____

3. The medical assistant administers immunizations to infants, children, and adults.

____

____

4. The medical assistant authorizes prescription refills for patients on long-term medication therapy.

____

____

5. The medical assistant obtains specimens of venous blood by finger-stick and phlebotomy and performs diagnostic tests using the blood specimens.

____

____

6. Discuss what a medical assistant should do if he or she notices that another medical assistant in the practice has performed a sterile procedure, such as catherization or starting an intravenous infusion, with no previous training in the procedure.

____

____

____

7. Look up the term "scope of practice" and provide a complete definition.

____

____

Notes

PRACTICE FOR COMPETENCY

Procedure 2-1: Locating and Defining a State's Legal Scope of Practice

A. Research the legal scope of practice for a medical assistant in your state and make notes in order to write a brief written report.

B. With a classmate, discuss the consequences for medical assistants and patients if the medical assistant performs activities that are not included in the legal scope of practice.

C. Role-play patient situations as needed to demonstrate performing within the scope of practice.

Notes

EVALUATION OF COMPETENCY

Procedure 2-1: Locating and Defining a State's Legal Scope of Practice

Name: ______________________________ Date: ______________

Evaluated By: ______________________________ Score: ______________

Performance Objective

Outcome:	Locate and define a specific state's legal scope of practice.
Conditions:	Given access to the Internet, computer, and printer.
Standards:	Time to complete role-play and discussion: 45 minutes. Student completed procedure in ________ minutes.
	Accuracy: Satisfactory score on the Performance Evaluation Checklist.

Performance Evaluation Checklist

Trial 1	Trial 2	Point Value	Performance Standards
		•	Researched the legal scope of practice for a medical assistant in own state.
		•	Wrote a paper summarizing the scope of practice and discussing the consequences for medical assistants and patients if the medical assistant performs activities that are not included in the legal scope of practice.
		•	Included a discussion that described and differentiated between procedures that can and cannot be delegated to a medical assistant by different health professionals (physician, nurse, physician assistant) in various healthcare settings.
		•	Summarized a situation on an index care where a medical assistant practices within thc legal scope of practice.
		•	Summarized a situation on an index card where a medical assistant performed outside the legal scope of practice.
		•	Participated in two role-play situations of a classmate related to activities within or outside the legal scope of practice for a medical assistant.
		*	Participated in a group discussion to identify which role play situations fell within and which were outside of the medical assistant scope of practice.
		*	Handed in a satisfactory report and two satisfactory situations on index cards to instructor.
		•	Completed the role play and group discussion within 45 minutes.
			TOTALS

Evaluation of Student Performance

EVALUATION CRITERIA			COMMENTS
Symbol	**Category**	**Point Value**	
*	Critical Step	16 points	
●	Essential Step	6 points	
Ⓐ	Affective Competency	6 points	
▷	Theory Question	2 points	
Score calculation: 100 points – ___ points missed ___ Score Satisfactory score: 85 or above			

2008 CAAHEP Competencies Achieved
Psychomotor (Skills) ☑ IX.2. Perform within scope of Practice ***Affective (Behavior)*** ☑ IX.2. Demonstrate awareness of the consequences of not working within the legal scope of practice.

2015 CAAHEP Competencies Achieved
Psychomotor (Skills) ☑ X.1. Locate a state's legal scope of practice for medical assistants.

ABHES Competencies Achieved
☑ 4. f. 1. Define scope of practice for the medical assistant within the state that the medical assistant is employed. ☑ 4. f. 2. Describe what procedures can and cannot be delegated to the medical assistant and by whom within various employment settings.

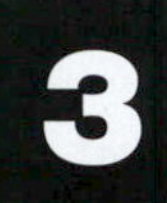

Ethics and Law for the Medical Office

CHAPTER ASSIGNMENTS

✓ After Completing	Date Due	Study Guide Page(s)	STUDY GUIDE ASSIGNMENTS (CTA: Critical Thinking Activity)	Possible Points	Points You Earned
		25	Pretest	10	
		 26 26-27	Term Key Term Assessment A. Ethics B. Law	 16 36	
		27-32	Evaluation of Learning questions	54	
		32	CTA A: Ethical Issues	20	
		32-33	CTA B: Patient Advocate	2	
		33	CTA C: Personal and Professional Ethics	14	
		33-34	CTA D: Patient Bill of Rights	5	
		34	CTA E: Negligence	4	
			Evolve Site: Apply Your Knowledge questions	10	
			Evolve Site: Quiz Show (Record points earned)		
		25	Posttest	10	
			ADDITIONAL ASSIGNMENTS		
			TOTAL POINTS		

✓ When Assigned by Your Instructor	Study Guide Page(s)	Practices Required	LABORATORY ASSIGNMENTS (Procedure Number and Name)	Score*
	35	3	**Practice for Competency** 3-1: Separating Personal and Professional Ethics Textbook reference: p. 42	
	37-38		**Evaluation of Competency** 3-1: Separating Personal and Professional Ethics	*
	35	3	**Practice for Competency** 3-2: Incorporating the Patient's Bill of Rights Textbook reference: p. 48	
	39-40		**Evaluation of Competency** 3-2: Incorporating the Patient's Bill of Rights	*
	35	3	**Practice for Competency** 3-3: Reporting Illegal Activities and Complying with Public Health Statutes Textbook reference: p. 56	
	41-42		**Evaluation of Competency** 3-3: Reporting Illegal Activities and Complying with Public Health Statutes	*
			ADDITIONAL ASSIGNMENTS	

Name ______________________________ Date ______________

PRETEST

True or False

_______ 1. Patients have the right to autonomy, which includes the right to refuse treatment.

_______ 2. Legal abortions and confidentiality are manifestations of the individual's right to privacy.

_______ 3. The branch of law that regulates interactions between individuals and groups is called criminal law.

_______ 4. To be enforceable, a contract must be written.

_______ 5. A physician cannot refuse to accept patients who seek treatment.

_______ 6. Written consent forms are usually used for surgery and other invasive procedures.

_______ 7. A wound infection after surgery is caused by negligence on the part of the physician.

_______ 8. If a patient is injured through the negligence of a medical assistant, a patient can sue the medical assistant and his or her physician employer.

_______ 9. If a trial is held for malpractice, it is only necessary to provide photocopies of the paper medical record.

_______ 10. A patient may begin a lawsuit for malpractice any time after an injury occurs.

POSTTEST

True or False

_______ 1. Physician-assisted suicide is illegal in all states because a federal law prohibits it.

_______ 2. Health professionals are considered to have a duty to be faithful to reasonable expectations of patients.

_______ 3. A serious crime committed with the intent to cause harm is called a felony.

_______ 4. For a contract to be valid, there must be a mutual agreement between the parties.

_______ 5. A physician can end a relationship with a patient, provided that the patient is notified in writing.

_______ 6. To give informed consent, a patient must understand the risks and benefits of a procedure.

_______ 7. When a physician fails to care for a patient correctly, causing injury to the patient, it is called professional negligence or malpractice.

_______ 8. Professional liability insurance only covers a physician for his or her own actions.

_______ 9. Most malpractice lawsuits are settled out of court, and no trial occurs.

_______ 10. The physician is not liable for injury to a patient if the patient refuses to follow medical advice.

Term KEY TERM ASSESSMENT: ETHICS

Directions: Match each key term with its definition.

_______ 1. Advocate
_______ 2. Autonomy
_______ 3. Beneficence
_______ 4. Cloning
_______ 5. DNR (do not resuscitate)
_______ 6. Duty
_______ 7. Ethics
_______ 8. Fidelity
_______ 9. Gene therapy
_______ 10. Genetic engineering
_______ 11. Health care proxy
_______ 12. Living will
_______ 13. Nonmalfeasance
_______ 14. Stem cells
_______ 15. Right
_______ 16. Veracity

A. Making, altering, or repairing genetic material
B. Cells that have the capacity to develop into various types of body tissue
C. Ability to make independent decisions without constraint or coercion from others
D. Truthfulness
E. Faithfulness
F. Ethical concept requiring that an action do no harm, or do less harm than good
G. Giving patients new genes or parts of genes to treat a disease or condition
H. A legal document that names an agent to make decisions about a person's medical care if he or she becomes unable to make wishes known
I. The branch of knowledge that deals with standards of behavior
J. Commitment to act in a certain way
K. Acting in the best possible way; performing good deeds
L. Producing genetically identical cells or individuals artificially
M. A legal document that specifies the kind of medical treatment a patient wants or does not want if he or she becomes incapacitated
N. A medical order signed by a physician that relieves health care personnel from the obligation to resuscitate a patient who stops breathing or whose heart stops
O. A claim that is expected to be honored
P. A person who intercedes on another person's behalf

Term KEY TERM ASSESSMENT: LAW

Directions: Match each key term with its definition.

_______ 1. Abandonment
_______ 2. Act
_______ 3. Arbitration
_______ 4. Assumption of risk
_______ 5. Case law
_______ 6. Common law
_______ 7. Contingency
_______ 8. Controlled substance
_______ 9. Defendant
_______ 10. Drug Enforcement Administration (DEA)
_______ 11. Embezzlement
_______ 12. Felony
_______ 13. Fraud
_______ 14. Informed consent
_______ 15. Larceny
_______ 16. Liability
_______ 17. License

A. A formal process in which the parties to a dispute agree to submit to the decision of a neutral party
B. Law established by decisions of previous court cases
C. Law enacted by a legislative body
D. Agreement to a medical procedure based on understanding of the procedure and its possible consequences and effects
E. Unwritten body of law based on general custom
F. Stealing another person's property or money without violence
G. Intentional deception resulting in injury or loss
H. A legal doctrine making an employer liable for the negligent acts of employees
I. The person or group against whom an action is brought in a court of law
J. Failing to perform an act that should have been performed
K. The person or group that makes the complaint in a lawsuit
L. Failure to continue to provide medical care to a patient without proper notification
M. Fraudulent appropriation of funds or property of an employer or client
N. Failure to act (or refrain from acting) as a reasonably prudent person would in similar circumstances
O. Performing a legal act in an improper way
P. A law limiting the time period for beginning a lawsuit
Q. A person under the age of 18 with the rights of an adult including the ability to consent to medical care

_______ 18. Litigation
_______ 19. Malfeasance
_______ 20. Malpractice
_______ 21. Mediation
_______ 22. Misdemeanor
_______ 23. Misfeasance
_______ 24. Negligence
_______ 25. Nonfeasance
_______ 26. Plaintiff
_______ 27. Prescription
_______ 28. Privilege
_______ 29. Prudent
_______ 30. Reciprocity
_______ 31. *Respondeat superior*
_______ 32. Standard of care
_______ 33. Statute of limitations
_______ 34. Statutory law
_______ 35. Subpoena *duces tecum*
_______ 36. Emancipated minor

R. The federal agency that enforces the Controlled Substances Act of 1970
S. A defense to a lawsuit that establishes that the plaintiff assumed the risk of whatever caused the injury
T. A less serious crime, punishable by a fine or imprisonment for less than 1 year
U. A court order to produce documents or records
V. A drug that has the potential for addiction or abuse
W. A bill or measure that has become law, often referring to legislation with several parts
X. Negotiation by a third party to help two parties resolve a dispute
Y. The process of taking a lawsuit through the courts
Z. A special immunity that protects against legal liability
AA. Using care or common sense
BB. Automatic issuing of a license in one state to the holder of a license in another state
CC. A crime or wrongdoing that is illegal or contrary to official obligation
DD. Legal responsibility
EE. A condition that must be met before a contract is binding
FF. Level of appropriate care required of a health professional
GG. Official permission to perform an activity or practice a profession
HH. A serious crime punishable by death or imprisonment
II. Negligence by a professional
JJ. An order to a pharmacist to dispense a supply of a medication

EVALUATION OF LEARNING

Directions: Fill in each blank with the correct answer.

1. Identify four reasons that medical assisting students can benefit from studying about ethics and bioethics.

____

____

2. Identify three sources of beliefs about the rights and duties of individuals and society as a whole.

____

____

____

3. Describe briefly what is included in each of the following ethical rights:

   a. Right to life_______________________________

   b. Right to privacy____________________________

   c. Right to autonomy___________________________

   d. Right to the means to sustain life_______________

4. Identify five duties of a health professional.

____

____

5. How does the medical assistant function as a patient advocate?

____

____

6. Why and how should a medical assistant report the illegal or unsafe behavior of another health professional?

____

____

____

7. Most states have a process to file a complaint against physicians whose illegal or unsafe activities threaten the health and safety of patients or others. What is the process in your state?

____

____

____

____

8. When does ethical conflict arise?

____

9. What are two issues that create conflict within society related to reproductive issues?

____

10. What is the current legal position with respect to stem cell research related to federal legislation?

____

____

11. Define the following terms:

a. Stem cell research______________________________

b. Genetic engineering______________________________

c. Cloning______________________________

d. Gene therapy______________________________

12. What are the general provisions of the Patient Self-Determination Act of 1990?

____

13. What is the difference between physician-assisted suicide and euthanasia? Is either legal in the United States?

____

____

14. Describe the difference between personal ethics and professional ethics, and explain which should take priority.

____

____

____

15. What are five recommended steps to make ethical decisions?

____

____

16. Describe the medical assistant's ethical responsibility related to patient care in the medical office.

____

17. What is a DNR order?

____

18. What is the difference between a living will and a health care proxy? Which is preferable?

____

____

19. What is the relationship between law and ethics?

____

20. Briefly describe the following three types of law:
   a. Criminal law_______________
   b. Civil law_______________
   c. Contract law_______________

21. Explain how an injury can result in both civil and criminal lawsuits.

____

22. Describe two classifications of crimes.

____

23. Describe each of the following crimes and identify how each might occur in a medical office:
   a. Manslaughter or criminal negligence_______________
   b. Embezzlement_______________
   c. Fraud_______________

24. What three elements are necessary for a legal contract?

____

____

25. Differentiate between an intentional tort and an unintentional tort.

____

26. Differentiate among a malfeasance, a misfeasance, and a nonfeasance.

____

____

27. Identify how the physician–patient relationship meets the definition of a contract.

____

____

____

28. Give examples of each of the following types of consent:
    a. Implied____
    b. Verbal____
    c. Written____

29. Identify four groups of people who cannot legally be party to a contract or give informed consent.

____

____

30. When can an individual who is not yet 18 consent to medical treatment?

____

____

31. When can a physician terminate care to a patient?

____

____

32. How should the physician notify the patient that he or she is terminating care? Why?

____

____

33. What does the term standard of care mean?

____

34. Why is informed consent usually verified by having the patient sign a consent form?

____

____

35. What is the medical assistant's role in obtaining a signature on a consent form?

____

36. What four elements must be proved in order to prove liability for professional negligence (malpractice)?

____

____

37. What does the doctrine of res ipsa loquitur refer to?

____

38. What are two reasons for physicians to purchase professional liability insurance?

____

39. If a physician believes that a patient is going to initiate a lawsuit, how should he or she respond?

____

40. What is a subpoena and a subpoena *duces tecum?*

____

41. Differentiate between mediation and arbitration.

____

42. Describe the following tort defenses:

a. Privilege_______________

b. Consent_______________

c. Self-defense_______________

d. Expiration of the statute of limitations_______________

e. Contributory negligence_______________

f. Comparative negligence_______________

g. Assumption of risk_______________

43. What are controlled substances, and what law regulates their use?

____

____

44. What are five measures to prevent misuse of prescription forms and tampering with written prescriptions?

____

____

45. What organization was created by the Health and Safety Act of 1970 to protect employees in the workplace?

____

46. What are two examples of measures to protect the health of employees in the medical office?

____

____

47. What employee rights are protected by the following laws?

a. Equal Opportunity Employment laws_______________

b. Americans with Disabilities Act and Amendments_______________

c. Family and Medical Leave Act_______________

d. Fair Labor Standards Act_______________

e. Employee Retirement Income Security Act_______________

48. What is the purpose of the Privacy Rule of the Health Insurance Portability and Accountability Act (HIPAA) of 1996?

____

49. What are four other rules included in HIPAA?

____

____

50. Describe what a mandated report is and give five examples of mandatory reporting for physicians.

____

____

51. What are the two elements of state medical practice acts?

____

____

____

52. What are grounds for suspending or revoking a license to practice medicine?

____

53. Which types of health care facilities usually require a state license?

____

54. Name two organizations that provide voluntary accreditation for physician's offices.

____

CRITICAL THINKING ACTIVITIES

A. Ethical Issues

Select one of the following topics for investigation. Do research about the topic to obtain information. Write a short paper giving information to describe the topic and demonstrate why it is controversial. Be sure to give credit for ideas and/or statistics that you have obtained from a book, journal article, or Internet article.

1. Genetically modified food products
2. Partial birth abortion
3. Federal funding for stem cell research
4. Physician-assisted suicide
5. Gene therapy

B. Patient Advocate

1. Describe the role of a medical assistant as a patient advocate.

____

____

____

2. Explain how a medical assistant might help a patient who has difficulty walking obtain a handicap placard in your state.

____

____

____

C. Personal and Professional Ethics

1. Write a one- to two-page plan for separation of personal and professional ethics (10 points).

2. Identify the conflicting values in each of the following situations, choose an action, and justify your action. Identify if you are guided by personal ethics, professional ethics, or both types of ethics.

   a. You find your brother, who is 12 years old, smoking a cigarette in the backyard.

   ____

   ____

   ____

   ____

   b. A patient tells you that she thinks she may be dependent on the narcotic analgesics she has been taking. Then she asks you not to tell the physician, because she still wants to get a refill for the prescription.

   ____

   ____

   ____

   ____

   c. An elderly relative whom you are extremely close to has a chronic condition causing muscle weakness. She begs you to help her "end everything."

   ____

   ____

   ____

   ____

   d. An expensive medication has been prescribed for a male relative by his personal physician. You mention that there are samples of that medication in your office. The relative asks you if you can get some for him.

   ____

   ____

   ____

   ____

D. Patient Bill of Rights

Using the summary of the Patient Bill of Rights in your textbook, give five examples of policies and procedures that a medical office might institute to protect patient rights.

a. ____

b. ____

c. ____

d. ______________________________

e. ______________________________

f. ______________________________

E. Negligence

Discuss with your classmates what a "reasonably prudent person" would be expected to do in the following situations.

1. Your elderly neighbor slips and falls on a patch of ice in your driveway. She appears unable to get up and complains of pain in her left hip.

   ____

   ____

2. You are in the washroom at work and you notice that the handle on the hot water tap is not working properly so that very hot water is constantly dripping into the sink.

   ____

   ____

3. You spill some coffee on a tile floor at your school.

   ____

   ____

4. You are in a restaurant, and you see another patron who appears to be starting to choke. The person is not coughing audibly, but he is clutching his throat and trying to cough.

   ____

   ____

PRACTICE FOR COMPETENCY

Procedure 3-1: Separating Personal and Professional Ethics

A. Discuss the difference between personal and professional ethics with a classmate and the requirements for professionalism when there is a conflict between personal and professional beliefs.

B. Role play situations with classmates where your personal beliefs may conflict with the beliefs of the patient and patient rights.

Procedure 3-2: Incorporating the Patient's Bill of Rights

A. Discuss the elements of the Patient's Bill of Rights from SimChart® for the Medical Office with a classmate.

B. Role-play activities that demonstrate preserving patient rights to privacy, choice of treatment, consent for treatment, and refusal of treatment in the medical office.

Procedure 3-3: Reporting Illegal Activities and Complying with Public Health Statutes

A. Research local, state and federal agencies to which criminal activity or abuse, theft or diversion of controlled substances, and public health threats such as communicable diseases or animal bites must be reported.

B. Role play making a verbal report of a criminal act, possible abuse, or a communicable disease.

Notes

EVALUATION OF COMPETENCY

Procedure 3-1: Separating Personal and Professional Ethics

Name: ____________________ Date: ____________

Evaluated By: ____________________ Score: ____________

Performance Objective

Outcome:	Develop a plan for separation of personal and professional ethics, and examine the impact personal ethics and morals have on the delivery of health care.
Conditions:	Given access to the Internet, computer, printer, index cards, and pen.
Standards:	Written report.
	Time to complete role play and group discussion: 30 minutes.
	Student completed procedure in ________ minutes.
	Accuracy: Satisfactory score on the Performance Evaluation Checklist.

Performance Evaluation Checklist

Trial 1	Trial 2	Point Value	Performance Standards
		●	Based on research identified conflicting values related to abortion, stem cell research, genetic engineering cloning, refusing/withholding treatment, or physician-assisted suicide.
		●	Determined own personal beliefs related to the issue identified.
		●	Created a written summary of the ethical issue, personal position, and the reasons for the personal position.
		●	Shared the information with a group of classmates.
		●	Created a possible situation involving a patient with a different personal position related to this ethical issue and described it on an index card.
		●	Participated with a classmate in role playing an interaction with conflict related to an ethical issue while maintaining a professional demeanor.
		●	Wrote a description of the effect of personal ethics on professional behavior and the delivery of health care, and prepared a plan to separate these.
		Ⓐ	Demonstrated an appropriate response to the ethical issue presented in the role play
		*	Handed in a satisfactory report and plan to separate personal and professional ethics to instructor.
		*	Completed the role play and group discussion within 30 minutes.
			TOTALS

Evaluation of Student Performance

<table>
<tr><th colspan="3">EVALUATION CRITERIA</th><th>COMMENTS</th></tr>
<tr><th>Symbol</th><th>Category</th><th>Point Value</th><td rowspan="6"></td></tr>
<tr><td>∗</td><td>Critical Step</td><td>16 points</td></tr>
<tr><td>●</td><td>Essential Step</td><td>6 points</td></tr>
<tr><td>Ⓐ</td><td>Affective Competency</td><td>6 points</td></tr>
<tr><td>▷</td><td>Theory Question</td><td>2 points</td></tr>
<tr><td colspan="3">Score calculation: 100 points
– ____ points missed
____ Score

Satisfactory score: 85 or above</td></tr>
</table>

2008 CAAHEP Competencies Achieved
Psychomotor (Skills)
☑ X.1. Develop a plan for separation of personal and professional ethics.
☑ X.2. Demonstrate appropriate response(s) to ethical issues.
Affective (Behavior)
☑ X.2. Examine the impact personal ethics and morals have on the individual's practice.

2015 CAAHEP Competencies Achieved
Psychomotor (Skills)
☑ XI.1. Develop a plan for separation of personal and professional ethics.
☑ XI.2 Demonstrate appropriate response(s) to ethical issues.
Affective (Behavior)
☑ XI.1. Examine the impact personal ethics and morals have on the delivery of health care.

ABHES Competency Achieved
☑ 4. g. Display compliance with the Code of Ethics of the profession.

EVALUATION OF COMPETENCY

Procedure 3-2: Incorporating the Patient's Bill of Rights

Name: ______________________________ Date: ______________

Evaluated By: ______________________________ Score: ______________

Performance Objective

Outcome:	Apply the Patient's Bill of Rights and HIPAA privacy rules
Conditions:	Given access to a computer, printer and role play cards (from instructor).
Standards:	Written list of policies or procedures to protect patient rights and descriptions of medical assistant behavior handed in.
	Time to complete role play on applying the Patient's Bill of Rights: 20 minutes.
	Student completed procedure in _________ minutes.
	Accuracy: Satisfactory score on the Performance Evaluation Checklist.

Performance Evaluation Checklist

Trial 1	Trial 2	Point Value	Performance Standards
		●	Made a list of policies or procedures a medical office should have in place to protect patient rights related to the right to choice of treatment, consent for treatment, refusal of treatment, and privacy.
		●	Included specific examples of ways a medical assistant should behave to preserve patient rights including privacy
		●	Included examples of how a medical assistant should respond if a patient refuses to have a diagnostic test or treatment.
		●	Included a discussion of HIPAA law related to privacy. Explained how patient rights might also be legally protected.
		●	Participated in role play situations with one or more classmates to apply the Patient's Bill of Rights to personal practice.
		●	Participated in at least one role play situation involving consent for or refusal of treatment.
		Ⓐ	In role play situations, demonstrated sensitivity to patient's rights.
		*	Handed in a satisfactory list and examples of medical assistant behavior to preserve patient rights to instructor.
		*	Completed the role play within 20 minutes.
			TOTALS

Evaluation of Student Performance

EVALUATION CRITERIA			COMMENTS
Symbol	**Category**	**Point Value**	
∗	Critical Step	16 points	
●	Essential Step	6 points	
Ⓐ	Affective Competency	6 points	
▷	Theory Question	2 points	
Score calculation: 100 points – ___ points missed ___ Score Satisfactory score: 85 or above			

2008 CAAHEP Competencies Achieved

Psychomotor (Skills)
☑ IX.3. Apply HIPAA rules in regard to privacy/release of information.
☑ IX.5. Incorporate the Patient's Bill of Rights into personal practice and medical office policies and procedures.

Affective (Behavior)
☑ IX.1. Demonstrate sensitivity to patient rights.

2015 CAAHEP Competencies Achieved

Psychomotor (Skills)
☑ X.2.a. Apply HIPAA rules in regard to privacy.
☑ X.4. a.b.c. Apply the Patient's Bill of Rights as it relates to choice of treatment, consent for treatment, and refusal of treatment.

Affective (Behavior)
☑ X.1. Demonstrate sensitivity to patient rights.

ABHES Competency Achieved

☑ 4. g. Display compliance with the Code of Ethics of the profession.

EVALUATION OF COMPETENCY

Procedure 3-3: Reporting Illegal Activities and Complying with Public Health Statutes

Name: ______________________________ Date: ______________

Evaluated By: ______________________________ Score: ______________

Performance Objective

Outcome:	Perform compliance reporting based on public health statutes and report illegal activities following proper protocol.
Conditions:	Given access to the Internet, computer, and printer.
Standards:	Written list, table, discussion, and sample report forms handed in.
	Time to complete role play of two verbal reports: 20 minutes.
	Student completed procedure in ________ minutes.
	Accuracy: Satisfactory score on the Performance Evaluation Checklist.

Performance Evaluation Checklist

Trial 1	Trial 2	Point Value	Performance Standards
		●	Based on research made a list of federal and state agencies to report theft or diversion of controlled substances, wounds or injuries that might be the result of criminal activity, possible abuse, and requirements for reporting public health threats based on public health statutes.
		●	Printed at least one report form from a government agency.
		●	Created a table with two columns identifying specific reportable conditions or actions and the agency or agencies to whom they must be reported.
		●	Wrote a one-page written discussion of the rights of patients when a legal report is mandated.
		●	Participated with a classmate in role playing making a verbal report of an illegal activity and a public health threat.
		Ⓐ	Participated in a role play explaining to a patient how and why a mandated report would be made that clarified the patient's rights in the situation.
		*	Handed in a satisfactory list, table, and one printed governmental report forms to instructor.
		*	Completed the role play within 20 minutes.
			TOTALS

Evaluation of Student Performance

EVALUATION CRITERIA			COMMENTS
Symbol	Category	Point Value	
✶	Critical Step	16 points	
●	Essential Step	6 points	
Ⓐ	Affective Competency	6 points	
▷	Theory Question	2 points	
Score calculation: 100 points − ___ points missed ___ Score Satisfactory score: 85 or above			

2008 CAAHEP Competencies Achieved
Psychomotor (Skills) ☑ X.1. Report illegal and/or unsafe activities and behaviors that affect health, safety, and welfare of others to proper authorities. ***Affective (Behavior)*** ☑ X.1. Apply ethical values, including honesty/integrity in performance of medical assisting practice.

2015 CAAHEP Competencies Achieved
Psychomotor (Skills) ☑ X.5. Perform compliance reporting based on public health statutes. ☑ X.6. Report an illegal activity in the healthcare setting following proper protocol. ***Affective (Behavior)*** ☑ X.1. Demonstrate sensitivity to patient rights.

ABHES Competency Achieved
☑ 4. g. Display compliance with the Code of Ethics of the profession.

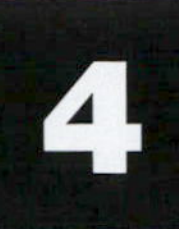

Interacting With Patients

CHAPTER ASSIGNMENTS

✓ After Completing	Date Due	Study Guide Page(s)	STUDY GUIDE ASSIGNMENTS (CTA: Critical Thinking Activity)	Possible Points	Points You Earned
		45	Pretest	10	
		46	Term Key Term Assessment A. Definitions B. Word Parts (Add 1 point for each medical term)	 25 7	
		47-50	Evaluation of Learning questions	31	
		50-52	CTA A: Nonverbal Cues	3	
		52-53	CTA B: Using Effective Communication Techniques	6	
		53	CTA C: Responses That Inhibit Communication	6	
		53	CTA D: Community Resources for Individuals With Terminal Illness	5	
			Evolve Site: Apply Your Knowledge questions	10	
		45	Posttest	10	
			ADDITIONAL ASSIGNMENTS		
			TOTAL POINTS		

✓ When Assigned by Your Instructor	Study Guide Page(s)	Practices Required	LABORATORY ASSIGNMENTS (Procedure Number and Name)	Score*
	55	3	**Practice for Competency** 4-1: Demonstrating Effective and Respectful Verbal and Nonverbal Communication Textbook reference: p. 71	
	57-58		**Evaluation of Competency** 4-1: Demonstrating Effective and Respectful Verbal and Nonverbal Communication	*
	55	3	**Practice for Competency** 4-2: Maintaining Boundaries and Demonstrating Respect for Boundaries in Communication Textbook reference: p. 73	
	59-60		**Evaluation of Competency** 4-2: Maintaining Boundaries and Demonstrating Respect for Boundaries in Communication	*
			ADDITIONAL ASSIGNMENTS	

Name ____ Date ____________________

PRETEST

True or False

_______ 1. The medical assistant communicates nonverbally using tone of voice and facial gestures.

_______ 2. A closed question expects a yes/no or very short answer.

_______ 3. Silence is an effective technique to encourage a patient to continue speaking.

_______ 4. A patient who is legally blind will be unable to distinguish light and shadow.

_______ 5. If a patient is not comfortable using English, translation must be done by a native speaker in person.

_______ 6. In Maslow's hierarchy of needs, the needs for safety and security are lower than the needs for esteem and recognition.

_______ 7. A patient experiencing moderate anxiety will have difficulty learning new information.

_______ 8. The patient is aware when he or she is relying on ego defense mechanisms like denial.

_______ 9. The medical assistant should remember that anger is often displaced from the true cause to another target.

_______ 10. If a patient believes that disease has a supernatural cause, the medical assistant should tell the patient tactfully that this is impossible.

POSTTEST

True or False

_______ 1. Internal factors that interfere with communication include excessive noise and lack of privacy.

_______ 2. Open questions encourage a patient to explain symptoms in his or her own way.

_______ 3. Paraphrasing is giving a short summary of a verbal communication.

_______ 4. The medical assistant uses both touch and words to guide a patient who is totally blind.

_______ 5. Both telephone and video translation services are available when patients are uncomfortable with English.

_______ 6. The needs depicted on the highest level of Maslow's hierarchy include oxygen, sleep, and adequate nutrition.

_______ 7. Hyperventilation may be a symptom of a full-blown anxiety attack.

_______ 8. Projection is an unconscious ego defense mechanism where an individual ascribes his or her own feelings to another.

_______ 9. If a patient is using denial as an ego defense mechanism, it is important to correct the patient as soon as possible.

_______ 10. A patient from a different culture may believe that changes in diet will help treat certain diseases.

KEY TERM ASSESSMENT

A. Definitions

Directions: Match each key term with its definition.

_______ 1. Acting out
_______ 2. Active listening
_______ 3. Anxiety
_______ 4. Body language
_______ 5. Chronic
_______ 6. Closed questions
_______ 7. Denial
_______ 8. Ego defense mechanism
_______ 9. Empathy
_______ 10. Hierarchy
_______ 11. Hospice
_______ 12. Judgmental
_______ 13. Nonverbal
_______ 14. Open questions
_______ 15. Oral
_______ 16. Paraphrasing
_______ 17. Physiologic
_______ 18. Projection
_______ 19. Reflecting
_______ 20. Self-actualization
_______ 21. Summarizing
_______ 22. Sympathy
_______ 23. Terminal
_______ 24. Verbal
_______ 25. Webcam

A. Existing over a long period of time
B. Expressing the meaning and emotion of another's words back to the person
C. Spoken; pertaining to the mouth
D. Unconscious mental process that offers psychological protection
E. The fulfillment of each individual's potential
F. Feeling the same emotions as another
G. Failure to acknowledge the reality of a situation
H. Making judgments about what is good or bad based on personal opinion
I. Using words to communicate
J. Translating unconscious emotions into inappropriate behavior
K. Objective awareness and sensitivity to the feelings and emotions of others
L. Questions that anticipate a yes/no or short answer
M. Pertaining to body processes
N. Small video camera attached to a computer that allows video to be transmitted on the Internet
O. Communication that occurs without words, such as through body posture or facial expression
P. Paying close attention to a speaker without thinking of anything else
Q. Classified according to rank or importance
R. Expressing the most important points of a conversation or written document
S. Communication that is expressed through facial expressions, body position, muscle activity, and other nonverbal means
T. Experiencing one's own emotions as those of another
U. A vague, unpleasant emotion of fear or dread often accompanied by restlessness or nervousness
V. A restatement of the words of another, often to clarify meaning
W. Questions that could have a variety of answers and encourage a personal response
X. The last stage of illness when death is expected to occur within 6 months
Y. An organization that manages care for dying patients

B. Word Parts

Directions: Indicate the meaning of each word part in the space provided. List as many medical terms as possible that incorporate the word part in the space provided.

Word Part	Meaning of Word Part	Medical Terms That Incorporate Word Part
1. non-		
2. verb/o		
3. -al		
4. os; or/o		
5. physi/o		
6. log/o; -logy		
7. -ic		

EVALUATION OF LEARNING

Directions: Fill in each blank with the correct answer.

1. Give four examples of different types of verbal communication.

2. Give four examples of nonverbal communication.

3. Identify and describe three examples of outside interference with effective communication.

4. Identify and describe three examples of inside interference with communication.

5. Describe active listening.

6. What are four listening techniques that facilitate good communication between medical assistants and patients?

7. How can the medical assistant use eye contact and body posture to facilitate communication?

8. Give two examples of how nonverbal communication is different in different cultures.

9. When is it appropriate to use closed questions during an interview?

10. When are open-ended questions more useful than closed questions?

11. Identify and describe six communication techniques that draw patients out and encourage them to keep talking.

a. ______________________________

b. ______________________________

c. ______________________________

d. ______________________________

e. ______________________________

f. ______________________________

12. What are three types of responses that inhibit communication or make the patient defensive?

____

____

13. How can the medical assistant improve communication with a patient whose understanding is impaired?

____

____

14. Differentiate between a patient who is totally blind and one who is legally blind.

____

15. How do patients who are totally blind usually prefer to be assisted in an unknown setting?

____

____

16. Differentiate between a patient who is deaf and a patient who is hearing impaired.

____

17. What measures will improve communication with a patient who is hearing impaired?

____

____

18. What measures should be implemented to communicate with a deaf patient?

____

____

19. What are three ways to provide translation services for a patient who is not comfortable communicating in English?

____

____

20. What are three things that patients often expect when they seek health care?

____

____

21. Identify the needs on each level of Maslow's hierarchy of needs.

a. Level 1 (lowest level): ____________________

b. Level 2: ____________________

c. Level 3: ____________________

d. Level 4: ____________________

e. Level 5 (highest level): ____________________

22. How do unmet needs affect a patient during illness?

____

23. Why is it important for medical assistants to identify the unmet needs of patients?

____

____

24. What are self-boundaries?

____

____

25. Give examples of appropriate ways for a medical assistant to maintain self-boundaries when a patient or other staff member appears to assume that a closer relationship exists than the medical assistant is comfortable with.

____

____

____

26. Differentiate between empathy and sympathy.

____

____

27. How can a medical assistant communicate caring to a patient?

____

____

28. Describe three ways to support a terminally ill patient in the grieving process.

____

____

____

29. What do individuals from other cultures sometimes believe is a cause of illness other than physiologic factors?

____

____

30. What is a general rule about accepting traditional medical practices that patients may use?

____

____

31. Identify and discuss two different cultural practices related to behavioral requirements for women and men.

____

____

CRITICAL THINKING ACTIVITIES

A. Nonverbal Cues

In any interaction, a significant part of communication is nonverbal and includes individual interpretation of nonverbal cues. Examine each of the following photographs and summarize your assumptions about each person in the photograph. Who is each person? What is he or she feeling? What might be happening between the two people in the photograph? How does the person's appearance affect your assessment? Distinguish between assumptions that you are sure of and those you would need more information to confirm.

1.

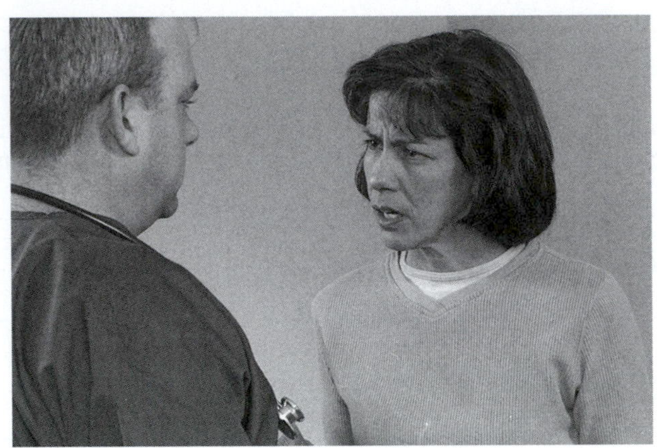

____

____

____

____

2.

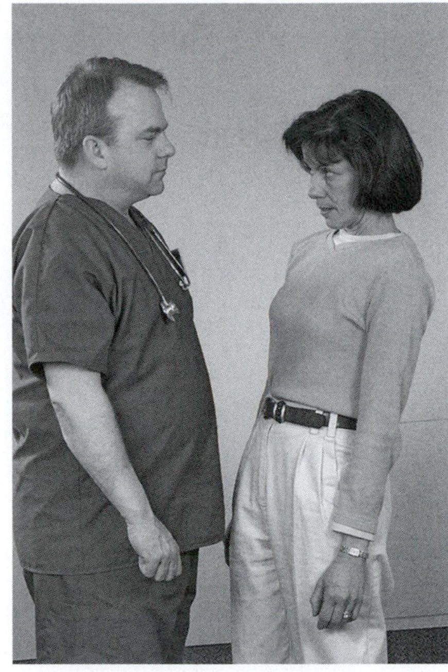

3.

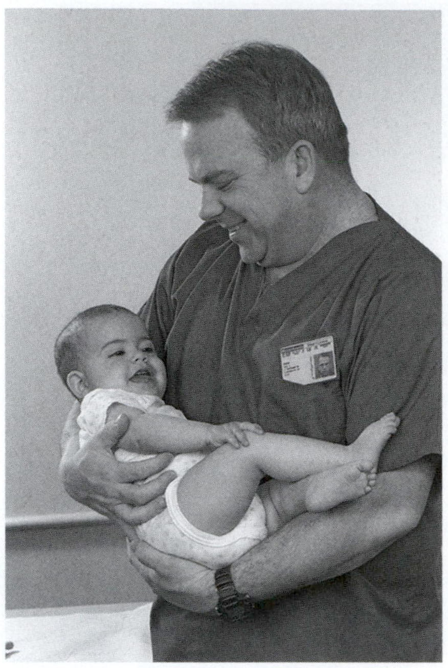

B. **Using Effective Communication Techniques**

After you have taken the vital signs of Valerie Hoffman, a 34-year-old teacher, she says, "I don't know if I'm sick or not. I mean, I hope that Dr. Hughes finds something wrong with me to explain why I feel so bad. I don't have any energy, you know. I get up in the morning, when I can finally get myself up, and in about 10 minutes I'm ready to go back to bed for a nap. Everything just seems like it takes so much effort."

Give an example of a response you could make that demonstrates each of the following communication techniques:

1. Paraphrasing

2. Translating a nonverbal message into words

3. Reflecting

4. Summarizing

5. Repeating or restating

6. Asking for clarification

C. Responses That Inhibit Communication

Refer to Table 4-2 in your textbook and identify how each response inhibits communication.

1. How do you know that bad spirits cause disease? Have you ever seen one?

2. The physician is very busy, you know, because some patients are very ill.

3. You are making a big fuss over a very small problem.

4. After your chemotherapy, you will feel fine in a few hours.

5. Why did you forget to take your blood pressure medication?

6. Your blood sugar is very high because you are not testing it often enough.

D. Community Resources for Individuals with Terminal Illness

1. What are the five steps of the grieving process as defined by Elizabeth Kübler-Ross?

2. List the names, addresses, and telephone numbers of at least five organizations in your community that can help patients and families struggling with a terminal illness.

Notes

PRACTICE FOR COMPETENCY

Procedure 4-1: Demonstrating Effective and Respectful Verbal and Nonverbal Communication

A. Role-play situations where medical assistants demonstrate empathy and active listening including empathy towards patients with a terminal illness.

B. Role-play situations where a medical assistant and a co-worker disagree while demonstrating empathy, active listening and respectful verbal and nonverbal communication.

Procedure 4-2: Maintaining Boundaries and Demonstrating Respect for Boundaries in Communication

A. Discuss the importance of self-boundaries in interactions between patients and medical assistants.

B. Role-play situations with classmates where the patient and medical assistant might have different interpretations of appropriate self-boundaries.

Notes

EVALUATION OF COMPETENCY

Procedure 4-1: Demonstrating Effective and Respectful Verbal and Nonverbal Communication

Name: ______________________ Date: ______________

Evaluated By: ______________________ Score: ______________

Performance Objective

Outcomes:	1. Responds to nonverbal communication 2. Demonstrates nonverbal communication, empathy, and active listening when communicating with patients, family and staff
Conditions:	Given a computer, printer, blank index cards, and a pen.
Standards:	Written description of role play situations handed in to instructor. Time to complete role play: 30 minutes. Student completed procedure in ________ minutes. Accuracy: Satisfactory score on the Performance Evaluation Checklist.

Performance Evaluation Checklist

Trial 1	Trial 2	Point Value	Performance Standards
		Ⓐ	Participated in three role play situations in groups of three (medical assistant, patient with a terminal illness, family member) and demonstrated empathy and active listening.
		•	Discussed with group members the nonverbal communication displayed after each role play situation, and evaluated the effectiveness of communication.
		Ⓐ	Participated in a role play situation between an medical assistant and a coworker to demonstrate active listening and empathy during a disagreement.
		•	Wrote a short description of the nonverbal communication that occurred during the role play situations including the nonvebal messages that were communicated.
		•	Included ways that empathy was communicated verbally and nonverbally in the role play situations.
		•	Included examples of active listening in the role play situations.
		•	Included places where nonverbal communication could have been improved in the role play situations.
		*	Handed in a satisfactory description of the role play situations to instructor.
		*	Completed the role play within 30 minutes.
			TOTALS

Evaluation of Student Performance

EVALUATION CRITERIA			COMMENTS
Symbol	Category	Point Value	
✶	Critical Step	16 points	
●	Essential Step	6 points	
Ⓐ	Affective Competency	6 points	
▷	Theory Question	2 points	
Score calculation: 100 points – ____ points missed ____ Score Satisfactory score: 85 or above			

2008 CAAHEP Competencies Achieved
Psychomotor (Skills) ☑ IV.1. Respond to nonverbal communication. ***Affective (Behavior)*** ☑ IV.1. Demonstrate empathy in communicating with patients, family, and staff. ☑ IV.3. Use appropriate body language and other nonverbal skills in communicating with patients, family, and staff.

2015 CAAHEP Competencies Achieved
Psychomotor (Skills) ☑ V.2. Respond to nonverbal communication. ***Affective (Behavior)*** ☑ V.1. Demonstrate a. empathy, b. active listening and c. nonverbal communication.

ABHES Competency Achieved
☑ 5. b.1. Use empathy when communicating with terminally ill patients.

EVALUATION OF COMPETENCY

Procedure 4-2: Maintaining Boundaries and demonstrating Respect for Boundaries in Communications

Name: ______________________________ Date: ______________

Evaluated By: ______________________________ Score: ______________

Performance Objective

Outcome:	Demonstrate awareness of self-boundaries and the effect of personal appearance, while protecting self-boundaries and demonstrating respect for individual diversity.
Conditions:	Given a computer and printer.
Standards:	Written report.
	Time to complete role play: 20 minutes.
	Accuracy: Satisfactory score on the Performance Evaluation Checklist.

Performance Evaluation Checklist

Trial 1	Trial 2	Point Value	Performance Standards
		●	Created three situations and wrote dialog for three specified situations where a medical assistant is taking vital signs and might respond to the patient's personal appearance.
		●	Analyzed each situation explaining how the apparance of the patient, territorial boundaries or personal bias might influence the interaction.
		●	Explained how the medical assistant should protect personal boundaries and demonstrate respect in each situation.
		Ⓐ	Participated in role play for each situation with a classmate.
		*	Completed role play within 20 minutes.
		*	Handed in a satisfactory written report with explanations of self-boundaries, influences of possible bias from appearance, and ways for a medical assistant to protect self-boundaries and demonstrate respect for invidual diversity including gender, race, religion, age, economic status, and appearance.
			TOTALS

Evaluation of Student Performance

<table>
<tr><th colspan="3">EVALUATION CRITERIA</th><th>COMMENTS</th></tr>
<tr><td>Symbol</td><td>Category</td><td>Point Value</td><td rowspan="6"></td></tr>
<tr><td>*</td><td>Critical Step</td><td>16 points</td></tr>
<tr><td>●</td><td>Essential Step</td><td>6 points</td></tr>
<tr><td>Ⓐ</td><td>Affective Competency</td><td>6 points</td></tr>
<tr><td>▷</td><td>Theory Question</td><td>2 points</td></tr>
<tr><td colspan="3">Score calculation: 100 points
– ____ points missed
____ Score

Satisfactory score: 85 or above</td></tr>
</table>

2008 CAAHEP Competencies Achieved
Affective (Behavior) ☑ IV.4. Demonstrate awareness of the territorial boundaries of the person with whom communicating. ☑ V.3. Demonstrate respect for individual diversity incorporating awareness of one's own biases including gender, race, religion, age, and economic status.

2015 CAAHEP Competencies Achieved
Affective (Behavior) ☑ V.2. Demonstrate the principles of self-boundaries. ☑ V.3. Demonstrate respect for individual diversity including: a. gender, b. race, c. religion, d. age, e. economic status, f. appearance.

ABHES Competency Achieved
☑ 5. 3.e. Analyze the effect of hereditary, cultural, and environmental influences on behavior.

Introduction to Anatomy and Physiology

CHAPTER ASSIGNMENTS

✓ After Completing	Date Due	Study Guide Page(s)	STUDY GUIDE ASSIGNMENTS (CTA: Critical Thinking Activity)	Possible Points	Points You Earned
		63	Pretest	10	
		 64 65	Key Term Assessment: A. Definitions B. Word Parts (Add 1 point for each key term)	 38 27	
		66-78	Evaluation of Learning questions The Human Body Cell Structure and Function Tissue and Membranes	 19 32 68	
		79	CTA A: Planes of the Body	3	
		79	CTA B: Cavities of the Body	8	
		80	CTA C: Abdominopelvic Quadrants	4	
		80	CTA D: Abdominopelvic Regions	9	
		81	Evolve Site: CTA E: Road to Recovery: Body Area Terms (Record points earned)		
		81	Evolve Site: CTA F: Body Spectrum: General Human Cell	10	
		81-82	CTA G: Cell Structure and Function	40	
		83	CTA H: Crossword Puzzle	25	
		63	Posttest	10	
			ADDITIONAL ASSIGNMENTS		
			TOTAL POINTS		

Notes

Name ______________________ Date ______________

PRETEST

True or False

_______ 1. The study of the shape and structure of the human body is known as *human anatomy.*

_______ 2. The integumentary system protects underlying tissue from injury.

_______ 3. The lungs are located in the pelvic cavity.

_______ 4. The nucleolus is the control center that directs the activities of the cell.

_______ 5. The function of lysosomes is to destroy cellular debris and foreign particles.

_______ 6. A human cell has 23 pairs of chromosomes.

_______ 7. Cytology is the microscopic study of tissues.

_______ 8. Fibroblasts secrete mucus.

_______ 9. Adipose tissue protects the body from invasion by pathogens.

_______ 10. Platelets initiate the blood clotting mechanism.

POSTTEST

True or False

_______ 1. An organ is made up of a group of tissues with a similar structure and function.

_______ 2. A frontal plane divides the body into right and left portions.

_______ 3. The plasma membrane determines what can enter or leave a cell.

_______ 4. Ribosomes are responsible for protein synthesis.

_______ 5. Microvilli are hairlike processes that move substances across the surface of a cell.

_______ 6. A red blood cell will hemolyze if it is placed in a hypertonic solution.

_______ 7. Capillary walls are made up of simple squamous epithelial tissue.

_______ 8. An endocrine gland secretes its product onto a free surface through a duct.

_______ 9. Skeletal muscle tissue is under involuntary control.

_______ 10. A mucous membrane lines a body cavity that opens to the outside.

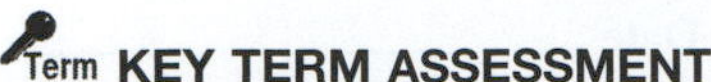

KEY TERM ASSESSMENT

A. Definitions

Directions: Match each key term with its definition.

_______ 1. Active transport	A. Division of the cell at the end of mitosis to form two separate daughter cells
_______ 2. Anatomic position	B. Connective tissue cell that produces fibers
_______ 3. Axon	C. The type of nuclear division in which the number of chromosomes is reduced to half the number found in a body cell; results in the formation of an egg or sperm
_______ 4. Chondrocyte	D. A response mechanism of the body in which a stimulus initiates reactions that reduces the stimulus
_______ 5. Collagenous fibers	E. The diffusion of water through a selectively permeable membrane.
_______ 6. Cutaneous membrane	F. The standard reference position for the body.
_______ 7. Cytokinesis	G. The movement of substances from a region of high concentration to a region of low concentration
_______ 8. Dendrites	H. Fibers composed of elastin that have a stretching quality
_______ 9. Diffusion	I. The study of the shape and structure of the human body and the relationship of its parts
_______ 10. Elastic fibers	J. Cells located in nervous tissue that provide support for neurons
_______ 11. Erythrocytes	K. A group of cells with a similar structure that are specialized to form a certain function
_______ 12. Fibroblast	L. Strong and flexible connective tissue fibers that contain collagen
_______ 13. Histology	M. The process that moves substances across or through a membrane and requires cellular energy
_______ 14. Homeostasis	N. The microscopic study of tissues
_______ 15. Human anatomy	O. The engulfing and destruction of foreign particles such as bacteria
_______ 16. Human physiology	P. The scientific study of the functions of the human body and its parts
_______ 17. Leukocytes	Q. A nerve cell
_______ 18. Macrophage	R. The formation of vesicles to transfer fluid droplets into a cell; cell drinking
_______ 19. Mast cell	S. A normal stable condition in which the body's internal environment remains the same
_______ 20. Meiosis	T. A cartilage cell
_______ 21. Meninges	U. A large phagocytic cell that cleans up cellular debris and foreign particles from the tissues
_______ 22. Mitosis	V. A connective tissue cell that produces heparin and histamine
_______ 23. Mucous membrane	W. The process by which the nucleus of a body cell divides to form two new (daughter) cells, each identical to the parent cell
_______ 24. Negative feedback	X. A mature bone cell
_______ 25. Neuroglia	Y. The process that moves substances across or through a membrane and does not require cellular energy
_______ 26. Neuron	Z. Efferent process of a neuron.
_______ 27. Osmosis	AA. A type of epithelial membrane; skin.
_______ 28. Osteocyte	BB. Treelike processes of a neuron; efferent processes
_______ 29. Passive transport	CC. Red blood cells
_______ 30. Pericardium	DD. White blood cells
_______ 31. Peritoneum	EE. Connective tissue membranes that cover the brain and spinal cord
_______ 32. Phagocytosis	FF. Epithelial membrane that lines body cavities that open directly to the exterior
_______ 33. Pinocytosis	GG. Membrane that surrounds the heart
_______ 34. Pleura	HH. Serous membrane associated with the abdominopelvic cavity
_______ 35. Serous membrane	II. Serous membrane that surrounds the lungs
_______ 36. Synovial membrane	JJ. Epithelial membrane that lines closed body cavities
_______ 37. Thrombocyte	KK. Membrane that lines the cavities of freely movable joints
_______ 38. Tissue	LL. A formed element of the blood that functions in blood clotting; platelet

B. Word Parts

Directions: Indicate the meaning of each word part in the space provided. List as many medical terms as possible that incorporate the word part in the space provided.

Word Part	Meaning of Word Part	Medical Terms That Incorporate Word Part
1. chondr/o		
2. -cyte		
3. cutane/o		
4. -ous		
5. -kinesis		
6. erythr/o		
7. fibr/o		
8. -blast		
9. hist/o		
10. -ology		
11. home/o		
12. -stasis		
13. physi/o		
14. leuk/o		
15. macro-		
16. phag/o		
17. mening/o		
18. neur/o		
19. -glia		
20. oste/o		
21. peri-		
22. cardi/o		
23. -osis		
24. pin/o		
25. pleur/o		
26. ser/o		
27. thromb/o		

EVALUATION OF LEARNING

Directions: Fill in each blank with the correct answer.

The Human Body

1. What is the difference between gross human anatomy and microscopic human anatomy?

____

____

2. What is the relationship between human anatomy and physiology?

____

____

3. What are the six levels of organization of the body?

____

____

4. What are the four main types of tissue found in the body?

____

____

5. What makes up an organ? List examples of organs.

____

____

6. What makes up a body system? List examples of body systems.

____

____

7. What makes up a total human organism?

____

8. What is the function of the following systems?

   a. Integumentary: ____

   ____

   b. Skeletal: ____

   ____

   c. Muscular: ____

   ____

   d. Nervous: ____

   ____

   e. Endocrine: ____

   ____

f. Cardiovascular: ______________________________

g. Lymphatic: ______________________________

h. Digestive: ______________________________

i. Respiratory: ______________________________

j. Urinary: ______________________________

k. Reproductive: ______________________________

9. What is homeostasis? Why is it important to the body?

10. How does the body maintain normal blood pressure using a negative feedback mechanism?

11. Describe the body in anatomic position.

12. Define the following body directions and provide an example of each:

    a. Superior: ______________________________

    b. Inferior: ______________________________

    c. Anterior: ______________________________

    d. Posterior: ______________________________

    e. Medial: ______________________________

f. Lateral: ______________________________

____

g. Proximal: ______________________________

____

h. Distal: ______________________________

____

i. Superficial: ______________________________

____

j. Deep: ______________________________

____

k. Visceral: ______________________________

____

l. Parietal: ______________________________

____

13. Define the following planes and sections of the body:

a. Sagittal plane: ______________________________

____

b. Midsagittal plane: ______________________________

____

c. Transverse plane: ______________________________

____

d. Frontal plane: ______________________________

____

14. What are the subdivisions of the dorsal cavity? ______________________________

____

15. What are the subdivisions of the ventral cavity? ______________________________

____

16. What structures are located in the thoracic cavity? ______________________________

____

17. What structures are located in the abdominal cavity? ______________________________

____

18. What structures are located in the pelvic cavity? ______________________________

____

19. What structures are located in the following regions of the body?

   a. Axial: ______

   b. Appendicular: ______

Cell Structure and Function

1. What is the function of the plasma membrane?

______

______

2. What is cytoplasm?

______

3. What are organelles?

______

4. What substances are dissolved in the intracellular fluid of the cytoplasm?

______

______

5. What is the function of the nucleus?

______

______

6. Where is the nucleolus located?

______

7. What is the function of the nucleolus?

______

______

8. What is the function of mitochondria?

______

______

9. What is the function of ribosomes?

______

10. What is the function of the endoplasmic reticulum?

______

______

11. What is the function of the Golgi apparatus?

______

______

12. What is the function of lysosomes?

____

____

13. What are cilia, and what is their function?

____

____

14. What is simple diffusion?

____

____

15. How does diffusion result in the exchange of oxygen and carbon dioxide in the lungs?

____

____

____

16. What is osmosis?

____

____

17. What occurs when a red blood cell is placed in an isotonic solution?

____

____

18. What occurs when a red blood cell is placed in a hypertonic solution? Explain the reason for your answer.

____

____

19. What occurs when a red blood cell is placed in a hypotonic solution? Explain the reason for your answer.

____

____

20. What process in the body relies on filtration?

____

21. What is active transport?

____

____

22. What process in the body relies on active transport?

____

____

23. What is endocytosis?

24. What occurs during phagocytosis?

25. What is exocytosis?

26. List two examples of exocytosis.

27. What is a somatic cell?

28. What is a gamete?

29. How many pairs of chromosomes are present in a human cell?

30. What are the two methods the body uses to reproduce cells?

31. What is mitosis?

32. What is meiosis?

Tissues and Membranes

1. What is histology?

2. What is the intercellular matrix?

3. What are the four main tissues of the body?

4. Where is epithelial tissue located?

5. What is the name of the structure that attaches epithelial cells to underlying connective tissue?

6. Describe the shape of the cell and its nucleus for each of the following types of epithelial cells:

   a. Squamous:

   b. Cuboidal:

   c. Columnar:

7. What is the difference between simple epithelium and stratified epithelium?

8. Describe the appearance of simple squamous epithelium. In the margin of this page, draw a sketch of simple -squamous epithelium.

9. Where is simple squamous epithelium located in the body?

10. Describe the appearance of simple cuboidal epithelium. In the margin of this page, draw a sketch of simple cuboidal epithelium.

11. Where is simple cuboidal epithelium located in the body?

12. Describe the appearance of simple columnar epithelium. In the margin of this page, draw a sketch of simple columnar epithelium.

____

____

13. Where is simple columnar epithelium located in the body?

____

14. What are microvilli? What is their purpose?

____

____

15. What is the purpose of goblet cells?

____

16. What is the appearance of pseudostratified columnar epithelium? In the margin of this page, draw a sketch of -pseudostratified columnar epithelium.

____

____

17. Where is pseudostratified columnar epithelium located in the body?

____

____

18. What is the appearance of stratified squamous epithelium? In the margin of this page, draw a sketch of stratified squamous epithelium.

____

____

19. Where is stratified squamous epithelium located in the body?

____

____

20. What special quality is present in transitional epithelium?

____

____

21. Where is transitional epithelium located in the body?

____

22. What is glandular epithelium?

____

____

23. What is the difference between an exocrine gland and an endocrine gland?

____

____

24. What are examples of exocrine glands?

____

25. What is the function of connective tissue?

____

____

26. What are the characteristics of collagenous fibers?

____

____

27. What structures are composed of collagenous fibers?

____

28. What are the characteristics of elastic fibers?

____

29. What three cells are most commonly found in connective tissue? List the function of each of these cells.

Cell	Function

30. What is the function of loose connective tissue?

____

____

31. What is the function of adipose tissue?

____

____

32. Describe the characteristics of dense fibrous connective tissue.

____

____

33. What is the function of tendons?

34. What is the function of ligaments?

35. What body structures are composed of elastic connective tissue?

36. What is the function of cartilage?

37. Describe the following components of cartilage:

Chondrocyte:

Perichondrium:

38. Where is hyaline cartilage located?

39. Where is fibrocartilage located in the body?

40. Where is elastic cartilage located in the body?

41. What is the function of bone?

42. Describe the following components of bone:

Osteons (haversian systems):

Osteonic canal (haversian canal):

Osteocyte:

Canaliculi:

43. What qualities do the following give to bone?

Collagenous fibers: ___

Calcium: ___

44. What is the function of the following blood components?

Erythrocytes: ___

___

Leukocytes: ___

___

Thrombocytes: ___

___

Plasma: ___

___

45. What is the function of muscle tissue?

___

___

46. Describe the appearance of skeletal muscle cells. In the margin of this page, draw a sketch of skeletal muscle cells.

___

___

47. What is the function of skeletal muscle in the body?

___

48. Describe the appearance of smooth muscle cells. In the margin of this page, draw a sketch of smooth muscle cells.

___

___

49. Where is smooth muscle located in the body?

___

50. What is the function of smooth muscle?

___

___

51. Describe the appearance of cardiac muscle cells. In the margin of this page, draw a sketch of cardiac muscle cells.

___

52. Where is cardiac muscle located in the body?

___

53. What is the function of cardiac muscle?

____

____

54. Where is nervous tissue located in the body?

____

55. What is the function of nervous tissue?

____

____

56. Describe the following components of nervous tissue:

Neuron:______________________________________

Nerve cell body:______________________________

Dendrites:___________________________________

Axons:______________________________________

Neuroglia:___________________________________

57. What is a mucous membrane?

____

____

58. Where are mucous membranes located in the body?

____

____

59. What is the function of mucus secreted by a mucous membrane?

____

60. What is a serous membrane?

____

____

61. What is the function of serous fluid?

____

____

62. Where are serous membranes located in the body?

____

____

63. What are synovial membranes?

64. Where are synovial membranes located in the body?

65. What is the function of synovial fluid?

66. What are the meninges?

67. What is the function of the meninges?

68. List and describe the three layers that make up the meninges.

Layer	Description

CRITICAL THINKING ACTIVITIES

A. Planes of the Body

Using Figure 5-3 in your textbook as a reference, label each of the planes of the body on the following diagram.

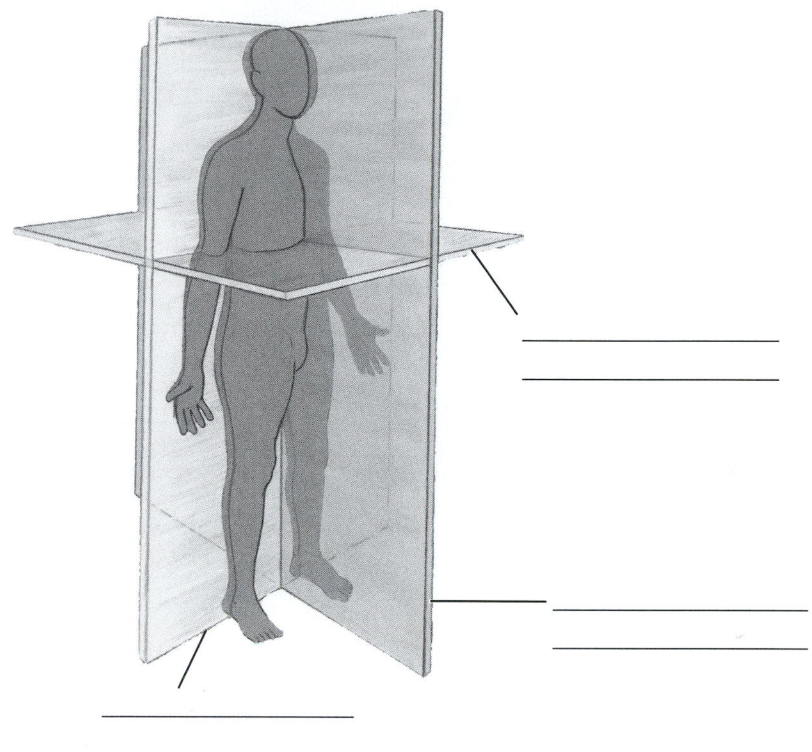

(Modified from Applegate E: *The anatomy and physiology learning system*, ed 4, St. Louis, 2011, Saunders.)

B. Cavities of the Body

Using Figure 5-4 in your textbook as a reference, label each of the cavities of the body on the following diagram.

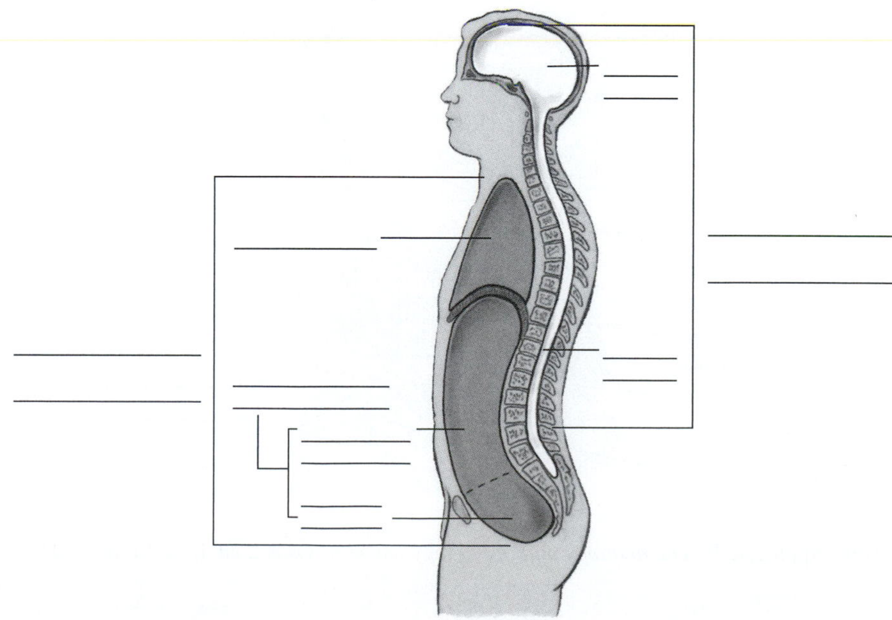

(Modified from Applegate E: *The anatomy and physiology learning system*, ed 4, St. Louis, 2011, Saunders.)

C. Abdominopelvic Quadrants

Using Figure 5-5 in your textbook as a reference, label each of the quadrants of the body on the following diagram.

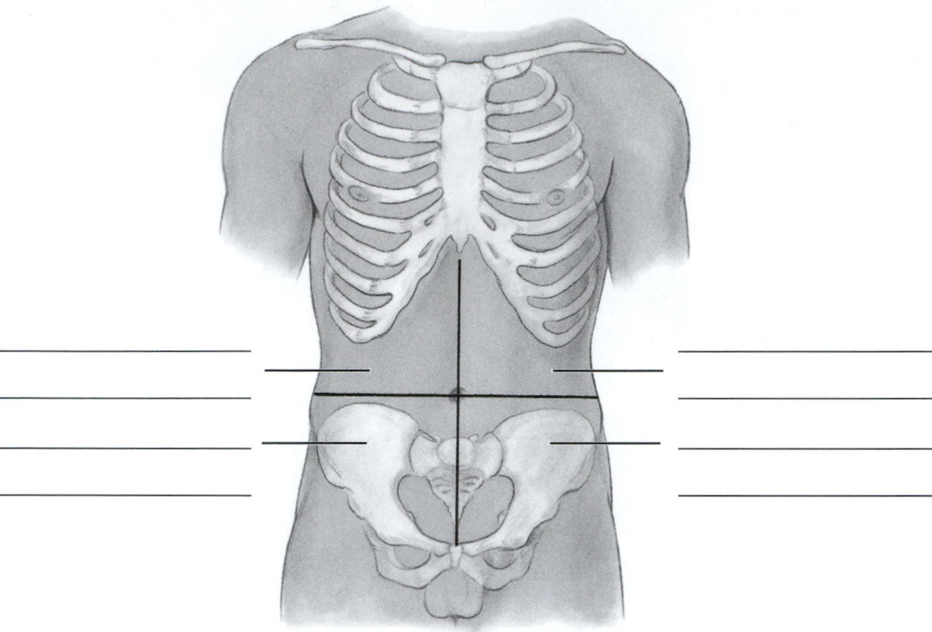

(Modified from Applegate E: *The anatomy and physiology learning system*, ed 4, St. Louis, 2011, Saunders.)

D. Abdominopelvic Regions

Using Figure 5-6 in your textbook as a reference, label each of the abdominopelvic regions of the body on the following diagram.

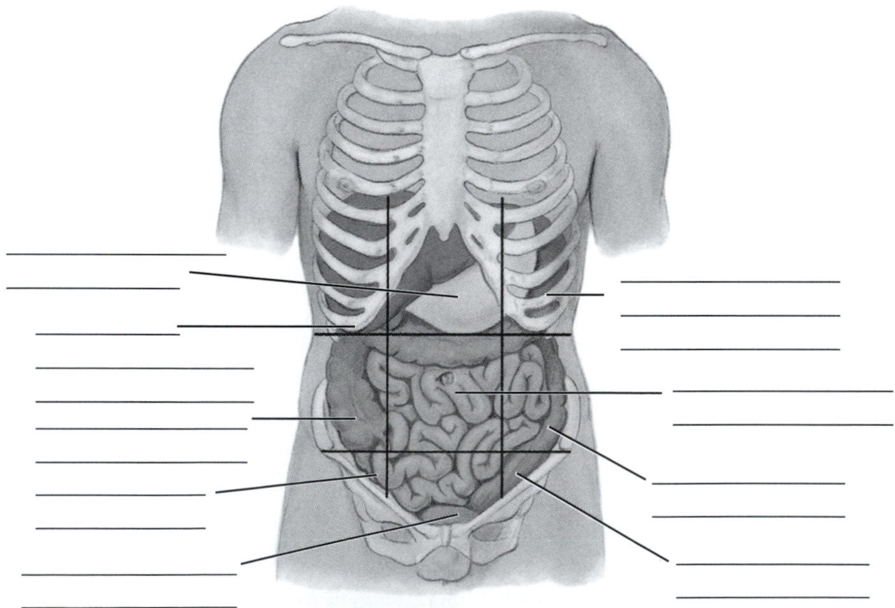

(Modified from Applegate E: *The anatomy and physiology learning system*, ed 4, St. Louis, 2011, Saunders.)

E. Evolve Site: Road to Recovery

Body Area Terms

Directions:

1. Review the body area terms presented in Table 5-2 of your textbook.
2. Access the Evolve site.
3. Play the Road to Recovery Game presented in Chapter 5.
4. Record your points on your assignment sheet.

F. Evolve Site: Body Spectrum

General Human Cell

Body Spectrum directions:

1. Access the Body Spectrum on the Evolve site.
2. If necessary, access the HELP screen for directions on using the Body Spectrum program.
3. Go to the *Contents* screen.
4. Select the following category from the *Contents* screen:
   Cell Structure
5. Select the following anatomic diagram:
   General Human Cell
6. Identify the structures on the diagram.
7. Print out the diagram.

G. Cell Structure and Function

You are an oxygen molecule that has just entered a body cell. In the space provided below, describe all of the structures you see in the cell. Also describe what function each structure is performing in the cell. Each of the following structures should be included in your discussion:

a. Plasma membrane
b. Cytoplasm
c. Nucleus
d. Nuclear membrane
e. Nucleolus
f. Mitochondria
g. Ribosomes
h. Rough endoplasmic reticulum
i. Smooth endoplasmic reticulum
j. Golgi apparatus
k. Lysosomes
l. Centrioles
m. Chromatin
n. Secretory vesicle

____

____

____

____

____

____

____

H. Crossword Puzzle: Introduction to Anatomy and Physiology

Directions: Complete the crossword puzzle using the clues provided.

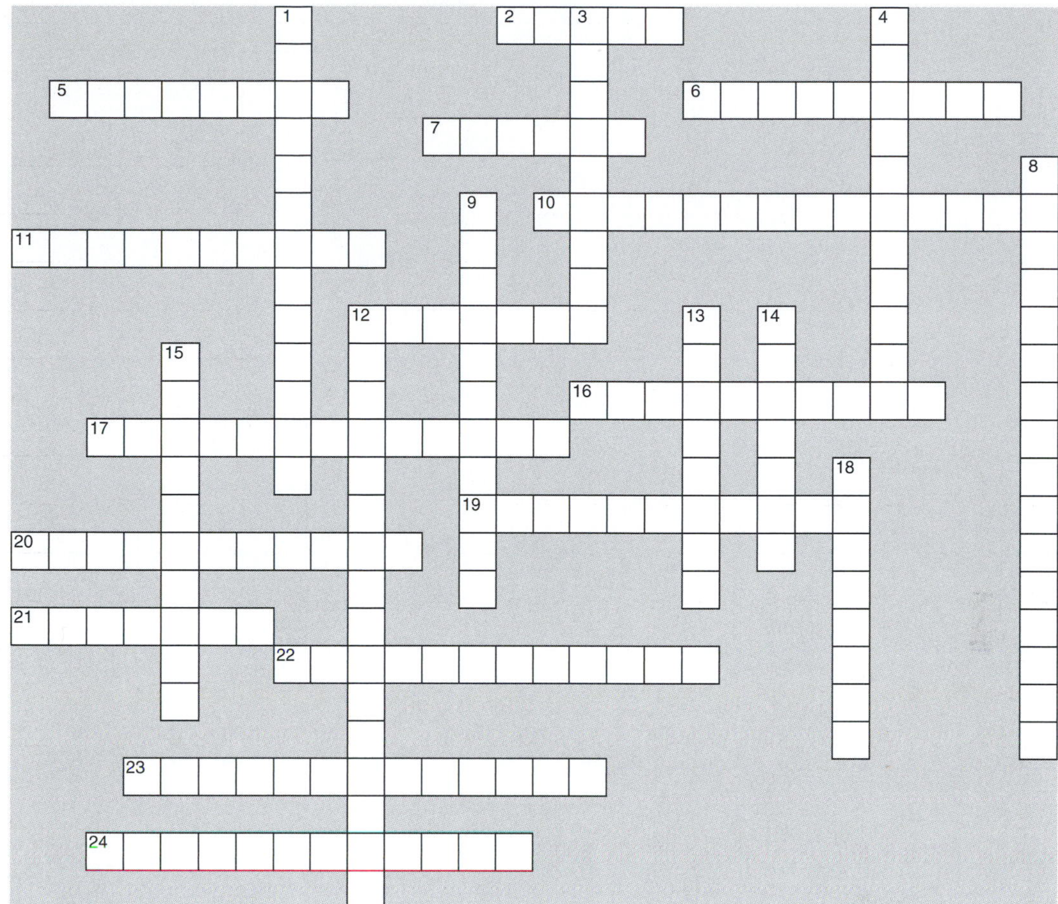

Across

2 Little hairs on cell membrane
5 Number of chromosomes in human cell
6 Synthesizes proteins
7 Connects muscle to bone
10 Packaging and shipping plant
11 Secretes mucus
12 Produces two daughter cells
16 Helps distribute chromosomes to daughter cells
17 Brain, spinal cord, and nerves
19 On or near the surface
20 Everything is "A-OK"
21 Cell's control center
22 Cell eating
23 Houses the brain
24 Power plant of cell

Down

1 Contains fat cells
3 Destroys cellular debris
4 Cartilage cell
8 Has same concentration as RBCs
9 Cell drinking
12 Divides body into right and left halves
13 Toward the front
14 Cell division that produces eggs and sperm
15 Lines abdominopelvic cavity
18 Sperm tail

Notes

6 Integumentary System

CHAPTER ASSIGNMENTS

✓ After Completing	Date Due	Study Guide Page(s)	STUDY GUIDE ASSIGNMENTS (CTA: Critical Thinking Activity)		
		87	Pretest	10	
		88	Key Term Assessment A. Definitions B. Word Parts (Add 1 point for each key term)	 16 12	
		89-92	Evaluation of Learning questions	43	
		92	Evolve Site: CTA A: Body Spectrum—Skin Structure	10	
		92	Evolve Site: CTA B: Body Spectrum—Glands of the Skin	10	
		92	Evolve Site: CTA C: Body Spectrum—Skin and Hypodermis	10	
		93	Evolve Site: CTA D: Body Spectrum—Hair Follicle	10	
		93	Evolve Site: CTA E: Body Spectrum—Hair Follicle Enlarged	10	
		93-95	CTA F: Inquiring Patients Want to Know	20	
		95	CTA G: Crossword Puzzle	22	
		87	Posttest	10	
			ADDITIONAL ASSIGNMENTS		
			TOTAL POINTS		

Notes

Name ______________________________ Date ______________

PRETEST

True or False

_______ 1. The nails are part of the integumentary system.

_______ 2. The thickest layer of the epidermis is the stratum corneum.

_______ 3. Cerumen provides waterproofing for the skin.

_______ 4. Sensory receptors allow the body to detect changes in the environment.

_______ 5. The subcutaneous layer cushions underlying organs.

_______ 6. The ultraviolet rays of the sun increase melanocyte activity.

_______ 7. The face does not contain hair.

_______ 8. Hair is produced by hair follicles.

_______ 9. The neck and chest have the most sweat glands.

_______ 10. Vitamin A is necessary for the absorption of calcium in the body.

POSTTEST

True or False

_______ 1. The epidermis consists of simple squamous epithelial tissue.

_______ 2. Skin cells grow and multiply in the stratum basale layer of the epidermis.

_______ 3. Melanocytes produce a yellow pigment.

_______ 4. Sebaceous glands are embedded in the dermis.

_______ 5. An individual with a large number of melanin granules in his or her skin will have dry skin.

_______ 6. The part of the hair that is visible is known as the *shaft.*

_______ 7. The outermost covering of the hair is known as the *cuticle.*

_______ 8. Shivering is caused by contraction of the arrector pili muscles.

_______ 9. Sebum keeps hair and skin soft and pliable.

_______ 10. Cerumen traps foreign material.

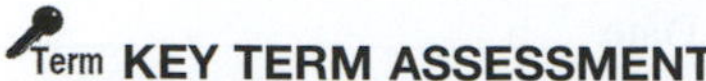

KEY TERM ASSESSMENT

A. Definitions

Directions: Match each key term with its definition.

_______ 1. Arrector pili
_______ 2. Ceruminous gland
_______ 3. Cutaneous membrane
_______ 4. Dermis
_______ 5. Epidermis
_______ 6. Hypodermis
_______ 7. Keratinization
_______ 8. Melanin
_______ 9. Melanocyte
_______ 10. Sebaceous gland
_______ 11. Sebum
_______ 12. Stratum corium
_______ 13. Stratum corneum
_______ 14. Subcutaneous layer
_______ 15. Sudoriferous gland
_______ 16. Sweat glands

A. A dark brown or black pigment found in parts of the body, especially skin and hair
B. A gland in the ear canal that produces cerumen or earwax
C. A gland in the skin that produces perspiration; also called sweat gland
D. An oil gland of the skin that produces sebum or body oil
E. Below the skin; a sheet of areolar connective tissue and adipose tissue beneath the dermis of the skin; also called *hypodermis* or *superficial fascia.*
F. Inner layer of the skin that contains the blood vessels, nerves, glands, and hair follicles
G. Muscle associated with hair follicles
H. Outermost layer of the skin
I. Process by which the cells of the epidermis become filled with keratin and move to the surface, where they are sloughed off
J. Another name for the skin
K. A sheet of areolar connective tissue and adipose beneath the dermis of the skin
L. A cell that produces the dark or black pigment melanin
M. Oily secretion from sebaceous glands
N. Another name for the dermis
O. Outermost layer of the epidermis
P. Glands in the skin that produce perspiration

B. Word Parts

Directions: Indicate the meaning of each word part in the space provided. List as many medical terms as possible that incorporate the word part in the space provided.

Word Part	Meaning of Word Part	Medical Terms That Incorporate Word Part
1. epi-		
2. kerat/o		
3. -ation		
4. melan/o		
5. seb/o		
6. -ous		
7. sub-		
8. cutane/o		
9. sud-		
10. pil/o		
11. derm/o		
12. strat-		

EVALUATION OF LEARNING

Directions: Fill in each blank with the correct answer.

1. What structures make up the integumentary system?

 ____

2. What is another name for the skin?

 ____

3. What occurs during keratinization?

 ____

 ____

4. Why do cells in the epidermis flatten out and die as they reach the surface of the skin?

 ____

 ____

5. What occurs in the stratum basale?

 ____

 ____

6. What are melanocytes?

 ____

 ____

7. What makes up the stratum corneum?

 ____

 ____

8. What is the function of keratin?

 ____

 ____

9. What is another name for the dermis?

 ____

10. What structures are embedded in the dermis?

 ____

11. What happens if the dermis is overstretched?

 ____

 ____

12. What is the function of sensory receptors?

____

____

13. What causes fingerprints and footprints?

____

____

14. What are two other terms for the subcutaneous layer?

____

15. What type of tissue is located in the subcutaneous layer?

____

16. What is the function of subcutaneous tissue?

____

____

17. What controls the activity of melanocytes?

____

____

18. What occurs when the body is unable to produce melanin?

____

19. What is the name of the pigment that results in a yellow tint of the skin?

____

20. What effect does ultraviolet light have on melanocyte activity?

____

21. What parts of the body do not grow hair?

____

22. What is the name given to the part of the hair that is visible?

____

23. Where is the root of the hair located?

____

24. What is the name of the outer covering of a hair? What makes up this covering?

____

____

25. What is the function of a hair follicle?

26. How is hair color determined?

27. What occurs when the arrector pili muscles contract?

28. What can cause the arrector pili muscles to contract?

29. What makes up a nail?

30. What is the name given to the visible portion of a nail?

31. What is another name for the cuticle of a nail?

32. Why do nails appear pink?

33. What is the function of sebum?

34. What parts of the body have the most sweat glands?

35. What is a sweat pore?

36. What causes perspiration to occur?

37. What is the function of cerumen?

38. List four ways in which the skin protects the body.

____

____

39. How does the skin regulate body temperature?

____

40. Vitamin D assists in the absorption of what minerals?

____

41. What are the functions of calcium and phosphorus in the body?

____

42. How does the skin produce vitamin D?

____

____

43. How do each of the following changes due to aging affect the skin?

a. Decrease in elastic fibers and adipose tissue:______________________

b. Loss of collagen fibers:______________________

c. Slower mitotic activity in the stratum basale:______________________

d. Reduced in sebaceous gland activity:______________________

e. Reduction in melanocyte activity:______________________

CRITICAL THINKING ACTIVITIES

A. Evolve Site: Body Spectrum

Integumentary: Skin Structure

Body Spectrum directions:

1. Access the Body Spectrum on the Evolve site.
2. If necessary, access the HELP screen for directions on using the Body Spectrum program.
3. Go to the *Contents* screen.
4. Select the following category from the *Contents* screen:
   Integumentary
5. Select the following anatomic diagram:
   Skin Structure
6. Identify the structures on the diagram.
7. Print out the diagram.

B. Evolve Site: Body Spectrum

Integumentary: Glands of the Skin

Directions: Identify the structures on this diagram following the Body Spectrum directions outlined under CTA A.

C. Evolve Site: Body Spectrum

Integumentary: Skin and Hypodermis

Directions: Identify the structures on this diagram following the Body Spectrum directions outlined under CTA A.

D. Evolve Site: Body Spectrum

Integumentary: Hair Follicle

Directions: Identify the structures on this diagram following the Body Spectrum directions outlined under CTA A.

E. Evolve Site: Body Spectrum

Integumentary: Hair Follicle Enlarged

Directions: Identify the structures on this diagram following the Body Spectrum directions outlined under CTA A.

F. Inquiring Patients Want to Know

You are working in a general practice medical office. Your patients ask you the following questions. In the space provided, indicate how you would respond to each question in terms the patient would understand.

1. What makes skin waterproof?

____

____

2. What causes a blister?

____

____

3. What causes blushing?

____

____

4. What causes curly hair?

____

____

5. Why does it not hurt when my hair is cut?

____

____

6. What causes split ends?

____

____

7. How does hair grow?

____

____

8. What causes freckles?

____

____

9. Why do I have red hair?

10. Why does my skinny friend get cold all the time?

11. What causes age spots?

12. What causes wrinkles?

13. What causes a person to tan?

14. What causes "goose bumps?"

15. What causes pimples?

16. What causes baldness?

17. What causes warts?

18. What causes itching?

19. What causes hair to turn white?

20. How does sunshine cause the body to produce vitamin D?

____

____

G. Crossword Puzzle: Integumentary System

Directions: Complete the crossword puzzle using the clues provided.

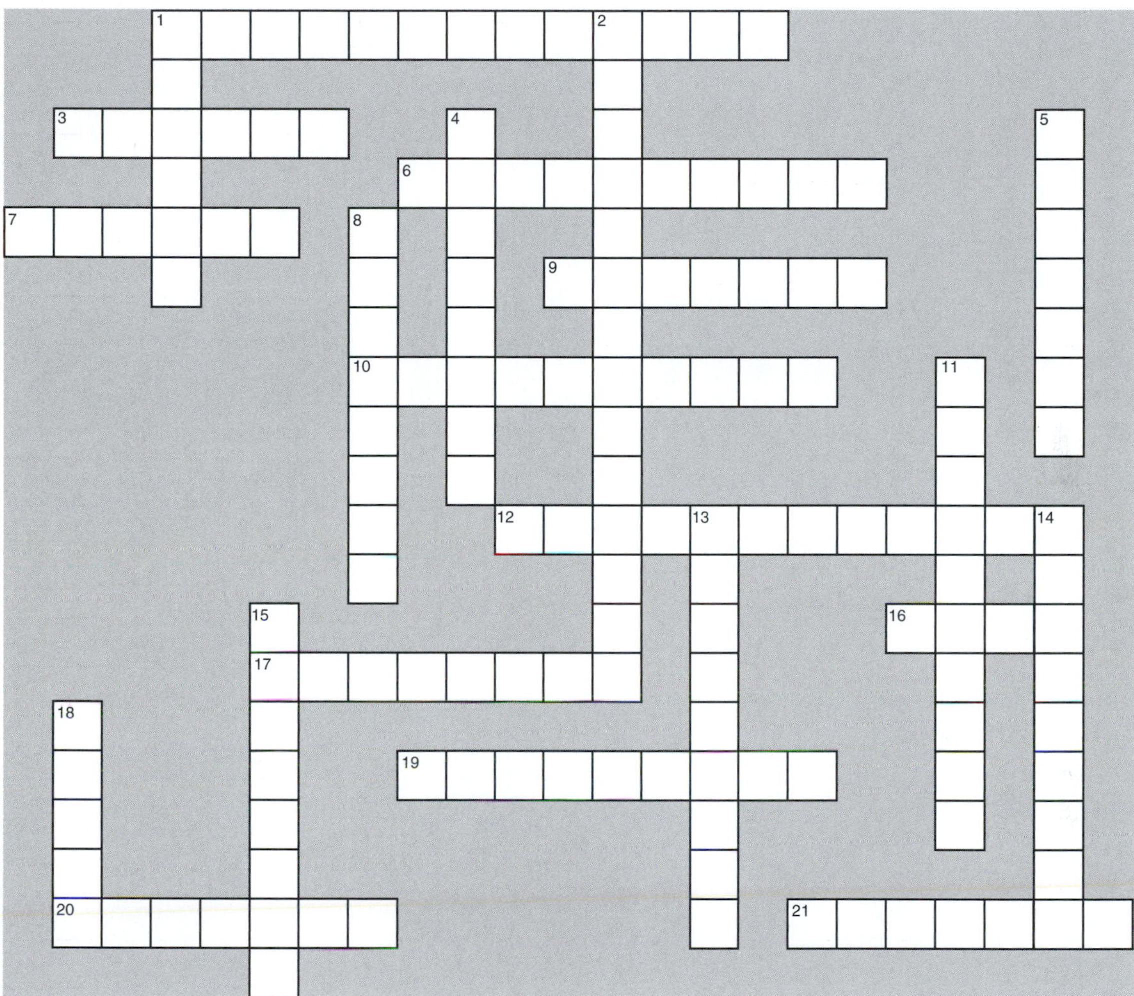

Across

1 Melanocytes live here
3 Inner skin layer
6 Inflammation of the skin
7 Converts precursor in skin to vitamin D
9 Outermost covering of hair
10 Function of skin
12 Caused by papillae
16 Teenager skin problem
17 Cannot produce melanin
19 Hives
20 Responsible for skin color
21 Earwax

Down

1 Stretch marks
2 Outermost layer of epidermis
4 Cancerous skin growth
5 Needed for vitamin D absorption
8 Baldness
11 Cuticle
13 Outer layer of skin
14 Skin opening of sweat gland
15 Yellowish pigment
18 Oily secretion

Notes

7 Skeletal System

CHAPTER ASSIGNMENTS

✓ After Completing	Date Due	Study Guide Page(s)	STUDY GUIDE ASSIGNMENTS (CTA: Critical Thinking Activity)	Possible Points	Points You Earned
		99	Pretest	10	
		100 100-101	Key Term Assessment A. Definitions B. Word Parts (Add 1 point for each key term)	23 14	
		101-106	Evaluation of Learning questions	64	
		107	Evolve Site: CTA A: Body Spectrum—Structure of Bone	10	
		108	CTA B: Long Bone	12	
		108	Evolve Site: CTA C: Body Spectrum—Skeleton Anterior	10	
		108	Evolve Site: CTA D: Body Spectrum—Skeleton Posterior	10	
		108	Evolve Site: CTA E: Body Spectrum—Skull Anterior	10	
		108	Evolve Site: CTA F: Body Spectrum—Skull Right Lateral	10	
		108	Evolve Site: CTA G: Body Spectrum—Paranasal Sinuses	40	
		108	Evolve Site: CTA H: Body Spectrum—Cranial Vault	10	
		108	Evolve Site: CTA I: Body Spectrum—Skull Inferior	10	
		108	Evolve Site: CTA J: Body Spectrum—Vertebral Column	10	
		108	Evolve Site: CTA K: Body Spectrum—Individual Vertebrae	10	
		108	Evolve Site: CTA L: Body Spectrum—Thorax and Ribs	10	
		108	Evolve Site: CTA M: Body Spectrum—Right Wrist and Hand	10	

✓ After Completing	Date Due	Study Guide Page(s)	STUDY GUIDE ASSIGNMENTS (CTA: Critical Thinking Activity)	Possible Points	Points You Earned
		108	ⓔ Evolve Site: CTA N: Body Spectrum—Male Pelvis	10	
		108	ⓔ Evolve Site: CTA O: Body Spectrum—Female Pelvis	10	
		109	ⓔ Evolve Site: CTA P: Body Spectrum—Right Foot	10	
		109	CTA Q: Synovial Joint	5	
		109-110	CTA R: Inquiring Patients Want to Know	10	
		111	CTA S: Crossword Puzzle	23	
		99	Posttest	10	
			ADDITIONAL ASSIGNMENTS		
			TOTAL POINTS		

Name ______________________________ Date ______________

PRETEST

True or False

_______ 1. The skeletal system provides a rigid framework for the body.

_______ 2. Blood cell formation takes place in the spleen.

_______ 3. Vertebrae are made up of flat bones.

_______ 4. Articular cartilage covers the ends of long bones.

_______ 5. Long bones grow in length at the epiphyseal line.

_______ 6. The maxillary bones form the upper jaw.

_______ 7. The sacrum makes up the small of the back.

_______ 8. The shoulder is an example of a hinge joint.

_______ 9. The patella is the kneecap.

_______ 10. The humerus makes up the thigh.

POSTTEST

True or False

_______ 1. The formation of blood cells is known as hemogenesis.

_______ 2. Osteons are the microscopic units of compact bone.

_______ 3. Calcium is located in an osteonic canal.

_______ 4. The shaft of a long bone is the diaphysis.

_______ 5. The endosteum is the tough fibrous connective tissue that covers a long bone.

_______ 6. A mature bone cell is an osteoblast.

_______ 7. The central indentation of the sternum is the jugular (suprasternal) notch.

_______ 8. The clavicle and scapula make up the pelvic girdle.

_______ 9. The ileum, ischium, and pubis make up the coxal bones.

_______ 10. The ulna is located on the lateral side of the forearm.

Term KEY TERM ASSESSMENT

A. Definitions

Directions: Match each key term with its definition.

_______ 1. Amphiarthrosis
_______ 2. Appendicular
_______ 3. Appositional growth
_______ 4. Articular cartilage
_______ 5. Articulation
_______ 6. Axial skeleton
_______ 7. Diaphysis
_______ 8. Diarthrosis
_______ 9. Endosteum
_______ 10. Epiphyseal plate
_______ 11. Epiphyseal plate
_______ 12. Epiphysis
_______ 13. Hematopoiesis
_______ 14. Osteoblast
_______ 15. Osteoclast
_______ 16. Osteocyte
_______ 17. Osteogenesis
_______ 18. Osteon
_______ 19. Pectoral girdle
_______ 20. Pelvic girdle
_______ 21. Periosteum
_______ 22. Sutures
_______ 23. Synarthrosis

A. A slightly movable joint
B. An immovable joint
C. Bone-forming cell
D. Cell that destroys or resorbs bone tissue
E. Freely movable joint characterized by a joint cavity; also called a *synovial joint*
F. Mature bone cell
G. Structural unit of bone; haversian system
H. The cartilaginous plate between the epiphysis and diaphysis of a bone; responsible for the lengthwise growth of a long bone
I. The end of a long bone
J. The long, straight shaft of a long bone
K. Production of blood or its cells
L. Bones that are attached to the body; upper and lower extremities
M. Thin layer of hyaline cartilage that covers the ends of long bones in joints
N. Membranous lining of a cavity within a bone
O. Growth resulting from material being deposited on the surface, such as growth in diameter of long bones
P. Bones of the head, neck, and trunk
Q. The remnant of the epiphyseal plate after the cartilage calcifies and growth ceases
R. A joint: area of contact between two bones
S. Formation of bone
T. Immovable fibrous joints between the flat bones of the skull
U. Attachment for the upper extremities in the chest region; clavicle and scapula
V. Attachment for the lower extremities: ilium, ischium, pubis
W. Tough white outer membrane that covers a bone.

B. Word Parts

Directions: Indicate the meaning of each word part in the space provided. List as many medical terms as possible that incorporate the word part in the space provided.

Word Part	Meaning of Word Part	Medical Terms That Incorporate Word Part
1. arthr/o		
2. -osis		
3. dia-		
4. end/o		
5. epi-		
6. -phys		
7. hem/		
8. oste/o		

Word Part	Meaning of Word Part	Medical Terms That Incorporate Word Part
9. -blast		
10. -clast		
11. -cyte		
12. -genesis		
13. pect/o		
14. syn-		

EVALUATION OF LEARNING

Directions: Fill in each blank with the correct answer.

1. What structures make up the skeletal system?

____

____

2. What are the five functions of the skeletal system?

____

____

3. How is the blood calcium level maintained in the body?

____

____

4. What is the function of red bone marrow?

____

5. Where is red bone marrow found in the adult?

____

____

6. What is an osteon?

____

7. Describe the following structures that make up an osteon:

   a. Osteonic canal (haversian canal): ______________________________

   ____

   b. Lamella: ______________________________

   ____

   c. Osteocytes: ______________________________

   d. Lacunae: ______________________________

   ____

e. Canaliculi: ___

8. What is the difference between spongy bone and compact bone?

___

9. List examples of each of the following classifications of bone:

a. Long bones: ___

b. Short bones: ___

c. Flat bones: ___

d. Irregular bones: ___

10. Describe each of the following structures that make up a long bone:

a. Diaphysis: ___

b. Medullary cavity: ___

c. Epiphysis: ___

d. Articular cartilage: ___

e. Periosteum: ___

f. Nutrient foramina: ___

g. Endosteum: ___

11. What is ossification?

___

12. What is the function of each of the following types of bone cells?

a. Osteoblast: ___

b. Osteocyte: ___

c. Osteoclast: ___

13. Where is the epiphyseal plate located in a long bone?

___

14. What type of cartilage is found in the epiphyseal plate?

___

15. How do long bones grow in length?

___

16. When does an individual stop growing in length?

___

17. What happens to the epiphyseal plate when long bones stop growing?

____

18. What influences bone growth in the body?

____

____

19. How many bones make up the skeleton of an adult?

____

20. What are the two divisions of the skeleton? What structures are included in each division?

____

____

21. How many bones make up the skull?

____

22. What is the function of the cranium?

____

23. What are sinuses and what is their function?

____

24. What bones make up the cranium?

____

____

25. What is the function of the facial bones?

____

____

26. What are the names of the three small bones located in the middle ear?

____

27. What is the function of the hyoid bone?

____

____

28. How many vertebrae make up the vertebral column?

____

29. What are the functions of the intervertebral disks?

____

____

30. What structures make up the vertebrae?

____

____

31. How many vertebrae are included in each of the following divisions of the vertebral column?

a. Cervical: ______________________________

b. Thoracic: ______________________________

c. Lumbar: ______________________________

32. Describe the following:

a. Sacrum: ______________________________

____

b. Coccyx: ______________________________

____

33. What are the functions of the thoracic cage?

____

____

34. What is the name of the central indentation in the superior margin of the sternum?

____

35. How many pairs of ribs are present in the human skeleton?

____

36. What is the difference between true ribs and false ribs?

____

____

37. What are floating ribs?

____

38. What is the function of the appendicular skeleton?

____

39. What two bones make up the pectoral girdle?

____

40. What is another name for the clavicle?

____

41. What is the name of the shallow depression on the scapula where the head of the humerus connects to the scapula?

____

42. What bone is located in the upper arm?

____

43. What bones are located in the forearm?

____

44. State the location of the following bones making up the hand:
    a. Carpal bones: ______________________________
    b. Metacarpal bones: ______________________________
    c. Phalanges: ______________________________

45. What are the functions of the pelvic girdle?

____

____

46. What three bones fuse to form a coxal bone?

____

47. What is the symphysis pubis?

____

48. What bone is located in the thigh?

____

49. What is the patella?

____

50. What is the function of the patella?

____

51. What bones are located in the leg?

____

52. What does the lateral malleolus do?

____

53. Describe the location of the following bones making up the foot:
    a. Tarsal bones:
    b. Calcaneus bone:
    c. Metatarsal bones:
    d. Phalanges:

54. What is an articulation?

____

55. What is a synarthrosis?

____

56. What is an example of a synarthrosis?

____

57. What is an amphiarthrosis?

____

58. What is an example of an amphiarthrosis?

____

59. What is a diarthrosis?

____

60. Describe the following parts of a diarthrosis:

   a. Articular cartilage: ______________________
   b. Joint cavity: ______________________
   c. Joint capsule: ______________________
   d. Synovial membrane: ______________________
   e. Synovial fluid: ______________________

61. What is the function of fibrocartilaginous pads located in the knee?

____

____

62. What are bursae?

____

63. What are the functions of bursae?

____

____

64. List examples of the following types of joints. What range of movement is possible with each of the following joints?

Joint	Examples	Range of Movement
a. Ball-and-socket		
b. Condyloid		
c. Saddle		
d. Pivot		
e. Hinge		
f. Gliding		

CRITICAL THINKING ACTIVITIES

A. Evolve Site: Body Spectrum

Skeletal: Structure of Bone

Body Spectrum directions:

1. Access the Body Spectrum program on the Evolve site.
2. If necessary, access the HELP screen for directions on using the Body Spectrum program.
3. Go to the Contents screen.
4. Select the following category from the Contents screen:
   Skeletal
5. Select the following anatomic diagram:
   Structure of Bone.
6. Identify the structures on the diagram.
7. Print out the diagram.

B. Long Bone

Using Figure 7-2 in your textbook as a reference, label each of the parts of a long bone on the following diagram.

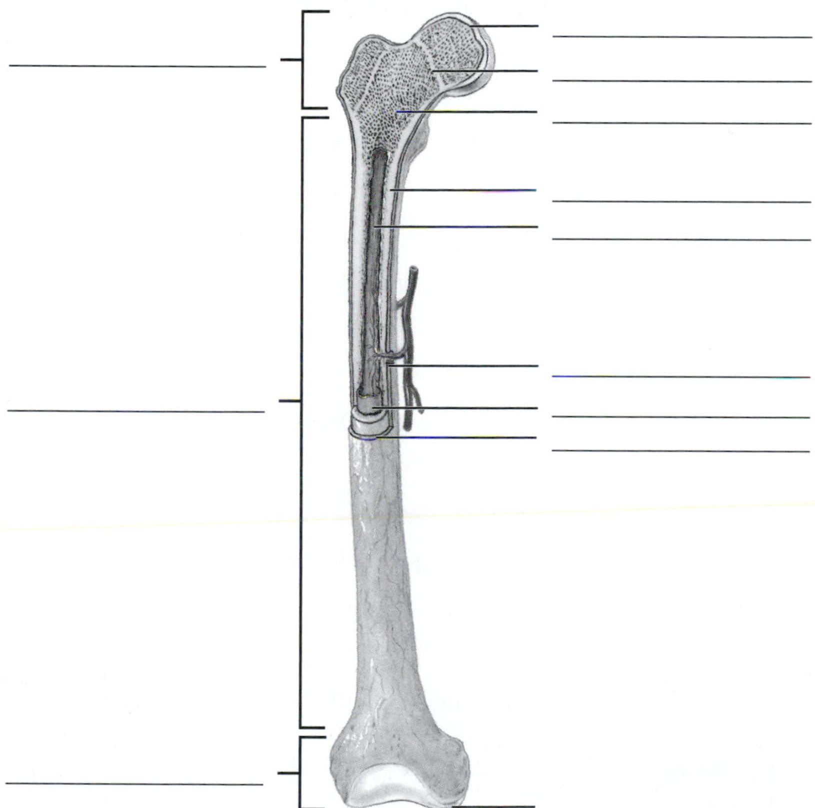

(Modified from Applegate E: *The anatomy and physiology learning system*, ed 4, St. Louis, 2011, Saunders.)

C. Evolve Site: Body Spectrum
Skeletal: Skeleton Anterior
Directions: Identify the structures on this diagram following the Body Spectrum directions outlined under CTA A.

D. Evolve Site: Body Spectrum
Skeletal: Skeleton Posterior
Directions: Identify the structures on this diagram following the Body Spectrum directions outlined under CTA A.

E. Evolve Site: Body Spectrum
Skeletal: Skull Anterior
Directions: Identify the structures on this diagram following the Body Spectrum directions outlined under CTA A.

F. Evolve Site: Body Spectrum
Skeletal: Skull Right Lateral
Directions: Identify the structures on this diagram following the Body Spectrum directions outlined under CTA A.

G. Evolve Site: Body Spectrum
Skeletal: Paranasal Sinuses
Directions: Identify the structures on this diagram following the Body Spectrum directions outlined under CTA A.

H. Evolve Site: Body Spectrum
Skeletal: Cranial Vault
Directions: Identify the structures on this diagram following the Body Spectrum directions outlined under CTA A.

I. Evolve Site: Body Spectrum
Skeletal: Skull Inferior
Directions: Identify the structures on this diagram following the Body Spectrum directions outlined under CTA A.

J. Evolve Site: Body Spectrum
Skeletal: Vertebral Column
Directions: Identify the structures on this diagram following the Body Spectrum directions outlined under CTA A.

K. Evolve Site: Body Spectrum
Skeletal: Individual Vertebrae
Directions: Identify the structures on this diagram following the Body Spectrum directions outlined under CTA A.

L. Evolve Site: Body Spectrum
Skeletal: Thorax and Ribs
Directions: Identify the structures on this diagram following the Body Spectrum directions outlined under CTA A.

M. Evolve Site: Body Spectrum
Skeletal: Right Wrist and Hand
Directions: Identify the structures on this diagram following the Body Spectrum directions outlined under CTA A.

N. Evolve Site: Body Spectrum
Skeletal: Male Pelvis
Directions: Identify the structures on this diagram following the Body Spectrum directions outlined under CTA A.

O. Evolve Site: Body Spectrum
Skeletal: Female Pelvis
Directions: Identify the structures on this diagram following the Body Spectrum directions outlined under CTA A.

P. Evolve Site: Body Spectrum

Skeletal: Right Foot

Directions: Identify the structures on this diagram following the Body Spectrum directions outlined under CTA A.

Q. Synovial Joint

Using Figure 7-17 in your textbook as a reference, label each of the parts of a synovial joint on the following diagram.

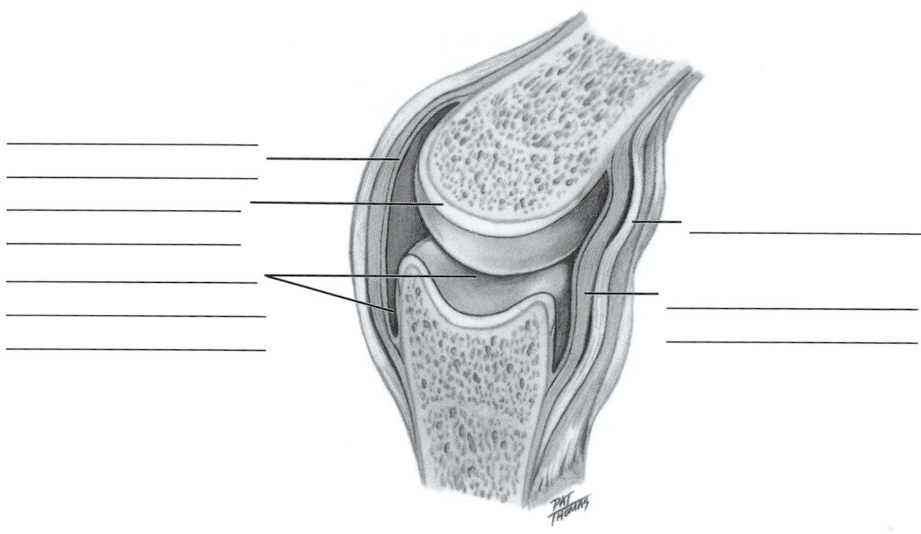

(Modified from Applegate E: *The anatomy and physiology learning system*, ed 4, St. Louis, 2011, Saunders.)

R. Inquiring Patients Want to Know

You are working in a general practice medical office. Your patients ask you the following questions. In the space provided, indicate how you would respond to each question in terms the patient would understand. Use your textbook and Internet resources to develop your responses.

1. What causes osteoporosis?

____

____

2. What causes my sinus headaches?

____

____

3. How does a baby get through the bones of the pelvis during childbirth?

____

____

4. What causes older people to break their hips?

____

____

5. What causes gout?

6. Why do people get shorter when they get older?

7. Why do babies have “soft spots” on their heads?

8. What is the difference between osteoarthritis and rheumatoid arthritis?

9. What happens when someone cracks his or her knuckles?

10. What is the difference between a strain and a sprain?

S. Crossword Puzzle: Skeletal System

Directions: Complete the crossword puzzle using the clues provided.

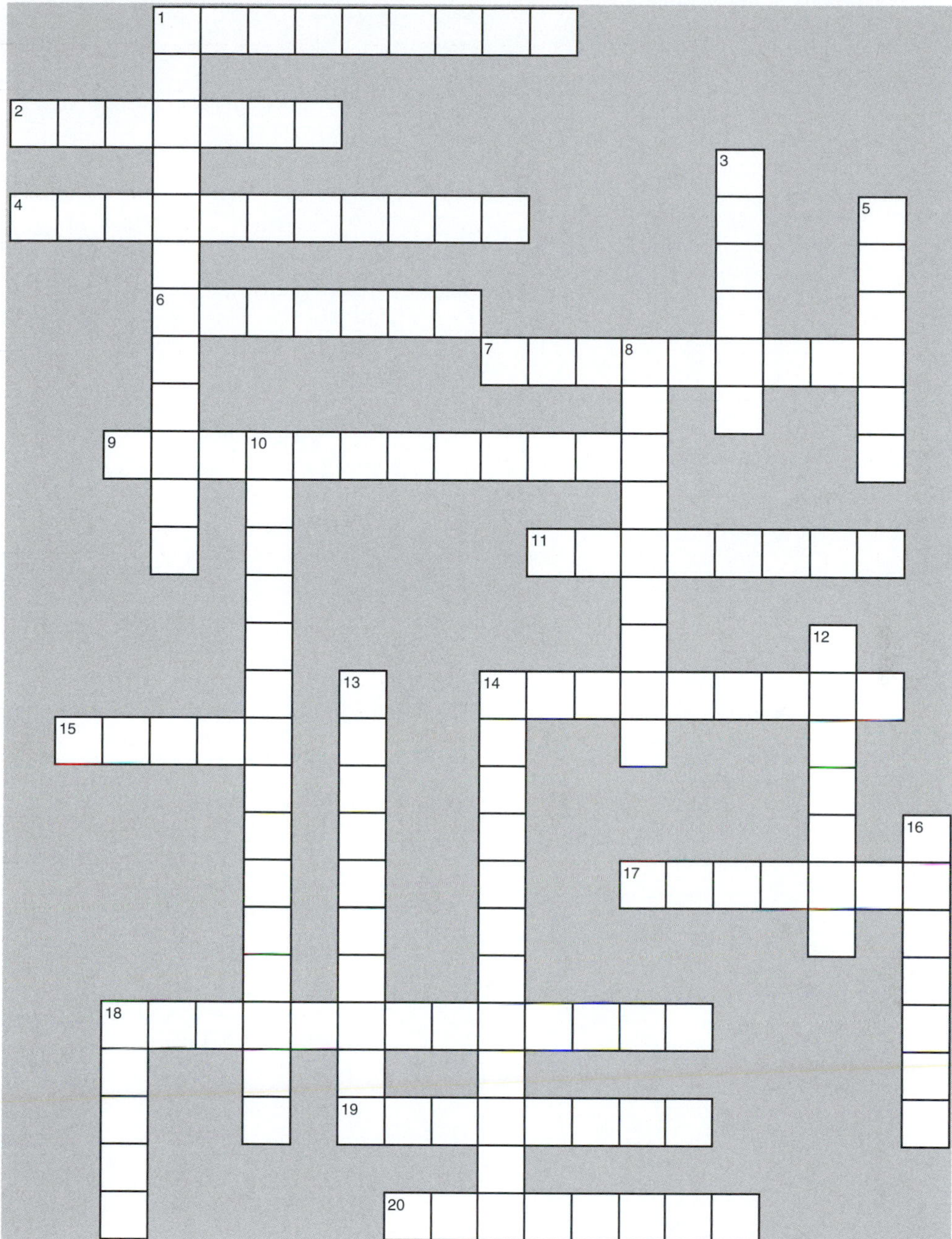

Across

1 Abnormal side-to-side spinal curvature
2 Bones that protect brain
4 Freely movable joint
6 Upper arm bone
7 Shaft of a long bone
9 Softening of bones
11 Collarbone
14 Bone cell
15 Air-filled cavity in the skull
17 Shoulder blade
18 Spinal cord passes through this part of the skull
19 Bones of the upper jaw
20 Lower jaw bones

Down

1 Immovable joint
3 Tailbone
5 Ankle
8 Finger bones
10 Where bones grow in length
12 Breastbone
13 Outer surface of a long bone
14 Process of bone formation
16 Kneecap
18 Thigh bone

Notes

8 Muscular System

CHAPTER ASSIGNMENTS

✓ After Completing	Date Due	Study Guide Page(s)	STUDY GUIDE ASSIGNMENTS (CTA: Critical Thinking Activity)	Possible Points	Points You Earned
		115	Pretest	10	
		116	Key Term Assessment A. Definitions B. Word Parts (Add 1 point for each key term)	17 10	
		117-121	Evaluation of Learning questions	46	
		121	Evolve Site: CTA A: Body Spectrum: Face—Lateral	10	
		121	Evolve Site: CTA B: Body Spectrum: Face—Anterior	10	
		121	Evolve Site: CTA C: Body Spectrum: Anterior Abdominal	10	
		121	Evolve Site: CTA D: Body Spectrum: Musculature—Anterior	10	
		121	Evolve Site: CTA E: Body Spectrum: Upper Chest—Superficial	10	
		121	Evolve Site: CTA F: Body Spectrum: Right Arm—Lateral	10	
		121	Evolve Site: CTA G: Body Spectrum: Musculature—Posterior	10	
		121-122	CTA H: Inquiring Patients Want to Know	10	
		123	CTA I: Crossword Puzzle	25	
		115	Posttest	10	
			ADDITIONAL ASSIGNMENTS		
			TOTAL POINTS		

Notes

Name ______________________________ Date ______________

PRETEST

True or False

_______ 1. Skeletal muscle is under involuntary control.

_______ 2. A ligament indirectly attaches skeletal muscle to bone.

_______ 3. The cytoplasm of a muscle fiber is the sarcolemma.

_______ 4. Calcium is a neurotransmitter responsible for muscle contractions.

_______ 5. Oxygen must be present for aerobic respiration to occur.

_______ 6. Bending the elbow is an example of flexion.

_______ 7. The orbicularis oculus is used to wink, blink, and squint.

_______ 8. The diaphragm forms a partition between the thorax and abdomen.

_______ 9. The deltoid muscle moves the shoulder and upper arm.

_______ 10. Another name for the calcaneal tendon is the ankle.

POSTTEST

True or False

_______ 1. Most of the heat produced in the body is through visceral muscle contractions.

_______ 2. The epimysium is a connective tissue sheath that surrounds a muscle.

_______ 3. The insertion is the end of a muscle that is attached to a relatively movable part.

_______ 4. An axon terminal meets a muscle fiber at the neuromuscular junction.

_______ 5. The products of anaerobic respiration are amino acids and carbon dioxide.

_______ 6. Moving the arm away from the body is an example of adduction.

_______ 7. The sternocleidomastoid muscle is located in the neck.

_______ 8. The internal intercostal muscles assist with inspiration.

_______ 9. The gluteus maximus muscle is used when an intramuscular injection is administered.

_______ 10. The quadriceps femoris muscle is used to extend the leg.

Term KEY TERM ASSESSMENT

Directions: Match each key term with its definition.

_______ 1. Acetylcholine
_______ 2. Acetylcholinesterase
_______ 3. Antagonist
_______ 4. Aponeurosis
_______ 5. Contractility
_______ 6. Elasticity
_______ 7. Epimysium
_______ 8. Excitability
_______ 9. Extensibility
_______ 10. Insertion
_______ 11. Motor unit
_______ 12. Neuromuscular junction
_______ 13. Neurotransmitter
_______ 14. Origin
_______ 15. Prime mover
_______ 16. Sarcolemma
_______ 17. Synergist

A. A chemical substance that is released at the axon terminals to stimulate a muscle fiber contraction or an impulse in another neuron
B. A muscle that assists a prime mover but is not capable of producing the movement by itself
C. A muscle that has an action opposite to the prime mover
D. A single neuron and all the muscle fibers it stimulates
E. The area of communication between the axon terminal of a motor neuron and the sarcolemma of a muscle fiber; also called a myoneural junction
F. The end of a muscle that is attached to a relatively immovable part; the end opposite the insertion
G. The end of a muscle that is attached to a relatively movable part; the end opposite the origin
H. The muscle that is mainly responsible for a particular body movement; also called agonist
I. The ability of muscle tissue to stretch when pulled
J. A broad flat sheet of connective tissue that connects one muscle to another
K. Fibrous connective tissue that surrounds a whole muscle
L. Covering of a muscle cell: the muscle cell membrane
M. A neurotransmitter at the neuromuscular junction
N. The ability of muscle and nerve tissue to receive and respond to stimuli
O. The ability of muscle cells to shorten to produce movement
P. An enzyme that inactivates acetylcholine
Q. The ability of tissue to return to its original shape after contraction or extension

B. Word Parts

Directions: Indicate the meaning of each word part in the space provided. List as many medical terms as possible that incorporate the word part in the space provided.

Word Part	Meaning of Word Part	Medical Terms That Incorporate Word Part
1. -ase		
2. anti-		
3. epi-		
4. mys		
5. neur/o		
6. trans-		
7. sarc/o		
8. lemm-		
9. syn-		
10. erg/o		

EVALUATION OF LEARNING

Directions: Fill in each blank with the correct answer.

1. What are the three types of muscle tissue?

2. How many skeletal muscles are found in the human body?

3. List and describe the four characteristics of skeletal muscle.

4. What four functions are provided to the body by muscle contractions?

5. What is the epimysium?

6. Describe the following parts of a muscle cell:
   a. Sarcolemma:
   b. Sarcoplasm:

7. Why does a muscle cell have numerous mitochondria?

8. List and describe the two ways in which skeletal muscle is attached to bone.
   a.
   b.

9. What is the name of the nerve cell that stimulates a skeletal muscle to contract?

10. What is a motor unit?

11. What is the neuromuscular junction?

12. What is a synaptic cleft?

13. What is the name of the neurotransmitter responsible for muscle contractions? Where is this neurotransmitter housed before being released?

14. What happens when a nerve impulse reaches its axon terminal?

15. What inactivates acetylcholine?

16. What is the function of ATP?

17. What is creatine phosphate?

18. What are the primary energy sources for muscles that are actively contracting for extended periods of time?

19. What must be available for aerobic respiration to occur?

20. What are the products of aerobic respiration?

21. What occurs when the muscles are contracting vigorously for long periods of time?

22. How does the body produce energy when it runs out of oxygen?

23. What happens when there is a buildup of lactic acid in the muscles?

24. What is oxygen debt? How is oxygen debt paid back?

___

___

___

25. Describe each of the following types of body movements, and give an example of each:

Type	Definition	Example
Flexion		
Extension		
Hyperextension		
Dorsiflexion		
Plantar flexion		
Abduction		
Adduction		
Rotation		
Supination		
Pronation		
Circumduction		
Inversion		
Eversion		

26. State the function of each of the following muscles involved with facial expressions:
   a. Frontalis: ___
   b. Orbicularis oris: ___
   c. Orbicularis oculi: ___
   d. Buccinator: ___
   e. Zygomaticus: ___

27. What are the names of the muscles responsible for chewing?

___

28. What is the function of the following neck muscles?
   a. Sternocleidomastoid: ___
   b. Trapezius: ___

29. What muscles located in the trunk are responsible for maintaining posture?

___

30. What is the function of the intercostal muscles?

___

31. Where is the diaphragm located?

____

32. What is the function of the diaphragm?

____

33. What are the four muscle pairs that make up the wall of the abdomen?

____

____

34. What muscles allow an individual to shrug his or her shoulders?

____

35. Where is the pectoralis major muscle located?

____

36. Where is the latissimus dorsi muscle located?

____

37. What is the name of the muscle in the arm that is used for administering an intramuscular injection?

____

38. What muscle is responsible for extending the forearm?

____

39. What muscle is responsible for flexing the forearm?

____

40. What thigh muscle is used to administer an intramuscular injection?

____

41. What muscles make up the quadriceps femoris?

____

____

42. What is the function of the quadriceps femoris?

____

43. What muscles are used to flex the leg?

____

44. What muscles allow an individual to stand on his or her tiptoes?

____

45. What is another name for the calcaneal tendon?

____

46. What are the best deterrents to prevent the loss of muscle mass and strength as an individual ages?

____

CRITICAL THINKING ACTIVITIES

A. Evolve Site: Body Spectrum

Muscular: Face—Lateral

Body Spectrum directions:

1. Access the Body Spectrum program on the Evolve site.
2. If necessary, access the HELP screen for directions on using the Body Spectrum program.
3. Go to the Contents screen.
4. Select the following category from the Contents screen:
   Muscular
5. Select the following anatomic diagram:
   Face—Lateral
6. Identify the structures on the diagram.
7. Print out the diagram.

B. Evolve Site: Body Spectrum

Muscular: Face—Anterior

Directions: Identify the structures on this diagram following the Body Spectrum directions outlined under CTA A.

C. Evolve Site: Body Spectrum

Muscular: Anterior Abdominal

Directions: Identify the structures on this diagram following the Body Spectrum directions outlined under CTA A.

D. Evolve Site: Body Spectrum

Muscular: Musculature—Anterior

Directions: Identify the structures on this diagram following the Body Spectrum directions outlined under CTA A.

E. Evolve Site: Body Spectrum

Muscular: Upper Chest—Superficial

Directions: Identify the structures on this diagram following the Body Spectrum directions outlined under CTA A.

F. Evolve Site: Body Spectrum

Muscular: Right Arm—Lateral

Directions: Identify the structures on this diagram following the Body Spectrum directions outlined under CTA A.

G. Evolve Site: Body Spectrum

Muscular: Musculature—Posterior

Directions: Identify the structures on this diagram following the Body Spectrum directions outlined under CTA A.

H. Inquiring Patients Want to Know

You are working in a general practice medical office. Your patients ask you the following questions. In the space provided, indicate how you would respond to each question in terms the patient would understand. Use your textbook and Internet resources to develop your responses.

1. What causes hiccups?

____

____

2. What causes menstrual cramps?

3. Why does someone get stiff and rigid after he or she dies?

4. What causes shin splints?

5. What causes an eye tic?

6. Why do my leg muscles burn when I run a 3-mile race?

7. Why do my muscles ache when I have the flu?

8. How does lifting weights make muscles bigger?

9. What causes shivering?

10. What happens to a muscle when it is torn?

I. Crossword Puzzle: Muscular System

Directions: Complete the crossword puzzle using the clues provided.

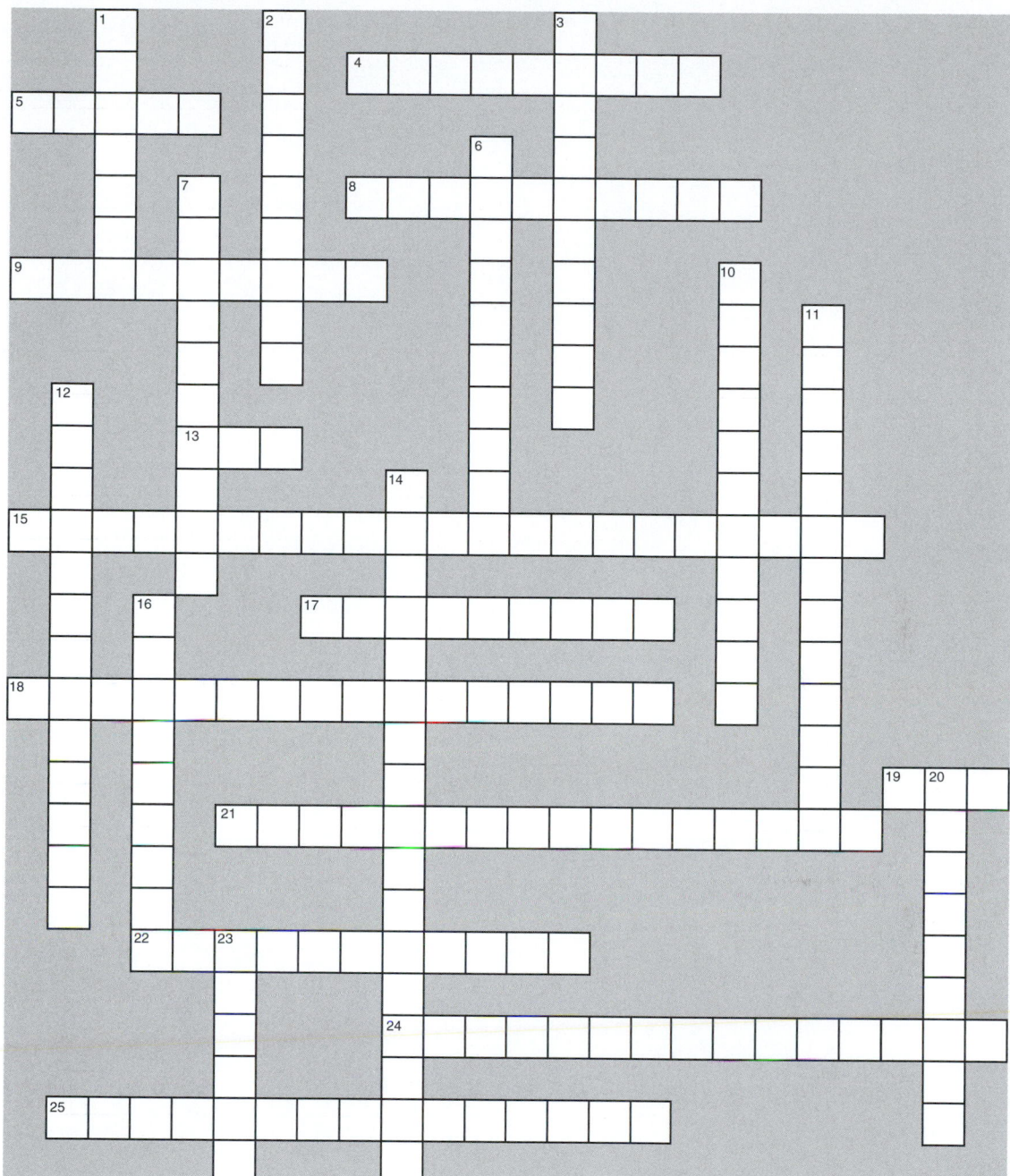

Across

4 Eyebrow-raising muscle
5 Muscle's fleshy part
8 Muscle that opposes a movement
9 Movement away from midline
13 Muscle-contraction neurotransmitter
15 Where an axon meets a muscle fiber
17 Movement toward midline
18 Winking muscle
19 Energy source for muscle contractions
21 Where ACh lives
22 Stimulates contraction of skeletal muscle
24 Kissing muscle
25 Chest muscle

Down

1 Abducts arm
2 Longest muscle in the body
3 Muscle fiber cytoplasm
6 Muscle fiber cell membrane
7 Cheek muscle
10 Smiling muscle
11 Extends vertebral column
12 Flexes forearm
14 Muscle group that extends leg
16 Sheath that surrounds a muscle
20 Shrugging shoulders muscle
23 Attaches muscle to bone

Notes

9 Nervous System

CHAPTER ASSIGNMENTS

✓ After Completing	Date Due	Study Guide Page(s)	STUDY GUIDE ASSIGNMENTS (CTA: Critical Thinking Activity)	Possible Points	Points You Earned
		127	Pretest	10	
		128 129	Term Key Term Assessment A. Definitions B. Word Parts (Add 1 point for each key term)	23 11	
		129-134	Evaluation of Learning questions	54	
		135	Evolve Site: CTA A: Body Spectrum: Structure of a Neuron	10	
		135	CTA B: Synapse	7	
		135	Evolve Site: CTA C: Body Spectrum: Brain—Meningeal Coverings	10	
		136	CTA D: Cerebrum	18	
		136	Evolve Site: CTA E: Body Spectrum: Spinal Cord	10	
		136	Evolve Site: CTA F: Body Spectrum: Brain—Inferior	10	
		136-137	CTA G: Inquiring Patients Want to Know	10	
		138	CTA H: Crossword Puzzle	27	
		127	Posttest	10	
			ADDITIONAL ASSIGNMENTS		
			TOTAL POINTS		

Notes

Name ______________________________ Date ______________

PRETEST

True or False

_______ 1. The function of a neuron is to transmit nerve impulses.

_______ 2. Neuroglia support and protect neurons.

_______ 3. Myelin is a white, fatty substance that surrounds nerve fibers.

_______ 4. Sneezing is an example of a reflex.

_______ 5. The central sulcus divides the cerebrum into two hemispheres.

_______ 6. The hypothalamus functions in the regulation of body temperature.

_______ 7. The pons functions in body coordination, posture, and balance.

_______ 8. The peripheral nervous system provides a communication network between the central nervous system (CNS) and the body.

_______ 9. Sensory nerves contain only efferent fibers.

_______ 10. The body has 12 pairs of cranial nerves.

POSTTEST

True or False

_______ 1. An axon transmits impulses toward a neuron cell body.

_______ 2. Gray matter is made up of myelinated fibers.

_______ 3. A myelin sheath is formed around axons within the CNS by Schwann cells.

_______ 4. Synapse is the name of the region of communication between two neurons.

_______ 5. The CNS is made up of cranial nerves and spinal nerves.

_______ 6. The cerebral cortex consists of gray matter.

_______ 7. The spinal cord extends from the base of the skull to the fourth lumbar vertebra.

_______ 8. The autonomic nervous system supplies motor impulses to visceral organs.

_______ 9. Nerves that carry both sensory and motor fibers are known as mixed nerves.

_______ 10. The sympathetic division of the autonomic nervous system prepares the body for fight or flight.

KEY TERM ASSESSMENT

A. Definitions

Directions: Match each key term with its definition.

_______ 1. Action potential
_______ 2. Axon
_______ 3. Basal ganglia
_______ 4. Brain stem
_______ 5. Central sulcus
_______ 6. Cerebellum
_______ 7. Cerebrospinal fluid
_______ 8. Cerebrum
_______ 9. Dendrites
_______ 10. Decussation
_______ 11. Diencephalon
_______ 12. Myelin
_______ 13. Neurilemma
_______ 14. Neuroglia
_______ 15. Neuron
_______ 16. Neurotransmitters
_______ 17. Nodes of Ranvier
_______ 18. Refractory period
_______ 19. Saltatory conduction
_______ 20. Somatomotor cortex
_______ 21. Somatosensory cortex
_______ 22. Synapse
_______ 23. Threshold stimulus

A. A nerve impulse; a rapid change in membrane potential that involves depolarization and repolarization
B. Minimum level of stimulation that is required to start a nerve impulse or muscle contraction; also called liminal stimulus
C. Part of the brain between the cerebral hemispheres and the midbrain; includes the thalamus, hypothalamus, and epithalamus
D. Process in which a nerve impulse travels along a myelinated nerve fiber by jumping from one node of Ranvier to the next
E. Second largest part of the human brain, located posterior to the pons and medulla oblongata, and involved in the coordination of muscular movements
F. The largest and uppermost part of the human brain; concerned with consciousness, learning, memory, sensations, and voluntary movements
G. The layer of cells that surrounds a nerve fiber in the peripheral nervous system and, in some cases, produces myelin
H. The portion of the brain between the diencephalon and spinal cord that contains the midbrain, pons, and medulla oblongata
I. The region of communication between two neurons
J. White, fatty substance that surrounds many nerve fibers
K. The branching afferent processes of a neuron that receive impulses from other neurons and transmit them to the cell body
L. Short spaces between segments of myelin in a myelinated nerve fiber
M. The groove or furrow between the frontal and parietal lobes of the cerebrum
N. A fluid that fills the subarachnoid space around the brain and spinal cord and is in the ventricles of the brain
O. Time during which an excitable cell cannot respond to a stimulus that is usually adequate to initiate an action potential
P. Supporting cells of nervous tissue
Q. Nerve cell including its processes
R. Paired regions of gray matter located within the white matter of the cerebrum
S. A crossing over
T. A chemical substance that is released from axon terminals to stimulate muscle fiber contraction or an impulse in another neuron;
U. The primary sensory area of the brain; receives sensory impulses from the body
V. The single efferent process of a neuron that carries impulses away from the cell body
W. The primary motor area of the brain; transmits motor impulses to the body

B. Word Parts

Directions: Indicate the meaning of each word part in the space provided. List as many medical terms as possible that incorporate the word part in the space provided.

Word Part	Meaning of Word Part	Medical Terms That Incorporate Word Part
1. act-		
2. gangli-		
3. cerebell/o		
4. cerebr/o		
5. cephal/o		
6. neur/o		
7. gli/a		
8. -lemma		
9. -tion		
10. somat/o		
11. syn-		

EVALUATION OF LEARNING

Directions: Fill in each blank with the correct answer.

1. What makes up the nervous system?

___

2. Describe the following three general functions of the nervous system:

   a. Sensory functions: ___

   b. Integrative functions: ___

   c. Motor functions: ___

3. What is an effector? What are two types of effectors?

___

___

4. What are the two main subdivisions of the nervous system?

___

5. What is the function of the following subdivisions of the peripheral nervous system?

   a. Afferent (sensory) division: ___

   b. Efferent (motor) division: ___

6. What function is performed by the following subdivisions of the efferent (motor) division?

   a. Somatic nervous system: ___

   b. Autonomic nervous system: ___

7. What are the two subdivisions of the autonomic nervous system?

____

8. What are the three basic parts of a neuron?

____

9. What is the function of a dendrite?

____

10. What is the function of an axon?

____

11. What is a myelin sheath?

____

12. What makes up the white matter in the central nervous system?

____

13. What makes up the gray matter in the central nervous system?

____

14. Describe the appearance of a node of Ranvier.

____

15. What is the neurilemma, and what is its function?

____

____

____

16. What is the function of oligodendrocytes?

____

17. Why can't nerve fibers in the central nervous system regenerate?

____

18. Describe the structure and function of the three types of neurons:

   a. Afferent (sensory) neurons: _______________

   ____

   b. Efferent (motor) neurons: _______________

   ____

   c. Interneurons: _______________

   ____

19. What is the function of neuroglia?

20. What is a resting membrane?

21. What happens to sodium ions when a neuron receives a stimulus?

22. Describe how a nerve impulse is propagated along the length of a neuron through an action potential.

23. What is a synapse?

24. How is a nerve impulse transmitted across a synapse?

25. What is a reflex?

26. What are some examples of reflexes that take place in the body?

27. What makes up the central nervous system?

28. What bones surround and protect the brain?

29. What three layers make up the meninges, starting with the outer layer?

30. What are the four parts of the human brain?

31. What is the function of the corpus callosum?

___

32. What five lobes make up the cerebral hemisphere?

___

___

33. Where is the cerebral cortex located? What makes up the cerebral cortex?

___

___

34. What functions are controlled by the cerebral cortex?

___

___

35. What is the function of the following structures making up the diencephalons?

a. Thalamus: ___

___

b. Hypothalamus: ___

___

c. Epithalamus: ___

___

36. What structures make up the brain stem?

___

37. List and explain the functions of the three control centers located in the medulla.

Control Center	Function
a.	
b.	
c.	

38. What is the function of the cerebellum?

___

___

39. What are ventricles?

___

40. What is the function of cerebrospinal fluid?

____

____

____

41. What is the starting point and ending point of the spinal cord?

____

42. How long is the spinal cord?

____

43. What surrounds the spinal cord?

____

44. How many pairs of spinal nerves are present in the human body?

____

45. What are the functions of the spinal cord?

____

____

46. What is the difference between ascending tracts and descending tracts of the spinal cord?

____

____

47. What makes up the peripheral nervous system?

____

48. What is the makeup and function of the somatic nervous system?

____

____

49. What is the makeup and function of the autonomic nervous system?

____

50. What type of nerve fibers make up each of the following?

a. Sensory nerves: _______________

b. Motor nerves: _______________

c. Mixed nerves: _______________

51. What are the names of the 12 cranial nerves, and what is the function of each?

Cranial Nerve	Name	Function
I.		
II.		
III.		
IV.		
V.		
VI.		
VII.		
VIII.		
IX.		
X.		
XI.		
XII.		

52. What are some examples of body functions controlled by the autonomic nervous system?

53. What are the functions of the following two divisions of the autonomic nervous system?

a. Sympathetic:

b. Parasympathetic:

54. How is memory affected as the nervous system ages?

CRITICAL THINKING ACTIVITES

A. Evolve Site: Body Spectrum

Nervous: Structure of a Neuron

Body Spectrum directions:

1. Access the Body Spectrum program on the Evolve site.
2. If necessary, access the HELP screen for directions on using the Body Spectrum program.
3. Go to the Contents screen.
4. Select the following category from the Contents screen:
   Nervous
5. Select the following anatomic diagram:
   Structure of a Neuron
6. Identify the structures on the diagram.
7. Print out the diagram.

B. Synapse

Using Figure 9-4 in your textbook as a reference, label each of the components of a synapse on the following diagram.

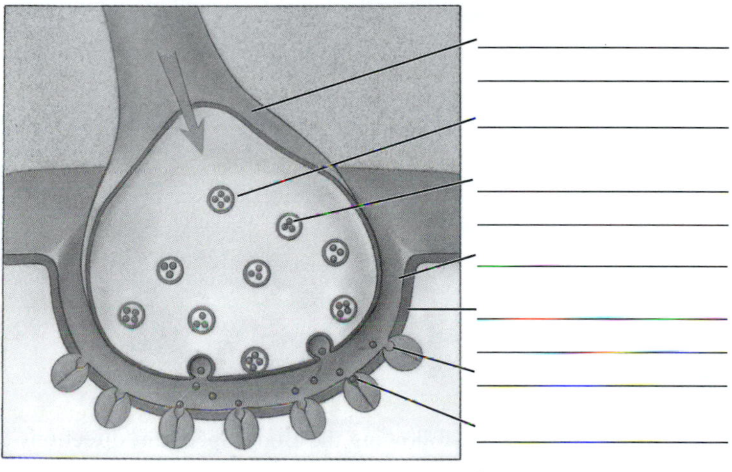

(Modified from Applegate E: *The anatomy and physiology learning system*, ed 4, St. Louis, 2011, Saunders.)

C. Evolve Site: Body Spectrum

Nervous: Brain—Meningeal Coverings

Directions: Identify the structures on this diagram following the Body Spectrum directions outlined under CTA A.

D. Cerebrum

Using Figure 9-8 in your textbook as a reference, label each of the lobes and functional areas of the cerebrum on the following diagram.

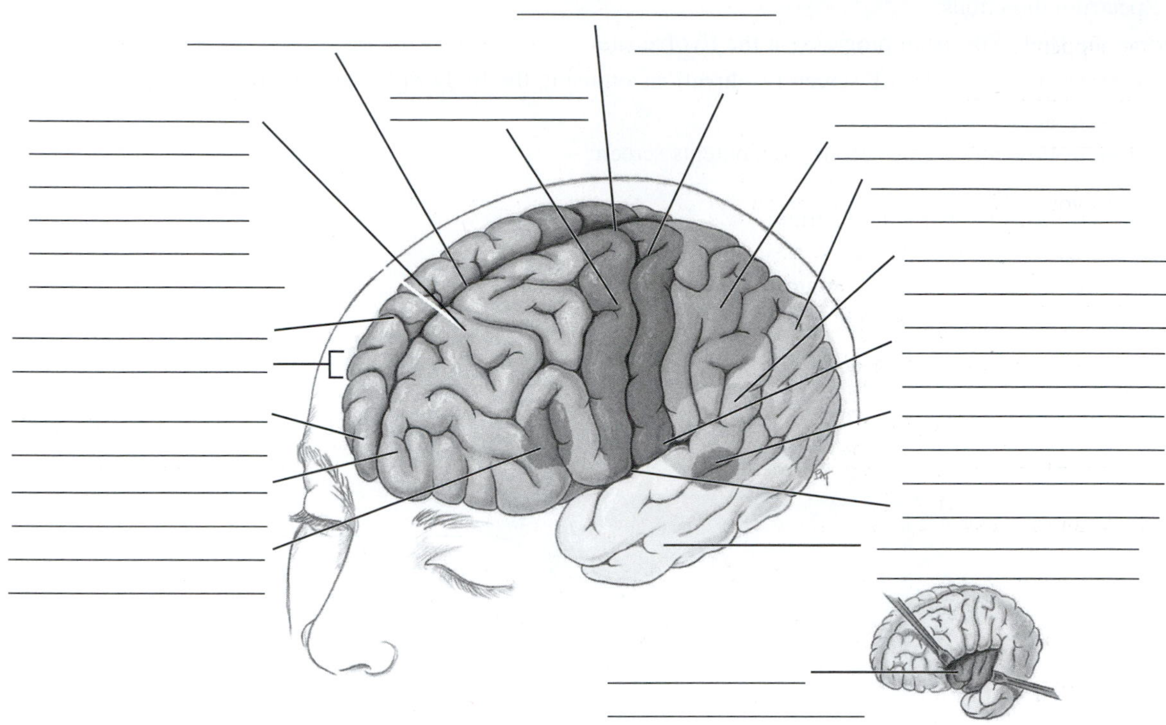

(Modified from Applegate E: *The anatomy and physiology learning system*, ed 4, St. Louis, 2011, Saunders.)

E. Evolve Site: Body Spectrum

Nervous: Spinal Cord

Directions: Identify the structures on this diagram following the Body Spectrum directions outlined under CTA A.

F. Evolve Site: Body Spectrum

Nervous: Brain—Inferior

Directions: Identify the structures on this diagram following the Body Spectrum directions outlined under CTA A.

G. Inquiring Patients Want to Know

You are working in a general practice medical office. Your patients ask you the following questions. In the space provided, indicate how you would respond to each question in terms the patient would understand. Use your textbook and Internet resources to develop your responses.

1. What causes cerebral palsy?

____

____

2. What sometimes causes a "brain freeze" when you eat ice cream?

____

____

3. What does it mean if someone is right-brained or left-brained?

4. What happens in the brain when someone has a migraine headache?

5. Why do you become permanently paralyzed from a spinal cord injury?

6. What makes someone left-handed?

7. How do antidepressants like Prozac work?

8. Is it possible to improve your memory?

9. Why does your knee jerk when the doctor hits it with a rubber hammer?

10. What happens in the brain of a person with Alzheimer's disease?

H. Crossword Puzzle: Nervous System

Directions: Complete the crossword puzzle using the clues provided.

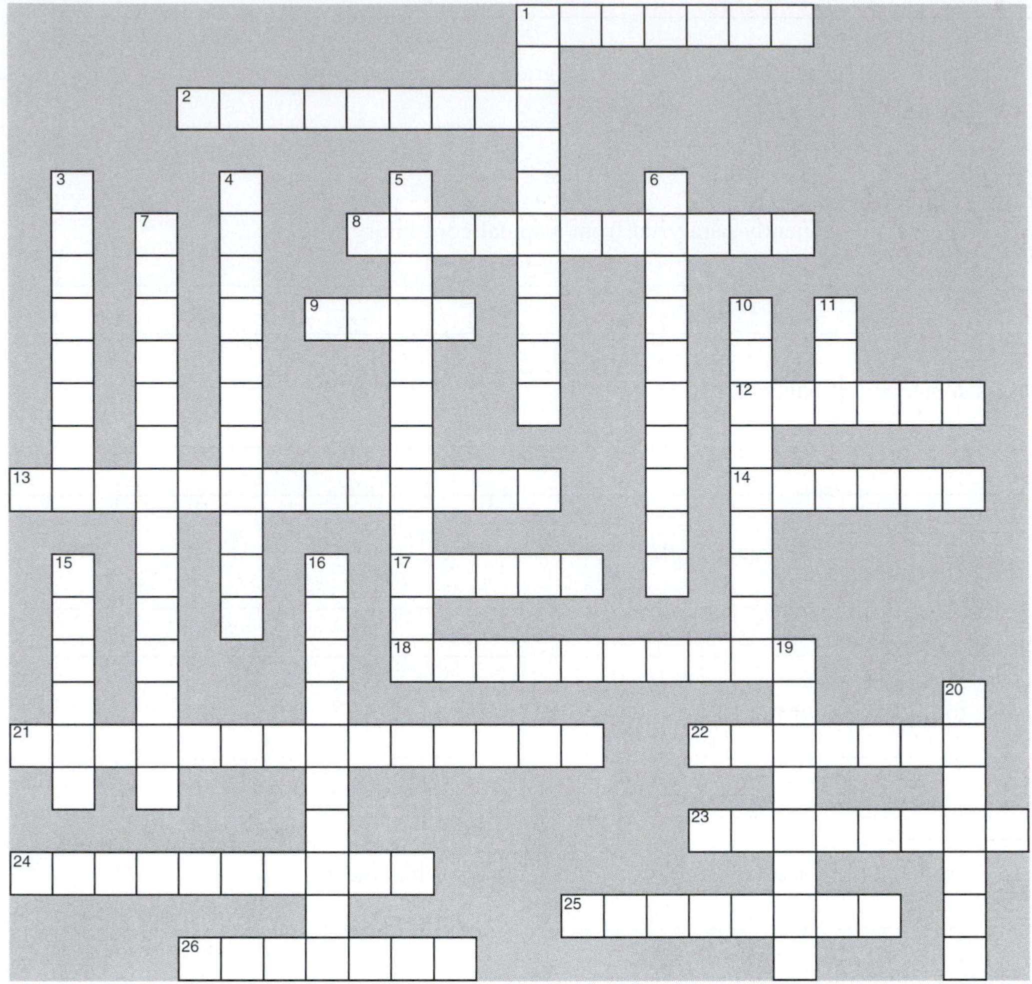

Across

1 Group of nerve cell bodies outside CNS
2 Support system for neurons
8 "Fight or flight" NS division
9 Carries impulses away from cell body
12 Automatic involuntary response
13 Space between neurons
14 White substance surrounding nerve fibers
17 Nerves that carry impulses away from CNS
18 Protected by vertebral column
21 Gaps in myelin
22 Communication region between neurons
23 Largest part of the brain
24 In charge of coordination, posture, and balance
25 Inner layer of meninges
26 Nerves that carry impulses toward CNS

Down

1 Cell bodies and unmyelinated fibers
3 Main part of neuron
4 Consists of myelinated nerve fibers
5 Regulates body temperature
6 Produces myelin in PNS
7 Outermost part of the cerebrum
10 Outer layer of meninges
11 Brain and spinal cord fluid
15 Nerve cell
16 Fluid-filled brain cavities
19 Transmits impulses to cell body
20 Respiratory center lives here

10 The Senses

CHAPTER ASSIGNMENTS

✓ After Completing	Date Due	Study Guide Page(s)	STUDY GUIDE ASSIGNMENTS (CTA: Critical Thinking Activity)	Possible Points	Points You Earned
		141	Pretest	10	
		142 142-143	Key Term Assessment A. Definitions B. Word Parts (Add 1 point for each key term)	20 17	
		143-148	Evaluation of Learning questions	65	
		148	Evolve Site: CTA A: Body Spectrum: Right Eye—Cross Section	10	
		148	Evolve Site: CTA B: Body Spectrum: Normal Structure of the Eye	10	
		149	Evolve Site: CTA C: Eye-Dentify (Record points earned)		
		149-150	CTA D: Light Ray	40	
		150	Evolve Site: CTA E: Body Spectrum: Ear—Cross Section	10	
		150	Evolve Site: CTA F: Body Spectrum: Muscles of the Middle Ear	10	
		150	Evolve Site: CTA G: Can You Hear Me Now? (Record points earned)		
		150-151	CTA H: Sound Wave	40	
		151-152	CTA I: Inquiring Patients Want to Know	10	

✓ After Completing	Date Due	Study Guide Page(s)	STUDY GUIDE ASSIGNMENTS (CTA: Critical Thinking Activity)	Possible Points	Points You Earned
		153	CTA J: Crossword Puzzle	28	
		141	Posttest	10	
			ADDITIONAL ASSIGNMENTS		
			TOTAL POINTS		

Name ______________________________ Date ______________

PRETEST

True or False

_______ 1. Special senses have receptors that are localized in a particular area.

_______ 2. Thermoreceptors are located in subcutaneous tissue.

_______ 3. There are more cold receptors in a given area than heat receptors.

_______ 4. The olfactory cortex interprets smell sensations.

_______ 5. The inner layer of the eye that contains rods and cones is the retina.

_______ 6. The region of the retina that produces the sharpest image is the optic disk.

_______ 7. Visual impulses are interpreted in the occipital lobe.

_______ 8. Cerumen helps prevent foreign substances from reaching the eardrum.

_______ 9. The range of frequencies for normal speech is 300 to 4000 vibrations per second.

_______ 10. The cochlea is a coiled structure in the inner ear that functions in hearing.

POSTTEST

True or False

_______ 1. Meissner corpuscles are stimulated by heavy pressure.

_______ 2. The sense of position or orientation is known as proprioception.

_______ 3. A nociceptor is stimulated by tissue damage.

_______ 4. Taste receptors are stimulated by the pressure of food on the tongue.

_______ 5. The white part of the eye is the choroid.

_______ 6. When the ciliary muscle contracts, the lens bulges for close vision.

_______ 7. Rhodopsin allows the eye to adapt to dim light.

_______ 8. Receptors for hearing are chemoreceptors.

_______ 9. The oval window equalizes the pressure between the outside and the middle ear.

_______ 10. The semicircular canals contain the sense organs for static equilibrium.

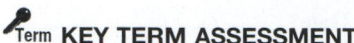

KEY TERM ASSESSMENT

A. Definitions

Directions: Match each key term with its definition.

_______ 1. Accommodation
_______ 2. Bulbus oculi
_______ 3. Chemoreceptor
_______ 4. Cochlea
_______ 5. Crista ampullaris
_______ 6. General senses
_______ 7. Gustatory sense
_______ 8. Lacrimal apparatus
_______ 9. Macula lutea
_______ 10. Mechanoreceptor
_______ 11. Nociceptor
_______ 12. Olfaction
_______ 13. Otoliths
_______ 14. Photoreceptor
_______ 15. Proprioception
_______ 16. Refraction
_______ 17. Rhodopsin
_______ 18. Sensory adaptation
_______ 19. Special senses
_______ 20. Thermoreceptor

A. A sensory receptor that detects changes in temperature
B. A sensory receptor that detects light; located in the retina of the eye
C. A sensory receptor that detects the presence of chemicals; responsible for taste, smell, and monitoring the concentration of certain chemicals in body fluids
D. A sensory receptor that responds to a bending or deformation of the cell; examples include receptors for touch, pressure, hearing, and equilibrium
E. A sensory receptor that responds to tissue damage; pain receptor
F. Mechanism that allows the eye to focus at various distances, primarily achieved by changing the curvature of the lens
G. Phenomenon in which some receptors respond when a stimulus is first applied but decrease their response if the stimulus is maintained; receptor sensitivity decreases with prolonged stimulation
H. The sense of body position and movements
I. Receptor organ located within the ampulla of the semicircular canals; functions in dynamic equilibrium
J. Yellowish depression on the retina
K. Little stones of calcium carbonate in the macula of the inner ear
L. The eyeball
M. Photosensitive pigment in the rods; also called visual purple
N. Spiral or snail-shaped portion of the inner ear
O. Senses with receptors localized in a particular area; taste, smell, vision, hearing, and equilibrium
P. The structures that produce and convey tears
Q. Sense of taste
R. Sense of smell
S. Senses that are located throughout the body; somatic senses
T. The bending of light as it passes from one medium to another

B. Word Parts

Directions: Indicate the meaning of each word part in the space provided. List as many medical terms as possible that incorporate the word part in the space provided.

Word Part	Meaning of Word Part	Medical Terms That Incorporate Word Part
1. ocul/o		
2. chem/o		
3. coch-		
4. gust-		
5. lacr-		
6. macul-		
7. lute-		
8. mechan/o		
9. noci-		
10. -ceptor		

Word Part	Meaning of Word Part	Medical Terms That Incorporate Word Part
11. olfact/o		
12. ot/o		
13. lith		
14. phot/o		
15. propri/o		
16. rhod/o		
17. therm/o		

EVALUATION OF LEARNING

Directions: Fill in each blank with the correct answer.

1. What is the difference between the general senses and the special senses?

____

____

2. What are the five types of sense receptors? List an example of each.

Type of Receptor	Example

3. What are the steps involved in perceiving sensation?

____

____

____

4. What is sensory adaptation?

____

____

5. What senses are classified as the general senses?

____

____

6. What type of stimulus activates a mechanoreceptor?

____

7. What is the function of each of the following mechanoreceptors involved with touch and pressure?
   a. Free nerve endings: ____
   ____
   b. Meissner corpuscles: ____
   ____
   c. Pacinian corpuscles: ____
   ____

8. What is proprioception?
   ____

9. What mechanoreceptors are involved with proprioception?
   ____

10. What are thermoreceptors located?
   ____

11. In which part of the body are thermoreceptors the most numerous? Where are they the least numerous?
   ____
   ____

12. How do the number of cold receptors compare with the number of heat receptors?
   ____

13. What type of receptors do extreme temperatures stimulate?
   ____

14. Describe the sensory adaptation that occurs with thermoreceptors.
   ____
   ____

15. What stimulates a nociceptor?
   ____

16. Where are nociceptors located?
   ____
   ____

17. How do nociceptors provide a protective function in the body?
   ____
   ____

18. What senses are classified as special senses?
   ____

19. What are the organs of taste?

___

20. What stimulates the receptors that determine taste?

___

21. What are the four different taste sensations?

___

22. What happens when taste hairs are stimulated?

___

___

23. What is olfaction?

___

24. What stimulates the receptors that distinguish smell?

___

25. What area of the brain interprets smell impulses?

___

26. What is the function of the following eye structures?
   a. Eyebrows: ___
   b. Eyelids: ___
   c. Eyelashes: ___
   d. Sebaceous glands: ___

27. What eye muscle performs the following?
   a. Closes the eye: ___
   b. Opens the eye: ___

28. Describe the location of the conjunctiva.

___

___

29. What is the purpose of mucus secreted by the eye?

___

30. What is a stye?

___

31. What structure produces tears?

___

32. What is the function of tears?

33. Describe the appearance of the sclera.

34. What are two functions of the choroid?

35. What effect does contraction of the ciliary muscle have on the lens of the eye?

36. How does the iris control the size of the pupil?

37. Where are the receptor cells of the eye located?

38. What is the optic disk, and why is it known as the "blind spot" of the eye?

39. Describe the location and appearance of the macula lutea.

40. What is the name of the eye structure that produces the sharpest image?

41. Where is the anterior cavity of the eye located?

42. What is the function of aqueous humor?

43. Where is the posterior cavity of the eye located?

44. What is the function of vitreous humor?

45. What is refraction?

____

46. What four structures of the eye function in refraction?

____

47. Describe the image that forms when light rays are refracted onto the retina.

____

48. What occurs in each of these structures during distance and close vision?

Vision	Ciliary Muscle	Suspensory Ligaments	Lens
a. Distance vision			
b. Close vision			

49. What is the function of rods?

____

50. What is the function of cones?

____

51. What is the function of rhodopsin?

____

52. What part of the brain interprets visual impulses?

____

53. What two functions are performed by the ear?

____

54. What is the function of the auricle?

____

____

55. What is the function of cerumen?

____

56. What effect do sound waves have on the tympanic membrane?

____

57. What is the function of the eustachian tube?

____

____

58. What are the names of the three auditory ossicles?

____

59. What structures in the inner ear function in equilibrium?

____

60. What structure in the inner ear functions in hearing?

____

61. What structure in the cochlea houses the sound receptors?

____

62. What is the range of frequencies of normal speech?

____

63. What nerve carries auditory impulses to the brain?

____

64. What is static equilibrium?

____

____

65. What is dynamic equilibrium?

____

____

CRITICAL THINKING ACTIVITIES

A. Evolve Site: Body Spectrum

Senses: Right Eye—Cross Section

Body Spectrum directions:

1. Access the Body Spectrum program on the Evolve site.
2. If necessary, access the HELP screen for directions on using the Body Spectrum program.
3. Go to the Contents screen.
4. Select the following category from the Contents screen:
   Senses
5. Select the following anatomic diagram:
   Right Eye—Cross Section
6. Identify the structures on the diagram.
7. Print out the diagram.

B. Evolve Site: Body Spectrum

Senses: Normal Structure of the Eye

Directions: Identify the structures on this diagram following the Body Spectrum directions outlined under CTA A.

C. Evolve Site: Eye-Dentify

Access the Evolve site to complete this activity. Record your points earned on your assignment sheet.

D. Light Ray

You are a ray of light that is getting ready to enter the eye where you will be converted into a nerve impulse and then travel to the brain for interpretation. In the space provided below, describe all of the structures you encounter on your way to the brain. Also describe what function each structure is performing in the eye. Each of the following structures should be included in your discussion:

a. Lacrimal apparatus
b. Conjunctiva
c. Sclera
d. Iris and pupil
e. Anterior cavity
f. Lens and suspensory ligaments
g. Ciliary muscle
h. Posterior cavity
i. Retina
j. Macula lutea
k. Rods and cones
l. Optic nerve
m. Optic chiasma
n. Thalamus
o. Occipital lobe

E. Evolve Site: Body Spectrum

Senses: Ear—Cross Section

Directions: Identify the structures on this diagram following the Body Spectrum directions outlined under CTA A.

F. Evolve Site: Body Spectrum

Senses: Muscles of the Middle Ear

Directions: Identify the structures on this diagram following the Body Spectrum directions outlined under CTA A.

G. Evolve Site: Can You Hear Me Now?

Access the Evolve site to complete this activity. Record your points earned on your assignment sheet.

H. Sound Wave

You are a sound wave that is getting ready to enter the ear where you will be converted into a nerve impulse and then travel to the brain for interpretation. In the space provided below, describe all of the structures you encounter on your way to the brain. Also describe what function each structure is performing in the ear. Each of the following structures should be included in your discussion:

a. Auricle
b. External auditory canal
c. Ceruminous glands
d. Tympanic membrane
e. Eustachian tube
f. Auditory ossicles
g. Oval window
h. Cochlea
i. Temporal lobe

I. Inquiring Patients Want to Know

You are working in a general practice medical office. Your patients ask you the following questions. In the space provided, indicate how you would respond to each question in terms the patient would understand. Use your textbook and Internet resources to develop your responses.

1. What causes an optical illusion?

2. How does LASIK surgery improve vision?

3. How does loud music damage hearing?

4. What is the reason for putting tubes in the eardrum?

5. What causes eye floaters?

6. Why do my ears get plugged when I am on an airplane?

7. What can cause an eardrum to rupture?

8. Why does a dog have a better sense of smell than a human?

9. Why can you not taste food when you have a bad cold?

10. Why do you feel dizzy when you spin around?

J. Crossword Puzzle: The Senses

Directions: Complete the crossword puzzle using the clues provided.

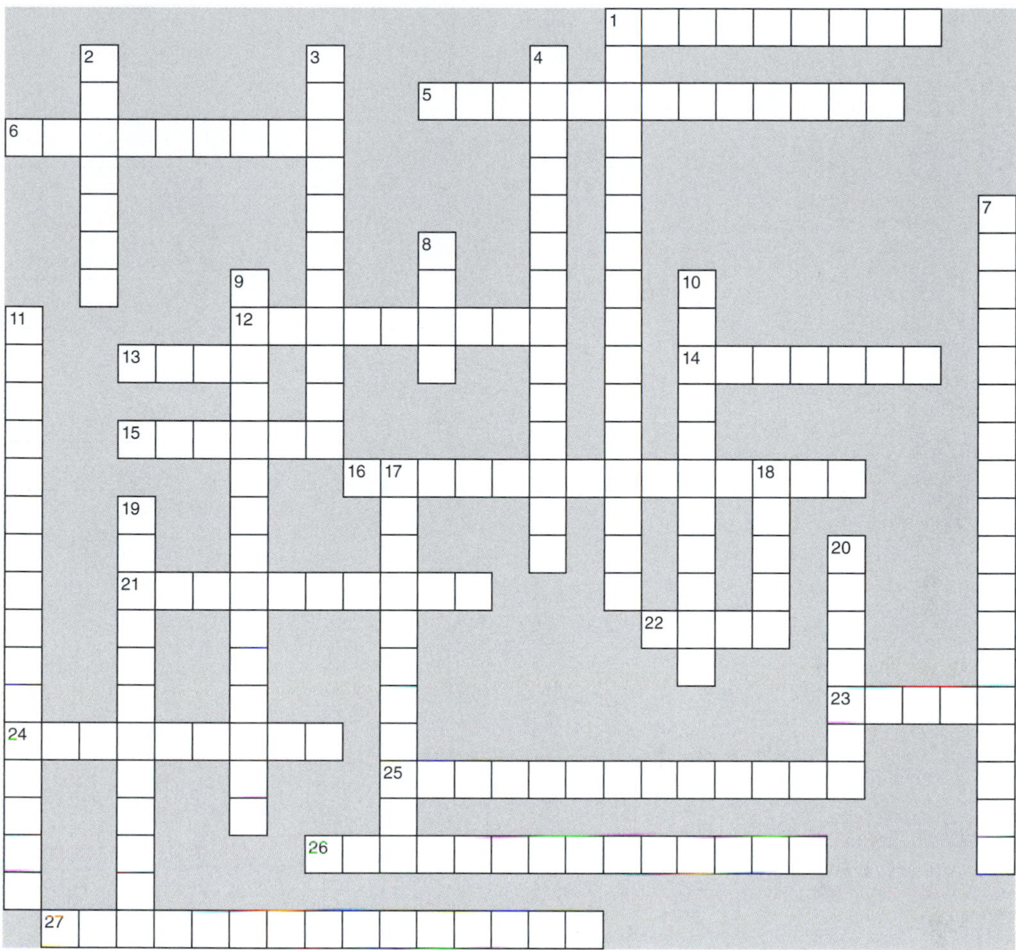

Across

1 Organs of taste
5 Produces tears
6 Visual purple
12 Blind spot
13 Colored part of eye
14 Earwax
15 White of the eye
16 Space between cornea and lens
21 Bending of light rays
22 This bulges for close vision
23 Receptors for color vision
24 Sense of smell
25 Where visual impulses are interpreted
26 Connects middle ear with throat
27 Stimulated by heat and cold

Down

1 Eardrum
2 Absorbs excess light rays
3 Covers front of eyeball except for cornea
4 Sense of position
7 Stimulated by heavy pressure
8 Sensitive to dim light
9 Contains vitreous humor
10 Yellow spot on retina
11 Muscle that closes the eye
17 Pain receptors
18 Auditory ossicle
19 Where taste impulses are interpreted
20 Collects sound waves

Notes

11 Endocrine System

CHAPTER ASSIGNMENTS

✓ After Completing	Date Due	Study Guide Page(s)	STUDY GUIDE ASSIGNMENTS (CTA: Critical Thinking Activity)	Possible Points	Points You Earned
		157	Pretest	10	
		158	Term Key Term Assessment A. Definitions B. Word Parts (Add 1 point for each key term)	 14 13	
		159-162	Evaluation of Learning questions	36	
		162	CTA A: Location of Endocrine Glands	20	
		162	CTA B: Pituitary Gland	20	
		163	CTA C: Inquiring Patients Want to Know	10	
		164	CTA D: Crossword Puzzle	24	
		157	Posttest	10	
			ADDITIONAL ASSIGNMENTS		
			TOTAL POINTS		

Notes

Name ______________________________ Date ______________

PRETEST

True or False

_______ 1. Endocrine glands have ducts that empty their secretions onto a surface.

_______ 2. Sex hormones are made up of proteins.

_______ 3. A target tissue is a tissue that has receptor sites for a particular hormone.

_______ 4. In an adult, an excess secretion of growth hormone can cause Down syndrome.

_______ 5. Oxytocin causes contraction of smooth muscle in the wall of the uterus.

_______ 6. Goiter results when there is a lack of iodine in the body.

_______ 7. Calcitonin functions by reducing the calcium level in the blood.

_______ 8. The adrenal glands are located above the kidneys.

_______ 9. Insulin is secreted by the beta cells of the pancreas.

_______ 10. Progesterone stimulates the production of milk in the lactating breast.

POSTTEST

True or False

_______ 1. Sebaceous glands are exocrine glands.

_______ 2. Luteinizing hormone is produced by the anterior pituitary gland.

_______ 3. Follicle-stimulating hormone stimulates development of eggs in the ovaries and sperm in the testes.

_______ 4. Diabetes mellitus results when there is not enough antidiuretic hormone secreted by the body.

_______ 5. The thyroid gland consists of two lobes located on each side of the trachea.

_______ 6. Aldosterone reduces the calcium level in the body.

_______ 7. The parathyroid glands are located on the anterior surface of the thyroid gland.

_______ 8. The function of insulin is to decrease the blood glucose concentration.

_______ 9. The function of glucagon is to raise blood glucose levels.

_______ 10. Melatonin is a hormone that regulates the sleep/wake cycle.

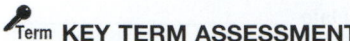

KEY TERM ASSESSMENT

A. Definitions

Directions: Match each key term with its definition.

_______ 1. Adenohypophysis
_______ 2. Androgens
_______ 3. Circadian rhythms
_______ 4. Endocrine gland
_______ 5. Endocrinology
_______ 6. Estrogens
_______ 7. Exocrine gland
_______ 8. Glucocorticoids
_______ 9. Gonadocorticoids
_______ 10. Hormone
_______ 11. Mineralocorticoids
_______ 12. Neurohypophysis
_______ 13. Pinealocytes
_______ 14. Target tissue

A. A substance secreted by an endocrine gland
B. A tissue (cells) that responds to a particular hormone because it has receptor sites for that hormone
C. Anterior portion of the pituitary gland
D. Gland that secretes its product directly into the blood
E. Gland that secretes its product to a surface or cavity through ducts
F. Posterior portion of the pituitary gland
G. Study of the endocrine glands
H. A group of hormones secreted by the adrenal cortex that regulates electrolyte balance in the body
I. Steroid hormones that promote male characteristics
J. Sex hormones from the adrenal cortex
K. Biological clock or a person's 24-hour rhythm such as a natural sleep-wake cycle
L. Secretory cells of the pineal gland; secrete melatonin
M. Group of hormones that stimulate the development of female secondary sex characteristics
N. Hormones from the adrenal cortex that raise blood sugar levels

B. Word Parts

Directions: Indicate the meaning of each word part in the space provided. List as many medical terms as possible that incorporate the word part in the space provided.

Word Part	Meaning of Word Part	Medical Terms That Incorporate Word Part
1. aden/o		
2. hypo-		
3. -physis		
4. andr/o		
5. endo-		
6. -crine		
7. exo-		
8. -ology		
9. gluc/o		
10. gonado/o		
11. hormon/o		
12. neur/o		
13. -cyte		

EVALUATION OF LEARNING

Directions: Fill in each blank with the correct answer.

1. How do the following systems regulate body activities?

   a. Nervous system: ______________________________

   b. Endocrine system: ______________________________

2. What are exocrine glands?

   ____

   ____

3. What are four examples of exocrine glands?

   ____

   ____

4. How does an endocrine gland function?

   ____

   ____

5. Why must insulin be administered by injection?

   ____

   ____

6. What hormones consist of steroids?

   ____

7. How do hormones exert their action on the body?

   ____

   ____

8. What is the function of the following hormones secreted by the anterior lobe of the pituitary gland?

   a. Growth hormone: ______________________________

   b. Thyroid stimulating hormone: ______________________________

      ____

   c. ACTH: ______________________________

      ____

   d. Follicle-stimulating hormone (FSH): ______________________________

   e. Luteinizing hormone:

      Female: ______________________________

      Male: ______________________________

   f. Prolactin: ______________________________

      ____

9. What is the function of the following hormones secreted by the posterior lobe of the pituitary gland?

 a. Antidiuretic hormone: ____

 b. Oxytocin: ____

10. What makes up the thyroid hormone?

11. Why does the adult thyroid gland enlarge when there is a lack of iodine in the body?

12. What effect do thyroid hormones have on the body?

13. What is the function of calcitonin?

14. Where are the parathyroid glands located?

15. What is the function of the parathyroid hormone?

16. Where are the adrenal glands located?

17. What is the function of mineralocorticoids secreted by the adrenal glands?

18. What is the name of the principal mineralocorticoid?

19. What is the function of glucocorticoids secreted by the adrenal cortex?

20. What is the principal glucocorticoid?

____

21. What is the name given to the sex hormones secreted by the adrenal cortex?

____

22. What causes the secretion of epinephrine and norepinephrine by the adrenal medulla?

____

23. What effect does the secretion of epinephrine and norepinephrine have on the body?

____

____

24. What is the location of the pancreas in relation to the stomach?

____

25. What are the names of the cells in the pancreas that secrete the following hormones?
    a. Glucagon: ____
    b. Insulin: ____

26. What is the function of glucagon?

____

27. What causes insulin to be secreted?

____

28. What is the function of insulin?

____

29. What are three factors that cause hypoactivity of insulin?

____

____

30. Why is it important for the body to maintain blood glucose levels within a normal range?

____

31. What are androgens?

____

32. What structure secretes testosterone?

____

33. What is the function of testosterone at the onset of puberty?

____

____

____

34. What are the functions of estrogen and progesterone at the onset of puberty?

____

____

____

35. What is the function of melatonin secreted by the pineal gland?

____

____

____

36. What is the function of the thymus gland?

____

____

____

CRITICAL THINKING ACTIVITIES

A. Location of Endocrine Glands

Using Figure 11-2 as a reference, sketch an outline of the human body. Draw, color, and label the major endocrine glands on your sketch.

B. Pituitary Gland

You are a pituitary gland and have control over your target tissues. In the chart provided, indicate what hormone you would secrete to stimulate each of the following target tissues. Also indicate what effect each hormone would have on its target tissue.

Target Tissue	What Hormone Would You Secrete to Stimulate This Target Tissue?	What Effect Would This Hormone Have on the Target Tissue?
Thyroid gland		
Adrenal cortex		
Ovarian follicles		
Seminiferous tubules		
Ovaries		
Testes		
Mammary glands		
Kidneys		
Uterus and mammary glands		
Most body tissues		

C. Inquiring Patients Want to Know

You are working in a general practice medical office. Your patients ask you the following questions. In the space provided, indicate how you would respond to each question in terms the patient would understand. Use your textbook and Internet resources to develop your responses.

1. Why does an adolescent girl with anorexia not have a menstrual period?

____

____

2. How is the insulin used for insulin injections made?

____

____

3. Why do some diabetics take medication orally?

____

____

4. How does an insulin pump work?

____

____

5. What are anabolic steroids, and why are they sometimes abused by athletes?

____

____

6. What side effects can occur from taking anabolic steroids?

____

____

7. What is an adrenaline rush?

____

____

8. Why do I feel so irritable when I am having trouble with hypoglycemia?

____

____

9. What is the best diet to follow for hypoglycemia?

____

____

10. Can hypoglycemia be cured?

____

____

D. Crossword Puzzle: Endocrine System

Directions: Complete the crossword puzzle using the clues provided.

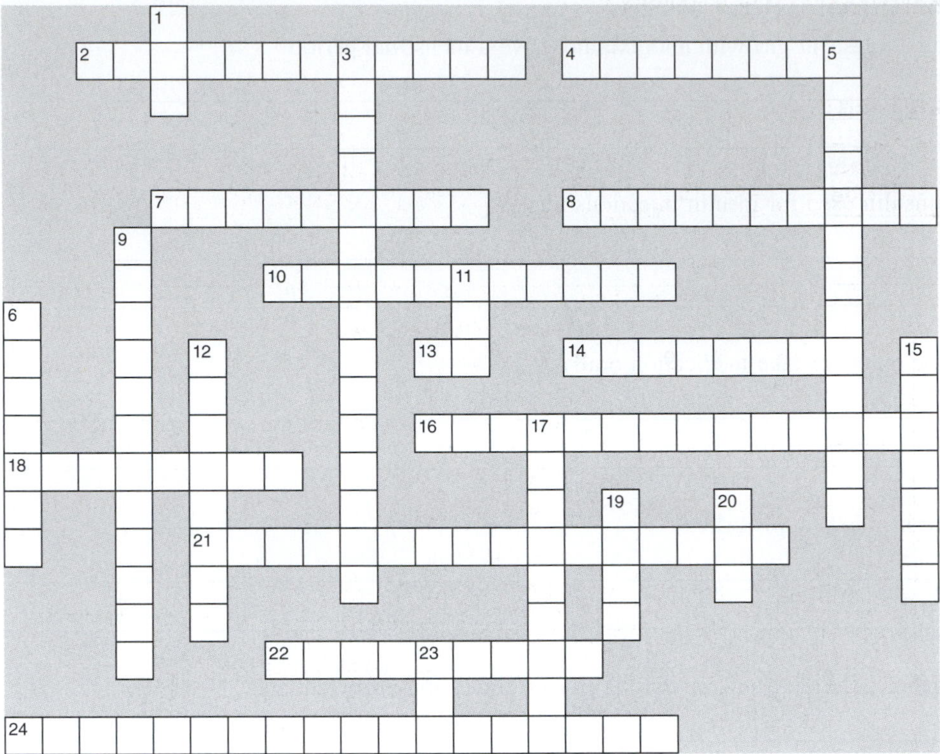

Across

2 Responsible for development of male reproductive structures
4 Thyroid hormone deficiency
7 Stimulates milk production by mammary gland
8 Reduces blood calcium level
10 Fight-or-flight hormone
13 Stimulates growth of bones and muscles
14 Glucocorticoid that counteracts inflammatory response
16 Glands with ducts
18 Causes uterus to contract
21 Sex hormones
22 Regulates circadian rhythms
24 Causes ovulation to occur

Down

1 Stimulates development of eggs and sperm
3 Glands that secrete hormones
5 Located on top of kidneys
6 Tumor of a gland
9 Causes uterus to thicken
11 Increases blood calcium levels
12 Raises blood glucose level
15 Decreases blood glucose level
17 Dwarfism with mental retardation
19 Stimulates adrenal gland to secrete cortisol
20 Promotes reabsorption of water by kidneys
23 Stimulates thyroid to secrete thyroid hormone

12 Circulatory System

CHAPTER ASSIGNMENTS

✓ After Completing	Date Due	Study Guide Page(s)	STUDY GUIDE ASSIGNMENTS (CTA: Critical Thinking Activity)	Possible Points	Points You Earned
		167	Pretest	15	
		168-169 169-170	Key Term Assessment A. Definitions B. Word Parts (Add 1 point for each key term)	42 30	
		170-179	Evaluation of Learning questions	97	
		180	Evolve Site: CTA A: Body Spectrum: Heart—Cross Section	10	
		180	Evolve Site: CTA B: Body Spectrum: Heart Circulation	10	
		180	Evolve Site: CTA C: Body Spectrum: Coronary Vessels	10	
		180	Evolve Site: CTA D: Name That Blood Cell (Record points earned)		
		180-181	CTA E: Blood Clotting	20	
		181-182	CTA F: Inquiring Patients Want to Know	10	
		183	CTA G: Crossword Puzzle	30	
		167	Posttest	15	
			ADDITIONAL ASSIGNMENTS		
			TOTAL POINTS		

Notes

Name ____ Date __________________

PRETEST

True or False

_______ 1. The pointed end of the heart is the apex.

_______ 2. The myocardium forms the bulk of the heart wall.

_______ 3. The coronary arteries branch off the aorta to supply the heart with oxygen and nutrients.

_______ 4. The SA node is located in the right atrium.

_______ 5. The adult male has 5 to 6 L of blood.

_______ 6. Erythrocytes lack a nucleus.

_______ 7. Vitamin K is necessary for the absorption of vitamin B_{12} from the intestines.

_______ 8. Leukocytes defend the body against disease.

_______ 9. Thrombocytes develop from large cells known as macrophages.

_______ 10. Veins carry blood toward the heart.

_______ 11. The function of the lymphatic system is to return excess interstitial fluid to the blood.

_______ 12. The liver is an example of a lymphatic organ.

_______ 13. Another name for pharyngeal tonsils are adenoids.

_______ 14. The spleen destroys old, worn-out red blood cells.

_______ 15. IgG antibodies are found in breast milk and provide immunity for the newborn.

POSTTEST

True or False

_______ 1. The peritoneum is the loose-fitting sac that encloses the heart.

_______ 2. The superior vena cava returns blood to the heart from the lower extremities.

_______ 3. The mitral valve is located between the right atrium and right ventricle.

_______ 4. When the ventricles are contracting, the atrioventricular (AV) valves are open.

_______ 5. The buffy coat is made up of white blood cells and platelets.

_______ 6. Neutrophils are the first leukocytes to respond to tissue damage.

_______ 7. Bile is the yellow pigment that results from the breakdown of red blood cells.

_______ 8. Acute infections cause an increase in the number of neutrophils.

_______ 9. Thrombin converts fibrinogen to fibrin.

_______ 10. Microscopic arteries are known as arterioles.

_______ 11. Lymphatic organs produce white blood cells.

_______ 12. The function of lymph nodes is to filter and cleanse lymph before it enters the blood.

_______ 13. The function of tonsils is to produce T cells.

_______ 14. Antibodies are an example of a non-specific defense mechanism.

_______ 15. Active artificial immunity develops when an individual receives a vaccination and produces immunity.

Term KEY TERM ASSESSMENT

A. Definitions

Directions: Match each key term with its definition.

Circulatory System

_______ 1. Agranulocytes
_______ 2. Atrioventricular valve
_______ 3. Atria
_______ 4. Cardiac cycle
_______ 5. Coagulation
_______ 6. Conduction myofibers
_______ 7. Diapedesis
_______ 8. Diastole
_______ 9. Endocardium
_______ 10. Epicardium
_______ 11. Erythrocyte
_______ 12. Erythropoiesis
_______ 13. Erythropoietin
_______ 14. Granulocytes
_______ 15. Hematopoiesis
_______ 16. Hemocytoblast
_______ 17. Hemoglobin
_______ 18. Hemostasis
_______ 19. Leukocyte
_______ 20. Macrophages
_______ 21. Megakaryocytes
_______ 22. Myocardium
_______ 23. Pericardial cavity
_______ 24. Pericardium
_______ 25. Pulmonary circulation
_______ 26. Renal erythropoietic factor
_______ 27. Semilunar valve
_______ 28. Systemic circulation
_______ 29. Systole
_______ 30. Thrombocyte
_______ 31. Ventricle

A. A complete heartbeat consisting of contraction and relaxation of both atria and both ventricles
B. A hormone released by the kidneys that stimulates red blood cell production
C. A stem cell in the bone marrow from which the blood cells arise
D. Blood cell production, which occurs in the red bone marrow
E. Cardiac muscle cells specialized for conducting action potentials to the myocardium; part of the conduction system of the heart; also called Purkinje fibers
F. Contraction phase of the cardiac cycle
G. One of the formed elements of the blood; functions in blood clotting
H. Red blood cell
I. Relaxation phase of the cardiac cycle
J. The process by which white blood cells squeeze between the cells in a vessel wall to enter the tissue spaces outside the blood vessel
K. The process of blood clotting
L. The process of red blood cell formation
M. Valve between a ventricle of the heart and the vessel that carries blood away from the ventricle
N. Valve between an atrium and a ventricle in the heart
O. White blood cell
P. Pathways that transport blood from the left side of the heart to all parts of the body and return the blood to the right atrium
Q. Membrane that surrounds the heart
R. Large phagocytic connective tissue cell that functions in immune responses
S. Small space around the heart between the parietal pericardium and visceral pericardium
T. The iron-containing protein in red blood cells responsible for transporting oxygen
U. The thin, smooth inner lining of each chamber of the heart
V. A large cell that contributes to the formation of platelets
W. A substance produced by the kidneys that activates erythropoietin to stimulate the production of red blood cells
X. Pumping chamber of the heart
Y. The outer layer of the heart wall
Z. White blood cells that lack granules in the cytoplasm
AA. Thin walled chambers of the heart that receive blood from veins
BB. White blood cells that have granules in the cytoplasm
CC. The control or stoppage of bleeding
DD. The pathway that takes blood from the right side of the heart to the lungs, and then returns it to the left side of the heart
EE. Middle layer of the heart wall composed of cardiac muscle tissue

Lymphatic System

_______ 1. Antibodies
_______ 2. Antibody-mediated immunity
_______ 3. Antigens
_______ 4. Cell-mediated immunity
_______ 5. Immunoglobulins
_______ 6. Non-specific defense mechanisms
_______ 7. Resistance
_______ 8. Right lymphatic duct
_______ 9. Specific defense mechanisms
_______ 10. Susceptibility
_______ 11. Thoracic duct

A. Immunity that is the result of T-cell action
B. Immunity that is the result of B-cell action and the production of antibodies
C. Substances produced by the body that inactivate or destroy other substances that are introduced into the body
D. Body's ability to counteract the effects of pathogens and other harmful agents
E. The primary collecting duct of the lymphatic system that collects lymph from all regions of the body except the upper right quadrant
F. Substances produced by the body that inactivate or destroy other substances that are introduced into the body
G. Body's ability to counteract all types of harmful agents
H. The collecting duct of the lymphatic system that collects lymph from the upper right quadrant of the body
I. Lack of resistance to disease
J. Substances that trigger an immune response when they are introduced into the body
K. Activities of the body that counteract only certain types of harmful agents

B. Word Parts

Directions: Indicate the meaning of each word part in the space provided. List as many medical terms as possible that incorporate the word part in the space provided.

Word Part	Meaning of Word Part	Medical Terms That Incorporate Word Part
1. anti		
2. atri/o		
3. ventricul/o		
4. coagul/o		
5. -tion		
6. my/o		
7. dia-		
8. card/i		
9. epi-		
10. -um		
11. erythr/o		
12. -cyte		
13. -poieses		
14. -poietin		
15. granul/o		
16. hem/o		
17. -blast		

Word Part	Meaning of Word Part	Medical Terms That Incorporate Word Part
18. -globin		
19. -stasis		
20. hemat/o		
21. immun/o		
22. leuk/o		
23. macr/o		
24. phag-		
25. mega		
26. kary/o		
27. peri-		
28. pulmon-		
29. ren/o		
30. thromb/o		

EVALUATION OF LEARNING

Directions: Fill in each blank with the correct answer.

Circulatory System

1. What makes up the following components of the circulatory system?

   a. Cardiovascular component:

   ____

   b. Lymphatic component:

   ____

2. What is the function of the heart?

   ____

   ____

3. How large is the average human heart?

   ____

4. Describe the following layers of the pericardium:

   a. Fibrous pericardium: ______________________________

   b. Parietal pericardium: ______________________________

   c. Visceral pericardium: ______________________________

5. What is the function of the epicardium?

6. What makes up the myocardium?

7. Why does the endocardium have a smooth surface?

8. What type of blood enters the right atrium?

9. The superior vena cava returns blood to the heart from what parts of the body?

10. The inferior vena cava returns blood to the heart from what parts of the body?

11. What is the interarterial septum?

12. What is the function of the right ventricle?

13. What is the function of the left ventricle?

14. Why does the left ventricle have a thicker myocardium than the right ventricle?

15. What is the interventricular septum?

16. Describe the location and function of each of the following valves:

Valve	Location	Function
a. Tricuspid valve		
b. Bicuspid valve		
c. Pulmonary semilunar valve		
d. Aortic semilunar valve		

17. Starting with the right atrium, trace the path of the blood through the heart.

______

______

______

______

18. What are the names of the vessels that supply the heart with oxygen?

______

19. What is the function of the SA node?

______

______

20. What is the function of the AV node?

______

______

21. What structures transmit the heart's impulse from the AV node to the ventricles?

______

22. What occurs with each of the following during atrial systole?
    a. AV valves: ______
    b. Atria: ______
    c. Ventricles: ______
    d. Semilunar valves: ______

23. What are each of the following structures doing during ventricular systole?
    a. AV valves: ______
    b. Atria: ______
    c. Ventricles: ______
    d. Semilunar valves: ______

24. What causes each of the following heart sounds?
    a. Lubb: ______
    b. Dupp: ______

25. What causes a heart murmur?

______

26. What is the total blood volume for a woman and a man?
    a. Woman:______
    b. Man:______

27. How does blood function as transportation in the body?

28. How does blood function to regulate the body?

29. How does blood function as protection for the body?

30. What percentage of the blood is made up of the following?
   a. Plasma:
   b. Red blood cells:

31. What makes up the buffy coat?

32. What is the function of the following plasma proteins?
   a. Albumins:
   b. Globulins:
   c. Fibrinogen:

33. What are the waste products of protein metabolism? How are these waste products excreted?

34. What seven cells develop from a hemocytoblast?

35. What is the normal range for a red blood count for the following?
   a. Adult male:
   b. Adult female:

36. Describe the appearance of a mature red blood cell.

____

37. What is the function of erythrocytes?

____

38. What is the name of the hormone that stimulates the red bone marrow to produce erythrocytes?

____

39. What vitamins and minerals are necessary for the production of red blood cells?

____

40. What is the function of the intrinsic factor?

____

41. What condition results when there is a lack of the intrinsic factor?

____

42. What is the life span of a red blood cell?

____

43. What happens when a red blood cell is worn out?

____

____

44. What is bilirubin?

____

45. What is the normal range for a white blood count?

____

46. Where do leukocytes do their work?

____

47. What is diapedesis?

____

48. What is the function of neutrophils? What causes an increase in neutrophils?

____

49. What is the function of eosinophils? What causes an increase in eosinophils?

____

50. What is the function of the following substances secreted by a basophil?

a. Histamine: _______________

b. Heparin: _______________

51. What is the function of lymphocytes? What causes an increase in lymphocytes?

____

52. What are macrophages, and what is their function?

____

____

53. Describe the appearance and list the normal range for each of the following:

a. Neutrophils: ____

____

b. Eosinohils: ____

____

c. Basophils: ____

____

d. Lymphocytes: ____

____

e. Monocytes: ____

____

54. What is another name for a thrombocyte?

____

55. What is a megakaryocyte?

____

56. What is the normal range for a platelet count?

____

57. What is the function of thrombocytes?

____

58. What is the term for the stoppage of bleeding?

____

59. What is the function of serotonin secreted by platelets when a blood vessel is torn or cut?

____

____

60. What is the function of a platelet plug?

____

61. What are procoagulants?

____

62. How does blood stay in a liquid form in the blood vessels?

63. What is necessary to convert inactive prothrombin to active thrombin?

64. What is the function of thrombin?

65. Why does a blood clot retract after it forms?

66. What antigens and antibodies occur with each of the following blood types?

Blood Type	Blood Antigens	Blood Antibodies
Type A		
Type B		
Type AB		
Type O		

67. What does it mean if someone is Rh positive? What does it mean if he or she is Rh negative?

68. What is the function of arteries?

69. What are the three layers that make up the wall of an artery?

70. What makes up the wall of a capillary?

71. What is the function of veins?

72. Why can veins hold more blood than arteries?

73. What is the function of venous valves?

74. What is the function of the pulmonary circuit?

75. What is the function of the systemic circuit?

76. What changes occur to the following parts of the circulatory system as an individual ages?

a. Left ventricle:

b. Endocardium:

c. Valves of the heart:

d. Dysrhythmias:

Lymphatic System

1. What are the three primary functions of the lymphatic system?

2. What is lymph? What is it derived from?

3. What are the characteristics of lymphatic organs?

4. List examples of lymphatic organs.

5. What is the function of lymph nodes?

6. Where is the location of the following clusters of lymph nodes?

a. Inguinal lymph nodes:

b. Axillary lymph nodes:

c. Cervical lymph nodes:

7. Where is the location of the following tonsils?

a. Pharyngeal tonsils:

b. Palatine tonsils:

c. Lingual tonsils:

8. What is the function of tonsils?

9. What is another name for the pharyngel tonsils?

10. What is the function of the spleen? Where is it located?

11. What is the function of the thymus gland? Where is it located?

12. What are non-specific defense mechanisms?

13. List examples of non-specific defense mechanisms?

14. What are the primary cells involved in immunity?

15. What are the characteristics of specific defense mechanisms?

16. What are the characteristics of cell-mediated immunity?

17. Cell-mediated immunity most effective against what agents?

18. What are the characteristics of antibody-mediated immunity?

___

___

___

19. Antibody-mediated immunity most effective against what agents?

___

20. What is the function of each of the following antibodies (immunoglobulins)?

a. IgG: ___

___

b. IgA: ___

___

c. IgM: ___

___

d. IgD: ___

___

e. IgE: ___

___

21. Explain how each of the following four types of immunity develop:

a. Active natural immunity:

___

___

b. Active artificial immunity:

___

___

c. Passive natural immunity:

___

___

d. Passive artificial immunity:

___

___

CRITICAL THINKING ACTIVITIES

A. Evolve Site: Body Spectrum

Circulatory: Heart—Cross Section

Body Spectrum directions:

1. Access the Body Spectrum program on the Evolve site.
2. If necessary, access the HELP screen for directions on using the Body Spectrum program.
3. Go to the Contents screen.
4. Select the following category from the Contents screen:
   Circulatory
5. Select the following anatomic diagram:
   Heart—Cross Section
6. Identify the structures on the diagram.
7. Print out the diagram.

B. Evolve Site: Body Spectrum

Circulatory: Heart Circulation

Directions: Identify the structures on this diagram following the Body Spectrum directions outlined under CTA A.

C. Evolve Site: Body Spectrum

Circulatory: Coronary Vessels

Directions: Identify the structures on this diagram following the Body Spectrum directions outlined under CTA A.

D. Evolve Site: Name That Blood Cell

Access the Evolve site to complete this activity. Record your points earned on your assignment sheet.

E. Blood Clotting

You are a blood vessel located in the finger of a human. Your human is cutting up vegetables and accidentally severs you with a knife. Describe what tasks are performed to heal you during each of the hemostatic processes listed below.

a. Vascular Constriction:

____

____

____

____

____

____

____

b. Platelet Plug Formation:

c. Coagulation:

F. Inquiring Patients Want to Know

You are working in a general practice medical office. Your patients ask you the following questions. In the space provided, indicate how you would respond to each question in terms the patient would understand. Use your textbook and Internet resources to develop your responses.

1. Why is blood red?

2. Why does a bruise eventually turn yellow?

3. What causes varicose veins?

4. What is the difference between iron-deficiency anemia and pernicious anemia?

5. How does a pacemaker work?

____

____

6. What happens in the body during carbon monoxide poisoning?

____

____

7. What is done with the plasma that is collected at plasma donor centers?

____

____

8. What happens to the heart when it is defibrillated?

____

____

9. How can poor circulation cause gangrene?

____

____

10. Why does the physician look at the blood vessels in my eye?

____

____

G. Crossword Puzzle: Circulatory System

Directions: Complete the crossword puzzle using the clues provided.

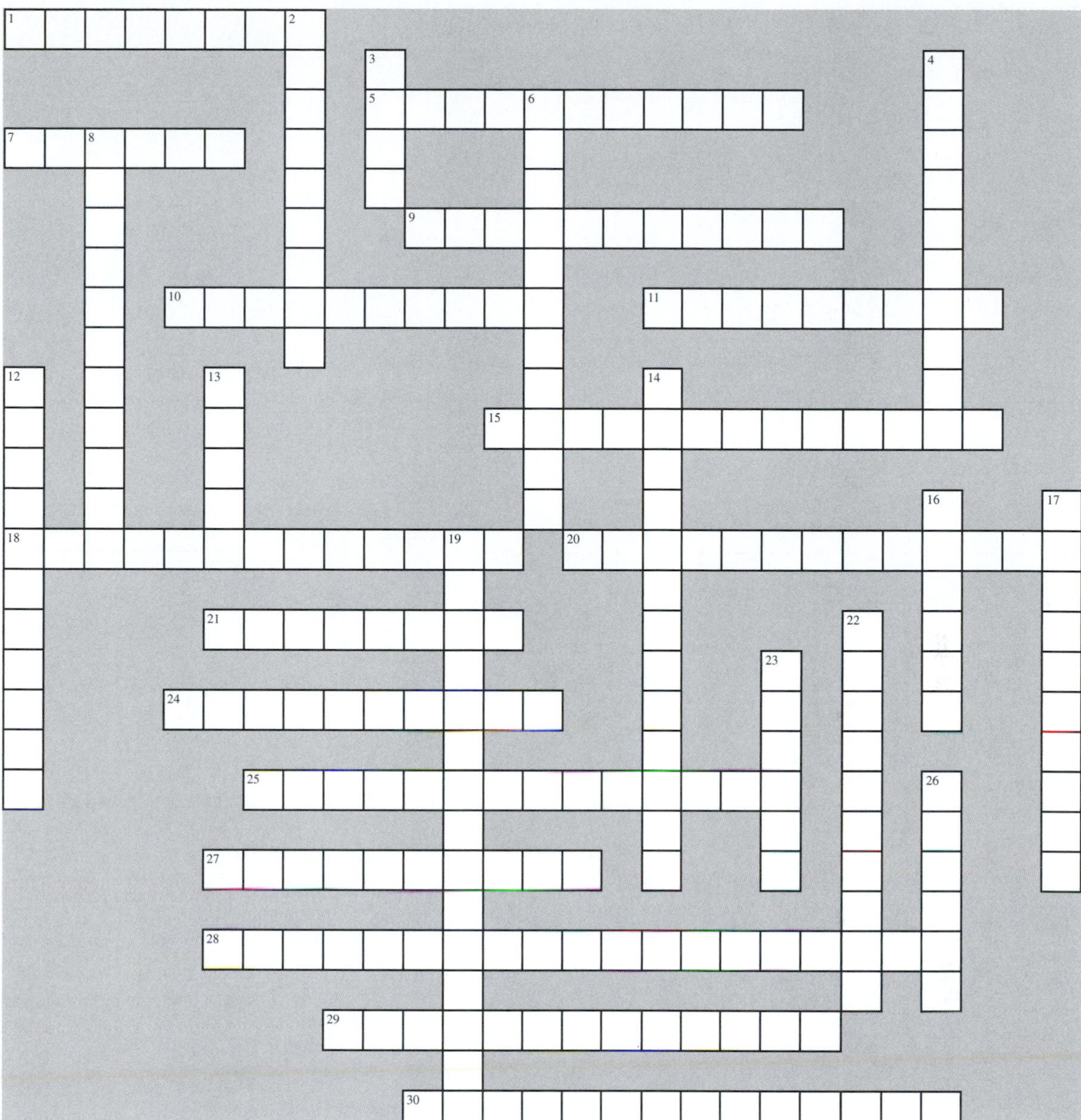

Across

1 Secretes histamine and heparin
5 Inner lining of heart wall
7 Abnormal heart sound
9 Sac that encloses the heart
10 Engulfs bacteria by phagocytosis
11 Consists of white blood cells and platelets
15 Shape of RBC
18 Production of blood cells
20 Between left atrium and left ventricle
21 Largest WBC
24 Forms bulk of heart wall
25 Between right atrium and right ventricle
27 Produces antibodies
28 Also known as the epicardium
29 Chamber that pumps blood to entire body
30 Stimulates RBC production

Down

2 White blood cell
3 Carries blood toward heart
4 Stoppage of bleeding
6 Tiny blood vessels
8 Receives deoxygenated blood
12 Red blood cell
13 No antigen blood
14 Inhibits clotting
16 Pacemaker of the heart
17 Receives oxygenated blood
19 Needed for absorption of vitamin B12
22 Transports oxygen
23 Carries blood away from heart
26 Liquid part of blood

Notes

13 Respiratory System

CHAPTER ASSIGNMENTS

✓ After Completing	Date Due	Study Guide Page(s)	STUDY GUIDE ASSIGNMENTS (CTA: Critical Thinking Activity)	Possible Points	Points You Earned
		187	Pretest	10	
		188	Term Key Term Assessment A. Definitions B. Word Parts (Add 1 point for each key term)	 20 8	
		189-191	Evaluation of Learning questions	34	
		192	Evolve Site: CTA A: Body Spectrum—Respiratory System	10	
		192	Evolve Site: CTA B: Body Spectrum—Nasal Cavity and Pharynx	10	
		192	Evolve Site: CTA C: Body Spectrum—Larynx and Upper Trachea	10	
		192-193	CTA D: Inquiring Patients Want to Know	10	
		194	CTA E: Crossword Puzzle	21	
		187	Posttest	10	
			ADDITIONAL ASSIGNMENTS		
			TOTAL POINTS		

Notes

Name ______________________________ Date ______________

PRETEST

True or False

_______ 1. The lungs are located in the lower respiratory tract.

_______ 2. The function of mucus in the respiratory tract is to destroy microorganisms.

_______ 3. The nasal septum divides the nose into two parts.

_______ 4. The auditory (eustachian) tubes open into the oropharynx.

_______ 5. The uvula is the posterior portion of the soft palate that helps direct food into the oropharynx.

_______ 6. The glottis prevents food and water from entering the trachea.

_______ 7. The vocal cords are made up of ligaments.

_______ 8. The right lung is divided into two lobes.

_______ 9. The process of taking air into the lungs is known as inhalation.

_______ 10. Sneezing is a nonrespiratory air movement.

POSTTEST

True or False

_______ 1. The exchange of gases between the blood and tissue cells is known as external respiration.

_______ 2. The paranasal sinuses are lined by a serous membrane.

_______ 3. Cilia propel mucus toward the pharynx.

_______ 4. The nasal conchae separate the nasal cavity from the oral cavity.

_______ 5. The oropharynx receives air, food, and water from the oral cavity.

_______ 6. The thyroid cartilage located in the larynx is commonly called the Adam's apple.

_______ 7. The larynx is supported by 15 to 20 C-shaped pieces of hyaline cartilage.

_______ 8. The pleura is a double-layered serous membrane that encloses the lungs.

_______ 9. Internal respiration is the exchange of gases between the tissue cells and the blood.

_______ 10. The respiratory center is located in the hypothalamus.

KEY TERM ASSESSMENT

Directions: Match each key term with its definition.

_______ 1. Alveoli
_______ 2. Bronchi
_______ 3. Bronchial tree
_______ 4. External respiration
_______ 5. Fauces
_______ 6. Internal respiration
_______ 7. Laryngopharynx
_______ 8. Larynx
_______ 9. Lower respiratory tract
_______ 10. Nasopharynx
_______ 11. Oropharynx
_______ 12. Pharynx
_______ 13. Pleura
_______ 14. Pleural cavity
_______ 15. Respiration
_______ 16. Respiratory membrane
_______ 17. Surfactant
_______ 18. Trachea
_______ 19. Upper respiratory tract
_______ 20. Ventilation

A. A substance, produced by certain cells in lung tissue, that reduces surface tension between fluid molecules that line the respiratory membrane and helps keep the alveolus from collapsing
B. Any surface in the lungs where diffusion occurs; consists of the layers that the gases must pass through to get into or out of the alveoli
C. Exchange of gases between the blood and tissue cells
D. Exchange of gases between the lungs and the blood
E. Microscopic dilations of terminal bronchioles in the lungs, where diffusion of gases occurs
F. Movement of air into and out of the lungs; breathing
G. The bronchi and all their branches that function as passageways between the trachea and the alveoli
H. Portion of the pharynx that is posterior to the nasal cavities; extends from the base of the skull to the uvula
I. Passageway for air that extends inferiorly to the carina where it branches into the bronchi (also known as the windpipe)
J. Opening from the oral cavity into the oropharynx
K. The small space between the parietal and visceral layers of the pleura
L. Passageway for air between the pharynx and trachea; (also known as the voice box)
M. The airways that are formed when the trachea branches
N. Passageway for air and food (also known as the throat)
O. Exchange of oxygen and carbon dioxide between the atmosphere and the body cells
P. Portion of the pharynx that is behind the larynx
Q. Serous membrane that lines the ribs and surrounds the lungs
R. Portion of the respiratory tract that includes the nose, pharynx, and larynx
S. Portion of the respiratory tract that is inferior to the larynx; includes the trachea, bronchial tree, and lungs
T. Portion of the pharynx that is posterior to the oral cavity

B. Word Parts

Directions: Indicate the meaning of each word part in the space provided. List as many medical terms as possible that incorporate the word part in the space provided.

Word Part	Meaning of Word Part	Medical Terms That Incorporate Word Part
1. alveol-		
2. bronchi-		
3. laryng/o		
4. nas/o		
5. or/o		
6. pharyng/o		
7. pleur/o		
8. respir/o		

EVALUATION OF LEARNING

Directions: Fill in each blank with the correct answer.

1. What are the functions of the respiratory system?

____

____

2. What is external respiration?

____

3. What is internal respiration?

____

4. What structures are located in the upper respiratory tract?

____

5. What structures are located in the lower respiratory tract?

____

6. Describe the following parts of the nose:

   a. Nasal cavity: ____

   b. Nasal septum: ____

   c. Nostrils: ____

   d. Internal nares: ____

   e. Palate: ____

   f. Uvula: ____

7. What is the difference between the hard palate and soft palate?

____

____

8. What are the functions of the nasal conchae?

____

____

9. What are the paranasal sinuses?

____

____

10. What are three functions of the paranasal sinuses?

____

____

11. What is the function of the mucus secreted by the mucous membrane of the nose?

12. What is the function of the cilia in the nasal cavity?

13. What is the nasopharynx?

14. What is the function of the eustachian tubes?

15. What is the oropharynx?

16. What is the laryngopharynx?

17. What is the layman's term for the thyroid cartilage?

18. What is the function of the epiglottis?

19. What are the functions of the following?
   a. False vocal cords: ______
   b. True vocal cords: ______

20. What is the glottis?

21. What holds the trachea open?

22. Describe the components of the bronchial tree.

23. Why do the walls of the alveolar ducts and alveoli consist of simple squamous epithelium?

24. Why are the lungs soft and spongy?

25. How does the right lung differ in appearance from the left lung?

26. What is the pleura?

27. What is another name for breathing?

28. What is included in one breath?

29. How does air move into the lungs during inhalation?

30. How does air move out of the lungs during exhalation?

31. Where is the respiratory center located?

32. What happens if there is an increase in carbon dioxide in the blood?

33. What are examples of nonrespiratory air movements?

34. What changes occur to the following parts of the respiratory system because of aging?
    a. Cartilage in the walls of the trachea and bronchi: __________
    b. Bronchioles: __________
    c. Alveoli: __________

CRITICAL THINKING ACTIVITIES

A. Evolve Site: Body Spectrum

Respiratory: Respiratory System

Body Spectrum directions:

1. Access the Body Spectrum program on the Evolve site.
2. If necessary, access the HELP screen for directions on using the Body Spectrum program.
3. Go to the Contents screen.
4. Select the following category from the Contents screen:
   Respiratory
5. Select the following anatomic diagram:
   Respiratory System
6. Identify the structures on the diagram.
7. Print out the diagram.

B. Evolve Site: Body Spectrum

Respiratory: Nasal Cavity and Pharynx

Directions: Identify the structures on this diagram following the Body Spectrum directions outlined under CTA A.

C. Evolve Site: Body Spectrum

Respiratory: Larynx and Upper Trachea

Directions: Identify the structures on this diagram following the Body Spectrum directions outlined under CTA A.

D. Inquiring Patients Want to Know

You are working in a general practice medical office. Your patients ask you the following questions. In the space provided, indicate how you would respond to each question in terms the patient would understand. Use your textbook and Internet resources to develop your responses.

1. What happens in the body when you sneeze?

____

____

2. Why do men have a deeper voice than women?

____

____

3. What do your tonsils do?

____

____

4. What damage does smoking do to the respiratory tract?

____

____

5. What do sinuses do?

6. Can you die from holding your breath?

7. What makes you yawn when someone else yawns?

8. Is it bad for you if you're drinking water and it goes down the wrong tube?

9. Why does your nose run when you have allergies?

10. Can you permanently lose your voice from laryngitis?

E. Crossword Puzzle: Respiratory System

Directions: Complete the crossword puzzle using the clues provided.

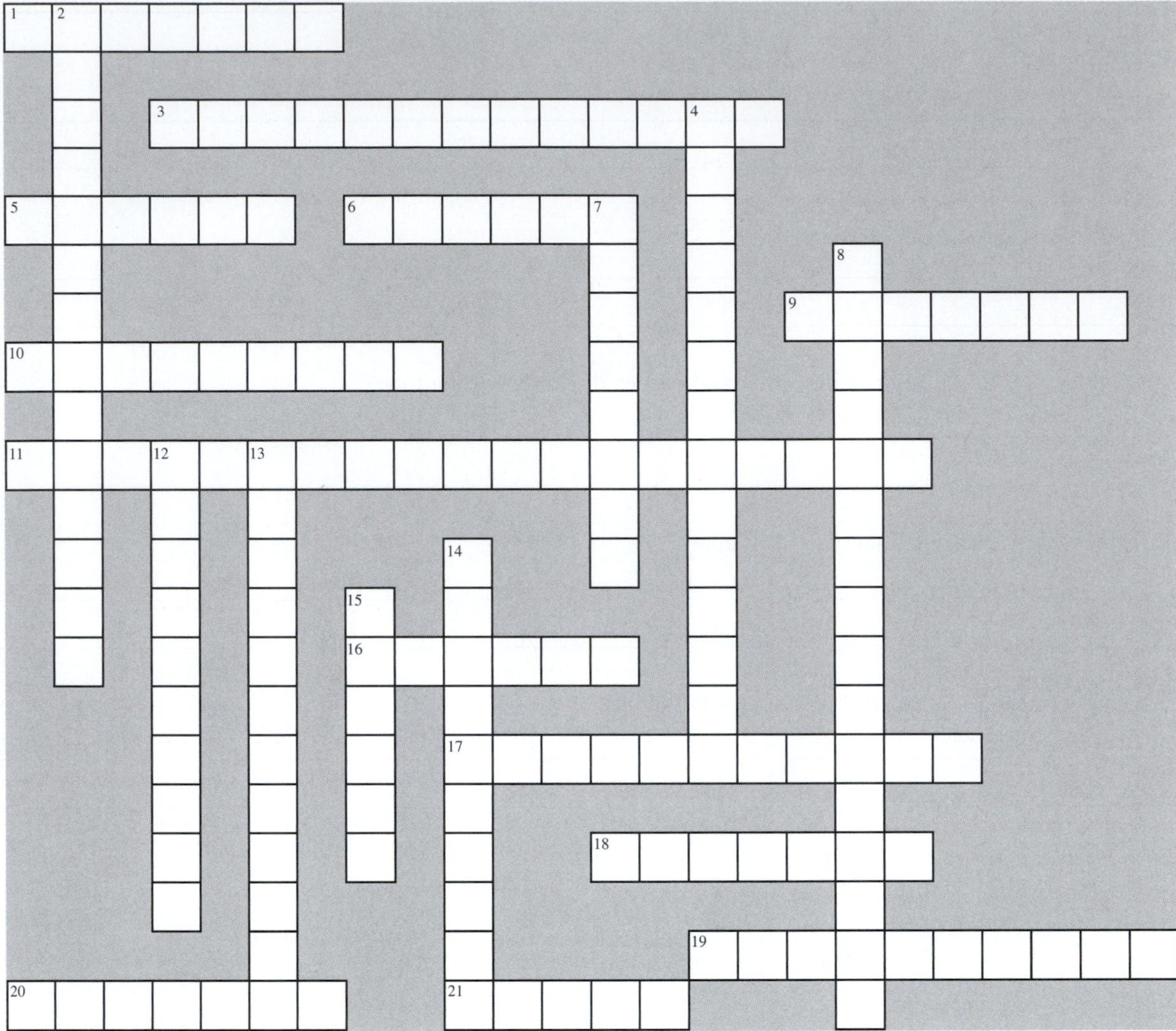

Across

1 Respiratory center
3 Contains serous fluid produced by the pleura
6 Separates nasal cavity from oral cavity
7 Opening between oral cavity and oropharynx
10 Throat
11 Has three lobes
12 Exchange of gases between tissues and blood
16 Voice box
17 Divides nose into two parts
18 Tiny air sacs
19 Prevents food from entering trachea
20 Windpipe
21 Air-filled cavity in skull

Down

2 Equalizes air pressure
4 Produces sound
7 Nonrespiratory air movement
8 Adam's apple
12 Expelling air from the lungs
13 Bony ridges that warm air
14 Inflammation of the vocal cords
15 Membrane around the lungs

14 Digestive System

CHAPTER ASSIGNMENTS

✓ After Completing	Date Due	Study Guide Page(s)	STUDY GUIDE ASSIGNMENTS (CTA: Critical Thinking Activity)	Possible Points	Points You Earned
		197	Pretest	10	
		198	Term Key Term Assessment A. Definitions B. Word Parts (Add 1 point for each key term)	 19 8	
		199-204	Evaluation of Learning questions	66	
		205	Evolve Site: CTA A: Body Spectrum: Digestive System	10	
		205	Evolve Site: CTA B: Body Spectrum: Teeth	10	
		205	CTA C: Structure of a Tooth	11	
		205	Evolve Site: CTA D: Body Spectrum: Salivary Glands	10	
		205	Evolve Site: CTA E: Body Spectrum: Anatomy of Large Intestine	10	
		205	Evolve Site: CTA F: Body Spectrum: Intestinal Secretion Sources	10	
		206	CTA G: Pizza Digestion	20	
		206-207	CTA H: Inquiring Patients Want to Know	10	
		208	CTA I: Crossword Puzzle	38	
		197	Posttest	10	
			ADDITIONAL ASSIGNMENTS		
			TOTAL POINTS		

Notes

Name ____ Date ____________________

PRETEST

True or False

_______ 1. The pancreas is an accessory organ of the digestive system.

_______ 2. Peristalsis consists of rhythmic waves of contractions that propel food particles through the digestive tract.

_______ 3. The buccinator muscle connects the tongue anteriorly to the floor of the mouth.

_______ 4. The total number of primary teeth is 32.

_______ 5. Saliva moistens and lubricates the food.

_______ 6. The esophagus provides a passageway for food between the pharynx and stomach.

_______ 7. The first part of the small intestine is the duodenum.

_______ 8. Hepatocytes are liver cells.

_______ 9. Iron is stored in the liver.

_______ 10. The function of the gallbladder is to produce bile.

POSTTEST

True or False

_______ 1. The taking in of food is known as mastication.

_______ 2. Mechanical digestion breaks down food into smaller particles through the mixing actions of the stomach.

_______ 3. The hard palate and uvula direct food away from the nasal cavity and into the oropharynx during swallowing.

_______ 4. Cuspids are teeth that have sharp edges used for biting food.

_______ 5. The cardiac sphincter acts as a valve between the stomach and small intestine.

_______ 6. The intrinsic factor aids in the absorption of vitamin B_{12} from the digestive tract.

_______ 7. Chyme is a semifluid that results when food is broken down in the stomach.

_______ 8. The large intestine functions in the absorption of nutrients.

_______ 9. Bile salts act as emulsifying agents to break down fat into small fat droplets.

_______ 10. The end product of protein digestion is glucose.

Term KEY TERM ASSESSMENT

Directions: Match each key term with its definition.

_______ 1. Absorption
_______ 2. Chyme
_______ 3. Defecation
_______ 4. Deglutition
_______ 5. Fauces
_______ 6. Gastric juice
_______ 7. Gastrin
_______ 8. Gingiva
_______ 9. Hydrolysis
_______ 10. Ileocecal valve
_______ 11. Lower esophageal sphincter
_______ 12. Mastication
_______ 13. Mesentery
_______ 14. Palate
_______ 15. Peristalsis
_______ 16. Plicae circulares
_______ 17. Pyloric sphincter
_______ 18. Rugae
_______ 19. Teniae coli

A. Circular folds in the mucosa and submucosa of the small intestine
B. Extensions of peritoneum that are associated with the intestine
C. Longitudinal folds in the mucosa of the stomach
D. Rhythmic contractions of the intestine that move food along the digestive tract
E. The passage of digestive end products from the gastrointestinal tract into the blood or lymph
F. The semifluid mixture of food and gastric juice that leaves the stomach through the pyloric sphincter
G. Roof of the mouth
H. Chemical breakdown of complex molecules by the addition of water
I. The process of swallowing
J. Bands of longitudinal muscle fibers in the large intestine
K. The secretions of the exocrine gastric glands
L. Valve between the esophagus and stomach
M. Soft tissue that covers the alveolar processes of the mandible and maxillae (also called gums)
N. The expulsion of indigestible wastes, or feces, through the anus
O. Valve between the stomach and first part of the small intestine
P. Opening from the oral cavity into the oropharynx
Q. The valve between the small intestine and large intestine
R. Hormone secreted by the endocrine glands in the stomach
S. The process of chewing

B. Word Parts

Directions: Indicate the meaning of each word part in the space provided. List as many medical terms as possible that incorporate the word part in the space provided.

Word Part	Meaning of Word Part	Medical Terms That Incorporate Word Part
1. gastr/o		
2. gingiv/o		
3. hydr/o		
4. -lysis		
5. ile/o		
6. -cee		
7. -stalsis		
8. col-		

EVALUATION OF LEARNING

Directions: Fill in each blank with the correct answer.

1. What are two other names for the digestive tract?

____

2. What structures make up the digestive tract?

____

____

3. What are the accessory organs of digestion?

____

____

4. What is ingestion?

____

5. What occurs during mechanical digestion?

____

____

6. What occurs during chemical digestion?

____

____

7. What is deglutition?

____

8. What is peristalsis?

____

____

9. What are the four layers of the digestive tract?

____

10. What are the functions of the sensory receptors located in the lips?

____

11. What muscle makes up the cheeks?

____

12. Describe the difference between the hard palate and soft palate.

____

____

____

13. What is the function of the uvula?

____

____

14. What is the lingual frenulum?

____

15. What are two functions of the papillae located on the tongue?

____

____

16. What is the function of the lingual tonsils?

____

17. What is the function of the tongue?

____

____

18. How many teeth make up the following?
    a. Primary teeth: ______________________
    b. Secondary teeth: ______________________

19. What are the functions of the following teeth?
    a. Incisors: ______________________
    b. Cuspids: ______________________
    c. Bicuspids and molars: ______________________

20. Describe the following three main parts of a tooth:
    a. Crown: ______________________
    b. Root: ______________________
    c. Neck: ______________________

21. Describe the following structures that make up a tooth:
    a. Pulp cavity: ______________________
    b. Pulp: ______________________
    c. Root canal: ______________________
    d. Apical foramen: ______________________
    e. Dentin: ______________________
    f. Cementum: ______________________
    g. Periodontal ligaments: ______________________
    h. Enamel: ______________________

22. What are the names and locations of the three salivary glands?

Name	Location

23. What is the function of saliva?

____

____

____

24. What are the three regions of the pharynx?

____

25. What is the function of the esophagus?

____

26. What is the function of the esophageal sphincter?

____

27. Describe the following structures that make up the stomach:

a. Cardiac region: ______________________________

b. Fundus: ______________________________

c. Body: ______________________________

d. Lesser curvature: ______________________________

e. Greater curvature: ______________________________

f. Pyloric region: ______________________________

g. Pyloric sphincter: ______________________________

28. What are rugae, and what is their function?

____

____

29. Indicate the type of gastric gland cells that produce the following gastric secretions and the function of each secretion.

Gastric Gland Secretion	Secreted by	Function
a. Thick and alkaline mucus		
b. Thin and watery mucus		
c. Hydrochloric acid		
d. Intrinsic factor		
e. Pepsinogen		

30. What is the function of pepsin?

31. How is inactive pepsinogen converted to active pepsin?

32. What is chyme?

33. What causes gastric juice to be released during the cephalic phase?

34. What causes gastric juice to be released during the gastric phase?

35. What triggers the intestinal phase of gastric secretion regulation?

36. What is the function of the small intestine?

37. What is the function of the plicae circulares?

38. Describe the appearance of the villi. What is the function of villi?

39. What are the three regions of the small intestine?

40. What is the function of the mesentery?

41. What are the functions of the following enzymes?
   a. Peptidase:
   b. Maltase, sucrose, and lactase:
   c. Intestinal lipase:

42. What is the ileocecal junction?

43. What are the four regions of the large intestine?

44. What are the four parts of the colon?

45. What is the function of the large intestine?

46. What is the function of the mucus secreted by the large intestine?

47. What is the function of the falciform ligament of the liver?

48. What are hepatocytes?

49. What substances are stored in the liver?

50. What is the function of Kupffer cells?

51. What makes up bile?

52. What are the functions of bile salts?

53. How are bile pigments produced?

54. What is the name of the principal bile pigment?

___

55. What is the function of the gallbladder?

___

56. What causes the release of cholecystokinin?

___

57. What is the function of cholecystokinin?

___

___

58. What is the function of the islets of Langerhans?

___

59. What is the function of pancreatic acinar cells?

___

___

60. What is the function of the pancreatic duct?

___

___

61. What digestive enzymes are found in pancreatic juice?

___

62. What effect does cholecystokinin have on the pancreas?

___

___

63. What are the end products of carbohydrate digestion?

___

64. What are the end products of protein digestion?

___

65. What are the end products of lipid digestion?

___

66. In what part of the small intestine does most absorption take place?

___

CRITICAL THINKING ACTIVITIES

A. Evolve Site: Body Spectrum

Digestive: Digestive System

Body Spectrum directions:

1. Access the Body Spectrum program on the Evolve site.
2. If necessary, access the HELP screen for directions on using the Body Spectrum program.
3. Go to the Contents screen.
4. Select the following category from the Contents screen:
   Digestive
5. Select the following anatomic diagram:
   Digestive System
6. Identify the structures on the diagram.
7. Print out the diagram.

B. Evolve Site: Body Spectrum

Digestive: Teeth

Directions: Identify the structures on this diagram following the Body Spectrum directions outlined under CTA A.

C. Structure of a Tooth

Using Figure 14-4 in your textbook as a reference, label each of the structures of a tooth on the following diagram.

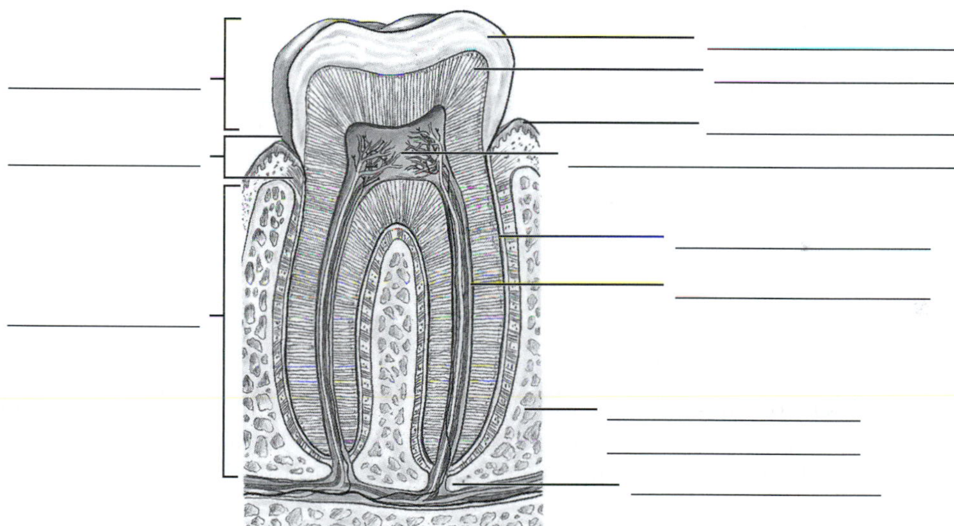

(Modified from Applegate E: *The anatomy and physiology learning system, ed* 4, St. Louis, 2011, Saunders.)

D. Evolve Site: Body Spectrum

Digestive: Salivary Glands

Directions: Identify the structures on this diagram following the Body Spectrum directions outlined under CTA A.

E. Evolve Site: Body Spectrum

Digestive: Anatomy of Large Intestine

Directions: Identify the structures on this diagram following the Body Spectrum directions outlined under CTA A.

F. Evolve Site: Body Spectrum

Digestive: Intestinal Secretion Sources

Directions: Identify the structures on this diagram following the Body Spectrum directions outlined under CTA A.

G. Pizza Digestion

You are a slice of pizza that has just been eaten by a human. Starting at the mouth, describe what you will go through during the digestive process.

H. Inquiring Patients Want to Know

You are working in a general practice medical office. Your patients ask you the following questions. In the space provided, indicate how you would respond to each question in terms the patient would understand. Use your textbook and Internet resources to develop your responses.

1. What is a cleft palate?

2. What causes cavities?

3. How does fluoride make your teeth stronger?

4. What causes heartburn?

5. What causes vomiting?

6. What causes someone to be lactose intolerant?

7. What is an ulcer?

8. What causes a hiatal hernia?

9. What causes gallstones?

10. How does drinking cause cirrhosis of the liver?

I. Crossword Puzzle: Digestive System

Directions: Complete the crossword puzzle using the clues provided.

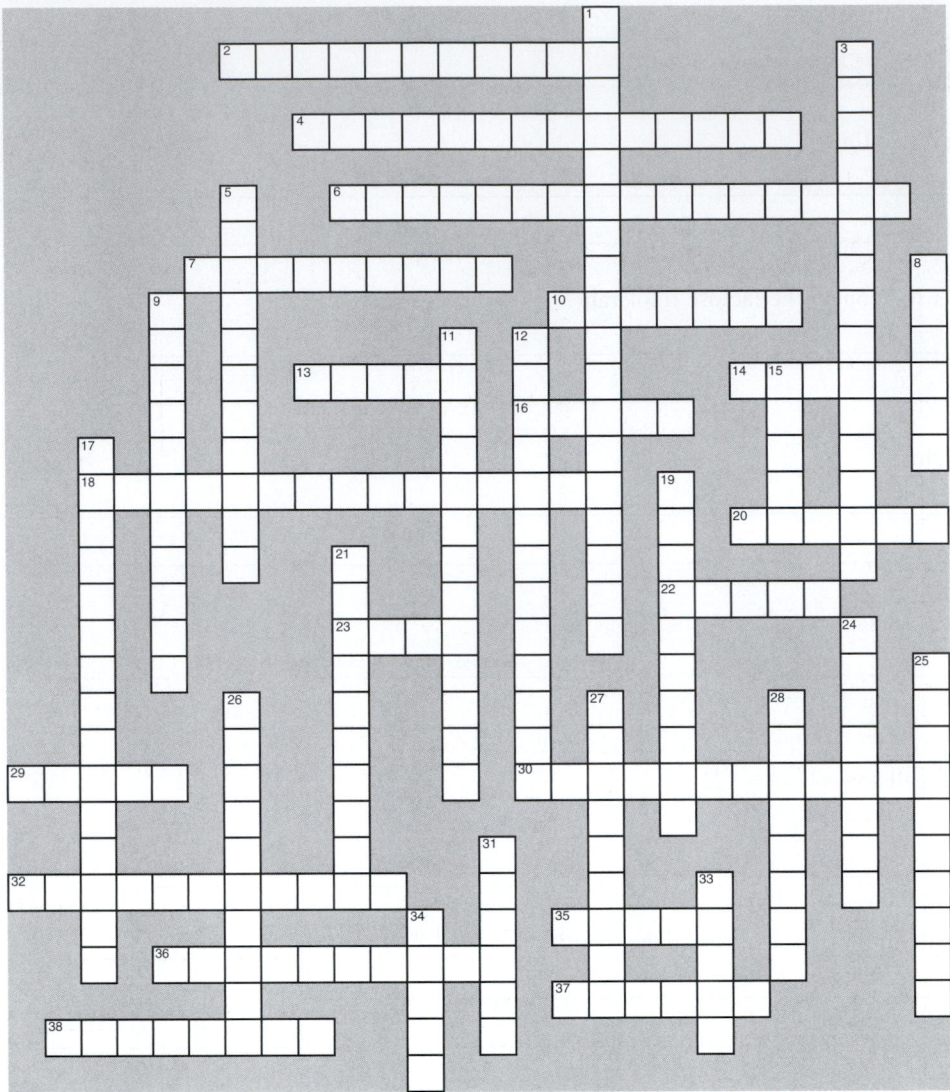

Across

2 Propels food through GI tract
4 Most food absorption occurs here
6 Valve between stomach and small intestine
7 Food tube
10 End product of carbohydrate digestion
13 Semifluid mixture of food and gastric juice
14 Innermost layer of GI tract
16 Allow stomach to expand
18 Aids in absorption of vitamin B_{12}
20 Moistens and lubricates food
22 Visible part of the tooth
23 Part of tooth that contains nerves and blood vessels
29 Last part of small intestine
30 S-shaped curve of large intestine
32 Stores bile
35 Increase surface area for food absorption
36 Length of GI tract
37 Hardest substance in the body
38 First part of small intestine

Down

1 Secrete insulin and glucagon
3 Causes gallbladder to contract
5 Chewing
8 Teeth used to crush and grind food
9 Swallowing
11 Triggered by seeing and smelling food
12 Largest salivary glands
15 Soft palate projection
17 Connects tongue to floor of mouth
19 Cheek muscle
21 Liver cell
24 Tongue projections that contain taste buds
25 End products of protein digestion
26 Removal of wastes through anus
27 Taking in of food
28 Teeth used to bite food
31 Forms bulk of tooth
33 Produces and secretes bile
34 Blind pouch in large intestine

15 Urinary System

CHAPTER ASSIGNMENTS

✓ After Completing	Date Due	Study Guide Page(s)	STUDY GUIDE ASSIGNMENTS (CTA: Critical Thinking Activity)	Possible Points	Points You Earned
		211	Pretest	10	
		212	Key Term Assessment A. Definitions B. Word Parts (Add 1 point for each key term)	 21 7	
		213-216	Evaluation of Learning questions	45	
		216	Evolve Site: CTA A: Body Spectrum: Urinary Tract	10	
		216	Evolve Site: CTA B: Body Spectrum: Kidney	10	
		217	CTA C: Nephron	9	
		217-218	CTA D: Inquiring Patients Want to Know	10	
		219	CTA E: Crossword Puzzle	31	
		211	Posttest	10	
			ADDITIONAL ASSIGNMENTS		
			TOTAL POINTS		

Notes

Name ______________________________ Date ______________

PRETEST

True or False

______ 1. The functional unit of the kidney is the nephron.

______ 2. The outer portion of the kidney is known as the renal medulla.

______ 3. The indentation in the kidney is known as the hilum.

______ 4. The glomerulus is made up of loose connective tissue.

______ 5. The glomerular capsule is also known as the Bowman's capsule.

______ 6. The ureters transport urine from the urinary bladder to the outside.

______ 7. Rugae located in the wall of the urinary bladder allow the bladder to expand.

______ 8. The urethra in a male functions only in the transport of urine.

______ 9. Glucose is reabsorbed into the body in the renal tubule.

______ 10. Micturition is the act of expelling urine.

POSTTEST

True or False

______ 1. The urinary system helps to regulate the blood pressure.

______ 2. The renal pelvis collects urine as it is produced.

______ 3. The nephron is made up of the glomerulus and Bowman's capsule.

______ 4. Blood enters the glomerulus through the efferent arteriole.

______ 5. The renal tubule carries fluid away from the Bowman's capsule toward a collecting duct.

______ 6. Urine is expelled from the urinary bladder through contraction of the detrusor muscle.

______ 7. The calyx is made up of three openings and is located in the floor of the urinary bladder.

______ 8. The urethral orifice controls the passage of urine through the urethra.

______ 9. Erythropoietin increases reabsorption of sodium and reduces urine output.

______ 10. In the absence of ADH, the urine is more dilute.

KEY TERM ASSESSMENT

Directions: Match each key term with its definition.

_______ 1. Detrusor muscle
_______ 2. Erythropoietin
_______ 3. Glomerular capsule
_______ 4. Glomerular filtration
_______ 5. Glomerulus
_______ 6. Juxtaglomerular apparatus
_______ 7. Micturition
_______ 8. Nephron
_______ 9. Nephron loop
_______ 10. Renal corpuscle
_______ 11. Renal cortex
_______ 12. Renal medulla
_______ 13. Renal pelvis
_______ 14. Renal tubule
_______ 15. Renin
_______ 16. Trigone
_______ 17. Tubular reabsorption
_______ 18. Tubular secretion
_______ 19. Ureter
_______ 20. Urethra
_______ 21. Urinary bladder

A. Complex of modified cells in the afferent arteriole and the ascending limb/distal tubule in the kidney; helps regulate blood pressure by secreting renin; consists of the macula densa and juxtaglomerular cells
B. Double-layered epithelial cup that surrounds the glomerulus in a nephron; also called Bowman capsule
C. Functional unit of the kidney consisting of a renal corpuscle and a renal tubule
D. Tubular portion of the nephron that carries the filtrate away from the glomerular capsule; site where tubular reabsorption and secretion occur
E. Act of expelling urine from the bladder
F. An enzyme secreted by the kidneys that functions in blood pressure regulation by stimulating the formation of angiotension
G. Storage reservoir for urine
H. The movement of blood plasma across the filtration membrane in the renal corpuscle
I. Inner portion of the kidney consisting of renal pyramids
J. Portion of the nephron where filtration occurs
K. The movement of substances from the blood into the renal tubules in response to the body's needs during urine formation
L. Passageway that conveys urine from the urinary bladder to the exterior
M. The smooth muscle in the wall of the urinary bladder
N. The movement of filtrate from the renal tubules back into the blood in response to the body's needs during urine formation
O. Cluster of capillaries in the nephron through which blood is filtered
P. Large cavity in the central region of the kidney that collects the urine as it is produced
Q. A hormone released by the kidneys that stimulates red blood cell production
R. Outer portion of the kidney that appears granular
S. The hairpin loop of the renal tubule that extends into the renal pyramids
T. Tubular structure that carries urine from the renal pelvis to the urinary bladder
U. Triangular area in the floor of the urinary bladder formed by the openings for the urethra and the two ureters

B. Word Parts

Directions: Indicate the meaning of each word part in the space provided. List as many medical terms as possible that incorporate the word part in the space provided.

Word Part	Meaning of Word Part	Medical Terms That Incorporate Word Part
1. erythr/o		
2. juxta-		
3. mict-		
4. nephr/o		
5. ren/o		
6. tri-		
7. ur-		

EVALUATION OF LEARNING

Directions: Fill in each blank with the correct answer.

1. What are the functions of the urinary system?

____

____

2. What is the function of erythropoietin?

____

____

3. What makes up the urinary system?

____

____

4. What are the functions of the kidneys?

____

____

5. What is renal fascia, and what is its function?

____

____

6. What is perirenal fat and what is its function?

____

____

7. What is the renal capsule, and what is its function?

____

____

8. Describe each of the following parts of the kidney:

   a. Hilum: ____

   b. Renal sinus: ____

   c. Renal cortex: ____

9. What makes up the renal medulla?

____

10. What do renal pyramids contain?

____

11. What are renal columns?

12. What is the function of the renal pelvis?

13. What is the function of a minor calyx?

14. What is a nephron?

15. What are the two parts of a nephron?

16. What makes up the glomerulus?

17. What is the name of the vessel that delivers blood to the glomerulus?

18. What vessel carries blood away from the glomerulus?

19. What is the function of the renal tubule?

20. What are the three regions of a renal tubule?

21. What is the function of renin?

22. What is the function of the ureters?

23. Where do the ureters enter the urinary bladder?

24. What is the function of the muscular layer of the ureter?

25. What is the function of the urinary bladder?

26. What is the function of the rugae located in the wall of the urinary bladder?

27. What is the function of the detrusor muscle?

28. What three openings are located in the trigone of the urinary bladder?

29. Where is the trigone located?

30. What is the function of the urethra?

31. What are the names of the sphincters that control the flow of urine through the urethra?

32. What is the external urethral orifice?

33. What two functions are served by the urethra in the male?

34. What are the three parts of the male urethra?

35. What are the three steps involved in the formation of urine?

36. What occurs during glomerular filtration?

37. What is tubular reabsorption?

38. What are examples of substances that are reabsorbed into the blood?

39. What is tubular secretion?

40. How do the following hormones influence urine concentration and volume?

a. Aldosterone: ______________________________

____

b. Presence of antidiuretic hormone: ______________________________

____

c. Absence of antidiuretic hormone: ______________________________

____

d. Atrial natriuretic hormone: ______________________________

____

41. What causes renin to be produced?

____

42. What effect does angiotensin II have on the blood pressure?

____

43. What is micturition?

____

44. What stimulates the micturition reflex?

____

____

45. What effect does aging have on the following parts of the urinary system?

A. Muscles in the wall of the urinary structures: ______________________________

B. Urinary bladder: ______________________________

C. Awareness of the need to urinate: ______________________________

CRITICAL THINKING ACTIVITIES

A. Evolve Site: Body Spectrum

Urinary: Urinary Tract

Body Spectrum directions:

1. Access the Body Spectrum program on the Evolve site.
2. If necessary, access the HELP screen for directions on using the Body Spectrum program.
3. Go to the Contents screen.
4. Select the following category from the Contents screen:
   Urinary
5. Select the following anatomic diagram:
   Urinary Tract
6. Identify the structures on the diagram.
7. Print out the diagram.

B. Evolve Site: Body Spectrum

Urinary: Kidney

Directions: Identify the structures on this diagram following the Body Spectrum directions outlined under CTA A.

C. Nephron

Using Figure 15-4 in your textbook as a reference, label each of the structures making up a nephron.

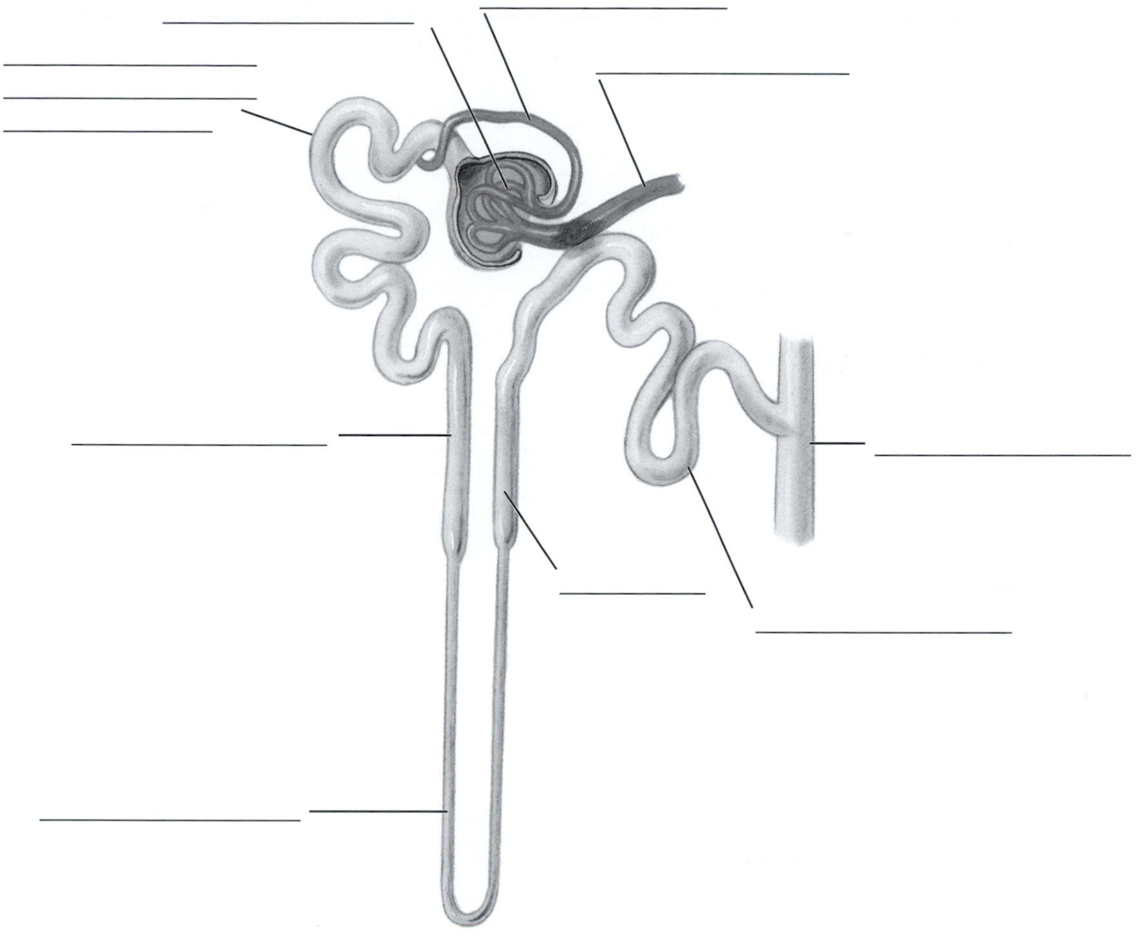

(Modified from Applegate E: *The anatomy and physiology learning system*, ed 4, St. Louis, 2011, Saunders.)

D. Inquiring Patients Want to Know

You are working in a general practice medical office. Your patients ask you the following questions. In the space provided, indicate how you would respond to each question in terms the patient would understand. Use your textbook and Internet resources to develop your responses.

1. Why is urine yellow?

____

____

2. Why do women have more urinary tract infections (UTIs) than men?

____

____

3. Is it safer to drink bottled water than tap water?

____

____

4. What causes kidney stones?

5. How are kidney stones removed?

6. Why is urine a darker yellow color in the morning?

7. What causes some older people to be incontinent?

8. Why should someone with a UTI drink cranberry juice?

9. What happens during kidney dialysis?

10. Do dialysis patients still urinate?

E. Crossword Puzzle: Urinary System

Directions: Complete the crossword puzzle using the clues provided.

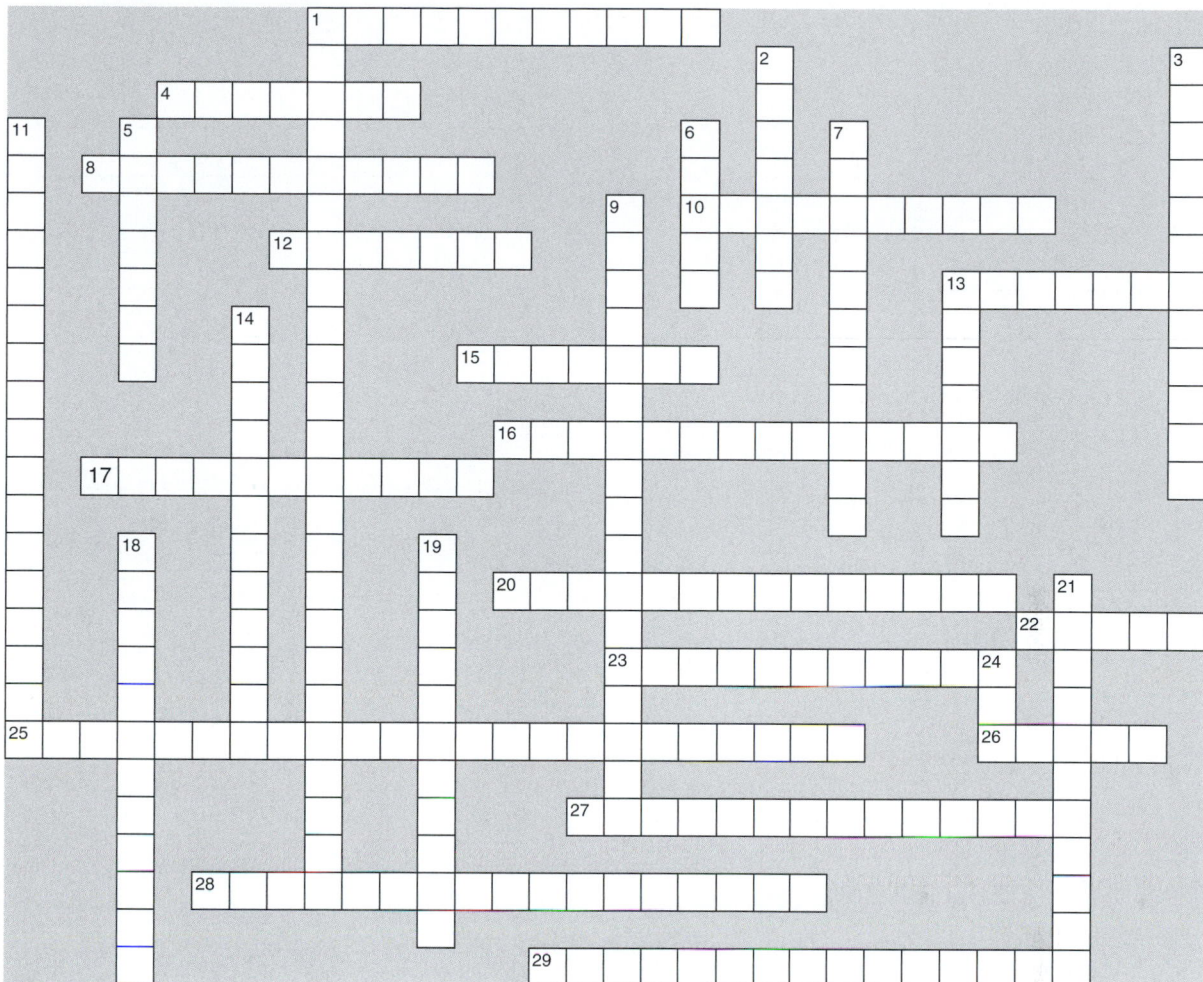

Across

1 How urine moves through ureter
4 Formed by three openings in urinary bladder
8 Act of expelling urine
10 Cluster of capillaries in nephron
12 Cuplike projections of renal pelvis
13 Transports urine from urinary bladder to outside
15 Functional unit of kidney
16 Stores urine
17 Outer region of kidney
20 Controls RBC production
22 Helps maintain normal BP
23 Hold kidney in place
25 Opening of urethra
26 Kidney indentation
27 Expels urine from bladder by contracting
28 Takes blood to glomerulus
29 Transports urine from nephron to minor calyces

Down

1 Where most of tubular reabsorption occurs
2 Substance that is reabsorbed by the kidney
3 Connective tissue that encases the kidney
5 Filters blood and removes wastes
6 Allows bladder to expand
7 Urinary bladder capacity in milliliters
9 Takes blood away from glomerulus
11 Epithelial cup that surrounds glomerulus
13 Transports urine from renal pelvis to urinary bladder
14 Inner region of kidney
18 Adipose tissue surrounding kidney
19 Hormone that increases reabsorption of sodium
21 Collects urine as it is produced
24 Hormone that increases reabsorption of water

Notes

16 Reproductive System

CHAPTER ASSIGNMENTS

✓ After Completing	Date Due	Study Guide Page(s)	STUDY GUIDE ASSIGNMENTS (CTA: Critical Thinking Activity)	Possible Points	Points You Earned
		223	Pretest	10	
		224 225	Key Term Assessment A. Definitions B. Word Parts (Add 1 point for each key term)	25 15	
		225-229 229-232	Evaluation of Learning questions: A. Male Reproductive System B. Female Reproductive System	44 38	
		232	Evolve Site: CTA A: Body Spectrum: Male Reproductive System	10	
		232	Evolve Site: CTA B: Body Spectrum: Female Reproductive System	10	
		232	Evolve Site: CTA C: Body Spectrum: Fertilization to Implantation	10	
		233	CTA D: Inquiring Patients Want to Know	10	
		234	CTA E: Crossword Puzzle	33	
		234	Posttest	10	
			ADDITIONAL ASSIGNMENTS		
			TOTAL POINTS		

Notes

Name ______________________________ Date ______________

PRETEST

True or False

_______ 1. The gonads include egg and sperm cells.

_______ 2. The head of a sperm contains 46 chromosomes.

_______ 3. Sperm are propelled through the ductus deferens by peristalsis.

_______ 4. The prostate gland encircles the urethra.

_______ 5. The scrotum is a pouch of skin and subcutaneous tissue that contains the testes.

_______ 6. The process of egg formation is known as oogenesis.

_______ 7. Fertilization usually takes place in the uterus.

_______ 8. The bulk of the uterine wall is made up of the myometrium.

_______ 9. The stratum functionale of the endometrium is shed from the uterine wall during the secretory phase of the uterine cycle.

_______ 10. The cessation of the female reproductive cycle is known as menarche.

POSTTEST

True or False

_______ 1. The interstitial cells in the testes produce male sex hormones.

_______ 2. Spermatogonia divide by mitosis.

_______ 3. The epididymis secretes a fluid containing fructose to provide an energy source for sperm.

_______ 4. Ejaculation is the forceful discharge of semen into the urethra.

_______ 5. The epididymis is a tightly coiled tube in which sperm complete the maturation process.

_______ 6. If fertilization does not take place, the corpus luteum continues to grow and enlarge.

_______ 7. Fimbriae help propel sperm through the uterus.

_______ 8. The growth of the ovarian follicle occurs during the follicular phase of the ovarian cycle.

_______ 9. In the female, luteinizing hormone (LH) is responsible for stimulating the growth and thickening of the endometrium.

_______ 10. The upper bulging surface of the uterus is the fundus.

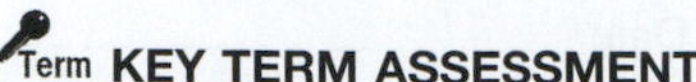

KEY TERM ASSESSMENT

A. Definitions

Directions: Match each key term with its definition.

_______ 1. Corpora cavernosa
_______ 2. Corpus albicans
_______ 3. Corpus luteum
_______ 4. Corpus spongiosum
_______ 5. Ductus deferens
_______ 6. Endometrium
_______ 7. Epididymis
_______ 8. Gametes
_______ 9. Gonads
_______ 10. Interstitial cells
_______ 11. Menarche
_______ 12. Myometrium
_______ 13. Oogenesis
_______ 14. Oogonia
_______ 15. Ovarian cycle
_______ 16. Ovarian follicle
_______ 17. Seminiferous tubules
_______ 18. Spermatogenesis
_______ 19. Spermatogonia
_______ 20. Spermiogenesis
_______ 21. Stratum basale
_______ 22. Stratum functionale
_______ 23. Uterine cycle
_______ 24. Uterine tubes
_______ 25. Vulvalute

A. An oocyte surrounded by one or more layers of cells within the ovaries
B. Monthly cycle of events that occur in the ovary from puberty to menopause; occurs concurrently with the uterine cycle
C. Monthly cycle of events that occur in the uterus from puberty to menopause; also called the menstrual cycle; occurs concurrently with the ovarian cycle
D. Morphologic changes that transform a spermatid into a mature sperm
E. Primary reproductive organs; organs that produce the gametes: testes in the male and ovaries in the female
F. Process of meiosis in the female in which one ovum and three polar bodies are produced from one primary oocyte
G. Process of meiosis in the male in which four spermatids are produced from one primary spermatocyte
H. Sex cells: sperm and ova
I. Tubular structure that is continuous with the epididymis which transports sperm to the ejaculatory duct
J. Two dorsal columns of erectile tissue found in the penis
K. Thick middle layer of the uterus composed of smooth muscle
L. Stem cells that give rise to sperm cells
M. Scar tissue in the ovary that forms when the corpus luteum degenerates
N. Innermost mucous membrane layer of the uterine wall
O. Cells between the seminiferous tubules in the testes which produce testosterone
P. Tightly coiled structures within which sperm are produced in the testes
Q. The tubes that extend laterally from the upper portion of the uterus (also known as fallopian tubes)
R. Tightly coiled tubule along the posterior margin of each testicle which functions in the maturation and storage of sperm
S. First period of menstrual bleeding at puberty
T. Portion of the endometrium that is sloughed off during menstruation
U. Bottom layer of the endometrium that is responsible for rebuilding the stratum functionale after menstruation
V. The yellow structure that develops from the mature follicle after ovulation
W. Collective term for the external accessory structures of the female reproductive system
X. Ventral column of erectile tissue found in the penis
Y. Stem cells that give rise to ova or egg cells

B. Word Parts

Directions: Indicate the meaning of each word part in the space provided. List as many medical terms as possible that incorporate the word part in the space provided.

Word Part	Meaning of Word Part	Medical Terms That Incorporate Word Part
1. corp/o		
2. lute/o		
3. duct/o		
4. men/o		
5. -arche		
6. my/o		
7. oo-		
8. -genesis		
9. ovary/o		
10. semin/i		
11. spermat/o		
12. spermi/o		
13. strat-		
14. uter/o		
15. vulv/o		

EVALUATION OF LEARNING

Directions: Fill in each blank with the correct answer.

Male Reproductive System

1. What are the four functions of the reproductive system?

____

____

2. What is another name for the primary reproductive organs?

____

3. What is another name for egg and sperm cells?

____

4. What is the function of the secondary reproductive organs?

____

____

5. Why are the testes located outside of the abdominal cavity?

6. What makes up the scrotum?

7. Describe the characteristics of the following:
   a. Tunica albuginea:
   b. Septa:
   c. Seminiferous tubules:

8. What is the function of the interstitial cells (cells of Leydig)?

9. Where in the testes does spermatogenesis take place?

10. What are spermatogonia?

11. What happens to spermatogonia at puberty? How many chromosomes do they have?

12. What occurs during meiosis I of spermatogenesis?

13. What occurs during meiosis II of spermatogenesis if fertilization occurs?

14. How many spermatids are eventually produced by each primary spermatocyte?

15. What occurs during spermiogenesis?

16. How many chromosomes are contained in the head of a sperm?

17. Where is the acrosome located, and what is its function?

18. What are the functions of the following parts of a mature sperm cell?

   a. Midpiece: ______________________________

   b. Tail: ______________________________

19. How long does it take for a mature sperm to be produced (starting with a primary spermatocyte)?

____

20. How long can sperm live in the female reproductive tract?

____

21. List the series of ducts that a sperm passes through to reach the outside of the body from the testes.

____

____

22. What occurs to sperm in the epididymis?

____

23. How are sperm moved through the ductus deferens?

____

24. What two ducts combine to form the ejaculatory duct?

____

25. Describe the location of each of the following parts of the male urethra:

   a. Prostatic: ______________________________

   b. Membranous: ______________________________

   c. Penile (spongy): ______________________________

26. What is the name of the opening of the penis to the outside?

____

27. What is contained in the fluid secreted by the seminal vesicles, and what is its function?

____

28. What structure does the prostate gland encircle?

____

29. What is the function of the fluid secreted by the prostate gland?

____

30. What are the three functions of the fluid secreted by the bulbourethral glands?

____

____

31. What is semen?

32. What is the usual number of sperm contained in each milliliter of semen?

33. What are the names and locations of the columns of erectile tissue located in the penis?

34. What are the three parts of the penis?

35. What is the prepuce (foreskin)?

36. What causes an erection of the penis?

37. What occurs during emission?

38. What occurs during ejaculation?

39. Why do the sphincters of the urinary bladder constrict during emission and ejaculation?

40. When does puberty usually begin in males? When does it usually end?

41. What hormone causes the pituitary gland to secrete LH and follicle-stimulating hormone (FSH)?

42. What is the function of LH in the male?

43. What two hormones are responsible for stimulating spermatogenesis?

44. What effect does testosterone have on the human male at puberty?

Female Reproductive System

1. What are the functions of the female reproductive organs?

2. Where are the ovaries located?

3. What is the tunica albuginea?

4. What is located in the cortex of the ovary?

5. What is the name for a female germ cell?

6. What structures are located in the medulla of the ovary?

7. What is oogenesis?

8. When do primitive germ cells in the female develop into primary oocytes?

9. How many chromosomes are present in a primary oocyte?

10. How many primary oocytes are present when a female infant is born?

11. What occurs during meiosis I of oogenesis?

12. What occurs during meiosis II of oogenesis if fertilization occurs?

13. What makes up an ovarian follicle?

____

____

14. What occurs during ovulation?

____

____

15. What happens to the secondary oocyte if it is not fertilized?

____

16. What happens to the secondary oocyte if it is fertilized?

____

____

17. What is the corpus luteum?

____

18. What hormones are secreted by the corpus luteum?

____

19. What happens to the corpus luteum if fertilization does not take place?

____

____

20. What happens to the corpus luteum if fertilization takes place?

____

____

21. Describe how an oocyte moves from the ovary and into the fallopian tube.

____

____

____

22. How long does it take an oocyte to move through a fallopian tube?

____

23. Where does fertilization usually occur?

____

24. Describe the following parts of the uterus:

a. Fundus: ____

b. Body: ____

c. Cervix: ____

d. Internal os: ______________________________

e. External os: ______________________________

25. What are the characteristics of the three layers that make up the wall of the uterus?

Wall of the Uterus	Characteristics
Perimetrium	
Myometrium	
Endometrium	

26. What are the functions of the vagina?

____

____

27. Describe the characteristics of the following structures that make up the external female genitalia.

Structure	Characteristics
Labia majora	
Mons pubis	
Labia minora	
Vestibule	
Clitoris	
Prepuce	
Paraurethral glands	
Greater vestibular glands	

28. What happens to the follicle during each of the phases of the ovarian cycle?

a. Follicular phase: ______________________________

b. Ovulatory phase: ______________________________

c. Luteal phase: ______________________________

29. What hormones are responsible for the following?

a. Growth of the ovarian follicle: ______________________________

b. Estrogen production by the ovaries: ______________________________

c. Rupture of the mature follicle out of the ovary: ______________________________

d. Stimulation of the corpus luteum to secrete estrogen and progesterone: ______________________________

30. What is the menstrual cycle?

____

____

31. What happens to the endometrium of the uterus during the following phases of the menstrual cycle?

a. Menstrual phase: ______

b. Proliferative phase: ______

c. Secretory phase: ______

32. What is menopause? ______

______

33. What is the function of the mammary glands?

______

34. What is the areola?

______

35. How many lobes of glandular tissue does each breast contain?

______

36. What determines the size and shape of the breasts?

______

37. What is the function of lactiferous ducts?

______

38. What effect do the following hormones have on the breasts?

a. Prolactin: ______

b. Oxytocin: ______

CRITICAL THINKING ACTIVITIES

A. Evolve Site: Body Spectrum

Reproductive: Male Reproductive System

Body Spectrum directions:

1. Access the Body Spectrum program on the Evolve site.
2. If necessary, access the HELP screen for directions on using the Body Spectrum program.
3. Go to the Contents screen.
4. Select the following category from the Contents screen:
   Reproductive
5. Select the following anatomic diagram:
   Male Reproductive System
6. Identify the structures on the diagram.
7. Print out the diagram.

B. Evolve Site: Body Spectrum

Reproductive: Female Reproductive System

Directions: Identify the structures on this diagram following the Body Spectrum directions outlined under CTA A.

C. Evolve Site: Body Spectrum

Reproductive: Fertilization to Implant

Directions: Identify the structures on this diagram following the Body Spectrum directions outlined under CTA A.

D. Inquiring Patients Want to Know

You are working in a general practice medical office. Your patients ask you the following questions. In the space provided, indicate how you would respond to each question in terms the patient would understand. Use your textbook and Internet resources to develop your responses.

1. How do birth control pills work?

____

____

2. What happens in the body during a hot flash?

____

____

3. Can you get pregnant during your menstrual period?

____

____

4. How does an erectile dysfunction drug work?

____

____

5. Is a vasectomy reversible?

____

____

6. Is it a good idea to douche?

____

____

7. How are embryos frozen?

____

____

8. What is a hymen?

____

____

9. What is the success rate for in vitro fertilization?

____

____

10. What causes PMS?

____

____

E. Crossword Puzzle: Reproductive System

Directions: Complete the crossword puzzle using the clues provided.

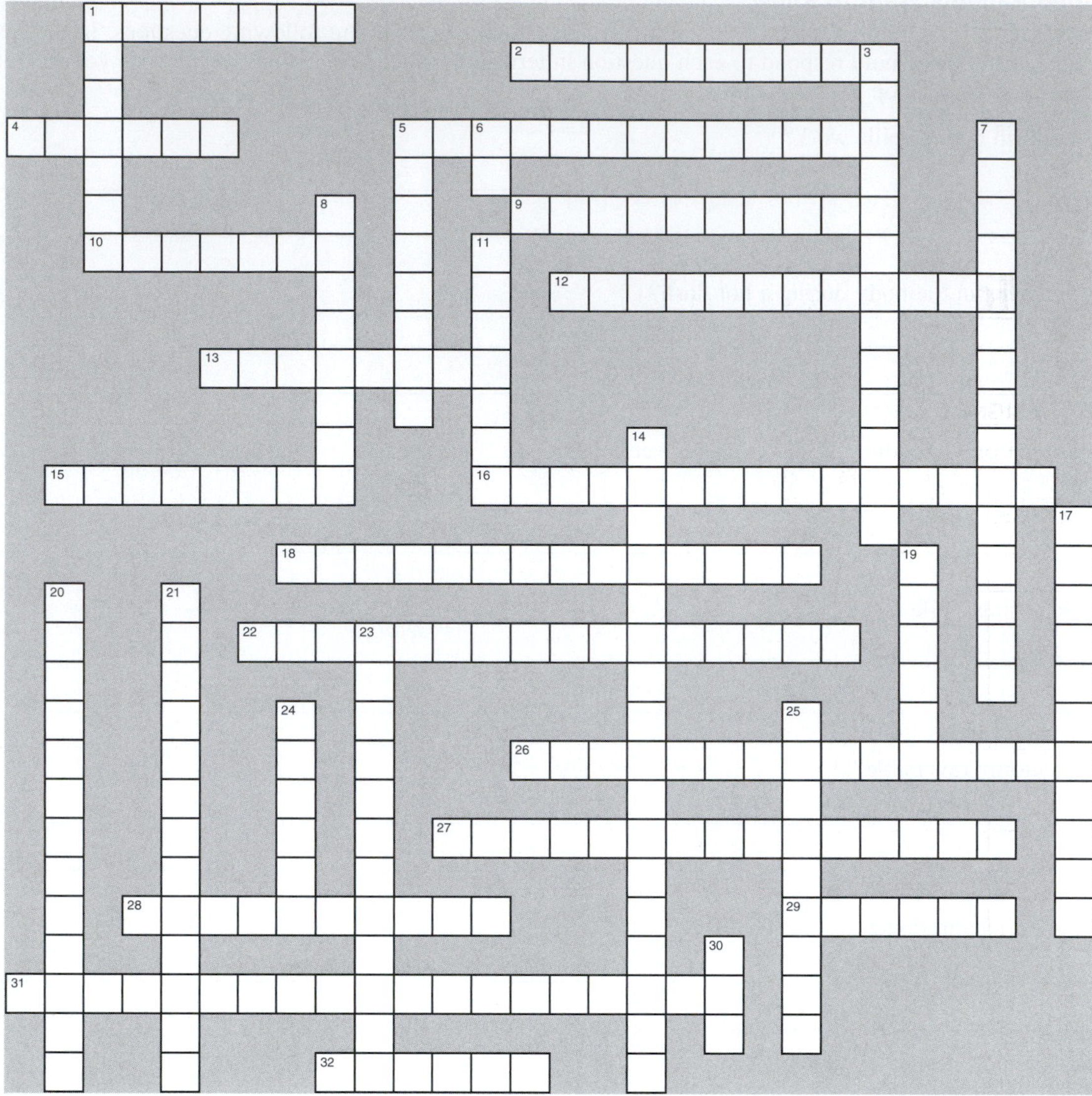

Across

1 Immature female germ cells
2 Where sperm mature
4 Part of uterus that projects into vagina
5 Tube that transports oocyte to uterus
9 Muscle layer of uterus
10 Contains the testes
12 Name of follicle after ovulation
13 Gland that encircles male urethra
15 Hormone that causes ejection of milk from mammary glands
16 Secrete fructose fluid to provide energy source for sperm
18 Transports sperm from epididymis to ejaculatory duct
22 Milk reservoir
26 Carries milk from lobule to nipple
27 Contains a developing oocyte
28 End of penis
29 Outer area of ovary
31 Produce sperm within the testes
32 Primary male reproductive organ

Down

1 Primary female reproductive organs
3 Immature male germ cells
5 Finger-like extensions of a fallopian tube
6 Stimulates ovulation to occur
7 Process of sperm formation
8 Discharge of semen into urethra
11 Egg and sperm cells
14 Produce male sex hormones
17 Outer layer of uterus
19 Provides growth environment for a fertilized egg
20 Holds uterus in place
21 Milk production organs
23 Hormone responsible for male secondary sex characteristics
24 Upper bulging surface of uterus
25 Hormone that stimulates milk production
30 Stimulates growth of ovarian follicle

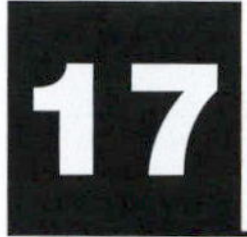

17 Medical Asepsis and the OSHA Standard

CHAPTER ASSIGNMENTS

✓ After Completing	Date Due	Study Guide Pages	STUDY GUIDE ASSIGNMENTS (CTA = Critical Thinking Activity)	Possible Points	Points You Earned
		239	Pretest	10	
		 240 241	Term Key Term Assessment A. Definitions B. Word Parts (Add 1 point for each key term)	 24 15	
		241-247	Evaluation of Learning questions	55	
		247	CTA A: Infection Process Cycle	5	
		248	CTA B: Handwashing	8	
		249	CTA C: Personal Protective Equipment: Gloves	8	
		249	CTA D: Personal Protective Equipment	30	
		249-250	CTA E: OSHA Standard	10	
		251	CTA F: Discarding Medical Waste	20	
			Evolve Site: Discard It!(Record points earned)		
		252	CTA G: Crossword Puzzle	25	
			Evolve Site: Quiz Show (Record points earned)		
			Evolve Site: Apply Your Knowledge questions (Record points earned)	10	

✓ After Completing	Date Due	Study Guide Pages	STUDY GUIDE ASSIGNMENTS (CTA = Critical Thinking Activity)	Possible Points	Points You Earned
			Evolve Site: Video Evaluation	56	
		239	Posttest	10	
			ADDITIONAL ASSIGNMENTS		
			TOTAL POINTS		

✓ When Assigned By Your Instructor	Study Guide Pages	Practices Required	LABORATORY ASSIGNMENTS (Procedure Number and Name)	Score*
	253	5	**Practice for Competency** 17-1: Handwashing Textbook reference: pp. 296-298	
	255-257		**Evaluation of Competency** 17-1: Handwashing	*
	253	4	**Practice for Competency** 17-2: Applying an Alcohol-Based Hand Rub Textbook reference: pp. 298-299	
	259-260		**Evaluation of Competency** 17-2: Applying an Alcohol-Based Hand Rub	*
	253	5	**Practice for Competency** 17-3: Application and Removal of Clean Disposable Gloves Textbook reference: pp. 300-301	
	261-262		**Evaluation of Competency** 17-3: Application and Removal of Clean Disposable Gloves	*
		3	**Evaluation of Competency** 17-A: Proper Use of a Sharps Container	*
		3	**Evaluation of Competency** 17-B: Disposal of Hazardous Material	*
			ADDITIONAL ASSIGNMENTS	

Notes

Name ______________________ Date ______________

PRETEST

True or False

_______ 1. A microorganism is a tiny living plant or animal that cannot be seen with the naked eye.

_______ 2. A disease-producing microorganism is known as a *nonpathogen*.

_______ 3. Microorganisms grow best in an acidic environment.

_______ 4. Coughing and sneezing help to force pathogens from the body.

_______ 5. An alcohol-based hand rub should be used to sanitize hands that are visibly soiled.

_______ 6. OSHA stands for *Occupational Safety and Health Administration*.

_______ 7. A biohazard warning label must be fluorescent orange or an orange-red color.

_______ 8. Prescription eyeglasses are acceptable eye protection when handling blood.

_______ 9. Hepatitis B is an infection of the liver caused by a virus.

_______ 10. AIDS cannot be transmitted through casual contact.

POSTTEST

True or False

_______ 1. Bacteria and viruses are examples of microorganisms.

_______ 2. An anaerobe can exist only in the presence of oxygen.

_______ 3. The optimum growth temperature is the temperature at which a microorganism grows the best.

_______ 4. Medical asepsis are practices that inhibit the growth and hinder the transmission of pathogenic microorganisms.

_______ 5. Resident flora are picked up in the course of daily activities and are usually pathogenic.

_______ 6. The purpose of the OSHA Standard is to prevent exposure of employees to bloodborne pathogens.

_______ 7. OSHA requires the Exposure Control Plan to be updated annually.

_______ 8. An engineering control includes all measures and devices that isolate or remove the bloodborne pathogens hazard from the workplace.

_______ 9. A reagent strip that has been used to test urine is an example of regulated medical waste.

_______ 10. Patients with chronic hepatitis B face an increased risk of developing pancreatitis.

Term KEY TERM ASSESSMENT

A. Definitions

Directions: Match each key term with its definition.

_______ 1. Aerobe
_______ 2. Anaerobe
_______ 3. Antiseptic
_______ 4. Bloodborne pathogens
_______ 5. Cilia
_______ 6. Contaminated
_______ 7. Exposure incident
_______ 8. Hand hygiene
_______ 9. Infection
_______ 10. Medical asepsis
_______ 11. Microorganism
_______ 12. Nonintact skin
_______ 13. Nonpathogen
_______ 14. Occupational exposure
_______ 15. Opportunistic infection
_______ 16. Optimal growth temperature
_______ 17. Pathogen
_______ 18. Parenteral
_______ 19. pH
_______ 20. Postexposure prophylaxis
_______ 21. Regulated medical waste
_______ 22. Reservoir host
_______ 23. Sharps
_______ 24. Transient flora

A. A disease-producing microorganism
B. Microorganisms that reside on the superficial skin layers and are picked up in the course of daily activities
C. A microorganism that needs oxygen to live and grow
D. Reasonably anticipated skin, eye, mucous membrane, or parenteral contact with bloodborne pathogens or other potentially infectious materials that may result from the performance of an employee's duties
E. Practices that are employed to inhibit the growth and hinder the transmission of pathogenic microorganisms
F. The piercing of the skin barrier or mucous membranes, such as through needlesticks, human bites, cuts, and abrasions
G. Skin that has a break in the surface
H. The temperature at which an organism grows best
I. The degree to which a solution is acidic or basic
J. A specific eye, mouth, other mucous membrane, nonintact skin, or parenteral contact with blood or other potentially infectious materials that results from an employee's duties
K. Pathogenic microorganisms capable of causing disease that are present in human blood
L. The condition in which the body, or part of it, is invaded by a pathogen
M. Any waste containing infectious material that may pose a threat to health and safety
N. Slender, hairlike processes that constantly beat toward the outside to remove microorganisms from the body
O. A microorganism that does not normally produce disease
P. A microscopic plant or animal
Q. A microorganism that grows best in the absence of oxygen
R. The presence or reasonably anticipated presence of blood or OPIM on an item or surface
S. The organism that becomes infected by a pathogen and also serves as a source of transfer of pathogens to others
T. An infection resulting from a defective immune system that cannot defend the body from pathogens normally found in the environment
U. An agent that inhibits the growth of or kills microorganisms
V. The process of cleaning or sanitizing the hands
W. Treatment administered to an individual after exposure to an infectious disease to prevent the disease
X. Objects that can penetrate the skin such as needles and lancets.

B. Word Parts

Directions: Indicate the meaning of each word part in the space provided. List as many medical terms as possible that incorporate the word part in the space provided.

Word Part	Meaning of Word Part	Medical Terms That Incorporate Word Part
1. aer/o		
2. an-		
3. anti-		
4. septic		
5. a-		
6. micro-		
7. non-		
8. path/o		
9. -gen		
10. para-		
11. enter/o		
12. -al		
13. post-		
14. pro-		
15. phylaxis		

EVALUATION OF LEARNING

Directions: Fill in each blank with the correct answer.

1. List four examples of types of microorganisms.

___

___

2. Define medical asepsis.

___

___

3. What type of microorganisms may remain on an object that is considered medically aseptic?

___

4. List the six growth requirements needed by microorganisms to survive.

___

___

___

5. What is the name given to the organism that uses organic or living substances for food?

___

6. Why do most microorganisms prefer a neutral pH?

7. List three examples of how a microorganism can be transmitted from one person to another.

8. List five examples of how microorganisms can enter the body.

9. List four examples of factors that would make a host more susceptible to the entrance of a pathogen.

10. List five protective devices of the body that prevent the entrance of microorganisms.

11. What is the difference between resident flora and transient flora?

12. List three examples of when handwashing should be performed in the medical office.

13. How does antiseptic handwashing sanitize the hands?

14. List five examples of when an alcohol-based hand rub may be used to sanitize the hands.

___

___

___

15. What are the advantages and disadvantages of alcohol-based hand rubs?

Advantages: ___

Disadvantages: ___

16. List six medical aseptic practices the medical assistant should follow in the medical office.

___

___

___

___

___

___

17. What are the advantages of latex gloves?

___

___

___

18. What are the symptoms of a mild and severe latex glove allergy?

a. Mild latex glove allergy: ___

___

b. Severe latex glove allergy: ___

___

19. What guidelines should be followed when working with gloves?

___

___

___

___

20. What can be done to prevent the development of latex allergies in the workplace?

___

___

___

___

21. What does the acronym *OSHA* stand for, and what is the purpose of OSHA?

____

____

22. What is the purpose of the OSHA Occupational Exposure to Bloodborne Pathogens Standard?

____

____

23. Who must follow the OSHA Bloodborne Pathogens Standard? List examples.

____

____

____

24. What is the purpose of the Needlestick Safety and Prevention Act?

____

____

25. What are sharps? List examples of sharps.

____

____

26. List five examples of other potentially infectious materials (OPIMs).

____

____

____

____

27. List examples of nonintact skin.

____

____

28. What is an exposure incident? List examples of exposure incidents.

____

____

____

29. What is the purpose of the exposure control plan (ECP)? How often must it be updated?

____

____

30. List three examples of items to which a biohazard warning label must be attached.

31. What is the purpose of a sharps injury log? What types of offices must maintain this log?

32. Define an engineering control, and list three examples of engineering controls.

33. What is a safer medical device?

34. What is a work practice control?

35. List examples of work practice controls required by the OSHA standard.

36. What should you do if you splash blood in your eyes?

37. What is personal protective equipment (PPE)? List examples of PPE.

38. List six guidelines that must be followed when using personal protective equipment (PPE).

39. List examples of housekeeping procedures required by the OSHA standard.

40. List four guidelines that must be followed with respect to biohazard sharps containers.

41. Who must be offered the hepatitis B vaccination?

42. When does an employer *not* have to offer the hepatitis B vaccine to medical office personnel?

43. What must be done if a medical office employee declines the hepatitis B vaccination?

44. What is regulated medical waste? What are examples of regulated medical waste?

45. Explain how to prepare regulated medical waste for pickup by a medical waste service.

46. How should regulated medical waste be stored while waiting for pickup by the medical waste service? Explain why.

47. What information is included on a regulated medical waste tracking form?

48. What is the most likely means of contracting hepatitis B in the health care setting?

49. What side effects may occur after the administration of a hepatitis B vaccine?

50. What postexposure prophylaxis (PEP) is recommended for an unvaccinated individual who has been exposed to hepatitis B?

51. What may eventually occur in a patient with chronic hepatitis C?

52. What is the difference between HIV and AIDS?

53. How is HIV transmitted? How is it not transmitted?

54. What is an opportunistic infection?

55. What are the characteristics of AIDS?

CRITICAL THINKING ACTIVITIES

A. Infection Process Cycle

Carefully review the infection process cycle and the requirements for growth needed by microorganisms. Create an environment in a medical office that would function to interrupt the infection process cycle and discourage the growth of pathogens.

B. Handwashing

Using the principles outlined in the handwashing procedure, explain what may happen under the following circumstances:

1. The medical assistant's uniform touches the sink during the handwashing procedure.

____

____

____

2. The hands are not held lower than the elbows during the handwashing procedure.

____

____

____

3. Friction is not used to wash the hands.

____

____

____

4. Water is splashed on the medical assistant's uniform during the handwashing procedure.

____

____

____

5. The medical assistant continually uses water that is too cold to wash hands.

____

____

____

6. The medical assistant turns off the running water with his or her bare hands.

____

____

____

7. The medical assistant does not clean his or her fingernails daily.

____

____

____

8. The medical assistant's skin becomes chapped.

____

____

____

C. Personal Protective Equipment: Gloves

In which of the following situations does OSHA require the use of clean disposable gloves? Indicate your answer by placing a checkmark in the space provided.

_______ 1. Performing a urinalysis on a urine specimen that contains blood.

_______ 2. Sanitizing operating scissors for sterilization.

_______ 3. Performing a finger puncture.

_______ 4. Performing a vision screening test on a school-aged child.

_______ 5. Cleaning up a blood spill on a laboratory work table.

_______ 6. Drawing blood from an elderly patient.

_______ 7. Measuring the weight of a college student.

_______ 8. Testing a blood specimen for glucose.

D. Personal Protective Equipment

Create a collage of items or articles that can and cannot be used as PPE following these guidelines:

1. Using items cut from a magazine, colored pencils, or markers, create a collage of items that are designated as PPE by OSHA.
2. On the reverse side of the sheet, create a collage of items or articles that are not permitted to be used as PPE.
3. In the classroom, choose a partner and trade sheets. For each PPE item, provide examples of the procedures or tasks that may require its use. For each item that is not PPE, explain why it should not be used as PPE.

Examples of PPE:

____

____

____

____

Not examples of PPE:

____

____

____

____

E. OSHA Standard

The following situations may occur in the medical office. For each situation, indicate an appropriate action to take that complies with the OSHA Bloodborne Pathogens Standard.

1. **Situation:** You just gave an injection to a patient, and after withdrawing the needle, you notice that there is no sharps container in the room.
   Action:

   ____

   ____

   ____

2. **Situation:** You are getting ready to apply gloves and notice that you have a cut on your finger.
Action:

3. **Situation:** You accidentally get some blood on your bare hands while removing your gloves.
Action:

4. **Situation:** A part-time clinical medical assistant was just hired. She is not immunized against hepatitis B.
Action:

5. **Situation:** A clinical medical assistant who has worked at the office for 5 years changes her mind and decides she wants the hepatitis B vaccine.
Action:

6. **Situation:** You are wearing a protective laboratory coat over your scrubs. While performing a laboratory test, some blood splashes onto your lab coat, but it does not penetrate through to your scrubs.
Action:

7. **Situation:** You go into an examining room and notice that the biohazard sharps container in that room is completely full.
Action:

8. **Situation:** Using glass tubes, you have collected three tubes of blood from a patient using glass tubes. You accidentally drop one of the blood tubes, and it breaks.
Action:

9. **Situation:** You are wearing a protective lab coat over your scrubs, and you are getting ready to leave for the day.
Action:

____

____

____

10. **Situation:** You remove your gloves after giving an injection to a patient and accidentally discard them into the biohazard sharps container.
Action:

____

____

____

F. Discarding Medical Waste

Indicate where each of the following (used) items should be discarded using these acronyms:
RWC: regular waste container
BSC: biohazard sharps container
BB: biohazard bag waste container

_______ 1. Urine testing strip

_______ 2. Lancet

_______ 3. Gloves with blood on them

_______ 4. Blood tube

_______ 5. Tongue depressor

_______ 6. Razor blade

_______ 7. Capillary pipet

_______ 8. Dressing saturated with blood

_______ 9. Patient drape

_______ 10. An empty urine container

_______ 11. Sutures caked with blood

_______ 12. Thermometer probe cover

_______ 13. Patient gown

_______ 14. Disposable diaper

_______ 15. Dressing saturated with a purulent discharge

_______ 16. Clean disposable gloves

_______ 17. Disposable vaginal speculum

_______ 18. An outdated vaccine

_______ 19. Syringe and needle

_______ 20. Examining table paper

G. Crossword Puzzle: Medical Asepsis and the OSHA Standard

Directions: Complete the crossword puzzle using the clues provided.

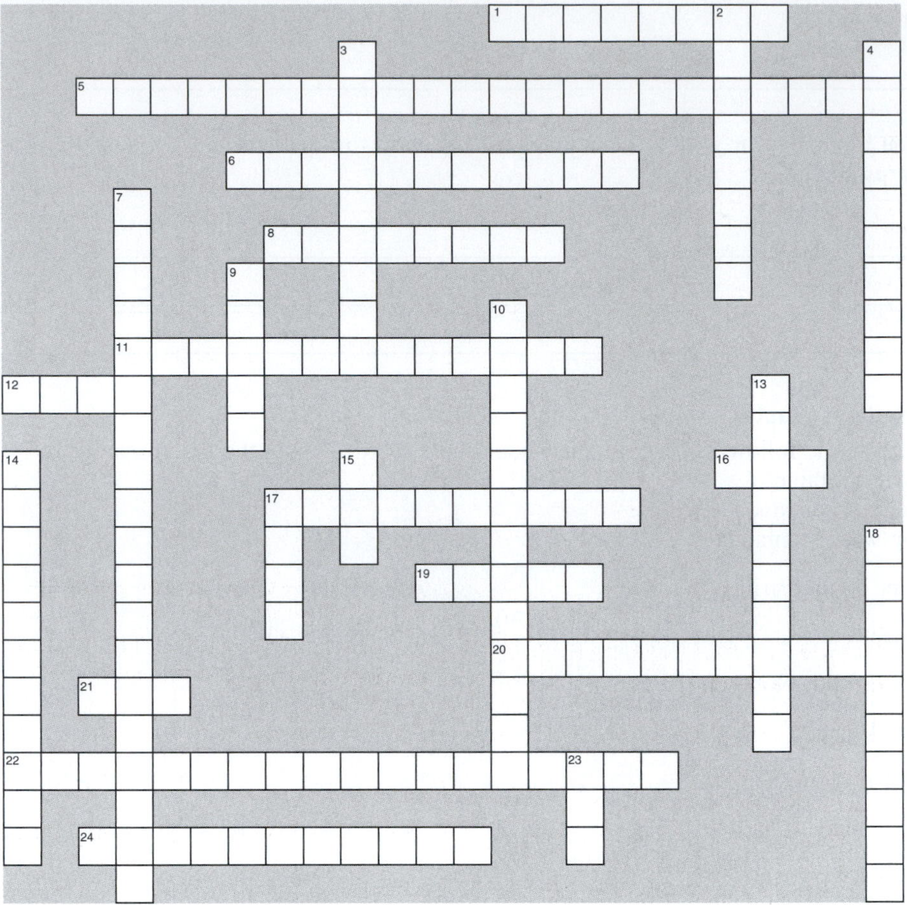

Across

1 Grows best without oxygen
5 Infection resulting from a defective immune system
6 HBV serious complication
8 Microorganism that causes disease
11 Normally live on the skin
12 Vaginal secretions (example)
16 Protector of public health
17 Can live dry for 1 week
19 Traps microorganisms
20 Low resistance
21 After exposure: may prevent disease
22 Isolates or removes bloodborne pathogens hazard
24 Eats "live stuff"

Down

2 Example of a microorganism
3 Body invasion by a pathogen
4 Found in antimicrobial soap
7 Way to prevent a needlestick injury
9 HIV screening test
10 Broken skin
13 #No. 1 chronic viral disease in the United States
14 #No. 1 aseptic practice
15 Scrubs are not this
17 Hepatitis B passive immunizing agent
18 Piercing of the skin barrier
23 Discard in a biohazard container

PRACTICE FOR COMPETENCY

Medical Asepsis

Procedure 17-1: Handwashing. Perform the handwashing procedure. List five medically aseptic steps that must be followed during this procedure.

1. ______________________________

____

2. ______________________________

____

3. ______________________________

____

4. ______________________________

____

5. ______________________________

____

Procedure 17-2: Applying an Alcohol-Based Hand Rub. Apply an alcohol-based hand rub. Practice applying a gel and a foam hand rub. List the brand names of the hand rubs you applied, and list the ingredients contained in them.

____

____

Procedure 17-3: Application and Removal of Clean Disposable Gloves. Apply and remove clean disposable gloves. What size gloves fit you best?

____

____

Procedure 17-A: Proper Use of A Sharps Container. Demonstrate the proper use of a sharps container by discarding contaminated sharps into the sharps container. In the space provided, indicate the items you discarded into the sharps container.

____

____

Procedure 17-B: Disposal of Hazardous Material. Handle and prepare regulated medical waste for pickup by a medical waste service.

____

____

Notes

EVALUATION OF COMPETENCY

Procedure 17-1: Handwashing

Name: ______________________ Date: ______________

Evaluated by: ______________________ Score: ______________

Performance Objective

Outcome:	Perform handwashing.
Conditions:	Using a sink.
	Given liquid soap and paper towels.
Standards:	Time: 5 minutes. Student completed procedure in ________ minutes.
	Accuracy: Satisfactory score on the performance evaluation checklist.

Performance Evaluation Checklist

Trial 1	Trial 2	Point Value	Performance Standards
		●	Removed watch or pushed it up on the forearm.
		●	Removed rings.
		▷	Stated the reason for removing rings.
		●	Stood at sink with clothing away from edge of sink.
		●	Turned on faucets with paper towel.
		▷	Explained the reason for turning on faucets with paper towel.
		●	Adjusted the water to a warm temperature.
		●	Discarded towel into trash can.
		●	Wet hands and forearms with water.
		●	Held hands lower than elbows at all times.
		▷	Explained why the hands should be held lower than elbows.
		●	Did not touch the inside of sink with hands.
		●	Applied soap to hands.
		●	Washed palms and backs of hands with 10 circular motions and friction.
		▷	Explained why circular motions and friction are needed to wash hands.
		●	Washed fingers with 10 circular motions.
		●	Washed fingers while interlaced using friction and circular motions.
		●	Rinsed well (keeping hands lower than elbows).

Trial 1	Trial 2	Point Value	Performance Standards
		●	Washed wrists and forearms using friction and circular motions.
		●	Cleaned fingernails using manicure stick.
		●	Rinsed arms and hands.
		●	Repeated handwashing procedure (if necessary).
		●	Dried hands gently and thoroughly.
		▷	Stated the reason for drying hands gently and thoroughly.
		●	Turned off faucets using paper towel.
		●	Did not touch sink area with bare hands.
		▷	Explained the reason for not touching sink area with bare hands.
		Ⓐ	Recognized the implications for failure to comply with Center for Disease Control (CDC) regulations in healthcare settings.
		✶	Completed the procedure within 5 minutes.
			TOTALS

Evaluation of Student Performance

EVALUATION CRITERIA			COMMENTS
Symbol	Category	Point Value	
✶	Critical Step	16 points	
●	Essential Step	6 points	
Ⓐ	Affective Competency	6 points	
▷	Theory Question	2 points	
Score calculation: 100 Points − ___ Points missed ___ Score Satisfactory score: 85 or above			

2008 CAAHEP Competencies Achieved
Psychomotor (Skills) ☑ III. 2. Practice Standard Precautions. ☑ III. 4. Perform handwashing. ☑ IX. 8. Apply local, state, and federal health care legislation and regulation appropriate to the medical assisting practice setting. ***Affective (Behavior)*** ☑ IX. 3. Recognize the importance of local, state, and federal legislation and regulations in the practice setting.

2015 CAAHEP Competencies Achieved
Psychomotor (Skills) ☑ III. 3. Perform handwashing. ***Affective (Behavior)*** ☑ III. 1. Recognize the implications for failure to comply with Center for Disease Control (CDC) regulations in healthcare settings.

ABHES Competencies Achieved
☑ 4. f. Comply with federal, state, and local health laws and regulations as they relate to healthcare settings. ☑ 9. a. Practice standard precautions and perform disinfection/sterilization techniques.

Notes

EVALUATION OF COMPETENCY

Procedure 17-2: Applying an Alcohol-Based Hand Rub

Name: ______________________ Date: ______________

Evaluated by: ______________________ Score: ______________

Performance Objective

Outcome:	Apply an alcohol-based hand rub.
Conditions:	Given an alcohol-based hand rub.
Standards:	Time: 2 minutes. Student completed procedure in ____ minutes.
	Accuracy: Satisfactory score on the performance evaluation checklist.

Performance Evaluation Checklist

Trial 1	Trial 2	Point Value	Performance Standards
		●	Inspected the hands to make sure they are not visibly soiled.
		▷	Stated the procedure to follow if the hands are visibly soiled.
		●	Removed watch or pushed it up on the forearm.
		●	Removed rings.
			Applied the alcohol-based hand rub to the palm of one hand as follows:
		●	***Gel or lotion:*** Applied an amount of gel or lotion approximately equal to the size of a dime.
		●	***Foam:*** Applied an amount of foam approximately equal to the size of a walnut.
		▷	Explained why it is important not to use more than the recommended amount of hand rub.
		●	Thoroughly spread the hand rub over the surface of both hands up to ½ inch above the wrist.
		●	Spread the hand rub around and under the fingernails.
		▷	Explained why it is important to cover the entire surface of the hands.
		●	Rubbed the hands together until they were dry.
		●	Did not touch anything until the hands were dry.
		Ⓐ	Recognized the implications for failure to comply with Center for Disease Control (CDC) regulations in healthcare settings.
		✶	Completed the procedure within 2 minutes.
			TOTALS

Evaluation of Student Performance

<table>
<tr><th colspan="3">EVALUATION CRITERIA</th><th>COMMENTS</th></tr>
<tr><td>Symbol</td><td>Category</td><td>Point Value</td><td rowspan="6"></td></tr>
<tr><td>*</td><td>Critical Step</td><td>16 points</td></tr>
<tr><td>●</td><td>Essential Step</td><td>6 points</td></tr>
<tr><td>Ⓐ</td><td>Affective Competency</td><td>6 points</td></tr>
<tr><td>▷</td><td>Theory Question</td><td>2 points</td></tr>
<tr><td colspan="3">Score calculation: 100 Points
– Points missed
____Score

Satisfactory score: 85 or above</td></tr>
</table>

2008 CAAHEP Competencies Achieved
Psychomotor (Skills) ☑ III. 2. Practice Standard Precautions. ☑ IX. 8. Apply local, state, and federal health care legislation and regulation appropriate to the medical assisting practice setting. ***Affective (Behavior)*** ☑ IX. 3. Recognize the importance of local, state, and federal legislation and regulations in the practice setting.

2015 CAAHEP Competencies Achieved
Psychomotor (Skills) ☑ III. 3. Perform handwashing. ***Affective (Behavior)*** ☑ III. 1. Recognize the implications for failure to comply with Center for Disease Control (CDC) regulations in healthcare settings.

ABHES Competencies Achieved
☑ 4. f. Comply with federal, state, and local health laws and regulations as they relate to healthcare settings. ☑ 9. a. Practice standard precautions and perform disinfection/sterilization techniques.

EVALUATION OF COMPETENCY

Procedure 17-3: Application and Removal of Clean Disposable Gloves

Name: ______________________________ Date: ______________

Evaluated by: ______________________________ Score: ______________

Performance Objective

Outcome:	Apply and remove clean disposable gloves.
Conditions:	Given the appropriate-sized clean disposable gloves.
Standards:	Time: 5 minutes. Student completed procedure in __________ minutes.
	Accuracy: Satisfactory score on the Performance Evaluation Checklist.

Performance Evaluation Checklist

Trial 1	Trial 2	Point Value	Performance Standards
			Application of Clean Gloves
		•	Removed all rings.
		▷	Stated why rings should be removed.
		•	Sanitized the hands.
		•	Chose the appropriate-sized gloves.
		▷	Explained what can happen if the gloves are too small or too large.
		•	Applied the gloves.
		•	Adjusted the gloves so that they fit comfortably.
		•	Inspected the gloves for tears.
		▷	Stated the procedure to follow if a glove is torn.
			Removal of Clean Gloves
		•	Grasped the outside of the left glove 1 to 2 inches from the top with the gloved right hand.
		•	Slowly pulled left glove off the hand.
		•	Pulled the left glove free, and scrunched it into a ball with the gloved right hand.
		•	Placed the index and middle fingers of the left hand on the inside of the right glove.
		•	Did not allow the clean hand to touch outside of the glove.
		•	Pulled the glove off the right hand, enclosing the balled-up left glove.
		•	Discarded both gloves in an appropriate waste container.
		▷	Stated when gloves should be discarded in a biohazardous waste container.

Trial 1	Trial 2	Point Value	Performance Standards
		●	Sanitized the hands.
		▷	Stated why the hands should be sanitized after removing gloves.
		Ⓐ	Recognized the implications for failure to comply with Center for Disease Control (CDC) regulations in healthcare settings.
		✶	Completed the procedure in 5 minutes.
			TOTALS

Evaluation of Student Performance

EVALUATION CRITERIA			COMMENTS
Symbol	**Category**	**Point Value**	
✶	Critical Step	16 points	
●	Essential Step	6 points	
Ⓐ	Affective Competency	6 points	
▷	Theory Question	2 points	
Score calculation: 100 Points − Points missed ___Score Satisfactory score: 85 or above			

2008 CAAHEP Competencies Achieved
Psychomotor (Skills) ☑ III. 2. Practice Standard Precautions. ☑ III. 3. Select appropriate barrier/personal protective equipment (PPE) for potentially infectious situations. ☑ IX. 8. Apply local, state, and federal health care legislation and regulation appropriate to the medical assisting practice setting. ***Affective (Behavior)*** ☑ IX. 3. Recognize the importance of local, state, and federal legislation and regulations in the practice setting.

2015 CAAHEP Competencies Achieved
Psychomotor (Skills) ☑ III. 2. Select appropriate barrier/personal protective equipment (PPE). ***Affective (Behavior)*** ☑ III. 1. Recognize the implications for failure to comply with Center for Disease Control (CDC) regulations in healthcare settings.

ABHES Competencies Achieved
☑ 4. f. Comply with federal, state, and local health laws and regulations as they relate to healthcare settings. ☑ 9. a. Practice standard precautions and perform disinfection/sterilization techniques.

EVALUATION OF COMPETENCY

Procedure 17-A: Proper Use of a Sharps Container

Name: ______________________________ Date: ______________

Evaluated by: ______________________________ Score: ______________

Performance Objective

Outcome:	Demonstrate the proper use of a sharps container.
Conditions:	Given the following: Sharps container and a contaminated sharp.
Standards:	Time: 3 minutes. Student completed procedure in ________ minutes.
	Accuracy: Satisfactory score on the performance evaluation checklist.

Performance Evaluation Checklist

Trial 1	Trial 2	Point Value	Performance Standards
		•	Ensured that the sharps container met the following OSHA Standards: a. Was closable b. Was puncture resistant c. Was leakproof d. Was labeled with a biohazard warning label e. Was color-coded in red
		•	Located the sharps container as close as possible to the area of use.
		▷	Stated why the sharps container should be located close to the area of use.
		•	Made sure the sharps container was maintained in an upright position.
		•	Immediately after use, placed the contaminated sharp in the sharps container.
		•	Dropped the contaminated sharp into the container without touching the sides of the container.
		•	Stated examples of items that must be discarded in a sharps container.
		•	Did not reach into the sharps container with the hands.
		•	Replaced the sharps container on a regular basis and did not allow it to overfill.
		▷	Stated when a sharps container should be replaced.
		Ⓐ	Recognized the implications for failure to comply with CDC and OSHA regulations in a healthcare setting.
		*	Completed the procedure within 5 minutes.
			TOTALS

Evaluation of Student Performance

EVALUATION CRITERIA			COMMENTS
Symbol	**Category**	**Point Value**	
∗	Critical Step	16 points	
●	Essential Step	6 points	
Ⓐ	Affective Competency	6 points	
▷	Theory Question	2 points	
Score calculation: 100 Points − ___ Points missed ___ Score Satisfactory score: 85 or above			

2008 CAAHEP Competencies Achieved

Psychomotor (Skills)

☑ III. 1. Participate in training on Standard Precautions.
☑ III. 2. Practice Standard Precautions.
☑ IX. 8. Apply local, state, and federal health care legislation and regulation appropriate to the medical assisting practice setting.
☑ XI. 5. Demonstrate proper use of the following equipment:
a. Eyewash
b. Fire extinguishers
c. Sharps disposal containers

Affective (Behavior)

☑ IX. 3. Recognize the importance of local, state, and federal legislation and regulations in the practice setting.

2015 CAAHEP Competencies Achieved

Psychomotor (Skills)

☑ III. 1. Participate in bloodborne pathogen training.
☑ III.10. Demonstrate proper disposal of biohazardous material
a. Sharps
b. Regulated waste
☑ X11. 2. Demonstrate proper use of:
d. Eyewash equipment
e. Fire extinguishers
f. Sharps disposal containers

Affective (Behavior)

☑ III. 1. Recognize the implications for failure to comply with Center for Disease Control CDC regulations in healthcare settings.

ABHES Competencies Achieved

☑ 4. f. Comply with federal, state, and local health laws and regulations as they relate to healthcare settings.
☑ 9. a. Practice standard precautions and perform disinfection/sterilization techniques.
☑ 10. c. Dispose of biohazardous materials.

EVALUATION OF COMPETENCY

Procedure 17-B: Disposal of Hazardous Material

Name: ______________________________ Date: ______________

Evaluated by: ______________________________ Score: ______________

Performance Objective

Outcome:	Handle and prepare regulated waste for pickup by a medical waste service.
Conditions:	Given the following: Disposable gloves, biohazard sharps container, biohazards bags, cardboard box with biohazard labels, packing tape, tracking record.
Standards:	Time: 5 minutes. Student completed procedure in __________ minutes.
	Accuracy: Satisfactory score on the performance evaluation checklist.

Performance Evaluation Checklist

Trial 1	Trial 2	Point Value	Performance Standards
			Handling regulated waste
		•	Sanitized hands and applied gloves.
		•	Closed and locked the lid of the full sharps container before removing it from the examining room.
		▷	Stated the reason for closing the lid of the sharps container before removing it from the examining room.
		•	Did not open, empty, or clean the sharps container.
		•	If the sharps container was leaking, placed it in a second container that is closable, leakproof, and appropriately labeled.
		•	Securely closed the full biohazard bag before removing it from an examining room.
		•	If required by the medical office policy, double-bag by placing the primary bag inside a second biohazard bag.
		•	Transported the biohazard containers to a secure area away from the general public.
			Preparing regulated waste for pickup by a medical waste service
		•	Placed sharps containers and biohazard bags into a cardboard box provided by the medical waste service.
		•	Removed gloves and sanitized the hands.
		•	Securely sealed the box with packing tape.
		•	Made sure that a biohazard warning label appeared on two-opposite sides of the box.
		•	Stored the biohazard box in a labeled locked room inside the facility or in a labeled locked collection container outside the facility.
		▷	Stated why biohazard boxes awaiting pickup must be stored in a locked storage area.

Trial 1	Trial 2	Point Value	Performance Standards
		●	Completed a tracking record, if required by your state.
		▷	Stated what information is included on a tracking record.
		Ⓐ	Recognized the implications for failure to comply with CDC and OSHA regulations in a healthcare setting.
		*	Completed the procedure within 5 minutes.
			TOTALS

Evaluation of Student Performance

EVALUATION CRITERIA			COMMENTS
Symbol	**Category**	**Point Value**	
*	Critical Step	16 points	
●	Essential Step	6 points	
Ⓐ	Affective Competency	6 points	
▷	Theory Question	2 points	
Score calculation: 100 Points – ____ Points missed ____ Score Satisfactory score: 85 or above			

2008 CAAHEP Competencies Achieved

Psychomotor (Skills)

☑ III. 1. Participate in training on Standard Precautions.
☑ III. 2. Practice Standard Precautions.
☑ IX. 8. Apply local, state, and federal health care legislation and regulation appropriate to the medical assisting practice setting.

Affective (Behavior)

☑ IX. 3. Recognize the importance of local, state, and federal legislation and regulations in the practice setting.

2015 CAAHEP Competencies Achieved

Psychomotor (Skills)

☑ III. 1. Participate in bloodborne pathogen training.
☑ III.10. Demonstrate proper disposal of biohazardous material
  c. Sharps
  d. Regulated waste

Affective (Behavior)

☑ III. 1. Recognize the implications for failure to comply with Center for Disease Control CDC regulations in healthcare settings.

ABHES Competencies Achieved

☑ 4. f. Comply with federal, state, and local health laws and regulations as they relate to healthcare settings.
☑ 9. a. Practice standard precautions and perform disinfection/sterilization techniques.
☑ 10. c. Dispose of biohazardous materials.

18 Sterilization and Disinfection

CHAPTER ASSIGNMENTS

✓ After Completing	Date Due	Study Guide Pages	STUDY GUIDE ASSIGNMENTS (CTA = Critical Thinking Activity)	Possible Points	Points You Earned
		271	Pretest	10	
		272	Term Key Term Assessment	17	
		272-278	Evaluation of Learning questions	53	
		278-279	CTA A: Safety Data Sheet	16	
		280-281	CTA B: Obtaining a Safety Data Sheet	18	
		282	CTA C: Sanitization	8	
		282-283	CTA D: Sterilization	10	
			Evolve Site: Chapter 18 What Happens Now? (Record points earned)		
			Evolve Site: Chapter 18 Quiz Show (Record points earned)		
			Evolve Site: Apply Your Knowledge questions (Record points earned)	10	
			Evolve Site: Video Evaluation	36	
		271	Posttest	10	
			ADDITIONAL ASSIGNMENTS		
			TOTAL POINTS		

Notes

✓ When Assigned By Your Instructor	Study Guide Pages	Practices Required	LABORATORY ASSIGNMENTS (Procedure Number and Name)	Score*
	285	3	**Practice for Competency** 18-1: Sanitization of Instruments Textbook reference: pp. 229-233	
	287-290		**Evaluation of Competency** 18-1: Sanitization of Instruments	*
	285	Paper: 3 Muslin: 3	**Practice for Competency** 18-2: Wrapping Instruments Using Paper or Muslin Textbook reference: pp. 342-343	
	291-292		**Evaluation of Competency** 18-2: Wrapping Instruments Using Paper or Muslin	*
	285	3	**Practice for Competency** 18-3: Wrapping Instruments Using a Pouch Textbook reference: p. 344	
	293-294		**Evaluation of Competency** 18-3: Wrapping Instruments Using a Pouch	*
	285	3	**Practice for Competency** 18-4: Sterilizing Articles in the Autoclave Textbook reference: pp. 345-347	
	295-297		**Evaluation of Competency** 18-4: Sterilizing Articles in the Autoclave	*
			ADDITIONAL ASSIGNMENTS	

Notes

Name ______________________________ Date ______________

PRETEST

True or False

_______ 1. A bacterial spore consists of a hard, thick-walled capsule that can resist adverse conditions.

_______ 2. The purpose of sanitization is to remove all microorganisms and spores from a contaminated article.

_______ 3. According to OSHA, gloves do not need to be worn during the sanitization process.

_______ 4. Glutaraldehyde (Cidex) is a high-level disinfectant.

_______ 5. High-level disinfection kills all microorganisms but not spores.

_______ 6. Sterilization is the process of destroying all forms of microbial life except for bacterial spores.

_______ 7. Autoclave tape indicates whether an autoclaved item is sterile.

_______ 8. The wrapper used to autoclave articles should prevent contaminants from getting in during handling and storage.

_______ 9. Tap water should be used in the autoclave.

_______ 10. The inside of the autoclave should be wiped every day with a damp cloth.

POSTTEST

True or False

_______ 1. The agent used to destroy microorganisms on an article depends on the size of the article.

_______ 2. The purpose of the Hazard Communications Standard is to make sure that employees do not use hazardous chemicals in the workplace.

_______ 3. The Hazard Communications Standard requires that the label of a hazardous chemical include GHS hazard pictograms.

_______ 4. Stethoscopes must be decontaminated using a high-level disinfectant.

_______ 5. The most common temperature and pressure for autoclaving is 212°F at 15 lb of pressure per square inch.

_______ 6. A sterilization strip should be positioned in the center of a wrapped pack.

_______ 7. The best means of determining the effectives of the sterilization process are biologic indicators.

_______ 8. The proper time for sterilizing an article in the autoclave depends on what is being autoclaved.

_______ 9. A pack that has been in the storage cupboard for 4 weeks should be resterilized.

_______ 10. Ethylene oxide gas is used by medical manufacturers to sterilize disposable items.

KEY TERM ASSESSMENT

Directions: Match each key term with its definition.

_______ 1. Autoclave
_______ 2. Critical item
_______ 3. Detergent
_______ 4. Disinfectant
_______ 5. Hazardous chemical
_______ 6. Incubate
_______ 7. Load
_______ 8. Noncritical item
_______ 9. Safety data sheet
_______ 10. Sanitization
_______ 11. Semicritical item
_______ 12. Spore
_______ 13. Sterilization
_______ 14. Thermolabile
_______ 15. Thermolabile

A. To provide proper conditions for growth and development
B. Easily affected or changed by heat
C. An item that comes in contact with intact skin but not mucous membranes
D. A hard, thick-walled capsule formed by some bacteria that contains only the essential parts of the protoplasm of the bacterial cell
E. An item that comes in contact with sterile tissue or the vascular system
F. An apparatus for the sterilization of materials, using steam under pressure
G. An agent that cleanses by emulsifying dirt and oil
H. An item that comes in contact with nonintact skin or intact mucous membranes
I. The articles that are being sterilized
J. An agent used to destroy pathogenic microorganisms but not their spores (usually applied to inanimate objects)
K. A sheet that provides information regarding a chemical and its hazards, and measures to take to avoid injury and illness when handling the chemical
L. A process to remove organic matter from an article and to lower the number of microorganisms to a safe level as determined by public health requirements
M. The process of destroying all forms of microbial life, including bacterial spores
N. Any chemical that is classified as a health or physical hazard.

EVALUATION OF LEARNING

Directions: Fill in each blank with the correct answer.

1. How does one determine what type of physical or chemical agent to use to destroy microorganisms on an article?

____

____

2. List two diseases that are caused by bacteria that produce spores.

____

____

3. What are the characteristics of bacterial spores?

____

____

4. What is the purpose of the Hazard Communication Standard?

____

____

5. What is the difference between a health hazard and a physical hazard?

____

____

6. What is the purpose of the Globally Harmonized System of Classification and Labeling of Chemicals (GHS)?

____

____

____

7. List four examples of hazardous chemicals that may be used in the medical office.

____

____

8. What information must be included on a hazardous chemical label?

____

____

____

9. What is the purpose of a GHS signal word?

____

____

10. What is the meaning of the following GHS signal words?
    a. Danger: ____
    b. Warning: ____

11. What is the difference between a GHS hazard statement and a GHS precautionary statement?

____

____

____

12. What is a GHS hazard pictogram and what is its purpose?

____

____

13. List and briefly describe the information that must be included on a Safety Data Sheet.

____
____
____
____
____
____
____
____

14. What is the purpose of sanitizing an article?

____
____

15. What is the advantage of using the ultrasound method to clean instruments?

____
____

16. Why should gloves be worn during the sanitization procedure?

____
____

17. Why should instruments be handled carefully?

____

18. Why should a chemical not be used past its expiration date?

____

19. Why must a cleaning agent with a neutral pH be used to sanitize instruments?

____
____

20. What type of brush should be used to clean the following parts of an instrument?
    a. Surface of an instrument: ____________________
    b. Grooves, crevices, or serrations: ____________________

21. How should each of the following be checked for defects and proper working condition?
    a. Blades of an instrument: ____________________
    b. Tips of an instrument: ____________________
    c. Instrument with a box lock: ____________________
    d. Cutting edge of a sharp instrument: ____________________
    e. Scissors: ____________________

22. What is the purpose of lubricating an instrument?

23. What is the definition of high-level disinfection?

24. List one example of an item that requires high-level disinfection. List one example of a high-level disinfectant.

25. List two examples of items that can be disinfected through intermediate-level disinfection. List one example of an intermediate-level disinfectant.

26. List two examples of items that are disinfected by low-level disinfection.

27. What is the purpose of sterilization?

28. What is a critical item? List examples of critical items.

29. What is the purpose of the pressure used in the autoclaving process?

30. Why is it important that all air be removed from the autoclave during the sterilization process?

31. What temperature and pressure are the most commonly used to sterilize materials with the autoclave?

32. What information does the Centers for Disease Control and Prevention (CDC) recommend be recorded in an autoclave log regarding each cycle?

____

____

____

33. What is the purpose of a sterilization indicator?

____

____

34. What should be done if a sterilization indicator does not change properly?

____

____

35. How should sterilization indicators be stored?

____

36. What are the advantages and disadvantages of autoclave tape?

____

____

37. How should a sterilization strip be placed in a wrapped pack?

____

38. How often should a biologic indicator be used to monitor an autoclave?

____

39. What is the purpose of wrapping articles to be autoclaved?

____

____

40. List two properties of a good wrapper for use in autoclaving.

____

____

41. List three examples of wrapping materials used for the autoclave and identify an advantage of each type.

____

____

____

42. What shouldn't tap water be used to fill the water reservoir of an autoclave?

____

____

43. How should the following be positioned in the autoclave?
   a. Small packs: ___
   b. Large packs: ___
   c. Jars and glassware: ___
   d. Sterilization pouches: ___

44. Why is more time needed to autoclave a large minor office surgery pack?

45. What determines the amount of time required to sterilize articles in the autoclave?

46. Why must a sterilized load be allowed to dry before it is removed from the autoclave?

47. What is event-related sterility?

48. How should sterilized packs be stored?

49. Describe the care an autoclave should receive on a daily basis.

50. Why is a longer exposure period needed to ensure sterilization when using the dry-heat oven?

51. What effect does moist heat have on instruments with sharp cutting edges?

52. How does the medical manufacturing industry use ethylene oxide gas sterilization?

53. What guidelines must be followed when using cold sterilization?

CRITICAL THINKING ACTIVITIES

A. Safety Data Sheet

Refer to the Safety Data Sheet (SDS) in the textbook (see Fig. 18-4), and answer the following questions.

1. What is the brand name of this chemical?

2. What is the recommended use of glutaraldehyde?

3. What is the GHS hazard classification of glutaraldehyde?

4. What is the signal word of glutaraldehyde?

5. What GHS hazard statements are associated with glutaraldehyde?

6. What are the first aid measures for glutaraldehyde for each of the following?
   a. Skin contact:
   b. Eye contact:
   c. Inhalation
   d. Ingestion

7. What should be done if glutaraldehyde is spilled?

8. How should glutaraldehyde be stored?

9. What type of personal protective equipment should be used with glutaraldehyde?

10. Describe the appearance and odor of glutaraldehyde.

11. What conditions should be avoided with glutaraldehyde?

12. What symptoms can occur from overexposure to glutaraldehyde for each of the following?

    a. Inhalation: _____

    b. Skin contact: _____

    c. Eye contact _____

    d. Ingestion _____

13. What medical conditions are aggravated by exposure to glutaraldehyde?

14. Does glutaraldehyde cause cancer?

15. What is the disposal method for glutaraldehyde?

16. When was the SDS last revised?

B. Obtaining a Safety Data Sheet

Obtain an SDS for one of the following hazardous chemicals, and answer the questions.

To locate an SDS on the Internet, enter the name of the chemical into a search engine with the abbreviation "SDS." (Example: Cidex SDS)

- Cidex
- MetriCide
- Cidex OPAn
- CaviCide
- MadaCide
- SaniZide
- Wavicide
- Biozide
- Sporox II
- Vesphene
- Envirocide
- Clorox bleach

1. What is the product name of this hazardous chemical?

____

2. What is brand or trade name of this chemical?

____

3. Who manufactures this chemical?

____

4. What number would you call if an emergency occurred with this chemical?

____

5. What is the recommended use of this chemical?

____

6. What is the GHS hazard classification of this chemical?

____

____

7. What is the signal word for this chemical?

____

8. What GHS hazard statements are associated with this chemical?

____

____

____

9. Sketch the GHS hazard pictograms associated with this chemical below:

10. What are the GHS precautionary statements associated with this chemical?

____

____

____

11. What are the first aid measures for this chemical?

____

____

____

12. What should be done if this chemical is spilled?

____

13. What are the precautions for safe handling of this chemical?

____

____

14. How should this chemical be stored?

____

15. What type of personal protective equipment should be used with this chemical?

____

____

16. What are the acute health hazards associated with this chemical?

____

____

____

17. What medical conditions are aggravated by exposure to this chemical?

____

____

18. What is the disposal method for this chemical?

____

____

C. Sanitization

For each of the following situations involving sanitization, write C if the technique is correct and I if the technique is incorrect. If the situation is correct, state the principle underlying the technique. If the situation is incorrect, explain what might happen if the technique were performed in the incorrect manner.

_______ 1. A contaminated surgical instrument is left in the examination room.

_______ 2. The medical assistant does not wear gloves when sanitizing surgical instruments.

_______ 3. The medical assistant piles instruments while preparing them for sanitization.

_______ 4. The medical assistant forgets to read the safety data sheet before decontaminating some surgical instruments in Cidex.

_______ 5. The medical assistant uses laundry detergent to sanitize surgical instruments.

_______ 6. Dried blood is not completely cleansed from hemostatic forceps before they are sterilized in the autoclave.

_______ 7. The medical assistant checks all instruments for proper working condition before sterilizing them.

_______ 8. The medical assistant lubricates hemostatic forceps with a steam-penetrable lubricant before sterilizing them.

D. Sterilization

For each of the following situations involving sterilization of articles in the autoclave, write C if the technique is correct, and I if the technique is incorrect. If the situation is correct, state the principle underlying the technique. If the situation is incorrect, explain what might happen if the technique were performed in the incorrect manner.

_______ 1. The medical assistant opens a hemostat before placing it in a sterilization pouch.

_______ 2. Tap water is used to fill the water reservoir of the autoclave.

____

____

_______ 3. When loading the autoclave, the medical assistant places glass jars in an upright position.

____

____

_______ 4. The medical assistant places four sterilization pouches on top of one another in the autoclave.

____

____

_______ 5. The medical assistant places small packs to be sterilized approximately 1 to 3 inches apart in the autoclave.

____

____

_______ 6. Spore strips are placed in the autoclave where steam will penetrate them most easily.

____

____

_______ 7. The medical assistant begins timing the load in the autoclave after the proper temperature of 250°F has been reached.

____

____

_______ 8. The medical assistant removes the load from the autoclave while it is still wet.

____

____

_______ 9. The medical assistant notices a tear in one of the wrappers while removing articles from the autoclave. He or she rewraps and resterilizes the article.

____

____

_______ 10. The medical assistant notices that a sterilized wrapped article stored on the storage shelf has opened up. He or she retapes the pack and places it back on the storage shelf.

____

____

Notes

PRACTICE FOR COMPETENCY

Procedure 18-1: Sanitization of Instruments

Sanitize instruments. In the space provided, indicate the following:

A. Name of the disinfectant ________________

B. Name of the instrument cleaner ________________

C. Names of instruments sanitized ________________

Procedures 18-2: Wrapping Instruments Using Paper or Muslin, and Procedure 18-3: Wrapping Instruments Using a Pouch

Wrap articles for autoclaving. In the space provided, list the information you indicated on the label of each pack that includes the contents of the pack, the date, and your initials.
Information indicated on the label of the wrapped article:

Procedure 18-4: Sterilizing Articles in the Autoclave

Sterilize articles in the autoclave. In the space provided, indicate the articles you sterilized.

Notes

EVALUATION OF COMPETENCY

Procedure 18-1: Sanitization of Instruments

Name: ______________________ Date: ______________

Evaluated by: ______________________ Score: ______________

Performance Objective

Outcome:	Sanitize instruments.
Conditions:	Given the following: disposable gloves, utility gloves, contaminated instruments, chemical disinfectant and SDS, disinfectant container, cleaning solution and SDS, basin, nylon brush, wire brush, paper towels, cloth towel, and instrument lubricant.
Standards:	Time: 10 minutes Student completed procedure in __________ minutes.
	Accuracy: Satisfactory score on the Performance Evaluation Checklist.

Performance Evaluation Checklist

Trial 1	Trial 2	Point Value	Performance Standards
		●	Reviewed the SDS for hazardous chemicals being used.
		●	Applied gloves.
		●	Transported the contaminated instruments to the cleaning area.
		●	Applied heavy-duty utility gloves over the disposable gloves.
		▷	Stated the purpose of the utility gloves.
		●	Separated sharp instruments and delicate instruments from other instruments.
		▷	Explained why instruments should be separated.
		●	Immediately rinsed the instruments thoroughly under warm running water.
		▷	Stated why the instruments should be rinsed immediately.
			Decontamination of the Instruments
		●	Checked the expiration date of the chemical disinfectant.
		▷	Explained why an expired disinfectant should not be used.
		●	Observed all personal safety precautions listed on the label.
		●	Followed label directions for proper mixing and use of the disinfectant.
		●	Labeled the disinfecting container with the name of the disinfectant and the reuse expiration date.
		●	Poured the disinfectant into the labeled container.

Trial 1	Trial 2	Point Value	Performance Standards
		●	Completely submerged the articles in the disinfectant.
		●	Covered the disinfectant container.
		▷	Stated the reason for covering the container.
		●	Disinfected the articles for 10 minutes.
		▷	Explained the reason for decontaminating the instruments.
			Cleaning the Instruments: Manual Method
		●	Checked the expiration date of the cleaning agent.
		●	Observed all personal safety precautions.
		●	Followed label directions for proper use and mixing of the cleaning agent.
		●	Removed articles from disinfectant and placed them in the cleaning solution.
		●	Cleaned the surface of the instruments with a nylon brush.
		●	Cleaned grooves, crevices, or serrations with a wire brush.
		●	Removed stains using commercial stain remover.
		●	Scrubbed the instruments until they were visibly clean.
		▷	Explained why all organic matter must be removed.
			Cleaning the Instruments: Ultrasound Method
		●	Prepared the cleaning solution in the ultrasonic cleaner.
		●	Observed all personal safety precautions listed on label.
		●	Removed the articles from the disinfectant.
		●	Separated instruments of dissimilar metals.
		●	Properly placed the instruments in the ultrasonic cleaner.
		●	Positioned hinged instruments in an open position.
		▷	Stated why hinged instruments must be in an open position.
		●	Ensured that sharp instruments did not touch other instruments.
		●	Checked to make sure all instruments were fully submerged.
		●	Placed the lid on the ultrasonic cleaner.
		●	Turned on the ultrasonic cleaner.
		●	Cleaned the instruments for the length of time recommended by the manufacturer.
		●	Removed the instruments from the machine.

Trial 1	Trial 2	Point Value	Performance Standards
		●	Rinsed each instrument thoroughly with warm water for 20 to 30 seconds.
		▷	Explained why instruments should be rinsed thoroughly.
		●	Dried each instrument with a paper towel.
			Completion of the Procedure
		●	Placed instrument on a towel for additional drying.
		▷	Stated the reason for drying the instruments.
		●	Checked each instrument for defects and proper working condition.
		●	Lubricated hinged instruments in an open position.
		●	Opened and closed the instrument to distribute the lubricant.
		●	Placed the lubricated instrument on a towel to drain.
		▷	Stated the reason for lubricating instruments.
		●	Disposed of the cleaning solution according to the manufacturer's instructions.
		●	Removed both sets of gloves.
		●	Sanitized hands.
		●	Wrapped the instruments.
		●	Sterilized the instruments in the autoclave.
		✶	Completed the procedure within 10 minutes.
			TOTALS

Evaluation of Student Performance

EVALUATION CRITERIA			COMMENTS
Symbol	Category	Point Value	
✶	Critical Step	16 points	
●	Essential Step	6 points	
Ⓐ	Affective Competency	6 points	
▷	Theory Question	2 points	
Score calculation: 100 Points − ___ Points missed ___ Score Satisfactory score: 85 or above			

2008 CAAHEP Competency Achieved
Psychomotor (Skills) ☑ III. 5. Prepare items for autoclaving.

2015 CAAHEP Competency Achieved
Psychomotor (Skills) ☑ III. 4. Prepare items for autoclaving.

ABHES Competency Achieved
☑ 9. a. Practice standard precautions and perform disinfection/sterilization techniques.

EVALUATION OF COMPETENCY

Procedure 18-2: Wrapping Instruments Using Paper or Muslin

Name: ______________________ Date: ______________

Evaluated by: ______________________ Score: ______________

Performance Objective

Outcome:	Wrap an instrument for autoclaving.
Conditions:	Given the following: sanitized instrument, wrapping material, sterilization indicator strip, autoclave tape, and a permanent marker.
	Time: 5 minutes. Student completed procedure in __________ minutes.
Standards:	Accuracy: Satisfactory score on the performance evaluation checklist.

Performance Evaluation Checklist

Trial 1	Trial 2	Point Value	Performance Standards
		●	Sanitized hands.
		●	Assembled equipment.
		●	Selected the appropriate-sized wrapping material.
		●	Checked the expiration date on the sterilization indicator box.
		▷	Stated why outdated strips should not be used.
		●	Placed wrapping material on clean, flat surface.
		●	Turned the wrap in a diagonal position.
		●	Placed instrument in the center of wrapping material.
		●	Placed instruments with movable joints in an open position.
		▷	Stated why instruments with movable joints must be placed in an open position.
		●	Placed a sterilization indicator in the center of the pack.
		●	Folded wrapping material up from the bottom and doubled back a small corner.
		●	Folded over one edge of wrapping material and doubled back the corner.
		●	Folded over the other edge of wrapping material and doubled back the corner.
		●	Folded the pack up from the bottom and secured with autoclave tape.
		●	Ensured that the pack was firm enough for handling, but loose enough to permit proper circulation of steam.
		▷	Stated why instruments are wrapped for autoclaving.

Trial 1	Trial 2	Point Value	Performance Standards
		●	Labeled and dated the pack. Included initials.
		▷	Stated the purpose of dating the pack.
		*	Completed the procedure within 5 minutes.
			TOTALS

Evaluation of Student Performance

EVALUATION CRITERIA			COMMENTS
Symbol	**Category**	**Point Value**	
*	Critical Step	16 points	
●	Essential Step	6 points	
Ⓐ	Affective Competency	6 points	
▷	Theory Question	2 points	
Score calculation: 100 Points − Points missed ____Score Satisfactory score: 85 or above			

2008 CAAHEP Competency Achieved
Psychomotor (Skills) ☑ III. 5. Prepare items for autoclaving.

2015 CAAHEP Competency Achieved
Psychomotor (Skills) ☑ III. 4. Prepare items for autoclaving.

ABHES Competency Achieved
☑ 9. a. Practice standard precautions and perform disinfection/ sterilization techniques.

EVALUATION OF COMPETENCY

Procedure 18-3: Wrapping Instruments Using a Pouch

Name: ______________________________ Date: ______________

Evaluated by: ______________________________ Score: ______________

Performance Objective

Outcome:	Wrap an instrument for autoclaving.
Conditions:	Given the following: sanitized instrument, sterilization pouch, and a permanent marker.
Standards:	Time: 5 minutes. Student completed procedure in __________ minutes.
	Accuracy: Satisfactory score on the performance evaluation checklist.

Performance Evaluation Checklist

Trial 1	Trial 2	Point Value	Performance Standards
		●	Sanitized hands.
		●	Assembled equipment.
		●	Selected the appropriate-sized pouch.
		●	Placed the pouch on a clean, flat surface.
		●	Labeled and dated the pack. Included initials.
		●	Inserted the instrument into the open end of the pouch.
		●	Sealed the pouch.
		●	Sterilized the pack in the autoclave.
		▷	Stated how long the pack is sterile once it has been autoclaved.
		*	Completed the procedure within 5 minutes.
			TOTALS

Evaluation of Student Performance

EVALUATION CRITERIA			COMMENTS
Symbol	**Category**	**Point Value**	
✶	Critical Step	16 points	
●	Essential Step	6 points	
Ⓐ	Affective Competency	6 points	
▷	Theory Question	2 points	
Score calculation: 100 Points – Points missed ____Score Satisfactory score: 85 or above			

2008 CAAHEP Competency Achieved
Psychomotor (Skills) ☑ III. 5. Prepare items for autoclaving.

2015 CAAHEP Competency Achieved
Psychomotor (Skills) ☑ III. 4. Prepare items for autoclaving.

ABHES Competency Achieved
☑ 9. a. Practice standard precautions and perform disinfection/sterilization techniques.

EVALUATION OF COMPETENCY

Procedure 18-4: Sterilizing Articles in the Autoclave

Name: ______________________________ Date: ______________

Evaluated by: ______________________________ Score: ______________

Performance Objective

Outcome:	Sterilize articles in the autoclave.
Conditions:	Using an autoclave.
	Time: 10 minutes. Student completed procedure in _______ minutes.
Standards:	Accuracy: Satisfactory score on the performance evaluation checklist.

Performance Evaluation Checklist

Trial 1	Trial 2	Point Value	Performance Standards
		●	Assembled equipment.
		●	Checked the water level in the autoclave.
		●	Properly loaded the autoclave.
		▷	Stated how far apart to place small packs and large packs.
		▷	Explained two ways for positioning pouches in the autoclave.
			Manual Operation of the Autoclave
		●	Determined the sterilizing time for the type of articles being autoclaved.
		●	Turned on the autoclave.
		●	Filled the chamber with water.
		●	Closed and latched the door.
		●	Set the timing control.
		▷	Stated when the timer should be set.
		●	Vented the chamber of steam.
		●	Dried the load.
		▷	Stated the reason for drying the load.
			Automatic operation of the Autoclave
		●	Closed and latched the door.
		●	Turned on the autoclave.
		●	Determined the sterilization program.
		●	Pressed the appropriate program button.

Trial 1	Trial 2	Point Value	Performance Standards
		●	Pressed the start button.
		▷	Stated the purpose of each control or indicator on the autoclave.
			Completion of the Procedure
		●	Turned off the autoclave.
		●	Removed the load with heat-resistant gloves.
		▷	Stated the reason for using heat-resistant gloves.
		●	Inspected the packs as they were removed for damage.
		▷	Explained what should be done if a pack is torn.
		●	Checked the sterilization indicators on the outside of the packs.
		●	Recorded information in the autoclave log.
		●	Stored the articles in a clean dust-proof area.
		●	Placed the most recently sterilized packs behind previously sterilized packs.
		●	Maintained appropriate daily care of the autoclave.
		▷	Described the care the autoclave should receive each day.
		Ⓐ	Recognized the implications for failure to comply with Center for Disease Control (CDC) regulations in healthcare settings.
		✶	Completed the procedure within 10 minutes.
			TOTALS

Evaluation of Student Performance

EVALUATION CRITERIA			COMMENTS
Symbol	**Category**	**Point Value**	
✶	Critical Step	16 points	
●	Essential Step	6 points	
Ⓐ	Affective Competency	6 points	
▷	Theory Question	2 points	
Score calculation: 100 Points – Points missed ____Score Satisfactory score: 85 or above			

2008 CAAHEP Competencies Achieved
Psychomotor (Skills) ☑ III. 6. Perform sterilization procedures. ***Affective (Behavior)*** ☑ IX. 3. Recognize the importance of local, state, and federal legislation and regulations in the practice setting.

2015 CAAHEP Competencies Achieved
Psychomotor (Skills) ☑ III. 5. Perform sterilization procedures. ☑ VI. 8. Perform routine maintenance of administrative or clinical equipment. ***Affective (Behavior)*** ☑ III. 1. Recognize the implications for failure to comply with Center for Disease Control (CDC) regulations in healthcare settings.

ABHES Competency Achieved
☑ 4. f. Comply with federal, state, and local health laws and regulations as they related to healthcare settings. ☑ 9. a. Practice standard precautions and perform disinfection/sterilization techniques.

Notes

19 Vital Signs

CHAPTER ASSIGNMENTS

✓ After Completing	Date Due	Study Guide Pages	STUDY GUIDE ASSIGNMENTS (CTA = Critical Thinking Activity)	Possible Points	Points You Earned
		303	Pretest	10	
		304-305 306	Key Term Assessment A. Definitions B. Word Parts (Add 1 point for each key term)	55 30	
		307-316	Evaluation of Learning questions	93	
		316-318	CTA A: Measurement of Body Temperature	17	
		318	CTA B: Alterations in Body Temperature	5	
		319	CTA C: Pulse Sites	6	
		319	CTA D: Pulse and Respiratory Rates	3	
		319-321	CTA E: Pulse Oximetry	18	
		321-322	CTA F: Blood Pressure Measurement	10	
		322	CTA G: Proper BP Cuff Selection	12	
		323	CTA H: Reading Blood Pressure Values	24	
			Evolve Site: Under Pressure (Record points earned)		
		324	CTA I: Interpreting Blood Pressure Readings	10	
		324	CTA J: Hypertension	20	
		325	CTA K: Crossword Puzzle	30	
			Evolve Site: Road to Recovery Game: Vital Signs Terminology (Record points earned)		
			Evolve Site: Apply Your Knowledge questions (Record points earned)	11	

✓ After Completing	Date Due	Study Guide Pages	STUDY GUIDE ASSIGNMENTS (CTA = Critical Thinking Activity)	Possible Points	Points You Earned
			Evolve Site: Video Evaluation	86	
		303	Posttest	10	
			ADDITIONAL ASSIGNMENTS		
			TOTAL POINTS		

✓ When Assigned By Your Instructor	Study Guide Pages	Practices Required	LABORATORY ASSIGNMENTS	Score*
	327-328	5	**Practice for Competency** 19-1: Measuring Oral Body Temperature—Electronic Thermometer Textbook reference: pp. 359-361	
	329-331		**Evaluation of Competency** 19-1: Measuring Oral Body Temperature—Electronic Thermometer	*
	327-328	3	**Practice for Competency** 19-2: Measuring Axillary Body Temperature—Electronic Thermometer Textbook reference: pp. 362-363	
	333-335		**Evaluation of Competency** 19-2: Measuring Axillary Body Temperature—Electronic Thermometer	*
	327-328	3	**Practice for Competency** 19-3: Measuring Rectal Body Temperature—Electronic Thermometer Textbook reference: pp. 363-364	
	337-339		**Evaluation of Competency** 19-3: Measuring Rectal Body Temperature—Electronic Thermometer	*
	327-328	5	**Practice for Competency** 19-4: Measuring Aural Body Temperature—Tympanic Membrane Thermometer Textbook reference: pp. 365-367	
	341-343		**Evaluation of Competency** 19-4: Measuring Aural Body Temperature—Tympanic Membrane Thermometer	*
	327-328	5	**Practice for Competency** 19-5: Measuring Temporal Body Temperature Textbook reference: pp. 367-369	
	345-347		**Evaluation of Competency** 19-5: Measuring Temporal Body Temperature	*
	327-328	10	**Practice for Competency** 19-6: Measuring Pulse and Respiration Textbook reference: pp. 374-375	
	349-351		**Evaluation of Competency** 19-6: Measuring Pulse and Respiration	*

✓ When Assigned By Your Instructor	Study Guide Pages	Practices Required	LABORATORY ASSIGNMENTS	Score*
	327-328	5	**Practice for Competency** 19-7: Measuring Apical Pulse Textbook reference: pp. 375-376	
	353-354		**Evaluation of Competency** 19-7: Measuring Apical Pulse	*
	327-328	5	**Practice for Competency** 19-8: Performing Pulse Oximetry Textbook reference: pp. 384-386	
	355-357		**Evaluation of Competency** 19-8: Performing Pulse Oximetry	*
	327-328	10	**Practice for Competency** 19-9: Measuring Blood Pressure Textbook reference: pp. 396-400	
	359-361		**Evaluation of Competency** 19-9: Measuring Blood Pressure	*
			ADDITIONAL ASSIGNMENTS	

Name ______________________________ Date ______________

PRETEST

True or False

_______ 1. The heat-regulating center of the body is the medulla.

_______ 2. A vague sense of body discomfort, weakness, and fatigue that often marks the onset of a disease is known as the blahs.

_______ 3. If an axillary temperature of 100° F was taken orally, it would register as 101° F.

_______ 4. If the lens of a tympanic membrane thermometer is dirty, the reading may be falsely low.

_______ 5. Chemical thermometers should be stored in the freezer.

_______ 6. The femoral pulse site can be used to assess circulation to the foot.

_______ 7. The term used to describe an irregularity in the heart's rhythm is dysrhythmia.

_______ 8. Pulse oximetry provides the physician with information on the amount of oxygen being delivered to the tissues.

_______ 9. Blood pressure measures the contraction and relaxation of the heart.

_______ 10. When taking blood pressure, the stethoscope is placed over the brachial artery.

POSTTEST

True or False

_______ 1. A temperature of 100° F is classified as a low-grade fever.

_______ 2. The rectal site should not be used to take the temperature of a newborn.

_______ 3. A tympanic membrane thermometer should not be used to measure temperature on a child younger than 6 years of age.

_______ 4. A temporal artery temperature reading is the same as an oral reading.

_______ 5. Excessive pressure should not be applied when measuring a pulse because it could obstruct the pulse.

_______ 6. A child has a faster pulse rate than an adult.

_______ 7. The normal respiratory rate of an adult ranges between 10 and 18 respirations per minute.

_______ 8. The term used to describe a bluish discoloration of the skin due to a lack of oxygen is hypoxia.

_______ 9. The oxygen saturation level of a healthy individual falls between 85% and 90%.

_______ 10. When measuring blood pressure, the patient's arm should be positioned above the level of the heart.

Term KEY TERM ASSESSMENT

A. Definitions

Temperature

Directions: Match each key term with its definition.

_______ 1. Afebrile
_______ 2. Antipyretic
_______ 3. Axilla
_______ 4. Celsius scale
_______ 5. Conduction
_______ 6. Convection
_______ 7. Crisis
_______ 8. Disinfectant
_______ 9. Fahrenheit scale
_______ 10. Febrile
_______ 11. Fever
_______ 12. Frenulum linguae
_______ 13. Hyperpyrexia
_______ 14. Hypothermia
_______ 15. Malaise
_______ 16. Radiation

A. An extremely high fever
B. An agent used to destroy disease-producing microorganisms but not necessarily their spores (usually applied to inanimate objects)
C. A body temperature that is below normal
D. The armpit
E. The transfer of energy, such as heat, through air currents
F. A body temperature that is above normal (pyrexia)
G. An agent that reduces fever
H. A temperature scale on which the freezing point of water is 32° and the boiling point of water is 212°
I. The transfer of energy, such as heat, in the form of waves
J. A temperature scale on which the freezing point of water is 0° and the boiling point is 100°
K. The midline fold that connects the undersurface of the tongue with the floor of the mouth
L. Pertaining to fever
M. The transfer of energy from one object to another by direct contact
N. A sudden falling of an elevated body temperature to normal
O. Without fever; the body temperature is normal
P. A vague sense of body discomfort, weakness, and fatigue often marking the onset of a disease and continuing through the course of the illness

Pulse

Directions: Match each key term with its definition.

_______ 1. Antecubital space
_______ 2. Aorta
_______ 3. Bounding pulse
_______ 4. Bradycardia
_______ 5. Dysrhythmia
_______ 6. Intercostal
_______ 7. Pulse rhythm
_______ 8. Pulse volume
_______ 9. Tachycardia
_______ 10. Thready pulse

A. Between the ribs
B. A pulse with an increased volume that feels very strong and full
C. The strength of the heartbeat
D. The space located at the front of the elbow
E. An abnormally fast heart rate (more than 100 beats per minute)
F. The major trunk of the arterial system of the body
G. The time interval between heartbeats
H. A pulse with a decreased volume that feels weak and thin
I. An irregular rhythm
J. An abnormally slow heart rate (less than 60 beats per minute)

Respiration and Pulse Oximetry

Directions: Match each key term with its definition.

_______ 1. Alveolus
_______ 2. Apnea
_______ 3. Bradypnea
_______ 4. Cyanosis
_______ 5. Dyspnea
_______ 6. Eupnea
_______ 7. Exhalation
_______ 8. Hyperpnea
_______ 9. Hyperventilation
_______ 10. Hypopnea
_______ 11. Hypoxemia
_______ 12. Hypoxia
_______ 13. Inhalation
_______ 14. Orthopnea
_______ 15. Pulse oximeter
_______ 16. Pulse oximetry
_______ 17. SaO_2
_______ 18. SpO_2
_______ 19. Tachypnea

A. The act of breathing out
B. A reduction in the oxygen supply to the tissues of the body
C. A decrease in the oxygen saturation of the blood; may lead to hypoxia
D. The temporary cessation of breathing
E. An abnormal increase in the respiratory rate of more than 20 respirations per minute
F. A computerized device consisting of a probe and monitor used to measure the oxygen saturation of arterial blood
G. An abnormal decrease in the rate and depth of respiration
H. A thin-walled air sac of the lungs in which the exchange of oxygen and carbon dioxide takes place
I. The use of a pulse oximeter to measure the oxygen saturation of arterial blood
J. The act of breathing in
K. A bluish discoloration of the skin and mucous membranes first observed in the nail beds and lips
L. Abbreviation for the percentage of hemoglobin that is saturated with oxygen in arterial blood
M. The condition in which breathing is easier when an individual is in a standing or sitting position
N. Shortness of breath or difficulty in breathing
O. Abbreviation for the percentage of hemoglobin that is saturated with oxygen in arterial blood as measured by a pulse oximeter
P. Normal respiration
Q. An abnormally fast and deep type of breathing usually associated with acute anxiety conditions
R. An abnormal decrease in the respiratory rate of less than 10 respirations per minute
S. An abnormal increase in the rate and depth of respiration

Blood Pressure

Directions: Match each key term with its definition.

_______ 1. Diastole
_______ 2. Diastolic pressure
_______ 3. Hypertension
_______ 4. Hypotension
_______ 5. Meniscus
_______ 6. Pulse pressure
_______ 7. Sphygmomanometer
_______ 8. Stethoscope
_______ 9. Systole
_______ 10. Systolic pressure

A. The curved surface on a column of liquid in a tube
B. High blood pressure
C. The point of maximum pressure on the arterial walls
D. The phase in the cardiac cycle in which the heart relaxes between contractions
E. An instrument for measuring arterial blood pressure
F. The point of lesser pressure on the arterial walls
G. Low blood pressure
H. The phase in the cardiac cycle in which the ventricles contract, sending blood out of the heart and into the aorta and pulmonary aorta
I. An instrument for amplifying and hearing sounds produced by the body
J. The difference between the systolic and diastolic pressures

B. Word Parts

Directions: Indicate the meaning of each word part in the space provided. List as many medical terms as possible that incorporate the word part in the space provided.

Word Part	Meaning of Word Part	Medical Terms That Incorporate Word Part
1. anti-		
2. pyr/o		
3. -ic		
4. -pnea		
5. brady-		
6. cardi/o		
7. -ia		
8. a-		
9. cyan/o		
10. -osis		
11. dys-		
12. eu-		
13. -ex		
14. hyper-		
15. hypo-		
16. tension		
17. therm/o		
18. ox/i		
19. in-		
20. inter-		
21. cost/o		
22. -al		
23. –mal		
24. –meter		
25. orth/o		
26. -metry		
27. sphygm/o		
28. steth/o		
29. -scope		
30. tachy-		

EVALUATION OF LEARNING

Temperature

Directions: Fill in each blank with the correct answer.

1. Define a vital sign.

2. What are the four vital signs?

3. What general guidelines should be followed when measuring vital signs?

4. List four ways in which heat is produced in the body.

5. List four ways in which heat is lost from the body.

6. What is the normal body temperature range? What is the average body temperature?

7. What is a fever?

8. How do diurnal variations affect body temperature?

9. How do emotional states affect the body temperature?

10. How does vigorous physical exercise affect body temperature?

11. What symptoms occur with a fever?

12. Describe the following fever patterns:
    a. Continuous fever

    b. Intermittent fever

    c. Remittent fever

13. What is the subsiding stage of a fever?

14. What five sites are used for taking body temperature?

15. List three instances in which the axillary site for taking body temperature would be preferred over the oral site.

16. Why does the rectal method for taking body temperature provide a very accurate temperature measurement?

17. When can the rectal method be used to take body temperature?

18. When can the aural method be used to take body temperature?

19. How does a temperature taken through the rectal and axillary methods compare (in terms of degrees) with a temperature taken through the oral method?

20. List and describe the four types of thermometers available for taking body temperature.

21. Describe the advantages of a tympanic membrane thermometer.

22. Explain how a tympanic membrane thermometer measures body temperature.

23. Explain how to clean the lens of a tympanic membrane thermometer.

24. What is the purpose of placing a probe cover on a tympanic membrane thermometer?

25. List three reasons why the temporal artery is a good site to measure body temperature.

26. How does the temperature obtained through the temporal site compare with oral, rectal, and axillary body temperatures?

27. List four factors that can result in an inaccurate temporal artery temperature reading.

28. Where should a chemical thermometer be stored? Explain why.

Pulse

Directions: Fill in each blank with the correct answer.

1. What causes the pulse to occur?

2. What is the unit of measurement for pulse rate?

3. How does physical activity affect the pulse rate?

4. What is the most common site for taking the pulse?

5. List two reasons for taking the pulse at the apical pulse site.

6. Where is the apex of the heart located?

7. When is the brachial artery used as a pulse site?

8. When is the carotid artery used as a pulse site?

9. When is the femoral artery used as a pulse site?

10. What two pulse sites can be used to assess circulation to the foot?

11. List two reasons for measuring the pulse rate.

____

____

12. State the normal range for a pulse rate for an adult.

____

13. What is the normal pulse range for the following age groups:
    a. Infant: ___________________________
    b. Toddler: ___________________________
    c. Preschooler: ___________________________
    d. School-age: ___________________________
    e. Adult after age 60: ___________________________

14. What is the normal pulse range for a well-trained athlete?

____

15. What may cause tachycardia?

____

16. How is an apical-radial pulse taken?

____

____

17. What is a pulse deficit?

____

18. If the rhythm and volume of a patient's pulse are normal, the medical assistant records the information as

____

Respiration

Directions: Fill in each blank with the correct answer.

1. What is the purpose of respiration?

____

____

2. What is the purpose of inhalation?

____

____

3. What is the purpose of exhalation?

____

____

4. What is included in one complete respiration?

____

____

5. The exchange of oxygen and carbon dioxide between the body cells and blood is known as

____

6. What is the name of the control center for involuntary respiration?

____

7. Why must respiration be measured without the patient's awareness?

____

8. What is the normal respiratory rate (range) for a normal adult?

____

9. What is the ratio of respirations to pulse beats?

____

10. List two factors that can increase the respiratory rate.

____

____

11. Describe a normal rhythm for respiration.

____

____

12. What can cause hyperventilation?

____

13. What type of patient may experience hypopnea?

____

14. Where is cyanosis first observed?

____

____

15. What can cause cyanosis?

____

16. What are two conditions in which dyspnea may occur?

____

____

17. Describe the character of normal breath sounds.

____

____

18. Describe the characters of the following abnormal breath sounds:

a. Crackles:

____

____

b. Rhonchi:

____

____

c. Wheezes:

____

____

Pulse Oximetry

Directions: Fill in each blank with the correct answer.

1. What is the purpose of pulse oximetry?

____

____

2. What is the function of hemoglobin?

____

3. What is the oxygen saturation level of a healthy individual?

____

4. What can occur if the oxygen saturation level falls between 85% and 90%?

____

____

5. List three patient conditions that can cause a decreased SpO_2 value.

____

____

____

6. When can pulse oximetry be used for the short-term continuous monitoring of a patient?

____

____

____

7. What is the purpose of the pulse oximeter power-on self-test (POST)?

8. What type of site must be used for applying a pulse oximeter probe?

9. How can dark fingernail polish cause a falsely low SpO_2 reading?

10. How can patient movement cause an inaccurate SpO_2 reading?

11. What type of patients may make it difficult to properly align the oximeter probe?

12. List three conditions that can cause poor peripheral blood flow.

13. Why must a reusable oximeter probe be free of all dirt and grime before it is used?

Blood Pressure

Directions: Fill in each blank with the correct answer.

1. What does blood pressure measure?

2. Why is the diastolic pressure lower than the systolic pressure?

3. What is considered normal blood pressure for an adult?

4. State the blood pressure range for each of the following:
   a. Prehypertension: ______
   b. Hypertension, stage 1: ______
   c. Hypertension, stage 2: ______
5. Why should blood pressure readings always be interpreted using the patient's baseline blood pressure?
6. How does age affect blood pressure?
7. How do diurnal variations affect blood pressure?
8. What are the two types of stethoscope chest pieces and the use of each?
9. What are the parts of a sphygmomanometer?
10. List the two types of sphygmomanometers.
11. When would each of the following cuffs be used to measure blood pressure?
   a. Child: ______
   b. Adult: ______
   c. Thigh: ______
12. Explain how to determine the proper cuff size for a patient.
13. What may occur if blood pressure is taken using a cuff that is too small or too large?

14. How should the blood pressure be measured if the patient's arm circumference is greater than 50 cm (20 inches)?

____

____

____

15. List the five phases included in Korotkoff's sounds, and describe what type of sound is heard during each phase.

____

____

____

____

____

16. List five advantages of an automated blood pressure monitor.

____

____

____

____

____

CRITICAL THINKING ACTIVITIES

A. Measurement of Body Temperature

For each of the following situations involving the measurement of body temperature, write C if the technique is correct and I if the technique is incorrect. If the situation is correct, state the principle underlying the technique. If the situation is incorrect, explain what might happen if the technique were performed in the incorrect manner.

Electronic Thermometer

_______ 1. The medical assistant takes a patient's oral temperature immediately after the patient has consumed a cup of coffee.

____

____

_______ 2. The medical assistant instructs the patient not to talk while his or her oral temperature is being measured.

____

____

_______ 3. The medical assistant forgets to lubricate the rectal probe before taking a patient's rectal temperature.

____

____

_______ 4. An axillary temperature reading is recorded as follows: 102.2° F.

____

____

_______ 5. The medical assistant discards a used rectal probe in a regular waste container.

____

____

_______ 6. The medical assistant's bare fingers accidentally touch a used oral probe cover while discarding it.

____

____

Tympanic Membrane Thermometer

_______ 1. A thermometer with a dirty probe lens is used to take the patient's temperature.

____

____

_______ 2. The ear canal is straightened before taking a patient's aural temperature.

____

____

_______ 3. The medical assistant does not seal the opening of the ear canal with the probe when taking aural temperature.

____

____

_______ 4. The probe is positioned toward the opposite temple when taking aural temperature.

____

____

_______ 5. The medical assistant waits 30 seconds before taking the patient's temperature in the same ear.

____

____

Temporal Artery Thermometer

_______ 1. The medical assistant checks to make sure the probe lens is clean and intact before using a temporal artery thermometer.

____

____

_______ 2. The medical assistant brushes hair away from the patient's forehead before measuring the patient's temperature.

____

____

_______ 3. The medical assistant slides the temporal artery probe across the patient's forehead while continually depressing the scan button.

____

____

_______ 4. The medical assistant quickly scans the patient's forehead during temporal artery temperature measurement.

____

____

_______ 5. After scanning the forehead, the medical assistant records the patient's temporal artery temperature reading.

____

____

_______ 6. The medical assistant cleans the temporal artery thermometer by immersing it in warm, sudsy water.

____

____

B. Alterations in Body Temperature

Label the following diagram with the terms that describe the body temperature alteration.

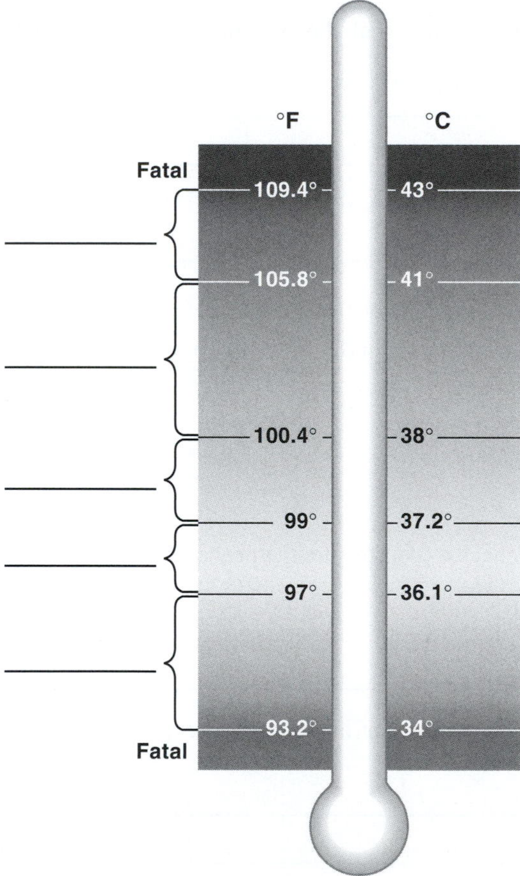

C. Pulse Sites

Locate the pulse at the following sites, and record the pulse rates below:

1. Brachial pulse __________
2. Temporal pulse __________
3. Carotid pulse __________
4. Femoral pulse __________
5. Popliteal pulse __________
6. Dorsalis pedis pulse __________

D. Pulse and Respiratory Rates

Take the pulse and respiration of a person before and after vigorous exercise, and record the results.

1. Before vigorous exercise

2. After vigorous exercise

3. Compare the results, and explain how exercise affects the pulse and respiratory rates.

E. Pulse Oximetry

Your physician asks you to measure the oxygen saturation level of the patients listed. For each situation, answer the following questions:

a. What would you do in each situation to prevent an inaccurate pulse oximetry reading?

b. What occurs with each of these situations and how does it affect the SpO_2 reading?

1. Kelly Collins, a patient with chronic bronchitis, is wearing navy blue nail polish.

2. Melvin Hosey has Parkinson's disease and is having difficulty controlling tremors in his hands.

3. Scott Kimes, a patient with emphysema, frequently experiences periods of prolonged coughing.

4. Nicole Lowe has returned to the office for a recheck of her viral pneumonia. You are getting ready to measure her oxygen saturation and notice that bright sunlight is coming through the window where she is seated and shining on her hand.

____

____

5. Rebecca Bensie, a patient on oxygen therapy, is morbidly obese, and you are having trouble properly aligning the oximeter probe on her finger.

____

____

6. Doug Habbershaw, a patient with peripheral vascular disease, has come to the office for a health checkup.

____

____

7. Emily Lacey has come to the office because she has been experiencing dyspnea. Her hands are very cold, and it is interfering with the pulse oximetry procedure.

____

____

8. Susan Boone, a patient with asthma, is wearing artificial fingernails.

____

____

9. Frank Stewart, a patient with congestive heart failure, is at the office to have a mole removed from his back. There are bright overhead lights in the room, and they cannot be turned off because the physician needs to have good lighting to perform the surgery.

____

____

10. Wanda Weaver is having a sebaceous cyst removed from her chest and has been sedated for the procedure. You have applied an automatic blood pressure cuff to her right arm. The physician asks you to apply an oximeter probe to Wanda's left finger to continuously monitor her oxygen saturation level during the procedure.

____

____

11. Which control, indicator, or display is involved when the following occurs:

    a. The oximeter is searching for a pulse.

    ____

    b. The oximeter cannot find a pulse.

    ____

    c. The oximeter is portraying the strength of the pulse.

    ____

d. The pulse is audibly broadcasted by a beeping sound.

e. The oximeter displays the oxygen saturation level.

f. The oximeter displays the pulse rate.

g. The battery is low.

h. You turn the oximeter off.

F. Blood Pressure Measurement

Using the principles outlined in your textbook, explain what happens under the following circumstances:

1. The blood pressure is taken on a patient who has just undergone vigorous physical exercise.

2. The blood pressure is taken on a patient with tight sleeves.

3. The blood pressure is taken on an apprehensive patient.

4. An adult cuff is used to measure blood pressure on a young child.

5. The blood pressure is taken over clothing.

6. The arm is below heart level during blood pressure measurement.

7. The patient's legs are crossed during blood pressure measurement.

8. The rubber bladder is not centered over the brachial artery.

___

___

9. The cuff is placed ½ inch above the bend in the elbows.

___

___

10. The manometer is viewed from a distance of 4 feet.

___

___

G. Proper BP Cuff Selection

Measurements of the arm circumference (in centimeters) are given for various patients. Using Table 19-9 on page 391 of your textbook, indicate what size of blood pressure cuff (child, small adult, adult, large adult, or adult thigh) should be used with each of these patients.

1. 47 cm: ___
2. 20 cm: ___
3. 32 cm: ___
4. 16 cm: ___
5. 38 cm: ___
6. 27 cm: ___
7. 52 cm: ___
8. 24 cm: ___

Measure the arm circumference of four classmates with a centimeter tape measure, and record the values below. Next to each value, indicate what size blood pressure cuff should be used with each of these individuals.

1. ___
2. ___
3. ___
4. ___

H. Reading Blood Pressure Values

Read and record the following blood pressure measurements in the space provided.

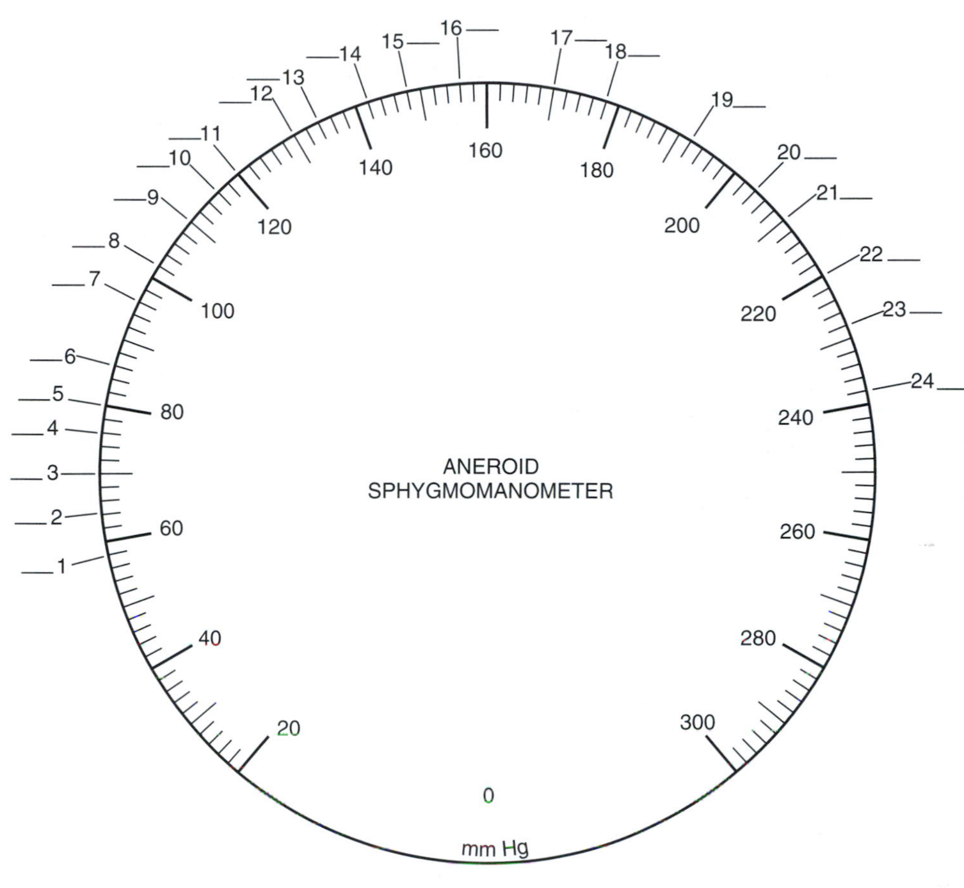

I. Interpreting Blood Pressure Readings

Classify each of the following blood pressure readings into its appropriate category. The readings are based on the average of two or more properly measured and seated blood pressure readings taken at each of two or more visits.

Normal

Prehypertension

Hypertension: Stage 1

Hypertension: Stage 2

1. 90/66: ______________________________
2. 126/76: ______________________________
3. 146/88: ______________________________
4. 120/88: ______________________________
5. 120/80: ______________________________
6. 158/102: ______________________________
7. 134/82: ______________________________
8. 180/106: ______________________________
9. 104/60: ______________________________
10. 148/94: ______________________________

J. Hypertension

Create a profile of an individual who is at risk for hypertension following these guidelines:

1. Using a blank piece of paper and colored pencils, crayons, or markers, draw a figure of an individual exhibiting risk factors for hypertension. Be as creative as possible.
2. Do not use any text in your drawing other than to label items you have drawn in your picture (e.g., cigarettes). A picture is worth a thousand words!
3. Include at least six risk factors for hypertension in your drawing. The Hypertension Patient Teaching Box in your textbook (page 389) can be used as a reference source).
4. In the classroom, choose a partner and trade drawings. Identify the risk factors for hypertension in your partner's drawing. Discuss with your partner what this person could do to lower his or her chances of developing hypertension.

K. Crossword Puzzle: Vital Signs

Directions: Complete the crossword puzzle using the clues provided.

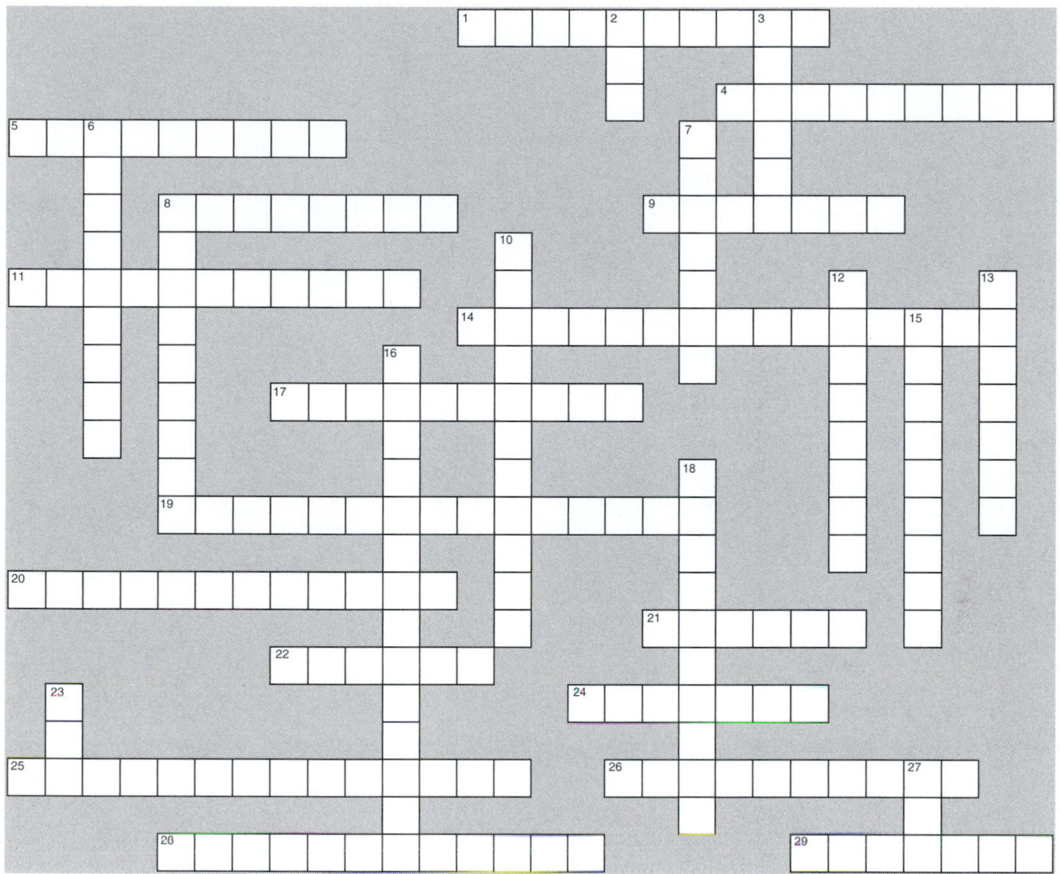

Across

1 Diaphragm or bell
4 Angled stethoscope earpieces
5 BP sounds
8 Has an S-shape
9 European temp measurement
11 Fever reducer
14 Fever increases this by 7% (for each ° F)
17 U.S. temp measurement
19 Lowers pulse rate over time
20 Above 140/90
21 High BP might cause this
22 2400 mg or less per day
24 Asthma breath sounds
25 Center BP cuff over this
26 Risk factor for high BP
28 Cools body
29 Cracked earpieces can cause this

Down

2 Pulse range for exercising
3 Body temperature increaser
6 Fever that occurs with the flu
7 Invented the stethoscope
8 COPD example
10 Profuse perspiration
12 Do this after aerobic exercise
13 Leading cause of COPD
15 Fever causer
16 Drug to help COPD
18 BP position for patient's arm
23 220 minus your age
27 Good cholesterol

Notes

PRACTICE FOR COMPETENCY

Measuring Body Temperature

Measure body temperature with each of the following types of thermometers, and record results in the chart provided.

Procedures 19-1, 19-2, and 19-3: Electronic Thermometer (Oral, Axillary, and Rectal)

Procedure 19-4: Tympanic Membrane Thermometer (Aural)

Procedure 19-5: Temporal Artery Thermometer

Measuring Pulse, Respiration, and Oxygen Saturation

Procedure 19-6: **Pulse and Respiration**. Measure the radial pulse and respiration. Describe the rhythm and volume of the pulse. Describe the rhythm and depth of the respirations. Record the results in the chart provided.

Procedure 19-7: Apical Pulse. Measure apical pulse. Describe the rhythm and volume of the pulse. Record the results in the chart provided.

Procedure 19-8: Pulse Oximetry. Measure the oxygen saturation level and record the results in the chart provided.

Measuring Blood Pressure

Procedure 19-9: Blood Pressure. Measure blood pressure. Record results in the chart provided.

CHART	
Date	

Chart

Date	

EVALUATION OF COMPETENCY

Procedure 19-1: Measuring Oral Body Temperature—Electronic Thermometer

Name: ______________________________ Date: ______________

Evaluated by: ______________________________ Score: ______________

Performance Objective

Outcome:	Measure oral body temperature.
Conditions:	Given the following: electronic thermometer and oral probe, probe cover, and a waste container.
Standards:	Time: 5 minutes. Student completed procedure in __________ minutes.
	Accuracy: Satisfactory score on the Performance Evaluation Checklist.

Performance Evaluation Checklist

Trial 1	Trial 2	Point Value	Performance Standards
		●	Sanitized hands.
		●	Assembled equipment.
		●	Removed thermometer from its storage base.
		●	Attached oral probe to thermometer unit.
		●	Inserted probe into the thermometer.
		●	Greeted the patient and introduced yourself.
		●	Identified the patient and explained the procedure.
		●	Asked the patient if he/she has ingested hot or cold -beverages.
		▷	Explained what to do if the patient has recently ingested a hot or cold beverage.
		●	Removed probe from the thermometer.
		▷	Explained what occurs when probe is removed from the thermometer.
		●	Attached probe cover to probe.
		▷	Stated the purpose of the probe cover.
		●	Correctly inserted the probe in patient's mouth.
		●	Instructed the patient to keep the mouth closed.
		▷	Explained why the mouth should be kept closed.
		●	Held probe in place until an audible tone was heard.
		●	Noted patient's temperature reading on display screen.
		●	Removed probe from patient's mouth.

Trial 1	Trial 2	Point Value	Performance Standards
		●	Discarded probe cover in a regular waste container.
		●	Did not allow fingers to come in contact with cover.
		●	Returned probe to the thermometer unit.
		▷	Stated what occurs when probe is returned to the thermometer.
		●	Returned the thermometer unit to its storage base.
		●	Sanitized hands.
		●	Charted the results correctly.
		*	The temperature recording was identical to the reading on the display screen.
		▷	Stated the normal body temperature range for an adult (97°F to 99°F).
		Ⓐ	Incorporated critical thinking skills when performing patient assessment.
		*	Completed the procedure within 5 minutes.
			TOTALS

CHART	
Date	

Evaluation of Student Performance

EVALUATION CRITERIA			COMMENTS
Symbol	**Category**	**Point Value**	
*	Critical Step	16 points	
●	Essential Step	6 points	
Ⓐ	Affective Competency	6 points	
▷	Theory Question	2 points	
Score calculation: 100 points – ____ points missed ____ Score Satisfactory score: 85 or above			

2008 CAAHEP Competencies Achieved
Psychomotor (Skills) ☑ I. 1. Obtain vital signs. ***Affective (Behavior)*** ☑ I. 1. Apply critical thinking skills in performing patient assessment and care.

2015 CAAHEP Competencies Achieved
Psychomotor (Skills) ☑ I. 1. b. Measure and record temperature. ***Affective (Behavior)*** ☑ I. 1. Incorporate critical thinking skills when performing patient assessment.

ABHES Competency Achieved
☑ 9. b. Obtain vital signs, obtain patient history, and formulate chief complaint.

Notes

EVALUATION OF COMPETENCY

Procedure 19-2: Measuring Axillary Body Temperature—Electronic Thermometer

Name: ______________________ Date: ______________

Evaluated by: ______________________ Score: ______________

Performance Objective

Outcome:	Measure axillary body temperature.
Conditions:	Given the following: electronic thermometer and oral probe, probe cover, and a waste container
Standards:	Time: 5 minutes. Student completed procedure in __________ minutes.
	Accuracy: Satisfactory score on the Performance Evaluation Checklist.

Performance Evaluation Checklist

Trial 1	Trial 2	Point Value	Performance Standards
		●	Sanitized hands.
		●	Assembled equipment.
		●	Removed thermometer from its storage base.
		●	Attached oral probe to thermometer unit.
		●	Inserted probe into the thermometer.
		●	Greeted the patient and introduced yourself.
		●	Identified the patient and explained the procedure.
		●	Removed clothing from patient's shoulder and arm.
		●	Made sure that the axilla was dry.
		●	Removed probe from the thermometer.
		●	Attached probe cover to probe.
		●	Placed probe in the center of the patient's axilla.
		●	Ensured that the arm was held close to the body.
		▷	Explained why the arm must be held close to the body.
		●	Held probe in place until an audible tone was heard.
		●	Removed probe from patient's axilla.
		●	Noted patient's temperature reading on display screen.
		●	Discarded probe cover in a regular waste container.
		●	Did not allow fingers to come in contact with cover.

Trial 1	Trial 2	Point Value	Performance Standards
		●	Returned probe to the thermometer unit.
		●	Returned the thermometer unit to its storage base.
		●	Sanitized hands.
		●	Charted the results correctly.
		*	Temperature recording was identical to the reading on the display screen.
		Ⓐ	Incorporated critical thinking skills when performing patient assessment.
		*	Completed the procedure within 5 minutes.
			TOTALS

CHART	
Date	

Evaluation of Student Performance

EVALUATION CRITERIA			COMMENTS
Symbol	**Category**	**Point Value**	
*	Critical Step	16 points	
●	Essential Step	6 points	
Ⓐ	Affective Competency	6 points	
▷	Theory Question	2 points	
Score calculation: 100 points − ___ points missed ___ Score Satisfactory score: 85 or above			

2008 CAAHEP Competencies Achieved
Psychomotor (Skills) ☑ I. 1. Obtain vital signs. ***Affective (Behavior)*** ☑ I. 1. Apply critical thinking skills in performing patient assessment and care.

2015 CAAHEP Competencies Achieved
Psychomotor (Skills) ☑ I. 1. b. Measure and record temperature. ***Affective (Behavior)*** ☑ I. 1. Incorporate critical thinking skills when performing patient assessment.

ABHES Competency Achieved
☑ 9. b. Obtain vital signs, obtain patient history, and formulate chief complaint.

Notes

EVALUATION OF COMPETENCY

Procedure 19-3: Measuring Rectal Body Temperature—Electronic Thermometer

Name: ______________________________ Date: ______________

Evaluated by: ______________________________ Score: ______________

Performance Objective

Outcome:	Measure rectal body temperature.
Conditions:	Given the following: electronic thermometer, rectal probe, probe cover, lubricant, disposable gloves, tissues, and a waste container.
Standards:	Time: 5 minutes. Student completed procedure in _____ minutes.
	Accuracy: Satisfactory score on the Performance Evaluation Checklist.

Performance Evaluation Checklist

Trial 1	Trial 2	Point Value	Performance Standards
		•	Sanitized hands.
		•	Assembled equipment.
		•	Removed thermometer from its storage base.
		•	Attached rectal probe to thermometer unit.
		•	Inserted probe into the thermometer.
		•	Greeted the patient and introduced yourself.
		•	Identified the patient and explained the procedure.
		•	Applied gloves.
		▷	Stated the reason for applying gloves.
		•	Positioned and draped the patient.
		▷	Explained how to position an adult and an infant.
		•	Removed probe from the thermometer.
		•	Attached probe cover to probe.
		•	Applied lubricant up to a level of 1 inch.
		▷	Stated the purpose of the lubricant.
		•	Instructed patient to lie still.
		•	Separated the buttocks and properly inserted the thermometer.
		▷	Stated how far the thermometer should be inserted for adults, children, and infants.
		•	Held probe in place until an audible tone was heard.

Trial 1	Trial 2	Point Value	Performance Standards
		●	Removed the probe in the same direction as it was inserted.
		●	Noted patient's temperature reading on display screen.
		●	Discarded probe cover in a regular waste container.
		▷	Explained why the cover can be discarded in a regular waste container.
		●	Returned probe to the thermometer unit.
		●	Returned the thermometer unit to its storage base.
		●	Wiped the anal area with tissues.
		●	Removed gloves and sanitized hands.
		●	Charted the results correctly.
		✶	The temperature recording was identical to the reading on the display screen.
		Ⓐ	Incorporated critical thinking skills when performing patient assessment.
		✶	Completed the procedure within 5 minutes.
			TOTALS

Chart	
Date	

Evaluation of Student Performance

EVALUATION CRITERIA			**COMMENTS**
Symbol	**Category**	**Point Value**	
✶	Critical Step	16 points	
●	Essential Step	6 points	
Ⓐ	Affective Competency	6 points	
▷	Theory Question	2 points	
Score calculation: 100 points – ___ points missed ____Score Satisfactory score: 85 or above			

2008 CAAHEP Competencies Achieved
Psychomotor (Skills) ☑ I. 1. Obtain vital signs. ***Affective (Behavior)*** ☑ I. 1. Apply critical thinking skills in performing patient assessment and care.

2015 CAAHEP Competencies Achieved
Psychomotor (Skills) ☑ I. 1. b. Measure and record temperature. ***Affective (Behavior)*** ☑ I. 1. Incorporate critical thinking skills when performing patient assessment.

ABHES Competency Achieved
☑ 9. b. Obtain vital signs, obtain patient history, and formulate chief complaint.

Notes

EVALUATION OF COMPETENCY

Procedure 19-4: Measuring Aural Body Temperature—Tympanic Membrane Thermometer

Name: ______________________ Date: ______________

Evaluated by: ______________________ Score: ______________

Performance Objective

Outcome:	Measure aural body temperature.
Conditions:	Given the following: tympanic membrane thermometer, probe cover, and a waste container.
Standards:	Time: 5 minutes. Student completed procedure in ________ minutes.
	Accuracy: Satisfactory score on the Performance Evaluation Checklist.

Performance Evaluation Checklist

Trial 1	Trial 2	Point Value	Performance Standards
		•	Sanitized hands.
		•	Assembled equipment.
		•	Greeted the patient and introduced yourself.
		•	Identified the patient and explained the procedure.
		•	Removed thermometer from its storage base.
		•	Checked to make sure the probe lens was clean and intact.
		▷	Stated what might occur if the lens was dirty.
		•	Attached a cover on the probe.
		▷	Explained the purpose of the probe cover.
		•	Observed the screen to determine if the thermometer is ready to use.
		•	Held the thermometer in the dominant hand.
		•	Straightened the patient's ear canal with the nondominant hand.
		▷	Explained the purpose of straightening the ear canal.
		•	Inserted the probe into the patient's ear canal and sealed the opening without causing the patient discomfort.
		•	Pointed the tip of the probe toward the opposite temple.
		▷	Stated the reason for pointing the probe toward the opposite temple.
		•	Asked the patient to remain still.
		•	Depressed the activation button for 1 full second or until an audible tone is heard.

Trial 1	Trial 2	Point Value	Performance Standards
		●	Removed the thermometer from the ear canal and noted the patient's temperature on the display screen.
		▷	Stated what should be done if the temperature seems too low.
		●	Disposed of the probe cover in a waste container.
		●	Replaced the thermometer in its storage base.
		▷	Explained the reason for storing the thermometer in its base.
		●	Sanitized hands.
		●	Charted the results correctly.
		*	The temperature recording was identical to the reading on the display screen.
		Ⓐ	Incorporated critical thinking skills when performing patient assessment.
		*	Completed the procedure within 5 minutes.
			TOTALS

CHART	
Date	

Evaluation of Student Performance

EVALUATION CRITERIA			COMMENTS
Symbol	**Category**	**Point Value**	
*	Critical Step	16 points	
●	Essential Step	6 points	
Ⓐ	Affective Competency	6 points	
▷	Theory Question	2 points	
Score calculation: 100 points − ___ points missed ___ Score Satisfactory score: 85 or above			

2008 CAAHEP Competencies Achieved
Psychomotor (Skills) ☑ I. 1. Obtain vital signs. ***Affective (Behavior)*** ☑ I. 1. Apply critical thinking skills in performing patient assessment and care.

2015 CAAHEP Competencies Achieved
Psychomotor (Skills) ☑ I. 1. b. Measure and record temperature. ***Affective (Behavior)*** ☑ I. 1. Incorporate critical thinking skills when performing patient assessment.

ABHES Competency Achieved
☑ 9. b. Obtain vital signs, obtain patient history, and formulate chief complaint.

Notes

EVALUATION OF COMPETENCY

Procedure 19-5: Measuring Temporal Body Temperature

Name: ______________________________ Date: ______________

Evaluated by: ______________________________ Score: ______________

Performance Objective

Outcome:	Measure temporal body temperature.
Conditions:	Given the following: temporal artery thermometer, disposable probe cover, antiseptic wipe, waste container.
Standards:	Time: 5 minutes. Student completed procedure in __________ minutes.
	Accuracy: Satisfactory score on the Performance Evaluation Checklist.

Performance Evaluation Checklist

Trial 1	Trial 2	Point Value	Performance Standards
		•	Sanitized the hands and assembled equipment.
		•	Greeted the patient and introduced yourself.
		•	Identified the patient and explained the procedure.
		•	Checked to make sure the probe lens is clean and intact.
		▷	Stated why the lens should be clean.
		•	Placed a disposable cover onto the probe or cleaned the probe with an antiseptic wipe and allowed it to dry.
		•	Selected an appropriate site (right or left side of the forehead)
		•	Brushed away any hair that is covering the scanning sites.
		▷	Explained why hair must be brushed away.
		•	Held the thermometer in the dominant hand with the thumb on the scan button.
		•	Gently positioned the probe of the thermometer on the center of the patient's forehead midway between the eyebrow and hairline.
		•	Depressed the scan button and kept it depressed for the entire measurement.
		▷	Stated why the scan button must be continually depressed.
		•	Slowly and gently slid the probe straight across the forehead midway between the eyebrow and the upper hairline.
		•	Continued until the hairline was reached making sure to keep the probe flush against the forehead.
		•	Keeping the button depressed, lifted the probe from the forehead and placed it behind the earlobe for 1 to 2 seconds.

Trial 1	Trial 2	Point Value	Performance Standards
		▷	Stated why the probe is placed behind the earlobe.
		●	Released the scan button and noted the temperature on the display screen.
		●	Disposed of the probe cover in a regular waste container.
		●	Wiped the probe with an antiseptic wipe and allowed it to dry.
		●	Sanitized hands.
		●	Charted the results correctly.
		*	The temperature recording was identical to the reading on the display screen.
		●	Stored the thermometer in a clean, dry area.
		Ⓐ	Incorporated critical thinking skills when performing patient assessment.
		*	Completed the procedure within 5 minutes.
			TOTALS

CHART	
Date	

Evaluation of Student Performance

EVALUATION CRITERIA			COMMENTS
Symbol	Category	Point Value	
*	Critical Step	16 points	
●	Essential Step	6 points	
Ⓐ	Affective Competency	6 points	
▷	Theory Question	2 points	
Score calculation: 100 points – ___ points missed ___ Score Satisfactory score: 85 or above			

2008 CAAHEP Competencies Achieved
Psychomotor (Skills) ☑ I. 1. Obtain vital signs. ***Affective (Behavior)*** ☑ I. 1. Apply critical thinking skills in performing patient assessment and care.

2015 CAAHEP Competencies Achieved
Psychomotor (Skills) ☑ I. 1. b. Measure and record temperature. ***Affective (Behavior)*** ☑ I. 1. Incorporate critical thinking skills when performing patient assessment.

ABHES Competencies Achieved
☑ 9. b. Obtain vital signs, obtain patient history, and formulate chief complaint.

Notes

EVALUATION OF COMPETENCY

Procedure 19-6: Measuring Pulse and Respiration

Name: ______________________ Date: ______________

Evaluated by: ______________________ Score: ______________

Performance Objective

Outcome:	Measure radial pulse and respiration.
Conditions:	Using a watch with a second hand.
Standards:	Time: 5 minutes. Student completed procedure in __________ minutes.
	Accuracy: Satisfactory score on the performance evaluation checklist.

Performance Evaluation Checklist

Trial 1	Trial 2	Point Value	Performance Standards
		●	Sanitized hands.
		●	Greeted the patient and introduced yourself.
		●	Identified the patient and explained the procedure.
		●	Observed patient for any signs that might affect the pulse rate or respiratory rate.
		▷	Stated two factors that would increase the pulse rate.
		●	Positioned the patient in a comfortable seated position.
		●	Placed three middle fingertips over the radial pulse site.
		▷	Explained why the pulse should not be taken with the thumb.
		●	Applied moderate, gentle pressure until the pulse was felt.
		▷	Stated what will occur if too much pressure is applied over the radial artery.
		●	Counted the pulse for 30 seconds and made a mental note of the number.
		●	Determined the rhythm and volume of the pulse.
		▷	Stated when the pulse should be measured for a full minute.
		●	Continued to hold the fingers on the patient's wrist.
		▷	Explained why respirations should be taken without the patient's awareness.
		●	Observed the rise and fall of patient's chest.
		●	Counted the number of respirations for 30 seconds and made a mental note of the number.
		▷	Stated what makes up one respiration.
		●	Determined the rhythm and depth of the respirations.

Trial 1	Trial 2	Point Value	Performance Standards
		●	Observed the patient's color.
		●	Sanitized hands.
		●	Multiplied the pulse and respiration values by 2.
		●	Charted the results correctly.
		✶	The pulse rate was within ± 2 beats of the evaluator's reading.
		✶	The respiratory rate was within 1 respiration of the evaluator's measurement.
		▷	Stated the normal adult range for the pulse rate (60 to 100 beats/min).
		▷	Stated the normal adult range for the respiratory rate (12 to 20 respirations/minute).
		Ⓐ	Incorporated critical thinking skills when performing patient assessment.
		✶	Completed the procedure within 5 minutes.
			TOTALS

CHART	
Date	

Evaluation of Student Performance

EVALUATION CRITERIA			COMMENTS
Symbol	**Category**	**Point Value**	
✶	Critical Step	16 points	
●	Essential Step	6 points	
Ⓐ	Affective Competency	6 points	
▷	Theory Question	2 points	
Score calculation: 100 points – ___points missed ___Score Satisfactory score: 85 or above			

2008 CAAHEP Competencies Achieved
Psychomotor (Skills) ☑ I. 1. Obtain vital signs. ***Affective (Behavior)*** ☑ I. 1. Apply critical thinking skills in performing patient assessment and care.

2015 CAAHEP Competencies Achieved
Psychomotor (Skills) ☑ I. 1. c. Measure and record pulse. ☑ I. 1. d. Measure and record respirations. ***Affective (Behavior)*** ☑ I. 1. Incorporate critical thinking skills when performing patient assessment.

ABHES Competency Achieved
☑ 9. b. Obtain vital signs, obtain patient history, and formulate chief complaint.

Notes

EVALUATION OF COMPETENCY

Procedure 19-7: Measuring Apical Pulse

Name: ______________________________ Date: ______________

Evaluated by: ______________________________ Score: ______________

Performance Objective

Outcome:	Measure apical pulse.
Conditions:	Given the following: stethoscope and antiseptic wipe.
Standards:	Using a watch with a second hand.
	Time: 5 minutes. Student completed procedure in __________ minutes.
	Accuracy: Satisfactory score on the Performance Evaluation Checklist.

Performance Evaluation Checklist

Trial 1	Trial 2	Point Value	Performance Standards
		●	Sanitized hands.
		●	Greeted the patient and introduced yourself.
		●	Identified the patient and explained the procedure.
		●	Observed the patient for any signs that might affect the pulse rate.
		●	Assembled equipment.
		●	Rotated the chest piece to the bell position.
		●	Cleaned earpieces and chest piece with antiseptic wipe.
		▷	Stated the reason for cleaning stethoscope with an -antiseptic.
		●	Asked the patient to unbutton or remove his or her shirt.
		●	Positioned patient in a sitting or lying position.
		●	Warmed chest piece of the stethoscope.
		▷	Explained the reason for warming chest piece.
		●	Inserted earpieces of stethoscope in a forward position in the ears.
		▷	Explained why the earpieces must be directed forward.
		●	Placed the chest piece over the apex of the heart.
		▷	Described the location of the apex of the heart.
		●	Counted the number of heartbeats for 30 seconds and multiplied by 2.
		*	The reading was within ±2 beats of the evaluator's -reading.
		●	Sanitized hands.

Trial 1	Trial 2	Point Value	Performance Standards
		●	Charted the results correctly.
		Ⓐ	Incorporated critical thinking skills when performing patient assessment.
		●	Cleaned earpieces and chest piece with an antiseptic wipe.
		*	Completed the procedure within 5 minutes.
			TOTALS

CHART	
Date	

Evaluation of Student Performance

EVALUATION CRITERIA			COMMENTS
Symbol	**Category**	**Point Value**	
*	Critical Step	16 points	
●	Essential Step	6 points	
Ⓐ	Affective Competency	6 points	
▷	Theory Question	2 points	
Score calculation: 100 points − ___ points missed ___ Score Satisfactory score: 85 or above			

2008 CAAHEP Competencies Achieved
Psychomotor (Skills) ☑ I. 1. Obtain vital signs. ***Affective (Behavior)*** ☑ I. 1. Apply critical thinking skills in performing patient assessment and care.

2015 CAAHEP Competencies Achieved
Psychomotor (Skills) ☑ I. 1. c. Measure and record pulse. ***Affective (Behavior)*** ☑ I. 1. Incorporate critical thinking skills when performing patient assessment.

ABHES Competency Achieved
☑ 9. b. Obtain vital signs, obtain patient history, and formulate chief complaint.

EVALUATION OF COMPETENCY

Procedure 19-8: Performing Pulse Oximetry

Name: ______________________ Date: ______________

Evaluated by: ______________________ Score: ______________

Performance Objective

Outcome:	Perform pulse oximetry.
Conditions:	Given the following: handheld pulse oximeter, reusable finger probe, and an antiseptic wipe.
Standards:	Time: 5 minutes. Student completed procedure in minutes.
	Accuracy: Satisfactory score on the Performance Evaluation Checklist.

Performance Evaluation Checklist

Trial 1	Trial 2	Point Value	Performance Standards
		●	Sanitized hands and assembled equipment.
		●	Ensured the probe opened and closed smoothly and that the windows were clean.
		●	Disinfected the probe windows and platforms and allowed them to dry.
		▷	Stated the purpose of disinfecting the probe windows.
		●	If necessary, connected the probe to the cable.
		●	Connected the cable to the monitor.
		●	Did not lift or carry the monitor by the cable.
		●	Greeted the patient and introduced yourself.
		●	Identified the patient and explained the procedure.
		●	Seated the patient in a chair with the lower arm supported and the palm facing down.
		▷	Explained why the arm should be supported.
		●	Selected an appropriate finger to apply the probe.
		●	Observed the patient's finger to make sure it is free of dark fingernail polish or an artificial nail.
		●	Checked to make sure the patient's fingertip is clean.
		●	Checked to make sure the patient's finger is not cold.
		▷	Explained what to do if the patient's finger is cold
		●	Made sure that ambient light will not interfere with the measurement.
		▷	Explained why ambient light should be avoided.

Trial 1	Trial 2	Point Value	Performance Standards
		●	Positioned the probe securely on the fingertip with the fleshy tip of the finger covering the window.
		●	Allowed the cable to lie across the back of the hand and parallel to the arm of the patient.
		●	Instructed the patient to remain still and to breathe -normally.
		▷	Stated why the patient must remain still.
		●	Turned on the pulse oximeter.
		●	Waited while the oximeter went through its power-on self-test (POST).
		▷	Explained the purpose of the POST.
		●	Allowed several seconds for the oximeter to detect the pulse and -calculate the oxygen saturation.
		●	Ensured that the pulse strength indicator fluctuates with each pulsation and that the pulse signal is strong.
		▷	Stated what should be done if the oximeter is unable to locate a pulse.
		●	Left the probe in place until the oximeter displayed a reading.
		●	Noted the oxygen saturation value and pulse rate.
		*	The reading was identical to the evaluator's reading.
		▷	Stated the normal oxygen saturation level of a healthy adult (95% to 99%).
		▷	Stated what should be done if the oxygen saturation is less than 95%.
		●	Removed the probe from the patient's finger and turned off the -oximeter.
		●	Sanitized hands.
		●	Charted the results correctly.
		●	Disconnected the cable from the monitor.
		●	Disinfected the probe with an antiseptic wipe.
		●	Properly stored the monitor in a clean dry area.
		Ⓐ	Incorporated critical thinking skills when performing patient assessment.
		*	Completed the procedure within 5 minutes.
			TOTALS

Chart	
Date	

Evaluation of Student Performance

EVALUATION CRITERIA			COMMENTS
Symbol	**Category**	**Point Value**	
✶	Critical Step	16 points	
●	Essential Step	6 points	
Ⓐ	Affective Competency	6 points	
▷	Theory Question	2 points	
Score calculation: 100 points – ___ points missed ___ Score Satisfactory score: 85 or above			

2008 CAAHEP Competencies Achieved
Psychomotor (Skills) ☑ I. 1. Obtain vital signs. ***Affective (Behavior)*** ☑ I. 1. Apply critical thinking skills in performing patient assessment and care.

2015 CAAHEP Competencies Achieved
Psychomotor (Skills) ☑ I. 1. i. Measure and record pulse oximetry. ***Affective (Behavior)*** ☑ I. 1. Incorporate critical thinking skills when performing patient assessment.

ABHES Competency Achieved
☑ 9. b. Obtain vital signs, obtain patient history, and formulate chief complaint.

Notes

EVALUATION OF COMPETENCY

Procedure 19-9: Measuring Blood Pressure

Name: ______________________________ Date: ______________

Evaluated by: ______________________________ Score: ______________

Performance Objective

Outcome:	Measure blood pressure.
Conditions:	Given the following: stethoscope, sphygmomanometer, and an antiseptic wipe.
Standards:	Time: 5 minutes. Student completed procedure in __________ minutes.
	Accuracy: Satisfactory score on the Performance Evaluation Checklist.

Performance Evaluation Checklist

Trial 1	Trial 2	Point Value	Performance Standards
		●	Sanitized hands.
		●	Assembled equipment.
		●	Rotated the chest piece to the diaphragm position.
		●	Cleaned earpieces and chest piece of stethoscope with an antiseptic wipe.
		●	Greeted the patient and introduced yourself.
		●	Identified the patient and explained the procedure.
		●	Observed patient for any signs that might influence the blood pressure reading.
		▷	Stated signs that would influence the blood pressure -reading.
		●	Determined how high to pump the cuff (palpated systolic pressure or checking the patient's chart).
		●	Positioned patient in a sitting position with the legs uncrossed.
		●	Made sure that the patient's arm was uncovered.
		▷	Explained why blood pressure should not be taken over clothing.
		●	Positioned patient's arm at heart level with the palm -facing up.
		●	Selected the proper cuff size.
		▷	Explained how to determine the proper cuff size.
		▷	Made sure the cuff was completely deflated and there was no residual air in the cuff.
		●	Located the brachial pulse with the fingertips.
		▷	Stated the location of the brachial pulse.
		●	Centered bladder over the brachial pulse site.

Trial 1	Trial 2	Point Value	Performance Standards
		▷	Explained why the bladder should be centered over the brachial pulse site.
		●	Placed cuff on patient's arm 1 to 2 inches above bend in elbow.
		●	Wrapped cuff smoothly and snugly around patient's arm and secured it.
		●	Positioned self and/or manometer for direct viewing and at a distance of no more than 3 feet.
		●	Instructed the patient not to talk.
		●	Inserted earpieces of stethoscope in a forward position in the ears.
		●	Located the brachial pulse again.
		●	Placed diaphragm of the stethoscope over the brachial pulse site to make a tight seal.
		▷	Explained why there should be good contact of the chest piece with the skin.
		●	Made sure chest piece was not touching cuff.
		▷	Explained why the chest piece should not touch the cuff.
		●	Closed valve on bulb by turning thumbscrew to the right.
		●	Rapidly pumped air into cuff up to a level approximately 30 mm Hg above the palpated or previously measured -systolic pressure.
		●	Did not overinflate the cuff.
		▷	Explained why the cuff should not be overinflated.
		●	Released pressure at a moderate, steady rate by turning thumbscrew to the left.
		●	Heard and noted the first clear tapping sound (systolic pressure).
		●	Continued to deflate the cuff for another 10 mm Hg.
		●	Heard and noted the point on the scale at which the sounds ceased (diastolic pressure).
		●	Quickly and completely deflated cuff to zero and removed earpieces from ears.
		▷	Stated how long to wait before taking the blood pressure again on the same arm.
		●	Carefully removed cuff from patient's arm.
		●	Sanitized hands.
		●	Charted the results correctly.
		*	The reading was within ± 2 mm Hg of the evaluator's reading.
		▷	Stated the normal blood pressure for an adult (less than 120/80 mm Hg).
		●	Cleaned earpieces and chest piece with an antiseptic wipe.
		Ⓐ	Incorporated critical thinking skills when performing patient assessment.
		*	Completed the procedure within 5 minutes.
			TOTALS

CHART	
Date	

Evaluation of Student Performance

EVALUATION CRITERIA			COMMENTS
Symbol	**Category**	**Point Value**	
✶	Critical Step	16 points	
●	Essential Step	6 points	
Ⓐ	Affective Competency	6 points	
▷	Theory Question	2 points	
Score calculation: 100 points – ___ points missed ___ Score Satisfactory score: 85 or above			

2008 CAAHEP Competencies Achieved
Psychomotor (Skills) ☑ I. 1. Obtain vital signs. ***Affective (Behavior)*** ☑ I. 1. Apply critical thinking skills in performing patient assessment and care.

2015 CAAHEP Competencies Achieved
Psychomotor (Skills) ☑ I. 1. a. Measure and record blood pressure. ***Affective (Behavior)*** ☑ I. 1. Incorporate critical thinking skills when performing patient assessment.

ABHES Competency Achieved
☑ 9. b. Obtain vital signs, obtain patient history, and formulate chief complaint.

Notes

20 The Physical Examination

CHAPTER ASSIGNMENTS

✓ After Completing	Date Due	Study Guide Pages	STUDY GUIDE ASSIGNMENTS (CTA = Critical Thinking Activity)	Possible Points	Points You Earned
		367	Pretest	10	
		368 368	Key Term Assessment A. Definitions B. Word Parts (Add 1 point for each key term)	17 9	
		369-372	Evaluation of Learning questions	31	
		372	CTA A: Preparation of the Examining Room	10	
		373	CTA B: Reading Weight Measurements	15	
			Evolve Site: By the Pound (Record points earned)		
		374	CTA C: Reading Height Measurements	11	
			Evolve Site: Feet and Inches (Record points earned)		
		375	CTA D: Calculating BMI	12	
		375	CTA E: Patient Positions	10	
			Evolve Site: Let's Get Physical (Record points earned)		
		376	CTA F: Examination Techniques	10	
		377	CTA G: Crossword Puzzle	25	
			Evolve Site: Apply Your Knowledge questions	10	

✓ After Completing	Date Due	Study Guide Pages	STUDY GUIDE ASSIGNMENTS (CTA = Critical Thinking Activity)	Possible Points	Points You Earned
			Evolve Site: Video Evaluation	54	
		367	Posttest	10	
			ADDITIONAL ASSIGNMENTS		
			TOTAL POINTS		

✓ When Assigned By Your Instructor	Study Guide Pages	Practices Required	LABORATORY ASSIGNMENTS (Procedure Number and Name)	Score*
	379-380	5	**Practice for Competency** 20-1: Measuring Weight and Height Textbook reference: pp. 415-416	
	381-383		**Evaluation of Competency** 20-1: Measuring Weight and Height	*
	379-380		**Practice for Competency** 20-A: Body Mechanics Textbook reference: pp. 418-420	
	385-387		**Evaluation of Competency** 20-A: Body Mechanics	*
	379-380	3	**Practice for Competency** 20-2: Sitting Position Textbook reference: p. 421	
	389-390		**Evaluation of Competency** 20-2: Sitting Position	*
	379-380	3	**Practice for Competency** 20-3: Supine Position Textbook reference: p. 422	
	391-392		**Evaluation of Competency** 20-3: Supine Position	*
	379-380	3	**Practice for Competency** 20-4: Prone Position Textbook reference: p. 423	
	393-395		**Evaluation of Competency** 20-4: Prone Position	*
	379-380	3	**Practice for Competency** 20-5: Dorsal Recumbent Position Textbook reference: p. 424	
	397-398		**Evaluation of Competency** 20-5: Dorsal Recumbent Position	*
	379-380	3	**Practice for Competency** 20-6: Lithotomy Position Textbook reference: pp. 425-426	
	399-401		**Evaluation of Competency** 20-6: Lithotomy Position	*
	379-380	3	**Practice for Competency** 20-7: Sims Position Textbook reference: pp. 426-427	
	403-405		**Evaluation of Competency** 20-7: Sims Position	*

✓ When Assigned By Your Instructor	Study Guide Pages	Practices Required	LABORATORY ASSIGNMENTS (Procedure Number and Name)	Score*
	379-380	3	**Practice for Competency** 20-8: Knee-Chest Position Textbook reference: pp. 427-428	
	407-409		**Evaluation of Competency** 20-8: Knee-Chest Position	*
	379-380	3	**Practice for Competency** 20-9: Fowler's Position Textbook reference: pp. 428-429	
	411-412		**Evaluation of Competency** 20-9: Fowler's Position	*
	379-380	3	**Practice for Competency** 20-10: Wheelchair Transfer Textbook reference: pp. 430-434	
	413-416		**Evaluation of Competency** 20-10: Wheelchair Transfer	*
	379-380	3	**Practice for Competency** 20-11: Assisting with the Physical Examination Textbook reference: pp. 436-438	
	417-420		**Evaluation of Competency** 20-11: Assisting with the Physical Examination	*
			ADDITIONAL ASSIGNMENTS	

Name ______________________________ Date ______________

PRETEST

True or False

_______ 1. A complete patient examination consists of a physical examination and laboratory tests.

_______ 2. Arthritis is an example of a chronic illness.

_______ 3. An otoscope is used to examine the eyes.

_______ 4. A patient should be identified by name and date of birth.

_______ 5. The reason for weighing a prenatal patient is to determine the baby's due date.

_______ 6. The height of an adult is measured during every office visit.

_______ 7. The lithotomy position is used to examine the vagina.

_______ 8. Inspection involves the observation of the patient for any signs of disease.

_______ 9. Measuring blood pressure is an example of auscultation.

_______ 10. The supine position is used to examine the back.

POSTTEST

True or False

_______ 1. The prognosis is what is wrong with the patient.

_______ 2. A risk factor means that a patient will develop a certain disease.

_______ 3. Electrocardiography is an example of a therapeutic procedure.

_______ 4. The function of a speculum is to open a body orifice for viewing.

_______ 5. The process of measuring the patient is called mensuration.

_______ 6. A reason for weighing a child is to determine drug dosage.

_______ 7. The purpose of draping a patient is to make it easier for the physician to examine the patient.

_______ 8. Sims' position is used for flexible sigmoidoscopy.

_______ 9. Measuring pulse is an example of percussion.

_______ 10. BMI is the acronym for *body mass index.*

Term KEY TERM ASSESSMENT

A. Definitions

Directions: Match each key term with its definition.

_______ 1. Audiometer
_______ 2. Auscultation
_______ 3. Bariatrics
_______ 4. Body mechanics
_______ 5. Clinical diagnosis
_______ 6. Diagnosis
_______ 7. Differential diagnosis
_______ 8. Inspection
_______ 9. Mensuration
_______ 10. Ophthalmoscope
_______ 11. Otoscope
_______ 12. Palpation
_______ 13. Percussion
_______ 14. Percussion hammer
_______ 15. Prognosis
_______ 16. Speculum
_______ 17. Symptom

A. An instrument for examining the interior of the eye
B. A tentative diagnosis obtained through the evaluation of the health history and the physical examination, without the benefit of laboratory or diagnostic tests
C. An instrument for opening a body orifice or cavity for viewing
D. An instrument used to measure hearing
E. The process of measuring a patient
F. The scientific method for determining and identifying a patient's condition
G. The process of tapping the body to detect signs of disease
H. The process of observing a patient to detect any signs of disease
I. Any change in the body or its functioning that indicates that a disease might be present
J. The process of listening to the sounds produced within the body to detect signs of disease
K. A determination of which of two or more diseases with similar symptoms is producing the patient's symptoms
L. An instrument for examining the external ear canal and tympanic membrane
M. The process of feeling with the hands to detect signs of disease
N. An instrument with a rubber head, used for testing reflexes
O. The probable course and outcome of a patient's condition and the patient's prospects for recovery
P. The branch of medicine that deals with the treatment and control of obesity and diseases associated with obesity
Q. Use of the correct muscles to maintain proper balance, posture, and body alignment to accomplish a task safely and efficiently.

B. Word Parts

Directions: Indicate the meaning of each word part in the space provided. List as many medical terms as possible that incorporate the word part in the space provided.

Word Part	Meaning of Word Part	Medical Terms That Incorporate Word Part
1. audi/o		
2. -meter		
3. bar/o		
4. -iatrics		
5. dia-		
6. -gnosis		
7. ophthalm/o		
8. -scope		
9. ot/o		

EVALUATION OF LEARNING

Directions: Fill in each blank with the correct answer.

1. What are the three parts of a complete patient examination?

____

____

2. List two functions of the physical examination.

____

____

3. What is the purpose of establishing a final diagnosis?

____

____

4. Why is there a space for indicating the clinical diagnosis on the laboratory request form?

____

____

5. What is a *risk factor*?

____

____

6. What is an acute illness? List two examples of acute illnesses.

____

____

7. What is a chronic illness? List two examples of chronic illnesses.

____

____

8. What is the difference between a therapeutic procedure and a diagnostic procedure?

____

____

____

9. How should a patient be identified?

____

____

10. Why is it important to properly identify the patient?

____

____

11. How can patient apprehension be reduced during a physical examination?

12. Why should patients be asked if they need to void before the physical examination?

13. What are two examples of locations for placing a paper-based patient record (PPR) for review by the physician?

14. What is the purpose for measuring weight?

15. Why is it important to use proper body mechanics?

16. What are the four curvatures of the vertebral column, and what is their purpose?

17. What body mechanics principles should be followed for each of the following?

    a. Physical condition of the body

    b. Reaching for something

    c. Working height

    d. Storing heavy and lighter items on shelves

    e. Retrieving an item from an overhead shelf

f. Lifting an object

g. Transferring a patient

h. Patient who starts to fall

i. You are unsure about your ability to lift a heavy object

18. What is the purpose of positioning and draping?

19. Indicate three types of examinations for which the supine position is used.

20. Indicate two types of examinations for which the lithotomy position is used.

21. Indicate one type of examination for which the knee-chest position is used.

22. What is the purpose of a wheelchair?

23. What is the purpose of a transfer belt for both the patient and the medical assistant?

24. What should the medical assistant do if he or she does not think it is possible to transfer a patient from a wheelchair to the examining table?

25. What is performed during a complete physical examination?

____

____

26. What is the advantage of using EMR software to record the results of a physical examination?

____

____

27. What are four types of assessments that can be made through inspection?

____

____

28. What are four types of assessments that can be made through palpation?

____

____

29. What can be assessed through the use of percussion?

____

____

30. What type of assessments can be made using auscultation?

____

____

31. What type of stethoscope chest piece should be used to assess the heart?

____

CRITICAL THINKING ACTIVITIES

A. Preparation of the Examining Room

For each of the following examining room preparation guidelines, indicate the problems that may result if the guideline is not followed.

	Preparation	Problems If Not Performed
1.	Ensure the examining room is well lit.	
2.	Restock supplies that are getting low.	
3.	Empty waste containers frequently.	
4.	Replace biohazard containers as necessary.	
5.	Make sure room is well ventilated.	
6.	Maintain room temperature that is comfortable for the patient.	
7.	Clean and disinfect examining table daily.	
8.	Change the examining table paper after each patient.	
9.	Check equipment and instruments to make sure they are in proper working condition.	
10.	Know how to operate and care for each piece of equipment and instrument.	

B. Reading Weight Measurements

The diagram is an illustration of a portion of the calibration bar of an upright balance beam scale. In the spaces provided, record the weight measurements indicated on the calibration bar. In all cases, assume that the lower weight is resting in the 100-lb notched groove.

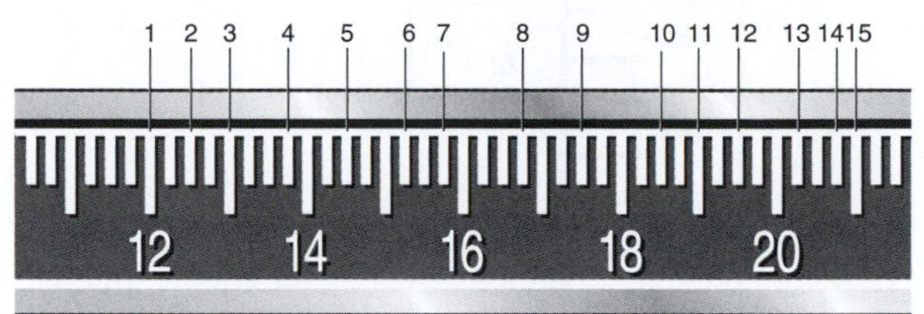

1. ____________________
2. ____________________
3. ____________________
4. ____________________
5. ____________________
6. ____________________
7. ____________________
8. ____________________
9. ____________________
10. ____________________
11. ____________________
12. ____________________
13. ____________________
14. ____________________
15. ____________________

C. Reading Height Measurements

The diagram is an illustration of a portion of the calibration rod of an upright balance beam scale. In the spaces provided, indicate the height measurements in feet and inches indicated on the calibration rod.

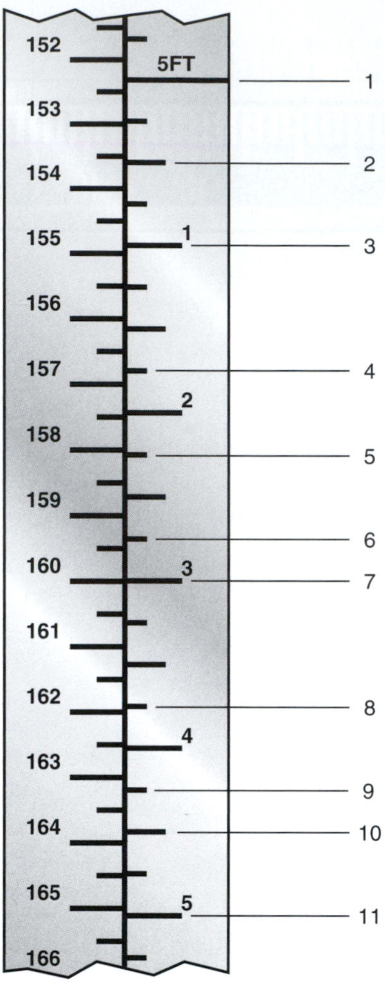

1. ____________________
2. ____________________
3. ____________________
4. ____________________
5. ____________________
6. ____________________
7. ____________________
8. ____________________
9. ____________________
10. ____________________
11. ____________________

D. Calculating Body Mass Index

1. Using the Highlight on Interpreting Body Weight box on page 360 of your textbook, calculate and interpret your BMI and record the results below.

____

2. Calculate the BMI of the following individuals, and record the value in the space provided. Interpret each BMI value according to the information indicated in Highlight on Interpreting Body Weight as follows: underweight, healthy weight, overweight, obesity (I), obesity (II), extreme obesity (III).

	Weight	Height	BMI	Interpretation of BMI
1.	146	5 ft 5 in		
2.	175	5 ft 6 in		
3.	110	5 ft 9 in		
4.	122	5 ft 1 in		
5.	260	6 ft		
6.	180	6 ft 8 in		
7.	330	5 ft 11 in		
8.	150	5 ft 4 in		
9.	170	5 ft 2 in		
10.	151	6 ft 4 in		

3. List the diseases that an individual with an above-normal BMI has an increased chance of developing.

____

____

____

____

E. Patient Positions

In which position would you place the patient for the following examinations or procedures?

1. Measurement of rectal temperature of an adult ______________________
2. Examination of the back ______________________
3. Measurement of vital signs ______________________
4. Pelvic examination ______________________
5. Examination of the upper extremities ______________________
6. Examination of the eyes, ears, nose, and throat ______________________
7. Examination of the breasts ______________________
8. Flexible sigmoidoscopy ______________________
9. Administration of an enema ______________________
10. Examination of the upper body of a patient with emphysema ______________________

F. Examination Techniques

List the examination technique (e.g., inspection, palpation, percussion, auscultation) that is used in each of the following situations.

1. A patient with a stutter ______
2. Taking the radial pulse ______
3. Finding the location of the apical pulse ______
4. Taking the apical pulse ______
5. Taking respiration (may be two answers, depending on method) ______
6. A patient with cracked lips ______
7. Checking for lumps in the breast ______
8. Checking reflexes ______
9. Obtaining the fetal heart rate ______
10. A patient with a fever (may be several methods) ______

G. Crossword Puzzle: The Physical Examination

Directions: Complete the crossword puzzle using the clues provided.

Across

1 Eye examiner
5 Ear examiner
7 BMI: 16 to 18.49
9 BMI: 25 to 29.9
10 "Listen to heart" position
14 Measuring the patient
16 I am listening
20 Metric unit of height
22 Metric unit of weight
23 Curative procedure
24 Reflex tester
25 Can cause premature death

Down

2 Hearing tester
3 Flex sigmoid position
4 Face-down
6 Orifice opener
8 What is the probable outcome?
11 What is wrong with you?
12 Before you measure weight
13 GYN position
15 Five feet in inches
17 Severe and intense condition
18 Provides warmth and modesty
19 Long-time illness
21 Face-up

Notes

PRACTICE FOR COMPETENCY

Procedure 20-1: Weight and Height. Take weight and height measurements. Record results in the chart provided.

Procedure 20-A: Body Mechanics. Demonstrate proper body mechanics while standing, sitting, and lifting an object.

Procedures 20-2 to 20-9: Positioning and Draping. Position and drape an individual in each of the following positions: sitting, supine, prone, dorsal recumbent, lithotomy, Sims', knee-chest, and Fowler's.

Procedure 20-10: Wheelchair Transfer. Transfer a patient from a wheelchair to the examining table and from the examining table to a wheelchair.

Procedure 20-11: Assisting with the Physical Examination. Prepare the patient and assist, with a physical examination. In the chart provided, record the results of the procedures you performed while assisting with the examination (e.g., vital signs, height, and weight).

Chart	
Date	

Chart	
Date	

EVALUATION OF COMPETENCY

Procedure 20-1: Measuring Weight and Height

Name: ______________________ Date: ______________

Evaluated by: ______________________ Score: ______________

Performance Objective

Outcome:	Measure weight and height.
Conditions:	Given a paper towel.
	Using an upright balance scale.
Standards:	Time: 5 minutes. Student completed procedure in _________ minutes.
	Accuracy: Satisfactory score on the performance evaluation checklist.

Performance Evaluation Checklist

Trial 1	Trial 2	Point Value	Performance Standards
			Weight
		•	Sanitized hands.
			Checked the balance scale for accuracy
		•	Verified that the upper and lower weights were on zero.
		•	Looked at the indicator point to make sure the scale is balanced.
		▷	Stated what will be observed if the scale is balanced.
		▷	Explained what to do if the indicator point rests below the center.
		▷	Explained what to do if the indicator point rests above the center.
		▷	Stated what occurs if the scale is not balanced.
		•	Greeted the patient and introduced yourself.
		•	Identified the patient and explained the procedure.
		•	Instructed patient to remove shoes and heavy outer clothing.
		•	Placed paper towel on the scale.
		•	Assisted patient onto the scale.
		•	Instructed patient not to move.
			Balanced the scale
		•	Moved the lower weight to the groove that did not cause the indicator point to drop to the bottom of the balance area.
		▷	Stated why the lower weight should be seated firmly in its groove.

Trial 1	Trial 2	Point Value	Performance Standards
		●	Slid the upper weight slowly until the indicator point came to a rest at the center of the balance area.
		●	Read the results to the nearest quarter pound. Jotted down this value or made a mental note of it.
		✱	The reading was identical to the evaluator's reading.
		●	Asked the patient to step off the scale.
			Height
		●	Slid the calibration rod until it was above the patient's height.
		●	Opened the measuring bar to its horizontal position.
		●	Instructed the patient to step onto the scale platform with his or her back to the scale.
		●	Instructed patient to stand erect and to look straight ahead.
		●	Carefully lowered the measuring bar until it rested gently on top of the patient's head.
		●	Verified that the bar was in a horizontal position.
		●	Instructed the patient to step down and put on his or her shoes.
		●	Read the marking to the nearest quarter inch. Jotted down this value or made a mental note of it.
		✱	The reading was identical to the evaluator's reading.
		●	Returned the measuring bar to its vertical position.
		●	Slid the calibration rod to its lowest position.
		●	Returned the weights to zero.
		●	Sanitized hands.
		●	Charted the results correctly.
		Ⓐ	Demonstrated a. empathy b. active listening c. nonverbal communication.
		Ⓐ	Demonstrated the principles of self-boundaries.
		✱	Completed the procedure within 5 minutes.
			TOTALS

CHART

Date	

Evaluation of Student Performance

EVALUATION CRITERIA			COMMENTS
Symbol	**Category**	**Point Value**	
✶	Critical Step	16 points	
●	Essential Step	6 points	
Ⓐ	Affective Competency	6 points	
▷	Theory Question	2 points	
Score calculation: 100 points – ____ points missed ____ Score Satisfactory score: 85 or above			

2008 CAAHEP Competencies Achieved
Psychomotor (Skills) ☑ IV. 6. Prepare a patient for procedures and/or treatments. ***Affective (Behavior)*** ☑ IV. 1. Demonstrate empathy in communicating with patients, family, and staff. ☑ IV. 9. Recognize and protect personal boundaries in communicating with others.

2015 CAAHEP Competencies Achieved
Psychomotor (Skills) ☑ I. 1. e. Measure and record height. ☑ I. 1. f. Measure and record weight. ***Affective (Behavior)*** ☑ V. 1. Demonstrate a. empathy b. active listening c. nonverbal communication. ☑ V. 2. Demonstrate the principles of self-boundaries.

ABHES Competencies Achieved
☑ 8. f. Display professionalism through written and verbal communication. ☑ 9. c. Assist provider with general/physical examination.

Notes

EVALUATION OF COMPETENCY

Procedure 20-A: Body Mechanics

Name: ______________________________ Date: ______________

Evaluated by: ______________________________ Score: ______________

Performance Objective

Outcome:	Demonstrate proper body mechanics while standing, sitting, and lifting an object.
Conditions:	Given the following: object for lifting.
	Using a chair.
Standards:	Time: 10 minutes. Student completed procedure in __________ minutes.
	Accuracy: Satisfactory score on the performance evaluation checklist.

Performance Evaluation Checklist

Trial 1	Trial 2	Point Value	Performance Standards
			Standing
		●	Wore comfortable low-heeled shoes that provide good support.
		●	Held the head erect at the midline of the body.
		●	Maintained the back as straight as possible with the pelvis tucked inward.
		●	The chest is forward with the shoulders back and the abdomen drawn in and kept flat.
		▷	Stated the purpose of standing correctly.
		●	Knees are slightly flexed.
		●	Feet are pointing forward and parallel to each other about 3 inches apart.
		▷	Explained the reason for proper positioning of the feet.
		●	Arms are positioned comfortably at the side.
		●	Weight of the body is evenly distributed over both feet.
			Sitting
		●	Sat in a chair with a firm back.
		●	Back and buttocks are supported against the back of the chair.
		●	Body weight is evenly distributed over the buttocks and thighs.
		●	A small pillow or rolled towel is used.
		▷	Stated the use of the pillow or rolled towel.
		●	Feet are flat on the floor.

Trial 1	Trial 2	Point Value	Performance Standards
		●	Knees are level with the hips.
		▷	Explained what to do if prolonged sitting is required.
			Lifting
		●	Determined the weight of the object.
		▷	Stated the purpose of determining the weight of an object before lifting it.
		●	Stood in front of the object with the feet 6 to 8 inches apart.
		●	The toes are pointed outward and one foot is slightly forward.
		●	Tightened the stomach and gluteal muscles in preparation for the lift.
		●	Bent the body at the knees and hips.
		▷	Stated the purpose of bending the body at the knees and hips.
		●	Grasped the object firmly with both hands.
		●	Lifted the object smoothly with the leg muscles while keeping the back straight.
		▷	Stated why the leg muscles and not the back muscles should be used to lift the object.
		●	Held the object as close to the body as possible at waist level.
		▷	Stated why the object should not be lifted higher than the chest.
		●	Turned by pivoting the whole body.
		●	Made sure the area of transport of the object is dry and free of clutter.
		●	Lowered the object slowly while bending from the knees.
		*	Completed the procedures within 10 minutes.
			TOTALS

Evaluation of Student Performance

EVALUATION CRITERIA			COMMENTS
Symbol	Category	Point Value	
*	Critical Step	16 points	
●	Essential Step	6 points	
Ⓐ	Affective Competency	6 points	
▷	Theory Question	2 points	
Score calculation: 100 points − ____ points missed ____ Score Satisfactory score: 85 or above			

2008 CAAHEP Competencies Achieved
Psychomotor (Skills) ☑ XI. 3. Develop a personal (patient and employee) safety plan. ☑ XI. 11. Use proper body mechanics.

2015 CAAHEP Competencies Achieved
Psychomotor (Skills) ☑ XII. 3. Use proper body mechanics.

ABHES Competencies Achieved
☑ 4. e. Perform risk management procedures.

Notes

EVALUATION OF COMPETENCY

Procedure 20-2: Sitting Position

Name: ______________________ Date: ______________

Evaluated by: ______________________ Score: ______________

Performance Objective

Outcome:	Position and drape an individual in the sitting position.
Conditions:	Given the following: a patient gown and a drape.
	Using an examining table.
Standards:	Time: 5 minutes. Student completed procedure in ________ minutes.
	Accuracy: Satisfactory score on the performance evaluation checklist.

Performance Evaluation Checklist

Trial 1	Trial 2	Point Value	Performance Standards
		•	Sanitized hands.
		•	Greeted the patient and introduced yourself.
		•	Identified the patient.
		•	Explained what type of examination or procedure will be performed.
		•	Provided patient with a patient gown.
		•	Instructed patient to remove clothing and to put on a patient gown with the opening in front.
		▷	Stated what qualities the disrobing facility should have.
		•	Pulled out the footrest and assisted the patient into a sitting position.
		•	The patient's buttocks and thighs were firmly supported on the edge of the table.
		•	Placed a drape over the patient's thighs and legs.
		•	Assisted the patient off the table after the examination.
		•	Returned the footrest to its normal position.
		•	Instructed the patient to get dressed.
		•	Discarded the gown and drape in a waste container.
		▷	Stated one use of the sitting position.
		Ⓐ	Demonstrated the principles of self-boundaries.
		*	Completed the procedure within 5 minutes.
			TOTALS

Evaluation of Student Performance

EVALUATION CRITERIA			COMMENTS
Symbol	Category	Point Value	
∗	Critical Step	16 points	
●	Essential Step	6 points	
Ⓐ	Affective Competency	6 points	
▷	Theory Question	2 points	
Score calculation: 100 points – ____ points missed ____ Score Satisfactory score: 85 or above			

2008 CAAHEP Competencies Achieved
Psychomotor (Skills) ☑ IV. 6. Prepare a patient for procedures and/or treatments. ☑ XI. 11. Use proper body mechanics. ***Affective (Behavior)*** ☑ IV. 4. Demonstrate awareness of the territorial boundaries of the person with whom communicating.

2015 CAAHEP Competencies Achieved
Psychomotor (Skills) ☑ I. 8. Instruct and prepare a patient for a procedure or a treatment. ☑ XII. 3. Use proper body mechanics. ***Affective (Behavior)*** ☑ V. 2. Demonstrate the principles of self-boundaries.

ABHES Competency Achieved
☑ 9. c. Assist provider with general/physical examination.

EVALUATION OF COMPETENCY

Procedure 20-3: Supine Position

Name: ______________________ Date: ______________

Evaluated by: ______________________ Score: ______________

Performance Objective

Outcome:	Position and drape an individual in the supine position.
Conditions:	Given the following: a patient gown and a drape.
	Using an examining table.
Standards:	Time: 5 minutes. Student completed procedure in ________ minutes.
	Accuracy: Satisfactory score on the performance evaluation checklist.

Performance Evaluation Checklist

Trial 1	Trial 2	Point Value	Performance Standards
		•	Sanitized hands.
		•	Greeted the patient and introduced yourself.
		•	Identified the patient.
		•	Explained what type of examination or procedure will be performed.
		•	Provided patient with a patient gown.
		•	Instructed patient to remove clothing and to put on a patient gown with the opening in front.
		•	Pulled out the footrest and assisted the patient into a sitting position.
		•	Placed a drape over the patient's thighs and legs.
		•	Asked the patient to move back on the table.
		•	Pulled out the table extension while supporting the patient's lower legs.
		•	Asked the patient to lie down on his or her back with the legs together.
		•	Placed the patient's arms above the head or alongside the body.
		•	Positioned the drape lengthwise over the patient.
		▷	Stated the purpose of the drape.
		•	Moved the drape according to the body parts being examined.
		•	Assisted the patient back into a sitting position after the examination.
		•	Slid the table extension back into place while supporting the patient's lower legs.
		•	Assisted the patient from the examining table.

Trial 1	Trial 2	Point Value	Performance Standards
		●	Returned the footrest to its normal position.
		●	Instructed the patient to get dressed.
		●	Discarded the gown and drape in a waste container.
		▷	Stated one use of the supine position.
		Ⓐ	Demonstrated the principles of self-boundaries.
		*	Completed the procedure within 5 minutes.
			TOTALS

Evaluation of Student Performance

EVALUATION CRITERIA			COMMENTS
Symbol	**Category**	**Point Value**	
*	Critical Step	16 points	
●	Essential Step	6 points	
Ⓐ	Affective Competency	6 points	
▷	Theory Question	2 points	
Score calculation: 100 points – ___ points missed ___ Score Satisfactory score: 85 or above			

2008 CAAHEP Competencies Achieved
Psychomotor (Skills) ☑ IV. 6. Prepare a patient for procedures and/or treatments. ☑ XI. 11. Use proper body mechanics. ***Affective (Behavior)*** ☑ IV. 4. Demonstrate awareness of the territorial boundaries of the person with whom communicating.

2015 CAAHEP Competencies Achieved
Psychomotor (Skills) ☑ I. 8. Instruct and prepare a patient for a procedure or a treatment. ☑ XII. 3. Use proper body mechanics. ***Affective (Behavior)*** ☑ V. 2. Demonstrate the principles of self-boundaries.

ABHES Competency Achieved
☑ 9. c. Assist provider with general/physical examination.

EVALUATION OF COMPETENCY

Procedure 20-4: Prone Position

Name: ______________________________ Date: ______________

Evaluated by: ______________________________ Score: ______________

Performance Objective

Outcome:	Position and drape an individual in the prone position.
Conditions:	Given the following: a patient gown and a drape.
	Using an examining table.
Standards:	Time: 5 minutes. Student completed procedure in __________ minutes.
	Accuracy: Satisfactory score on the performance evaluation checklist.

Performance Evaluation Checklist

Trial 1	Trial 2	Point Value	Performance Standards
		●	Sanitized hands.
		●	Greeted the patient and introduced yourself.
		●	Identified the patient.
		●	Explained what type of examination or procedure will be performed.
		●	Provided patient with a patient gown.
		●	Instructed patient to remove clothing and to put on a patient gown with the opening in back.
		●	Pulled out the footrest and assisted the patient into a sitting position.
		●	Placed a drape over the patient's thighs and legs.
		●	Asked the patient to move back on the table.
		●	Pulled out the table extension while supporting the patient's lower legs.
		●	Asked the patient to lie down on his or her back.
		●	Positioned the drape lengthwise over the patient.
		●	Asked the patient to turn onto his or her stomach by rolling toward you.
		●	Provided assistance.
		▷	Stated the reason for providing assistance.
		●	Positioned the patient with his or her legs together and the head turned to one side.
		●	Placed the patient's arms above the head or alongside the body.
		●	Adjusted the drape as needed.

Trial 1	Trial 2	Point Value	Performance Standards
		●	Moved the drape according to the body parts being examined.
		●	Assisted the patient into the supine position after the examination.
		●	Assisted the patient into a sitting position.
		●	Slid the table extension back into place while supporting the patient's lower legs.
		●	Assisted the patient from the examining table.
		●	Returned the footrest to its normal position.
		●	Instructed the patient to get dressed.
		●	Discarded the gown and drape in a waste container.
		▷	Stated one use of the prone position.
		Ⓐ	Demonstrated the principles of self-boundaries.
		*	Completed the procedure within 5 minutes.
			TOTALS

Evaluation of Student Performance

EVALUATION CRITERIA			COMMENTS
Symbol	**Category**	**Point Value**	
*	Critical Step	16 points	
●	Essential Step	6 points	
Ⓐ	Affective Competency	6 points	
▷	Theory Question	2 points	
Score calculation: 100 points – ___ points missed ___ Score Satisfactory score: 85 or above			

2008 CAAHEP Competencies Achieved
Psychomotor (Skills) ☑ IV. 6. Prepare a patient for procedures and/or treatments. ☑ XI. 11. Use proper body mechanics. ***Affective (Behavior)*** ☑ IV. 4. Demonstrate awareness of the territorial boundaries of the person with whom communicating.

2015 CAAHEP Competencies Achieved
Psychomotor (Skills) ☑ I. 8. Instruct and prepare a patient for a procedure or a treatment. ☑ XII. 3. Use proper body mechanics. ***Affective (Behavior)*** ☑ V. 2. Demonstrate the principles of self-boundaries.

ABHES Competency Achieved
☑ 9. c. Assist provider with general/physical examination.

Notes

EVALUATION OF COMPETENCY

Procedure 20-5: Dorsal Recumbent Position

Name: ________________________________ Date: ____________________

Evaluated by: ____________________________ Score: ____________________

Performance Objective

Outcome:	Position and drape an individual in the dorsal recumbent position.
Conditions:	Given the following: a patient gown and a drape. Using an examining table.
Standards:	Time: 5 minutes. Student completed procedure in ________ minutes. Accuracy: Satisfactory score on the performance evaluation checklist.

Performance Evaluation Checklist

Trial 1	Trial 2	Point Value	Performance Standards
		•	Sanitized hands.
		•	Greeted the patient and introduced yourself.
		•	Identified the patient.
		•	Explained what type of examination or procedure will be performed.
		•	Provided patient with a patient gown.
		•	Instructed patient to remove clothing and to put on a patient gown with the opening in front.
		•	Pulled out the footrest and assisted the patient into a sitting position.
		•	Placed a drape over the patient's thighs and legs.
		•	Asked the patient to move back on the table.
		•	Pulled out the table extension while supporting the patient's lower legs.
		•	Asked the patient to lie down on his or her back.
		•	Placed the patient's arms above their head or alongside the body.
		•	Positioned the drape diagonally over the patient.
		•	Asked the patient to bend the knees and place each foot at the edge of the table with the soles of the feet flat on the table.
		•	Provided assistance.
		•	Pushed in the table extension and the footrest.
		•	Adjusted the drape as needed.
		•	Folded back the center corner of the drape when the physician was ready to examine the patient.
		•	Pulled out the footrest and the table extension after the examination.

Trial 1	Trial 2	Point Value	Performance Standards
		●	Assisted the patient back into a supine position and then into a sitting position.
		●	Slid the table extension back into place while supporting the patient's lower legs.
		●	Assisted the patient from the examining table.
		●	Returned the footrest to its normal position.
		●	Instructed the patient to get dressed.
		●	Discarded the gown and drape in a waste container.
		▷	Stated one use of the dorsal recumbent position.
		Ⓐ	Demonstrated the principles of self-boundaries.
		✶	Completed the procedure within 5 minutes.
			TOTALS

Evaluation of Student Performance

EVALUATION CRITERIA			COMMENTS
Symbol	**Category**	**Point Value**	
✶	Critical Step	16 points	
●	Essential Step	6 points	
Ⓐ	Affective Competency	6 points	
▷	Theory Question	2 points	
Score calculation: 100 points – ___ points missed ___ Score Satisfactory score: 85 or above			

2008 CAAHEP Competencies Achieved
Psychomotor (Skills) ☑ IV. 6. Prepare a patient for procedures and/or treatments. ☑ XI. 11. Use proper body mechanics. ***Affective (Behavior)*** ☑ IV. 4. Demonstrate awareness of the territorial boundaries of the person with whom communicating.

2015 CAAHEP Competencies Achieved
Psychomotor (Skills) ☑ I. 8. Instruct and prepare a patient for a procedure or a treatment. ☑ XII. 3. Use proper body mechanics. ***Affective (Behavior)*** ☑ V. 2. Demonstrate the principles of self-boundaries.

ABHES Competency Achieved
☑ 9. c. Assist provider with general/physical examination.

EVALUATION OF COMPETENCY

Procedure 20-6: Lithotomy Position

Name: ______________________________ Date: ______________

Evaluated by: ______________________________ Score: ______________

Performance Objective

Outcome:	Position and drape an individual in the lithotomy position.
Conditions:	Given the following: a patient gown and a drape.
	Using an examining table.
Standards:	Time: 5 minutes. Student completed procedure in ________ minutes.
	Accuracy: Satisfactory score on the performance evaluation checklist.

Performance Evaluation Checklist

Trial 1	Trial 2	Point Value	Performance Standards
		•	Sanitized hands.
		•	Greeted the patient and introduced yourself.
		•	Identified the patient.
		•	Explained what type of examination or procedure will be performed.
		•	Provided patient with a patient gown.
		•	Instructed patient to remove clothing and to put on a patient gown with the opening in front.
		•	Pulled out the footrest and assisted the patient into a sitting position.
		•	Placed a drape over the patient's thighs and legs.
		•	Asked the patient to move back on the table.
		•	Pulled out the table extension while supporting the patient's lower legs.
		•	Asked the patient to lie down on his or her back.
		•	Placed the patient's arms above head or alongside body.
		•	Positioned the drape diagonally over the patient.
		•	Pulled out the stirrups and positioned them at an angle.
		•	Positioned the stirrups so that they were level with the examining table and pulled out approximately 1 foot from the edge of the table.
		•	Asked the patient to bend the knees and place each foot into a stirrup.
		•	Provided assistance.

Trial 1	Trial 2	Point Value	Performance Standards
		●	Pushed in the table extension and the footrest.
		●	Instructed the patient to slide buttocks to the edge of the table and to rotate thighs outward as far as is comfortable.
		●	Repositioned the drape as needed.
		●	Folded back the center corner of the drape when the physician was ready to examine the genital area.
		●	After completion of the examination, pulled out the footrest and the table extension.
		●	Asked the patient to slide the buttocks back from the end of the table.
		●	Lifted the patient's legs out of the stirrups at the same time and placed them on the table extension.
		▷	Stated why both legs should be lifted at the same time.
		●	Returned stirrups to the normal position.
		●	Assisted the patient back into a sitting position.
		●	Slid the table extension back into place while supporting the patient's lower legs.
		●	Assisted the patient from the examining table.
		●	Returned the footrest to its normal position.
		●	Instructed the patient to get dressed.
		●	Discarded the gown and drape in a waste container.
		▷	Stated one use of the lithotomy position.
		Ⓐ	Demonstrated the principles of self-boundaries.
		✶	Completed the procedure within 5 minutes.
			TOTALS

Evaluation of Student Performance

EVALUATION CRITERIA			COMMENTS
Symbol	**Category**	**Point Value**	
✶	Critical Step	16 points	
●	Essential Step	6 points	
Ⓐ	Affective Competency	6 points	
▷	Theory Question	2 points	
Score calculation: 100 points – ___ points missed ___ Score Satisfactory score: 85 or above			

2008 CAAHEP Competencies Achieved
Psychomotor (Skills) ☑ IV. 6. Prepare a patient for procedures and/or treatments. ☑ XI. 11. Use proper body mechanics. ***Affective (Behavior)*** ☑ IV. 4. Demonstrate awareness of the territorial boundaries of the person with whom communicating.

2015 CAAHEP Competencies Achieved
Psychomotor (Skills) ☑ I. 8. Instruct and prepare a patient for a procedure or a treatment. ☑ XII. 3. Use proper body mechanics. ***Affective (Behavior)*** ☑ V. 2. Demonstrate the principles of self-boundaries.

ABHES Competency Achieved
☑ 9. c. Assist provider with general/physical examination.

Notes

EVALUATION OF COMPETENCY

Procedure 20-7: Sims Position

Name: ______________________ Date: ______________

Evaluated by: ______________________ Score: ______________

Performance Objective

Outcome:	Position and drape an individual in the Sims position.
Conditions:	Given the following: a patient gown and a drape.
	Using an examining table.
Standards:	Time: 5 minutes. Student completed procedure in ________ minutes.
	Accuracy: Satisfactory score on the performance evaluation checklist.

Performance Evaluation Checklist

Trial 1	Trial 2	Point Value	Performance Standards
		•	Sanitized hands.
		•	Greeted the patient and introduced yourself.
		•	Identified the patient.
		•	Explained what type of examination or procedure will be performed.
		•	Provided patient with a patient gown.
		•	Instructed patient to remove clothing and to put on a patient gown with the opening in back.
		•	Pulled out the footrest and assisted the patient into a sitting position.
		•	Placed a drape over the patient's thighs and legs.
		•	Asked the patient to move back on the table.
		•	Pulled out the table extension while supporting the patient's lower legs.
		•	Asked the patient to lie down on his or her back.
		•	Positioned the drape lengthwise over the patient.
		•	Asked the patient to turn onto the left side.
		•	Provided assistance.
		•	Positioned the left arm behind the body and the right arm forward with the elbow bent.
		•	Assisted the patient in flexing the legs with the right leg flexed sharply and the left leg flexed slightly.

Trial 1	Trial 2	Point Value	Performance Standards
		●	Adjusted the drape by folding back the drape to expose the anal area when the physician was ready to examine the patient.
		●	Assisted the patient into a supine position and then into a sitting position following the examination.
		●	Slid the table extension back into place while supporting the patient's lower legs.
		●	Assisted the patient from the examining table.
		●	Returned the footrest to its normal position.
		●	Instructed the patient to get dressed.
		●	Discarded the gown and drape in a waste container.
		▷	Stated one use of the Sims position.
		Ⓐ	Demonstrated the principles of self-boundaries.
		✶	Completed the procedure within 5 minutes.
			TOTALS

Evaluation of Student Performance

EVALUATION CRITERIA			COMMENTS
Symbol	**Category**	**Point Value**	
✶	Critical Step	16 points	
●	Essential Step	6 points	
Ⓐ	Affective Competency	6 points	
▷	Theory Question	2 points	
Score calculation: 100 points – ___ points missed ___ Score Satisfactory score: 85 or above			

2008 CAAHEP Competencies Achieved
Psychomotor (Skills) ☑ IV. 6. Prepare a patient for procedures and/or treatments. ☑ XI. 11. Use proper body mechanics. ***Affective (Behavior)*** ☑ IV. 4. Demonstrate awareness of the territorial boundaries of the person with whom communicating.

2015 CAAHEP Competencies Achieved
Psychomotor (Skills) ☑ I. 8. Instruct and prepare a patient for a procedure or a treatment. ☑ XII. 3. Use proper body mechanics. ***Affective (Behavior)*** ☑ V. 2. Demonstrate the principles of self-boundaries.

ABHES Competency Achieved
☑ 9. c. Assist provider with general/physical examination.

Notes

EVALUATION OF COMPETENCY

Procedure 20-8: Knee-Chest Position

Name: ______________________ Date: ______________

Evaluated by: ______________________ Score: ______________

Performance Objective

Outcome:	Position and drape an individual in the knee-chest position.
Conditions:	Given the following: a patient gown and a drape.
	Using an examining table.
Standards:	Time: 5 minutes. Student completed procedure in ________ minutes.
	Accuracy: Satisfactory score on the performance evaluation checklist.

Performance Evaluation Checklist

Trial 1	Trial 2	Point Value	Performance Standards
		•	Sanitized hands.
		•	Greeted the patient and introduced yourself.
		•	Identified the patient.
		•	Explained what type of examination or procedure will be performed.
		•	Provided patient with a patient gown.
		•	Instructed patient to remove clothing and to put on a patient gown with the opening in back.
		•	Pulled out the footrest and assisted the patient into a sitting position.
		•	Placed a drape over the patient's thighs and legs.
		•	Asked the patient to move back on the table.
		•	Pulled out the table extension while supporting the patient's lower legs.
		•	Assisted the patient into the supine position and then into the prone position.
		•	Positioned the drape diagonally over the patient.
		•	Asked the patient to bend the arms at the elbows and rest them alongside the head.
		•	Asked the patient to elevate the buttocks while keeping the back straight.
		•	Turned the patient's head to one side, with the weight of the body supported by the chest.
		•	Used a pillow for additional support, if needed.
		•	Separated the knees and lower legs approximately 12 inches.

Trial 1	Trial 2	Point Value	Performance Standards
		●	Adjusted the drape diagonally as needed.
		●	Folded back a small portion of the drape to expose the anal area when the physician was ready to examine the patient.
		●	Assisted the patient into a prone position and then into a supine position after the examination.
		●	Allowed the patient to rest in a supine position before sitting up.
		▷	Stated why the patient should be allowed to rest.
		●	Assisted the patient into a sitting position.
		●	Slid the table extension back into place while supporting the patient's lower legs.
		●	Assisted the patient from the examining table.
		●	Returned the footrest to its normal position.
		●	Instructed the patient to get dressed.
		●	Discarded the gown and drape in a waste container.
		▷	Stated one use of the knee-chest position.
		Ⓐ	Demonstrated the principles of self-boundaries.
		*	Completed the procedure within 5 minutes.
			TOTALS

Evaluation of Student Performance

EVALUATION CRITERIA			COMMENTS
Symbol	**Category**	**Point Value**	
*	Critical Step	16 points	
●	Essential Step	6 points	
Ⓐ	Affective Competency	6 points	
▷	Theory Question	2 points	
Score calculation: 100 points – ___ points missed ___ Score Satisfactory score: 85 or above			

2008 CAAHEP Competencies Achieved
Psychomotor (Skills) ☑ IV. 6. Prepare a patient for procedures and/or treatments. ☑ XI. 11. Use proper body mechanics. ***Affective (Behavior)*** ☑ IV. 4. Demonstrate awareness of the territorial boundaries of the person with whom communicating.

2015 CAAHEP Competencies Achieved
Psychomotor (Skills) ☑ I. 8. Instruct and prepare a patient for a procedure or a treatment. ☑ XII. 3. Use proper body mechanics. ***Affective (Behavior)*** ☑ V. 2. Demonstrate the principles of self-boundaries.

ABHES Competency Achieved
☑ 9. c. Assist provider with general/physical examination.

Notes

EVALUATION OF COMPETENCY

Procedure 20-9: Fowler's Position

Name: ______________________ Date: ______________

Evaluated by: ______________________ Score: ______________

Performance Objective

Outcome:	Position and drape an individual in the Fowler's position.
Conditions:	Given the following: a patient gown and a drape. Using an examining table.
Standards:	Time: 5 minutes. Student completed procedure in ________ minutes. Accuracy: Satisfactory score on the performance evaluation checklist.

Performance Evaluation Checklist

Trial 1	Trial 2	Point Value	Performance Standards
		•	Sanitized hands.
		•	Greeted the patient and introduced yourself.
		•	Identified the patient.
		•	Explained what type of examination or procedure will be performed.
		•	Provided patient with a patient gown.
		•	Instructed patient to remove clothing and to put on a patient gown with the opening in front.
		•	Positioned the head of the table at a 45-degree angle for a -semi-Fowler's position or at a 90-degree angle for a full Fowler's position.
		•	Pulled out the footrest and assisted the patient into a sitting position.
		•	Placed a drape over the patient's thighs and legs.
		•	Pulled out the table extension while supporting the patient's lower legs.
		•	Asked the patient to lean back against the table head.
		•	Provided assistance.
		•	Positioned the drape lengthwise over the patient.
		•	Moved the drape according to the body parts being examined.
		•	Assisted the patient into a sitting position after the examination.
		•	Slid the table extension back into place while supporting the patient's lower legs.
		•	Assisted the patient from the examining table.

Trial 1	Trial 2	Point Value	Performance Standards
		●	Instructed the patient to get dressed.
		●	Returned the head of the table and the footrest to their normal positions.
		●	Discarded the gown and drape in a waste container.
		▷	Stated one use of the Fowler's position.
		Ⓐ	Demonstrated the principles of self-boundaries.
		✶	Completed the procedure within 5 minutes.
			TOTALS

Evaluation of Student Performance

EVALUATION CRITERIA			COMMENTS
Symbol	**Category**	**Point Value**	
✶	Critical Step	16 points	
●	Essential Step	6 points	
Ⓐ	Affective Competency	6 points	
▷	Theory Question	2 points	
Score calculation: 100 points – ____ points missed ____ Score Satisfactory score: 85 or above			

2008 CAAHEP Competencies Achieved
Psychomotor (Skills) ☑ IV. 6. Prepare a patient for procedures and/or treatments. ☑ XI. 11. Use proper body mechanics. ***Affective (Behavior)*** ☑ IV. 4. Demonstrate awareness of the territorial boundaries of the person with whom communicating.

2015 CAAHEP Competencies Achieved
Psychomotor (Skills) ☑ I. 8. Instruct and prepare a patient for a procedure or a treatment. ☑ XII. 3. Use proper body mechanics. ***Affective (Behavior)*** ☑ V. 2. Demonstrate the principles of self-boundaries.

ABHES Competency Achieved
☑ 9. c. Assist provider with general/physical examination.

EVALUATION OF COMPETENCY

Procedure 20-10: Wheelchair Transfer

Name: _______________ Date: _______________

Evaluated by: _______________ Score: _______________

Performance Objective

Outcome:	Transfer a patient from a wheelchair to the examining table and from the examining table to a wheelchair.
Conditions:	Given the following: transfer belt.
	Using an examining table and a wheelchair.
Standards:	Time: 10 minutes. Student completed procedure in _______ minutes.
	Accuracy: Satisfactory score on the performance evaluation checklist.

Performance Evaluation Checklist

Trial 1	Trial 2	Point Value	Performance Standards
			Transferring to the examining table:
		•	Sanitized hands.
		•	Greeted the patient and introduced yourself.
		•	Identified the patient and explained the procedure.
		•	Determined whether the patient has the mental and physical capability to perform the transfer.
		•	Estimated the weight of the patient and whether he or she can assist in the transfer.
		•	Assessed your ability to safely make the transfer.
		▷	Stated factors that would prevent you from making the transfer.
		•	Wrapped the transfer belt around the patient's waist and fastened it.
		•	The belt was snug with just enough space to allow the fingers to be inserted comfortably.
		▷	Stated why the belt should be snug.
		•	With the patient's stronger side next to the table, positioned the wheelchair at a 45-degree angle to the end of the examining table.
		•	If the table is height-adjustable, adjusted it to the same height as the wheelchair or slightly lower.
		•	If the table is not height-adjustable, pulled out the footrest.
		•	Locked the brakes of the wheelchair.
		▷	Stated why the brakes should be locked.

Trial 1	Trial 2	Point Value	Performance Standards
		●	Folded back the wheelchair footrests.
		●	Informed the patient what to do during the transfer.
		●	Made sure the patient's feet were flat on the floor.
		●	Stood in front of the patient with the feet 6 to 8 inches apart, with one foot slightly forward and the knees bent.
		●	Asked the patient to place his or her arms on the armrests of the wheelchair and to lean forward.
		●	Grasped the transfer belt on either side of the patient's waist using an underhand grasp.
		▷	Stated the purpose of the transfer belt.
		●	Instructed the patient to push off the armrests and into a standing position on the count of 3.
		●	Straightened the knees and assisted the patient to a standing position by pulling upward on the transfer belt.
		●	Kept the back straight lifted with the knees, arms, and legs, and not the back.
		●	Pivoted and positioned the patient's buttocks and back of the legs toward the examining table.
		●	Instructed the patient to step backward onto the footrest, one foot at a time.
		●	Gradually lowered the patient into a sitting position on the examining table.
		●	Removed the transfer belt.
		●	Unlocked the wheelchair and moved it out of the way.
		●	Pushed in the footrest of the examining table.
		●	Stayed with the patient to prevent falls.
			Transferring to the wheelchair:
		●	Wrapped the transfer belt snugly around the patient's waist and fastened it.
		●	Positioned the wheelchair at a 45-degree angle to the end of the examining table.
		●	If the table is height-adjustable, adjusted it to the same height as the wheelchair or slightly lower.
		●	If the table is not height-adjustable, pulled out the footrest.
		●	Locked the wheelchair in place and folded back the footrests, if needed.
		●	Informed the patient what to do during the transfer.
		●	Stood in front of the patient with the feet 6 to 8 inches apart, with one foot slightly forward and the knees bent.
		●	Asked the patient to place his or her arms on your shoulders.
		●	Did not allow the patient to place his or her arms around your neck.

Trial 1	Trial 2	Point Value	Performance Standards
		●	Grasped the transfer belt on either side of the patient's waist using an underhand grasp.
		●	Instructed the patient to stand on the count of 3.
		●	Straightened your knees and assisted the patient to a standing position by pulling upward on the transfer belt.
		●	Instructed the patient to step down from the footrest, one foot at a time.
		●	Pivoted the patient until the back of the legs are against the seat of the wheelchair.
		●	Asked the patient to grasp the armrests of the wheelchair.
		●	Gradually lowered the patient into the wheelchair by bending at the knees.
		●	Removed the transfer belt and made sure the patient was -comfortable.
		●	Repositioned the wheelchair footrests and assisted the patient in placing his or her feet in them.
		●	Unlocked the wheelchair.
		●	Pushed in the footrest of the examining table.
		Ⓐ	Demonstrated the principles of self-boundaries.
		*	Completed the procedure within 10 minutes.
			TOTALS

Evaluation of Student Performance

EVALUATION CRITERIA			COMMENTS
Symbol	**Category**	**Point Value**	
*	Critical Step	16 points	
●	Essential Step	6 points	
Ⓐ	Affective Competency	6 points	
▷	Theory Question	2 points	
Score calculation: 100 points − ___ points missed ___ Score Satisfactory score: 85 or above			

2008 CAAHEP Competencies Achieved
Psychomotor (Skills) ☑ IV. 6. Prepare a patient for procedures and/or treatments. ☑ XI. 11. Use proper body mechanics. ***Affective (Behavior)*** ☑ IV. 4. Demonstrate awareness of the territorial boundaries of the person with whom communicating.

2015 CAAHEP Competencies Achieved
Psychomotor (Skills) ☑ I. 8. Instruct and prepare a patient for a procedure or a treatment. ☑ XII. 3. Use proper body mechanics. ***Affective (Behavior)*** ☑ V. 2. Demonstrate the principles of self-boundaries.

ABHES Competencies Achieved
☑ 9. c. Assist provider with general/physical examination. ☑ 9. j. Make adaptations with patients with special needs.

EVALUATION OF COMPETENCY

Procedure 20-11: Assisting with the Physical Examination

Name: ______________________ Date: ______________

Evaluated by: ______________________ Score: ______________

Performance Objective

Outcome:	Prepare the patient and assist with a physical examination.
Conditions:	Given the following: equipment for the type of examination to be performed, patient examination gown, and drapes. Using an examining table.
Standards:	Time: 20 minutes. Student completed procedure in __________ minutes. Accuracy: Satisfactory score on the performance evaluation checklist.

Performance Evaluation Checklist

Trial 1	Trial 2	Point Value	Performance Standards
		●	Prepared examination room.
		●	Sanitized hands.
		●	Assembled all necessary equipment.
		●	Arranged instruments in a neat and orderly manner.
		●	Obtained the patient's medical record.
		●	Went to the waiting room, and asked the patient to come back.
		●	Escorted the patient to the examination room.
		●	Asked the patient to be seated.
		●	Greeted the patient and introduced yourself.
		●	Identified the patient by full name and date of birth.
		▷	Stated why a calm and friendly manner should be used.
		●	Seated yourself facing the patient at a distance of 3 to 4 feet.
		●	Obtained and documented essential patient information on patient allergies, current medications, and patient symptoms.
		●	Measured vital signs and charted results.
		▷	Stated the adult normal range for temperature (97°F to 99°F), pulse (60 to 100 beats/min), respiration (12 to 20 breaths/min), and blood pressure (<120/80 mm Hg).
		●	Measured weight and height, and charted results.

Trial 1	Trial 2	Point Value	Performance Standards
		●	Asked patient if he or she needs to void.
		▷	Stated why the patient should be asked to void.
		●	Instructed patient to remove all clothing and put on an examining gown.
		●	Informed the patient that the physician will be in soon.
		●	Left the room to provide patient with privacy.
		●	Made patient's medical record available to the physician (if using a PPR).
		●	Checked to make sure patient is ready to be seen.
		●	Informed physician that the patient is ready.
			Assisted the physician:
		●	Ensured the patient was in a sitting position on examination table.
		●	Handed the ophthalmoscope to the physician when requested.
		●	Dimmed the lights when the physician was ready to use the ophthalmoscope.
		▷	Stated why the lights are dimmed.
		▷	Stated the proper use of the ophthalmoscope.
		●	Handed the otoscope to the examiner when requested.
		▷	Stated the proper use of the otoscope.
		●	Is able to change the speculum and bulb in the otoscope.
		●	Handed the tongue depressor to the examiner when requested.
		●	Offered reassurance to patient as needed.
		●	Positioned patient as required for examination of the remaining body systems.
			Assisted and instructed patient:
		●	Allowed patient to rest in a sitting position before getting off the examining table.
		▷	Stated why the patient should be allowed to rest before getting off the table.
		●	Assisted patient off the examining table.
		●	Instructed patient to get dressed.
		●	Provided patient with any necessary instructions.
		▷	Stated what type of instructions may need to be relayed to the patient.
		●	Sanitized hands and charted any instructions given to the patient.
		●	Escorted the patient to the reception area.
			Cleaned the examination room:
		●	Discarded paper on the examining table and unrolled a fresh length.

Trial 1	Trial 2	Point Value	Performance Standards
		●	Discarded all disposable supplies into an appropriate waste container.
		●	Checked to make sure ample supplies are available.
		●	Removed reusable equipment for sanitization, sterilization, or disinfection.
		Ⓐ	Incorporated critical thinking skills when performing patient assessment.
		Ⓐ	Incorporated critical thinking skills when performing patient care.
		Ⓐ	Showed awareness of a patient's concerns related to the procedure being performed.
		Ⓐ	Demonstrated respect for individual diversity including a. gender. b. race. c. religion d. age e. economic status f. appearance.
		Ⓐ	Demonstrated sensitivity to patient rights.
		Ⓐ	Protected the integrity of the medical record.
		✶	Completed the procedure within 20 minutes.
			TOTALS

CHART	
Date	

Evaluation of Student Performance

EVALUATION CRITERIA			COMMENTS
Symbol	**Category**	**Point Value**	
✶	Critical Step	16 points	
●	Essential Step	6 points	
Ⓐ	Affective Competency	6 points	
▷	Theory Question	2 points	
Score calculation: 100 points – ___ points missed ___ Score Satisfactory score: 85 or above			

2008 CAAHEP Competencies Achieved

Psychomotor (Skills)
☑ I. 6. Perform patient screening using established protocols.
☑ I. 10. Assist physician with patient care.
☑ IV. 5. Instruct patients according to their needs to promote health maintenance and disease prevention.
☑ IV. 6. Prepare a patient for procedures and/or treatments.
☑ IV. 12. Develop and maintain a current list of community resources related to patients' health care needs.
☑ V. 9. Perform routine maintenance of office equipment with documentation.
☑ IX. 7. Document accurately in the patient record.
☑ XI. 11. Use proper body mechanics.

Affective (Behavior)
☑ I. 3. Demonstrate respect for diversity in approaching patients and families.
☑ IV. 2. Apply active listening skills.
☑ IV. 3. Use appropriate body language and other nonverbal skills in communicating with patients, family, and staff.
☑ IV. 8. Analyze communications in providing appropriate responses or feedback.
☑ IV. 10. Demonstrate respect for individual diversity, incorporating awareness of one's own biases in areas including gender, race, religion, age, and economic status.
☑ X. 3. Demonstrate awareness of diversity in providing patient care.

2015 CAAHEP Competencies Achieved

Psychomotor (Skills)
☑ I. 3. Perform patient screening using established protocols.
☑ I. 8. Instruct and prepare a patient for a procedure or a treatment.
☑ I. 9. Assist provider with a patient exam.
☑ V. 1. Use feedback techniques to obtain patient information including: a reflection b. restatement c. clarification.
☑ V. 4. Coach patients regarding: a. office policy b. health maintenance c. disease prevention d. treatment plan.
☑ V. 9. Develop a current list of community resources related to patients' healthcare needs.
☑ V. 11. Report relevant information concisely and accurately.
☑ X. 1. Apply HIPAA rules in regard to: a. privacy b. release of information.
☑ X. 3. Document patient care accurately in the medical record.
☑ XII. 3. Use proper body mechanics.

Affective (Behavior)
☑ I. 1. Incorporate critical thinking skills when performing patient assessment.
☑ I. 2. Incorporate critical thinking skills when performing patient care.
☑ I. 3. Show awareness of a patient's concerns related to the procedure being performed.
☑ V. 1. Demonstrate a. empathy b. active listening c. nonverbal communication.
☑ V. 3. Demonstrate respect for individual diversity including a. gender. b. race. c. religion d. age e. economic status f. appearance.
☑ X. 1. Demonstrate sensitivity to patient rights.
☑ X. 2. Protect the integrity of the medical record.

ABHES Competencies Achieved

☑ 4. a. Follow documentation guidelines.
☑ 5. e. Analyze the effect of hereditary, cultural, and environmental influences on behavior.
☑ 8. e. Maintain inventory of equipment and supplies.
☑ 8. f. Display professionalism through written and verbal communications.
☑ 9. b. Obtain vital signs, obtain patient history, and formulate chief complaint.
☑ 9. c. Assist provider with general/physical examination.
☑ 9. h. Teach self-examination, disease management and health promotion.
☑ 9. i. Identify community resources and Complementary and Alternative Medicine practices (CAM).

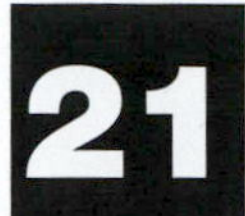

Eye and Ear Assessment and Procedures

CHAPTER ASSIGNMENTS

✓ After Completing	Date Due	Study Guide Pages	STUDY GUIDE ASSIGNMENTS (CTA = Critical Thinking Activity)	Possible Points	Points You Earned
		425	Pretest	10	
			Term Key Term Assessment		
		426	A. Definitions	13	
		426	B. Word Parts	11	
			(Add 1 point for each key term)		
		426-429	Evaluation of Learning questions	22	
		429	CTA A: Measuring Distance Visual Acuity	6	
		429	CTA B: Interpreting Visual Acuity Results	4	
		430	CTA C: Charting Visual Acuity Results	4	
		430-431	CTA D: Ear Procedures	8	
		431	CTA E: Dear Gabby	10	
		432	CTA F: Crossword Puzzle	19	
		433-436	CTA G: Eye and Ear Conditions	40	
			Evolve Site: Apply Your Knowledge questions	10	
			Evolve Site: Video Evaluation	70	
		425	Posttest	10	
			ADDITIONAL ASSIGNMENTS		
			TOTAL POINTS		

Notes

✓ When Assigned By Your Instructor	Study Guide Pages	Practices Required	LABORATORY ASSIGNMENTS (Procedure Number and Name)	Score*
	437-439	5	**Practice for Competency** 21-1: Assessing Distance Visual Acuity—Snellen Chart Textbook reference: pp. 447-448	
	441-443		**Evaluation of Competency** 21-1: Assessing Distance Visual Acuity—Snellen Chart	*
	437-439	3	**Practice for Competency** 21-2: Assessing Color Vision: Ishihara Test Textbook reference: pp. 449-450	
	445-447		**Evaluation of Competency** 21-2: Assessing Color Vision: Ishihara Test	*
	437-439	3	**Practice for Competency** 21-3: Performing an Eye Irrigation Textbook reference: pp. 451-453	
	449-451		**Evaluation of Competency** 21-3: Performing an Eye Irrigation	*
	437-439	3	**Practice for Competency** 21-4: Performing an Eye Instillation Textbook reference: pp. 453-455	
	453-455		**Evaluation of Competency** 21-4: Performing an Eye Instillation	*
	437-439	3	**Practice for Competency** 21-5: Performing an Ear Irrigation Textbook reference: pp. 460-462	
	457-459		**Evaluation of Competency** 21-5: Performing an Ear Irrigation	*
	437-439	3	**Practice for Competency** 21-6: Performing an Ear Instillation Textbook reference: pp. 463-464	
	461-463		**Evaluation of Competency** 21-6: Performing an Ear Instillation	*
			ADDITIONAL ASSIGNMENTS	

Notes

Name ______________________________ Date ______________

PRETEST

True or False

_______ 1. Refraction refers to the bending of light rays so that they can be focused on the retina.

_______ 2. A person who is farsighted has a condition known as myopia.

_______ 3. An optometrist can perform eye surgery.

_______ 4. The Snellen eye test is conducted at a distance of 20 feet.

_______ 5. The Snellen eye chart should be positioned at the medical assistant's eye level.

_______ 6. An eye instillation may be performed to treat an eye infection.

_______ 7. Conjunctivitis caused by a bacterium is not contagious.

_______ 8. The most specific type of hearing test is the tuning fork test.

_______ 9. Serous otitis media can result in a conductive hearing loss.

_______ 10. An ear instillation may be performed to treat an ear infection.

POSTTEST

True or False

_______ 1. A person who cannot see objects close up has a condition known as amblyopia.

_______ 2. Visual acuity refers to sharpness of vision.

_______ 3. Presbyopia is a decrease in the elasticity of the lens due to the aging process.

_______ 4. An optician fills prescriptions for eyeglasses.

_______ 5. The Snellen Big E chart is used with school-aged children.

_______ 6. The most common color vision defects are congenital in nature.

_______ 7. The external auditory canal of an adult is straightened by pulling the ear downward and backward.

_______ 8. The range of frequencies for normal speech is 300 to 4000 Hz.

_______ 9. Intense noise can result in a sensorineural hearing loss.

_______ 10. Tympanometry is used to diagnose patients with auditory nerve damage.

Term KEY TERM ASSESSMENT

A. Definitions

Directions: Match each key term with its definition.

_______ 1. Astigmatism
_______ 2. Audiometer
_______ 3. Canthus
_______ 4. Cerumen
_______ 5. Hyperopia
_______ 6. Impacted
_______ 7. Instillation
_______ 8. Irrigation
_______ 9. Myopia
_______ 10. Otoscope
_______ 11. Presbyopia
_______ 12. Refraction
_______ 13. Tympanic membrane

A. The washing of a body canal with a flowing solution
B. A decrease in the elasticity of the lens that occurs with aging, resulting in a decreased ability to focus on close objects
C. Farsightedness
D. The deflection or bending of light rays by a lens
E. The junction of the eyelids at either corner of the eye
F. Nearsightedness
G. The dropping of a liquid into a body cavity
H. An instrument for examining the external ear canal and tympanic membrane
I. Earwax
J. An instrument used to quantitatively measure hearing acuity for the various frequencies of sound waves
K. A thin, semitransparent membrane located between the external ear canal and the middle ear that receives and transmits sound waves
L. A refractive error that causes distorted and blurred vision for both near and far objects due to a cornea that is oval shaped
M. Wedged firmly together so as to be immovable

B. Word Parts

Directions: Indicate the meaning of each word part in the space provided. List as many medical terms as possible that incorporate the word part in the space provided.

Word Part	Meaning of Word Part	Medical Terms That Incorporate Word Part
1. a-		
2. stigma/a		
3. -ism		
4. audi/o		
5. -meter		
6. hyper-		
7. -opia		
8. ot/o		
9. -scope		
10. tympan/o		
11. -ic		

EVALUATION OF LEARNING

Directions: Fill in each blank with the correct answer.

1. What is visual acuity?

____

____

2. What type of symptoms might be experienced with myopia?

3. What methods can be used to correct myopia?

4. What causes an individual with astigmatism to have distorted and blurred vision?

5. What is each of the following eye professionals qualified to perform?

    a. Ophthalmologist

    b. Optometrist

    c. Optician

6. What condition can be detected by measuring distance visual acuity?

7. What type of patient would warrant use of the Snellen Big E eye chart? (Give two examples.)

8. Explain the significance of the top number and bottom number next to each line of letters on the Snellen eye chart.

9. List two conditions that can be detected by measuring near visual acuity.

10. Explain the difference between congenital and acquired color vision defects.

11. What is a polychromatic plate?

12. List three reasons for performing eye irrigation.

13. List three reasons for performing eye instillation.

14. What is the range of frequencies for normal speech?

15. List five conditions that may cause conductive hearing loss.

16. List four conditions that may result in sensorineural hearing loss.

17. What information is obtained through audiometry?

18. What information is obtained through tympanometry?

19. List three reasons for performing ear irrigation.

20. List three reasons for performing ear instillation.

____

21. Explain how impacted cerumen is removed from the ear.

____

____

____

22. Explain how to straighten the external auditory canal in an adult and in children 3 years old or younger.

____

____

____

CRITICAL THINKING ACTIVITIES

A. Measuring Distance Visual Acuity

For each of the following situations, write C if the technique is correct and I if the technique is incorrect.

_______ 1. The patient is not given an opportunity to study the Snellen chart before beginning the test.

_______ 2. The Snellen chart is positioned at the medical assistant's eye level.

_______ 3. The patient is instructed to use his or her hand to cover the eye that is not being tested.

_______ 4. The medical assistant instructs the patient to close the eye that is not being tested.

_______ 5. The first line that the medical assistant asks the patient to identify is the 20/20 line.

_______ 6. The medical assistant observes the patient for signs of squinting or leaning forward during the test.

B. Interpreting Visual Acuity Results

1. A patient has a distance visual acuity reading of 20/30 in the right eye. Using this information, answer the following questions:

   a. How far was the patient from the eye chart?

   ____

   b. At what distance would a person with normal acuity be able to read this line?

   ____

2. A patient has a distance visual acuity reading of 20/10 in the left eye. Using this information, answer the following questions:

   a. How far was the patient from the eye chart?

   ____

   b. At what distance would a person with normal acuity be able to read this line?

   ____

C. Charting Visual Acuity Results

Properly chart the distance visual acuity results in the spaces provided. In all cases, the line indicated is the smallest line the patient could read at a distance of 20 feet.

1. The patient read the line marked 20/30 with the right eye with two errors; with the left eye, the patient read the line marked 20/30 with one error. The patient was wearing corrective lenses.

____

____

2. The patient read the line marked 20/20 with the right eye with one error; with the left eye, the patient read the line marked 20/20 with no errors. The patient was wearing corrective lenses.

____

____

3. The patient read the line marked 20/40 with the right eye with two errors; with the left eye, the patient read the line marked 20/30 with one error. The patient exhibited squinting and frowning during the test. The patient was not wearing corrective lenses.

____

____

4. The patient read the line marked 20/15 with the right eye with no errors; with the left eye, the patient read the line marked 20/20 with one error. The patient was not wearing corrective lenses.

____

____

D. Ear Procedures

Explain the principle for each of the following procedures.

Ear Irrigation

1. Positioning the patient's head so that it is tilted toward the affected ear

____

____

2. Cleansing the outer ear before irrigating

____

____

3. Straightening the external auditory canal

____

____

4. Injecting the irrigating solution toward the roof of the ear canal

____

____

5. Making sure not to obstruct the canal opening

____

____

Ear Instillation

6. Positioning the patient's head so that it is tilted toward the unaffected ear

____

____

7. Instructing the patient to lie on the unaffected side after the instillation

____

____

8. Placing a cotton wick in the patient's ear

____

____

E. Dear Gabby

Gabby has a middle ear infection and is not feeling well. She wants you to fill in for her. In the space provided, respond to the following letter.

Dear Gabby:
I am dating the sweetest and dearest man. "Mike" has only one flaw. He likes loud music. He had those big boom boxes installed in his car. When we drive somewhere in his car, he blasts the music. Sometimes, when we are driving down a street, people even turn around to see where the loud music is coming from. The music hurts my ears, and I cannot think straight. My ears even start ringing when we go on a trip. When I am talking to Mike, he says I mumble, and I have to speak extra loud around him. I keep telling Mike that the loud music is going to damage our hearing, but he says that we are way too young for that and that only old people have trouble hearing. Please help me Gabby, because I love going on trips with Mike, but not if my ears hurt afterward.

Signed, Ears Are Ringing

____

____

____

____

____

____

____

____

____

____

____

F. Crossword Puzzle: Eye and Ear

Directions: Complete the crossword puzzle using the clues provided.

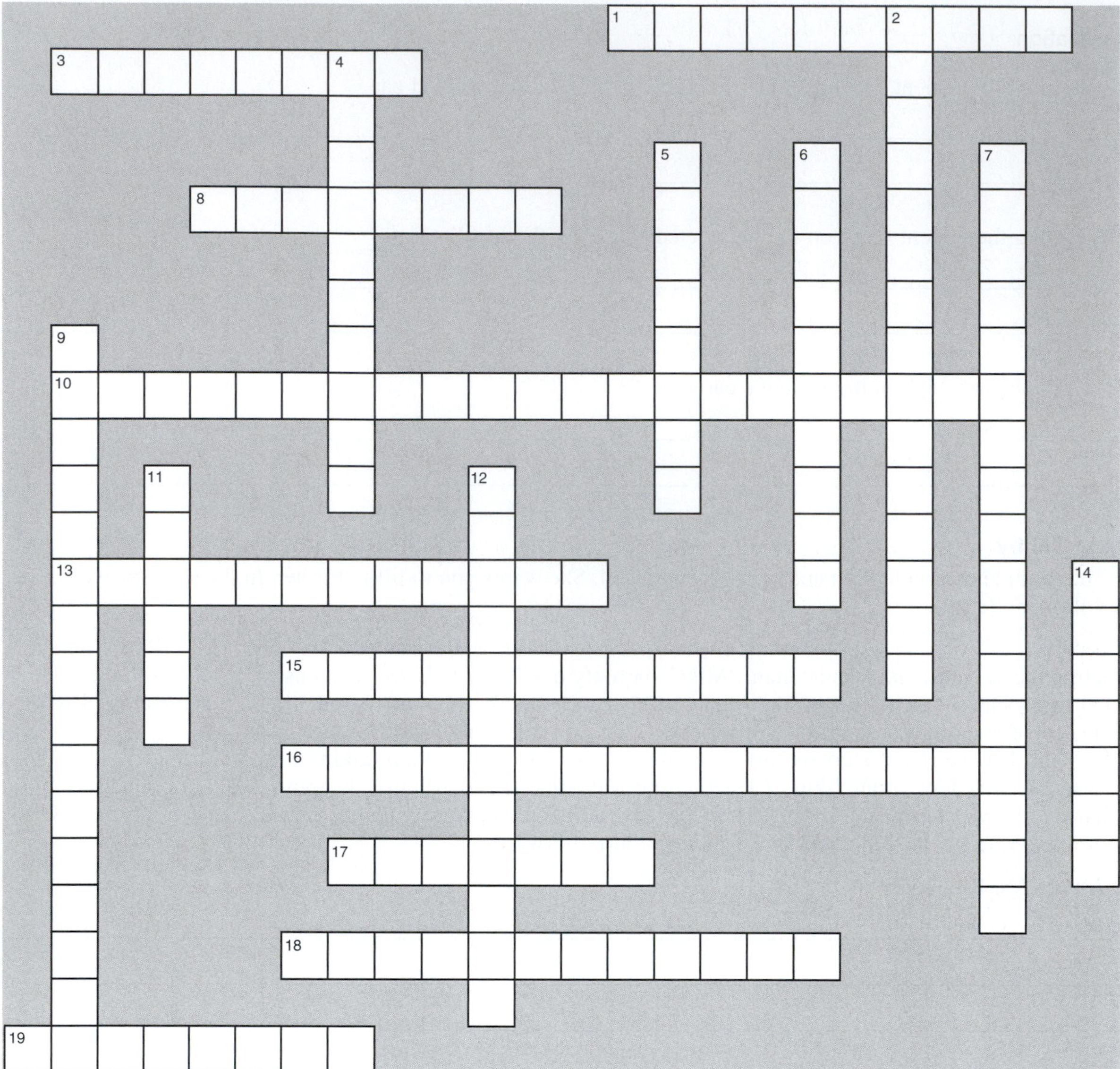

Across

1 Decreased lens elasticity
3 Fills eyeglasses prescriptions
8 Color blind test
10 Impacted cerumen may cause this
13 Fixed stapes
15 Assesses mobility of eardrum
16 Drum in your ear
17 Earwax
18 Normal DVA
19 Straighten this before ear irrigation

Down

2 Physician who diagnoses and treats eye disorders
4 Instrument that measures hearing
5 A cause of pink eye
6 Caught it!
7 Fluid in middle ear
9 Middle ear infection
11 Cannot see far away
12 Sharpness of vision
14 Loudness of sound measurement

G. Eye and Ear Conditions

1. You and your classmates work at a large clinic. It is National Eye and Ear Week. The physicians at your clinic ask you to develop for their patients informative, creative, and colorful brochures about eye and ear conditions. Choose a condition, and design a brochure using the blank Frequently Asked Questions (FAQ) brochure provided on the following page. Each student in the class should select a different topic. On a separate sheet of paper, write three true or false questions related to the information in your brochure.

2. Present your brochure to the class. After all the brochures have been presented, each student should ask three -questions to the entire class to see how well the class understands eye and ear conditions. (Note: You can take notes during the presentations and refer to them when answering the questions.)

Eye

1. Amblyopia (lazy eye)
2. Age-related macular degeneration
3. Astigmatism
4. Blepharitis
5. Cataracts
6. CMV retinitis
7. Corneal ulcer
8. Corneal abrasion
9. Strabismus (crossed-eyed)
10. Diabetic retinopathy
11. Drooping eyelids (ptosis)
12. Dry eyes
13. Floaters and spots
14. Glaucoma
15. Keratoconus
16. Ocular hypertension
17. Presbycusis
18. Retinal detachment
19. Retinitis pigmentosa
20. Stye

Ear

1. Acute mastoiditis
2. External otitis
3. Meniere's disease
4. Noise-induced hearing loss
5. Serous otitis media

Notes

FAQ on:

Q:

A:

Q:

A:

Q:

A:

Q:

A:

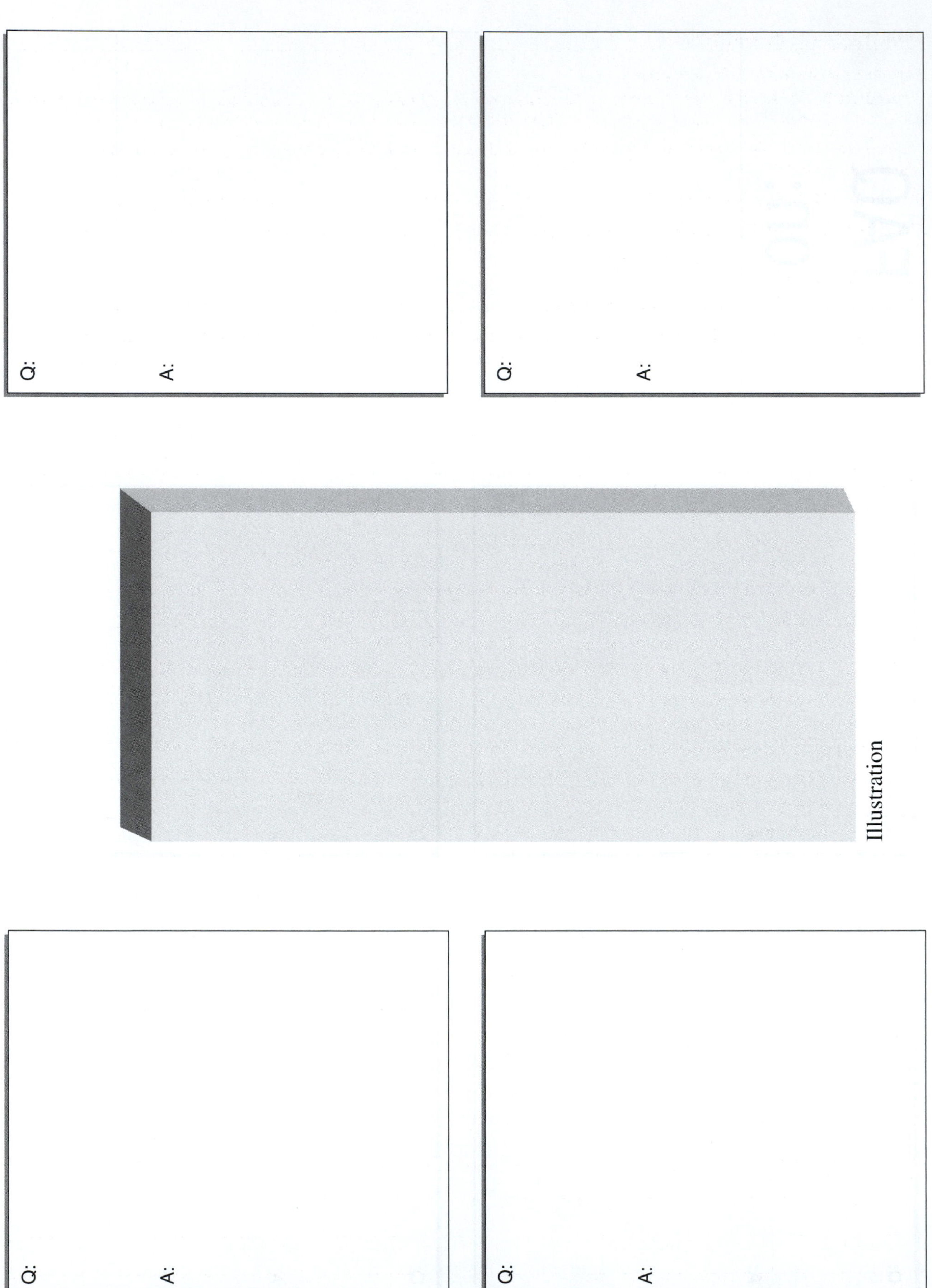
Q:
A:
Q:
A:
Illustration
Q:
A:
Q:
A:

PRACTICE FOR COMPETENCY

Eye Assessment and Procedures

Procedure 21-1: Distance Visual Acuity. Assess distance visual acuity using a Snellen eye chart, and record results in the chart provided. Circle any readings that indicate distance visual acuity above or below average.

Procedure 21-2: Color Vision. Assess color vision, and record results in the Ishihara charting gridprovided. Circle any abnormal results.

Procedure 21-3: Eye Irrigation. Perform an eye irrigation, and record the procedure in the chart provided.

Procedure 21-4: Eye Instillation. Perform an eye instillation, and record the procedure in the chart provided.

Ear Procedures

Procedure 21-5: Ear Irrigation. Perform an ear irrigation, and record the procedure in the chart provided.

Procedure 21-6: Ear Instillation. Perform an ear instillation, and record the procedure in the chart provided.

CHART	
Date	

Chart	
Date	

CHART		
Plate No.	Normal Person	Results
1	12	
2	8	
3	5	
4	29	
5	74	
6	7	
7	45	
8	2	
9	X	
10	16	
11	Traceable	
Date:		
Evaluated by :		

CHART		
Plate No.	Normal Person	Results
1	12	
2	8	
3	5	
4	29	
5	74	
6	7	
7	45	
8	2	
9	X	
10	16	
11	Traceable	
Date:		
Evaluated by:		

Notes

EVALUATION OF COMPETENCY

Procedure 21-1: Assessing Distance Visual Acuity—Snellen Chart

Name: ______________________________ Date: ______________

Evaluated by: ______________________________ Score: ______________

Performance Objective

Outcome:	Assess distance visual acuity.
Conditions:	Given the following: Snellen eye chart, eye occluder, and an antiseptic wipe.
	Time: 5 minutes. Student completed procedure in __________ minutes.
Standards:	Accuracy: Satisfactory score on the performance evaluation checklist.

Performance Evaluation Checklist

Trial 1	Trial 2	Point Value	Performance Standards
		•	Sanitized hands.
		•	Assembled equipment.
		•	Disinfected the eye occluder with an antiseptic wipe.
		•	Greeted the patient and introduced yourself.
		•	Identified the patient and explained the procedure.
		•	Determined if patient wears corrective lenses and instructed patient to leave them on during the test.
		•	Positioned patient 20 feet from the eye chart.
		•	Positioned the center of the eye chart at patient's eye level.
		•	Instructed patient to cover the left eye with the occluder and to keep the left eye open.
		▷	Stated how the occluder should be positioned if the patient wears glasses.
		▷	Explained why the patient's left eye should remain open.
		•	Instructed patient not to squint during the test.
		▷	Explained why the patient should not squint during the test.
		•	Asked patient to identify the 20/70 line, using the right eye.
		▷	Stated why the test should begin with a line that is above the 20/20 line.
		•	Proceeded down the chart if the patient identified the 20/70 line or proceeded up the chart if the patient was unable to identify the 20/70 line.
		•	Continued until the smallest line of letters that the patient could read was reached.
		•	Observed patient for any unusual symptoms.

Trial 1	Trial 2	Point Value	Performance Standards
		●	Jotted down the numbers next to the smallest line read by the patient.
		●	Asked patient to cover the right eye and to keep the right eye open.
		●	Measured visual acuity in the left eye.
		●	Jotted down the numbers next to the smallest line read by the patient.
		*	The visual acuity measurements were identical to the evaluator's measurements.
		●	Charted the results correctly.
		●	Disinfected the occluder with an antiseptic wipe.
		●	Sanitized hands.
		Ⓐ	Incorporated critical thinking skills when performing patient assessment.
		*	Completed the procedure within 5 minutes.
			TOTALS

CHART	
Date	

Evaluation of Student Performance

EVALUATION CRITERIA			COMMENTS
Symbol	Category	Point Value	
*	Critical Step	16 points	
●	Essential Step	6 points	
Ⓐ	Affective Competency	6 points	
▷	Theory Question	2 points	
Score calculation: 100 points – ___ points missed ___ Score Satisfactory score: 85 or above			

2008 CAAHEP Competencies Achieved
Psychomotor (Skills) ☑ IV. 6. Prepare a patient for procedures and/or treatments. ***Affective (Behavior)*** ☑ I. 2. Use language/verbal skills that enable patient's understanding. ☑ IV. 7. Demonstrate recognition of the patient's level of understanding in communications.

2015 CAAHEP Competencies Achieved
Psychomotor (Skills) ☑ I. 8. Instruct and prepare a patient for a procedure or a treatment. ***Affective (Behavior)*** ☑ I. 1. Incorporate critical thinking skills when performing patient assessment.

ABHES Competencies Achieved
☑ 4. a. Follow documentation guidelines. ☑ 9. e. Perform specialty procedures, but not limited to minor surgery, cardiac, respiratory, OB-GYN, neurological, gastroenterology.

Notes

EVALUATION OF COMPETENCY

Procedure 21-2: Assessing Color Vision—Ishihara Test

Name: ______________________ Date: ______________

Evaluated by: ______________________ Score: ______________

Performance Objective

Outcome:	Assess color vision.
Conditions:	Given an Ishihara book of color plates and a cotton swab.
Standards:	Time: 10 minutes. Student completed procedure in ________ minutes.
	Accuracy: Satisfactory score on the performance evaluation checklist.

Performance Evaluation Checklist

Trial 1	Trial 2	Point Value	Performance Standards
		●	Sanitized hands.
		●	Assembled equipment.
		●	Conducted the test in a quiet room illuminated by natural daylight.
		▷	Stated why natural daylight should be used.
		●	Greeted the patient and introduced yourself.
		●	Identified the patient.
		●	Explained the procedure using the practice plate.
		▷	Stated the purpose of the practice plate.
		●	Held the first plate 30 inches from the patient at a right angle to the patient's line of vision.
		●	Instructed patient to keep both eyes open.
		●	Told patient that he or she would have 3 seconds to identify each plate.
		●	Asked the patient to identify the number on the plate.
		●	Asked the patient to trace plates that have a winding line with a cotton swab.
		▷	Stated why a cotton swab should be used to make the tracing.
		●	Recorded the results after identification of each plate.
		●	Continued until the patient viewed all plates.
		●	Charted the results correctly.
		*	The results were identical to the evaluator's results.
		●	Returned the Ishihara book to its proper place, storing it in a closed position.

Trial 1	Trial 2	Point Value	Performance Standards
		▷	Explained why the book should be stored in a closed position.
		Ⓐ	Incorporated critical thinking skills when performing patient assessment.
		*	Completed the procedure within 10 minutes.
			TOTALS

CHART	
Date	

CHART		
Plate No.	Normal Person	Results
1	12	
2	8	
3	5	
4	29	
5	74	
6	7	
7	45	
8	2	
9	X	
10	16	
11	Traceable	
Date:		
Evaluated by :		

Evaluation of Student Performance

EVALUATION CRITERIA			COMMENTS
Symbol	Category	Point Value	
∗	Critical Step	16 points	
●	Essential Step	6 points	
Ⓐ	Affective Competency	6 points	
▷	Theory Question	2 points	
Score calculation: 100 points − ___ points missed ___ Score Satisfactory score: 85 or above			

2008 CAAHEP Competencies Achieved
Psychomotor (Skills) ☑ IV. 6. Prepare a patient for procedures and/or treatments. ***Affective (Behavior)*** ☑ I. 2. Use language/verbal skills that enable patients' understanding. ☑ IV. 7. Demonstrate recognition of the patient's level of understanding in communications.

2015 CAAHEP Competencies Achieved
Psychomotor (Skills) ☑ I. 8. Instruct and prepare a patient for a procedure or a treatment. ***Affective (Behavior)*** ☑ I. 1. Incorporate critical thinking skills when performing patient assessment.

ABHES Competencies Achieved
☑ 4. a. Follow documentation guidelines. ☑ 9. e. Perform specialty procedures, but not limited to minor surgery, cardiac, respiratory, OB-GYN, neurological, gastroenterology.

Notes

EVALUATION OF COMPETENCY

Procedure 21-3: Performing an Eye Irrigation

Name: ______________________ Date: ______________

Evaluated by: ______________________ Score: ______________

Performance Objective

Outcome:	Perform an eye irrigation.
Conditions:	Given the following: disposable (nonpowdered) gloves, irrigating solution, solution container, disposable rubber bulb syringe, basin, moisture-resistant towel, and sterile gauze pads.
Standards:	Time: 5 minutes. Student completed procedure in ________ minutes.
	Accuracy: Satisfactory score on the Performance Evaluation Checklist.

Performance Evaluation Checklist

Trial 1	Trial 2	Point Value	Performance Standards
		●	Sanitized hands.
		●	Assembled equipment.
		●	Checked the solution label with the physician's instructions.
		●	Checked expiration date of the solution.
		▷	Stated the reason for checking the expiration date.
		●	Warmed the irrigating solution to body temperature.
		▷	Explained why the solution should be at body temperature.
		●	Checked the label a second time and poured the solution into a basin.
		●	Checked the label a third time before returning the container to storage.
		●	Greeted the patient and introduced yourself.
		●	Identified the patient and explained the procedure.
		●	Asked patient to remove glasses or contact lenses.
		●	Positioned patient in a lying or sitting position.
		●	Placed a moisture-resistant towel on the patient's shoulder.
		●	Positioned a basin tightly against the patient's cheek under the affected eye.
		●	Asked patient to tilt head in the direction of the affected eye and hold the basin in place.
		▷	Explained why patient's head is turned in the direction of the affected eye.
		●	Applied nonpowdered gloves.

Trial 1	Trial 2	Point Value	Performance Standards
		▷	Stated why nonpowdered gloves should be used.
		●	Cleansed the eyelids from inner to outer canthus.
		▷	Stated why eyelids are cleansed.
		●	Filled irrigating syringe.
		●	Instructed patient to keep both eyes open and to look at a focal point.
		▷	Stated the reason for looking at a focal point.
		●	Separated eyelids.
		●	Held tip of syringe 1 inch above the eye at the inner canthus.
		●	Allowed solution to flow over the eye at a moderate rate from the inner canthus to the outer canthus and directed solution to the lower conjunctiva.
		▷	Explained why the syringe should be directed toward the lower conjunctiva.
		●	Did not allow syringe to touch the eye.
		●	Refilled the syringe and continued irrigating until the desired results were obtained or all the solution was used.
		●	Dried eyelids with gauze pad from inner to outer canthus.
		●	Removed gloves and sanitized hands.
		●	Charted the procedure correctly.
		●	Returned equipment.
		Ⓐ	Incorporated critical thinking skills when performing patient care.
		Ⓐ	Showed awareness of a patient's concerns related to the procedure being performed.
		Ⓐ	Explained to a patient the rationale for performance of a procedure.
		✶	Completed the procedure within 5 minutes.
			TOTALS

CHART	
Date	

Evaluation of Student Performance

EVALUATION CRITERIA			COMMENTS
Symbol	**Category**	**Point Value**	
∗	Critical Step	16 points	
●	Essential Step	6 points	
Ⓐ	Affective Competency	6 points	
▷	Theory Question	2 points	
Score calculation: 100 points – ___ points missed ___ Score Satisfactory score: 85 or above			

2008 CAAHEP Competencies Achieved
Psychomotor (Skills) ☑ II. 1. Prepare proper dosages of medication for administration. ☑ IV. 6. Prepare a patient for procedures and/or treatments. ***Affective (Behavior)*** ☑ II. 1. Verify ordered doses/dosages prior to administration. ☑ IV. 5. Demonstrate sensitivity appropriate to the message being delivered.

2015 CAAHEP Competencies Achieved
Psychomotor (Skills) ☑ I. 8. Instruct and prepare a patient for a procedure or a treatment. ☑ II. 1. Calculate proper dosages of medication for administration. ☑ X.3. Document patient care accurately in the medical record. ***Affective (Behavior)*** ☑ I. 2. Incorporate critical thinking skills when performing patient care. ☑ I. 3. Show awareness of a patient's concerns related to the procedure being performed. ☑ V. 4. Explain to a patient the rationale for performance of a procedure.

ABHES Competencies Achieved
☑ 2. c. Identify diagnostic and treatment modalities as they relate to each body system. ☑ 4. a. Follow documentation guidelines. ☑ 9. e. Perform specialty procedures, but not limited to minor surgery, cardiac, respiratory, OB-GYN, neurological, gastroenterology.

Notes

EVALUATION OF COMPETENCY

Procedure 21-4: Performing an Eye Instillation

Name: ______________________________ Date: ____________________

Evaluated by: ______________________________ Score: ____________________

Performance Objective

Outcome:	Perform an eye instillation.
Conditions:	Given the following: disposable (nonpowdered) gloves, ophthalmic medication, tissues, and gauze pads.
Standards:	Time: 5 minutes. Student completed procedure in __________ minutes.
	Accuracy: Satisfactory score on the Performance Evaluation Checklist.

Performance Evaluation Checklist

Trial 1	Trial 2	Point Value	Performance Standards
		●	Sanitized hands.
		●	Assembled equipment.
		●	Checked the drug label when removing it from storage.
		▷	Stated what word must appear on the medication label.
		●	Checked drug label and dosage against the physician's instructions.
		●	Checked the expiration date of the medication.
		●	Greeted the patient and introduced yourself.
		●	Identified the patient and explained the procedure.
		●	Positioned patient in a sitting or supine position.
		●	Applied nonpowdered gloves.
		●	Prepared the medication.
		●	Checked the drug label and removed the cap.
		●	Asked patient to look up and exposed the lower conjunctival sac.
		▷	Explained the reason for asking patient to look up.
		●	Drew the skin of the cheek downward and exposed the conjunctival sac.
		●	Inserted the medication correctly.
		▷	Explained how to instill eyedrops and ointment.
		●	Instructed patient to close eyes gently and move eyeballs.
		▷	Stated the reason for closing the eyes and moving the eyeballs.

Trial 1	Trial 2	Point Value	Performance Standards
		●	Told patient that the instillation may temporarily blur vision.
		●	Dried eyelids with a gauze pad from inner to outer canthus.
		●	Removed gloves and sanitized hands.
		●	Charted the procedure correctly.
		●	Returned equipment.
		Ⓐ	Incorporated critical thinking skills when performing patient care.
		Ⓐ	Showed awareness of a patient's concerns related to the procedure being performed.
		Ⓐ	Explained to a patient the rationale for performance of a procedure.
		*	Completed the procedure within 5 minutes.
			TOTALS

CHART	
Date	

Evaluation of Student Performance

EVALUATION CRITERIA			COMMENTS
Symbol	Category	Point Value	
*	Critical Step	16 points	
●	Essential Step	6 points	
Ⓐ	Affective Competency	6 points	
▷	Theory Question	2 points	
Score calculation: 100 points – ___ points missed ___ Score Satisfactory score: 85 or above			

2008 CAAHEP Competencies Achieved
Psychomotor (Skills) ☑ II. 1. Prepare proper dosages of medication for administration. ☑ IV. 6. Prepare a patient for procedures and/or treatments. *Affective (Behavior)* ☑ II. 1. Verify ordered doses/dosages prior to administration. ☑ IV. 5. Demonstrate sensitivity appropriate to the message being delivered.

2015 CAAHEP Competencies Achieved

Psychomotor (Skills)

☑ I. 8. Instruct and prepare a patient for a procedure or a treatment.
☑ II. 1. Calculate proper dosages of medication for administration.
☑ X.3. Document patient care accurately in the medical record.

Affective (Behavior)

☑ I. 2. Incorporate critical thinking skills when performing patient care.
☑ I. 3. Show awareness of a patient's concerns related to the procedure being performed.
☑ V. 4. Explain to a patient the rationale for performance of a procedure.

ABHES Competencies Achieved

☑ 2. c. Identify diagnostic and treatment modalities as they relate to each body system.
☑ 4. a. Follow documentation guidelines.
☑ 9. e. Perform specialty procedures, but not limited to minor surgery, cardiac, respiratory, OB-GYN, neurological, gastroenterology.

Notes

EVALUATION OF COMPETENCY

Procedure 21-5: Performing an Ear Irrigation

Name: ______________________ Date: ______________

Evaluated by: ______________________ Score: ______________

Performance Objective

Outcome:	Perform an ear irrigation.
Conditions:	Given the following: disposable gloves, irrigating solution, solution container, irrigating syringe, ear basin, moisture-resistant towel, gauze pads, and ear wick.
Standards:	Time: 10 minutes. Student completed procedure in ________ minutes.
	Accuracy: Satisfactory score on the performance evaluation checklist.

Performance Evaluation Checklist

Trial 1	Trial 2	Point Value	Performance Standards
		•	Sanitized hands.
		•	Assembled equipment.
		•	Checked the label of the irrigating solution with the physician's instructions.
		•	Checked expiration date of the solution.
		•	Warmed the irrigating solution to body temperature.
		▷	Stated the reason for warming the irrigating solution.
		•	Checked the label a second time and poured the solution into a basin.
		•	Checked the label a third time before returning the container to storage.
		•	Greeted the patient and introduced yourself.
		•	Identified the patient and explained the procedure.
		•	Positioned patient in a sitting position.
		•	Placed a towel on patient's shoulder under ear to be irrigated.
		•	Positioned basin under affected ear and asked patient to hold it in place.
		•	Asked patient to tilt head toward the affected ear.
		▷	Explained why the head should be tilted toward the affected ear.
		•	Applied gloves.
		•	Cleansed the outer ear.
		▷	Explained why the outer ear should be cleansed.
		•	Filled the irrigating syringe.

Trial 1	Trial 2	Point Value	Performance Standards
		●	Expelled air from syringe.
		▷	Explained why air should be expelled from syringe.
		●	Properly straightened the ear canal.
		▷	Stated why the canal must be straightened.
		●	Inserted syringe tip into the ear.
		●	Did not insert the syringe too deeply.
		●	Made sure that tip of syringe did not obstruct the canal opening.
		▷	Stated why the canal should not be obstructed.
		●	Injected the irrigating solution toward the roof of the ear canal.
		▷	Stated why solution should be injected toward roof of the canal.
		●	Refilled the syringe and continued irrigating until the desired results were obtained or all the solution was used.
		●	Observed the returning solution to note the material present and the amount.
		●	Dried outside of the ear with a gauze pad.
		●	Informed patient that the ear will feel sensitive.
		●	Instructed patient to lie on the affected side on treatment table.
		▷	Explained why patient should lie on the affected side.
		●	Inserted a cotton wick loosely in the ear canal for 15 minutes.
		▷	Stated the purpose of the cotton wick.
		●	Removed gloves and sanitized hands.
		●	Charted the procedure correctly.
		●	Returned equipment.
		Ⓐ	Incorporated critical thinking skills when performing patient care.
		Ⓐ	Showed awareness of a patient's concerns related to the procedure being performed.
		Ⓐ	Explained to a patient the rationale for performance of a procedure.
		✶	Completed the procedure within 10 minutes.
			TOTALS

CHART	
Date	

Evaluation of Student Performance

EVALUATION CRITERIA			COMMENTS
Symbol	**Category**	**Point Value**	
∗	Critical Step	16 points	
●	Essential Step	6 points	
Ⓐ	Affective Competency	6 points	
▷	Theory Question	2 points	
Score calculation: 100 points – ___ points missed ___ Score Satisfactory score: 85 or above			

2008 CAAHEP Competencies Achieved
Psychomotor (Skills) ☑ II. 1. Prepare proper dosages of medication for administration. ☑ IV. 6. Prepare a patient for procedures and/or treatments. ***Affective (Behavior)*** ☑ II. 1. Verify ordered doses/dosages prior to administration. ☑ IV. 5. Demonstrate sensitivity appropriate to the message being delivered.

2015 CAAHEP Competencies Achieved
Psychomotor (Skills) ☑ I. 8. Instruct and prepare a patient for a procedure or a treatment. ☑ II. 1. Calculate proper dosages of medication for administration. ☑ X.3. Document patient care accurately in the medical record. ***Affective (Behavior)*** ☑ I. 2. Incorporate critical thinking skills when performing patient care. ☑ I. 3. Show awareness of a patient's concerns related to the procedure being performed. ☑ V. 4. Explain to a patient the rationale for performance of a procedure.

ABHES Competencies Achieved
☑ 2. c. Identify diagnostic and treatment modalities as they relate to each body system. ☑ 4. a. Follow documentation guidelines. ☑ 9. e. Perform specialty procedures, but not limited to minor surgery, cardiac, respiratory, OB-GYN, neurological, gastroenterology.

Notes

EVALUATION OF COMPETENCY

Procedure 21-6: Performing an Ear Instillation

Name: ______________________________ Date: ______________

Evaluated by: ______________________________ Score: ______________

Performance Objective

Outcome:	Perform an ear instillation.
Conditions:	Given the following: disposable gloves, otic medication, and gauze pad.
Standards:	Time: 5 minutes. Student completed procedure in ________ minutes.
	Accuracy: Satisfactory score on the Performance Evaluation Checklist.

Performance Evaluation Checklist

Trial 1	Trial 2	Point Value	Performance Standards
		●	Sanitized hands.
		●	Assembled equipment.
		●	Checked the drug label when removing the medication from storage.
		▷	Stated what word must appear on the medication label.
		●	Checked the drug label and dosage against the physician's instructions.
		●	Checked the expiration date of the medication.
		▷	Explained what might occur if the medication is outdated.
		●	Greeted the patient and introduced yourself.
		●	Identified the patient and explained the procedure.
		●	Positioned patient in a sitting position.
		●	Warmed the eardrops with your hands.
		●	Applied gloves.
		●	Mixed medication if required, by shaking the container.
		●	Checked the drug label and removed the cap.
		●	Asked the patient to tilt the head in the direction of the unaffected ear.
		●	Properly straightened the ear canal.
		▷	Stated the reason for straightening the canal.
		●	Placed tip of dropper at the opening of the ear canal and inserted the proper amount of medication.
		●	Instructed patient to lie on the unaffected side for 2 to 3 minutes.

Trial 1	Trial 2	Point Value	Performance Standards
		▷	Explained why patient should lie on the unaffected side.
		●	Placed a moistened cotton wick loosely in the ear canal for 15 minutes.
		▷	Stated the reason for moistening the wick.
		●	Removed gloves and sanitized hands.
		●	Charted the procedure correctly.
		●	Returned equipment.
		Ⓐ	Incorporated critical thinking skills when performing patient care.
		Ⓐ	Showed awareness of a patient's concerns related to the procedure being performed.
		Ⓐ	Explained to a patient the rationale for performance of a procedure.
		*	Completed the procedure within 5 minutes.
			TOTALS

CHART	
Date	

Evaluation of Student Performance

EVALUATION CRITERIA			COMMENTS
Symbol	**Category**	**Point Value**	
*	Critical Step	16 points	
●	Essential Step	6 points	
Ⓐ	Affective Competency	6 points	
▷	Theory Question	2 points	
Score calculation: 100 points – ___ points missed ___ Score Satisfactory score: 85 or above			

2008 CAAHEP Competencies Achieved

Psychomotor (Skills)

☑ II. 1. Prepare proper dosages of medication for administration.
☑ IV. 6. Prepare a patient for procedures and/or treatments.

Affective (Behavior)

☑ II. 1. Verify ordered doses/dosages prior to administration.
☑ IV. 5. Demonstrate sensitivity appropriate to the message being delivered.

2015 CAAHEP Competencies Achieved
Psychomotor (Skills) ☑ I. 8. Instruct and prepare a patient for a procedure or a treatment. ☑ II. 1. Calculate proper dosages of medication for administration. ☑ X.3. Document patient care accurately in the medical record. ***Affective (Behavior)*** ☑ I. 2. Incorporate critical thinking skills when performing patient care. ☑ I. 3. Show awareness of a patient's concerns related to the procedure being performed. ☑ V. 4. Explain to a patient the rationale for performance of a procedure.

ABHES Competencies Achieved
☑ 2. c. Identify diagnostic and treatment modalities as they relate to each body system. ☑ 4. a. Follow documentation guidelines. ☑ 9. e. Perform specialty procedures, but not limited to minor surgery, cardiac, respiratory, OB-GYN, neurological, gastroenterology.

Notes

22 Physical Agents to Promote Tissue Healing

CHAPTER ASSIGNMENTS

✓ After Completing	Date Due	Study Guide Pages	STUDY GUIDE ASSIGNMENTS (CTA = Critical Thinking Activity)	Possible Points	Points You Earned
		469	Pretest	10	
		470	Term Key Term Assessment	9	
		470-472	Evaluation of Learning questions	15	
		472-473	CTA A: Dear Gabby	10	
		473	CTA B: Crutch Guidelines	8	
		474	CTA C: Accessibility for Physical Disabilities	7	
		475	CTA D: Crossword Puzzle	25	
		476-478	CTA E: Bone and Joint Conditions	40	
			Evolve Site: Quiz Show (Record points earned)		
			Evolve Site: Apply Your Knowledge questions	10	
			Evolve Site: Video Evaluation	63	
		469	Posttest	10	
			ADDITIONAL ASSIGNMENTS		
			TOTAL POINTS		

Notes

✓ When Assigned By Your Instructor	Study Guide Page(s)	Practices Required	LABORATORY ASSIGNMENTS (Procedure Number and Name)	Score*
	479-480	3	**Practice for Competency** 22-1: Applying a Heating Pad Textbook reference: p. 471	
	481-482		**Evaluation of Competency** 22-1: Applying a Heating Pad	*
	479-480	3	**Practice for Competency** 22-2: Applying a Hot Soak Textbook reference: p. 472	
	483-485		**Evaluation of Competency** 22-2: Applying a Hot Soak	*
	479-480	3	**Practice for Competency** 22-3: Applying a Hot Compress Textbook reference: pp. 473-474	
	487-489		**Evaluation of Competency** 22-3: Applying a Hot Compress	*
	479-480	3	**Practice for Competency** 22-4: Applying an Ice Bag Textbook reference: pp. 474-475	
	491-493		**Evaluation of Competency** 22-4: Applying an Ice Bag	*
	479-480	3	**Practice for Competency** 22-5: Applying a Cold Compress Textbook reference: pp. 475-476	
	495-497		**Evaluation of Competency** 22-5: Applying a Cold Compress	*
	479-480	3	**Practice for Competency** 22-6: Applying a Chemical Pack Textbook reference: p. 476	
	499-500		**Evaluation of Competency** 22-6: Applying a Chemical Pack	*
	479-480	3	**Practice for Competency** 22-7: Measuring for Axillary Crutches Textbook reference: p. 480	
	501-502		**Evaluation of Competency** 22-7: Measuring for Axillary Crutches	*
	479-480	3 × for each gait	**Practice for Competency** 22-8: Instructing a Patient in Crutch Gaits Textbook reference: pp. 481-483	
	503-505		**Evaluation of Competency** 22-8: Instructing a Patient in Crutch Gaits	*

✓ When Assigned By Your Instructor	Study Guide Page(s)	Practices Required	LABORATORY ASSIGNMENTS (Procedure Number and Name)	Score*
	479-480	Cane: 3 Walker: 3	**Practice for Competency** 22-9 and 22-10: Instructing a Patient in the Use of a Cane and Walker Textbook reference: p. 484	
	507-508		**Evaluation of Competency** 22-9 and 22-10: Instructing a Patient in the Use of a Cane and Walker	*
			ADDITIONAL ASSIGNMENTS	

Name ____ Date ______________

PRETEST

True or False

_______ 1. A hot compress is an example of moist heat.

_______ 2. Erythema is redness of the skin caused by dilation of superficial blood vessels.

_______ 3. The local application of cold may be used to relieve muscle spasms.

_______ 4. Heat is often prescribed by the physician for black eyes.

_______ 5. The medical assistant should instruct the patient to adjust the heating pad to a higher setting if it no longer feels warm.

_______ 6. Chemical cold packs should be stored in the refrigerator.

_______ 7. Forearm crutches are often used by patients with cerebral palsy.

_______ 8. The three-point gait is the most stable and slowest crutch gait.

_______ 9. Ambulation refers to the inability to walk.

_______ 10. A patient using crutches should be instructed to support his or her weight against the axilla.

POSTTEST

True or False

_______ 1. The recommended time for the application of heat is 15 to 30 minutes.

_______ 2. The local application of heat results in constriction of blood vessels in the area where it is applied.

_______ 3. An exudate is a discharge produced by the body's tissues.

_______ 4. After immersing a patient's foot in a hot soak, the medical assistant should add crushed ice to the soak.

_______ 5. A patient with diabetes mellitus may have more than usual sensitivity to the local application of heat.

_______ 6. An ice bag should be filled with large pieces of ice.

_______ 7. If axillary crutches have been fitted properly, the elbow will be flexed at an angle of 30 degrees.

_______ 8. Walkers are primarily used by pediatric patients.

_______ 9. Incorrectly fitted crutches may cause crutch palsy.

_______ 10. A cane should be held on the strong side of the body.

Term KEY TERM ASSESSMENT

Directions: Match each key term with its definition.

_______ 1. Ambulation
_______ 2. Compress
_______ 3. Edema
_______ 4. Erythema
_______ 5. Exudate
_______ 6. Soak
_______ 7. Sprain
_______ 8. Strain
_______ 9. Suppuration

A. A discharge produced by the body's tissues
B. An overstretching of a muscle caused by trauma
C. A soft, moist, absorbent cloth that is folded in several layers and applied to a part of the body in the local application of heat or cold
D. Walking or moving from one place to another
E. The direct immersion of a body part in water or a medicated solution
F. The retention of fluid in the tissues, resulting in swelling
G. Reddening of the skin caused by dilation of superficial blood vessels in the skin
H. Trauma to a joint that causes injury to the ligaments
I. The process of pus formation

EVALUATION OF LEARNING

Directions: Fill in each blank with the correct answer.

1. State whether the following is an example of dry heat, moist heat, dry cold, or moist cold.
   a. Hot compress
   ____
   b. Ice bag
   ____
   c. Heating pad
   ____
   d. Chemical hot pack
   ____
   e. Cold compress
   ____

2. List three factors that must be taken into consideration when applying heat or cold.
   ____
   ____

3. How does the local application of heat to an affected area for a short period of time influence the following?
   a. The diameter of the blood vessels in the affected area
   ____
   b. The blood supply to the affected area
   ____
   c. Tissue metabolism in the affected area
   ____

4. What happens to the diameter of blood vessels if heat is applied for a prolonged period (more than 1 hour)?

5. List three reasons for applying heat locally.

6. How does the local application of cold for a short period of time to an affected area influence the following?
   a. The diameter of the blood vessels in the affected area
   b. The blood supply to the affected area
   c. Tissue metabolism in the affected area

7. List two reasons for applying cold locally.

8. What factors does the physician take into consideration when prescribing an ambulatory assistive device?

9. Describe one advantage of the forearm crutch.

10. What may occur if axillary crutches are not fitted properly?

11. List eight guidelines that must be followed during crutch use to ensure safety.

12. List one use for each of the following crutch gaits:

a. Four-point gait ____

b. Three-point gait ____

c. Swing-to gait ____

13. List and describe the three types of canes.

14. List two reasons for prescribing a cane.

15. List two reasons for prescribing a walker.

CRITICAL THINKING ACTIVITIES

A. Dear Gabby

Gabby was called out of town unexpectedly and wants you to fill in for her. In the space provided, respond to the following letter.

Dear Gabby:

I am 15 years old and in the 10th grade. I need your help. I have a backpack; my dad weighed it and said it was 40 pounds. I only weigh 105 pounds. My back and neck hurt from lugging it around. I have to walk almost one-half mile to the bus stop. I do not have time to use my locker between classes because it is down a flight of stairs and at the end of the hall. Once, when I started using my locker, my science teacher got mad at me because I was late getting to class. Gabby, what should I do?

Signed,

Pain in the Neck

B. Crutch Guidelines

Each of the following patients is wearing a long leg cast because of a broken tibia and is using wooden axillary crutches to ambulate. Evaluate the crutch technique being practiced by each patient. Write C if the technique is correct and I if the technique is incorrect. If the technique is correct, explain why it should be performed this way. If incorrect, indicate what may happen from performing the technique in this manner.

1. Andy Morris wears Nike sports shoes when ambulating with his crutches.

2. Juliet Wright does not stand up straight when using her crutches.

3. Miguel Saldivia puts his weight on the axilla when getting around on his crutches.

4. Lindy Campbell has a lot of decorative throw rugs in her house, and she does not want to remove them.

5. Andrew Spence likes to move quickly on his crutches so he advances them forward about 20 inches with each step when using the swing-through gait.

6. Hanna Romes has tingling in her hands but thinks it is just part of what happens when one uses crutches.

7. Tamra Hetrick pads both the shoulder rests and the handgrips of her crutches.

8. Erica Anderson's crutch tips get wet but she does not take the time to dry them before going into a shopping mall.

C. Accessibility for Physical Disabilities

Next to each of the following facilities, list the features you have observed that facilitate accessibility of individuals with a physical disability.

1. Schools

2. Grocery stores

3. Shopping malls

4. Movie theaters

5. Restaurants

6. Doctors' offices

7. Community parks

D. Crossword Puzzle: Physical Agents to Promote Tissue Healing

Directions: Complete the crossword puzzle using the clues provided.

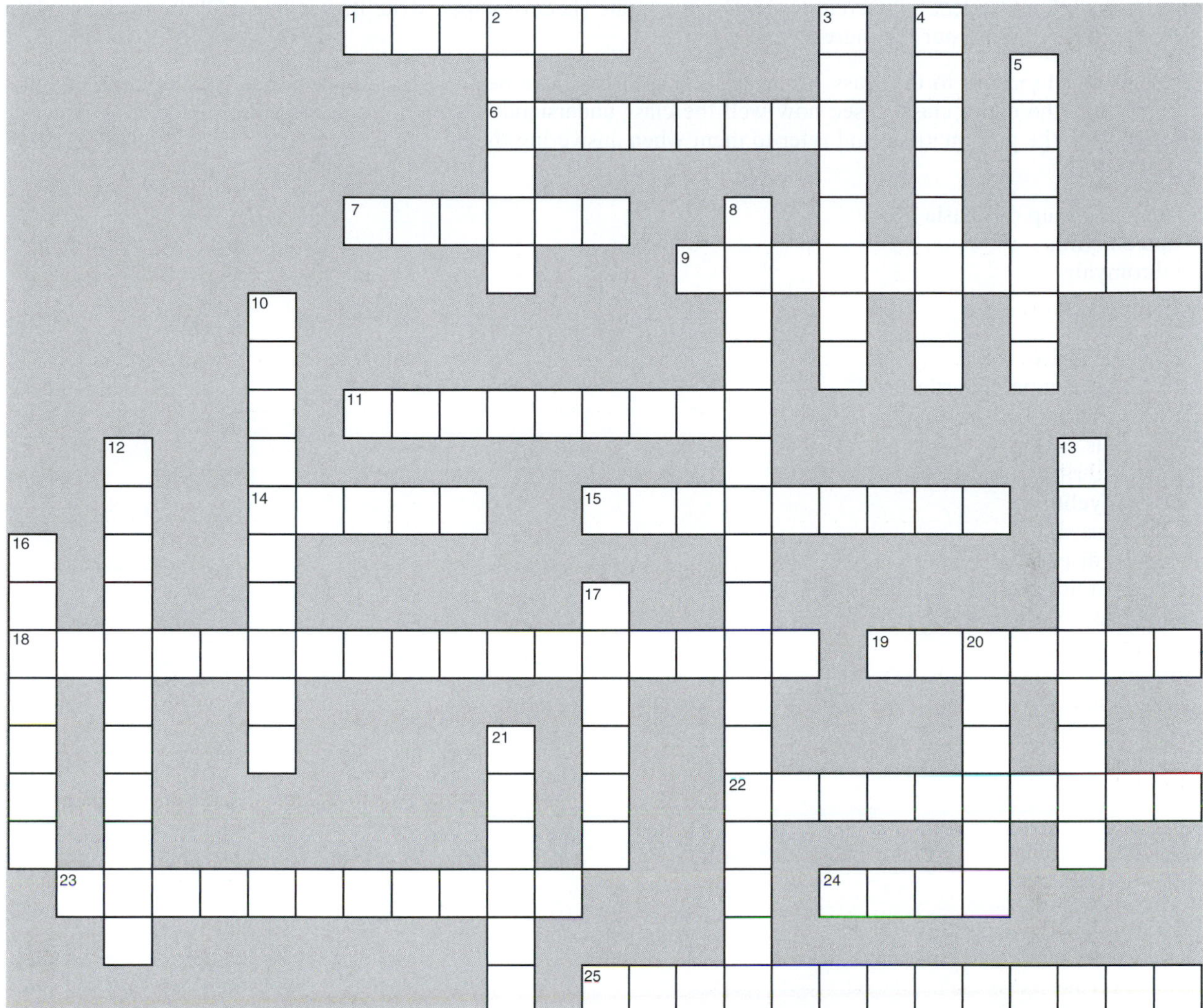

Across

1 Cold prescribed for this condition
6 Red skin
7 Overstretching of a muscle
9 "Too long" crutches may cause this
11 Cold blood vessels do this
14 Retention of fluid
15 Slow crutch gait
18 Do not use heat for this condition
19 Are more sensitive to cold
22 Walking
23 Crutch guideline for maintaining body balance
24 Examples: standard, tripod, or quad
25 Elbow flexion for crutches

Down

2 Example of dry cold
3 Condition that causes impaired circulation
4 Transfers weight from legs to arms
5 Discharge
8 Cane handle should be level with this
10 Broken leg crutch gait
12 Pus formation
13 Heat often prescribed for this condition
16 Application of heat promotes this
17 Needed after knee replacement
20 Warm blood vessels do this
21 Maximum minutes for heat application

E. Bone and Joint Conditions

1. It is National Bone and Joint Week. The mayor has asked you and your classmates to develop informative, creative, and colorful brochures for the community about bone and joint conditions. Choose a condition below and design a brochure using the blank Frequently Asked Questions (FAQs) brochure provided on the following page. Each student in the class should select a different topic. On a separate sheet of paper, write three true or false questions relating to the information in your brochure.

2. Present your brochure to the class. After all the brochures have been presented, each student should ask the three questions to the entire class to see how well the class understands bone and joint conditions. (Note: You can take notes during the presentations and refer to them when answering the questions.)

1. Bursitis
2. Congenital hip dysplasia
3. Epicondylitis
4. Fibromyalgia
5. Gout
6. Hammer toe
7. Herniated disk
8. Juvenile rheumatoid arthritis
9. Knee replacement surgery
10. Kyphosis
11. Osteoarthritis
12. Osteomyelitis
13. Osteoporosis
14. Paget's disease
15. Rheumatoid arthritis
16. Scoliosis
17. Sprain
18. Strain
19. Tendonitis

FAQ on:

Q:

A:

Q:

A:

Q:

A:

Q:

A:

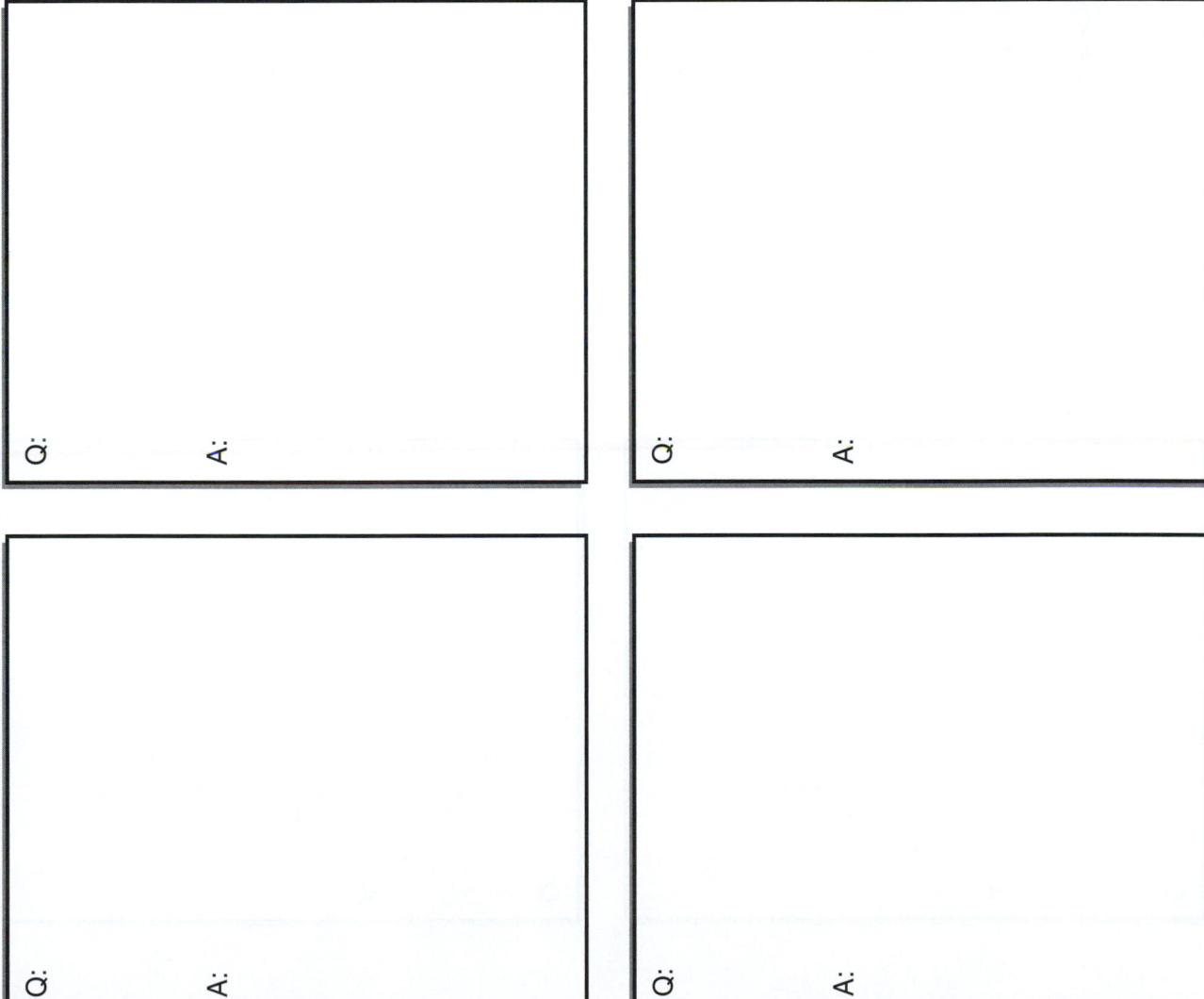

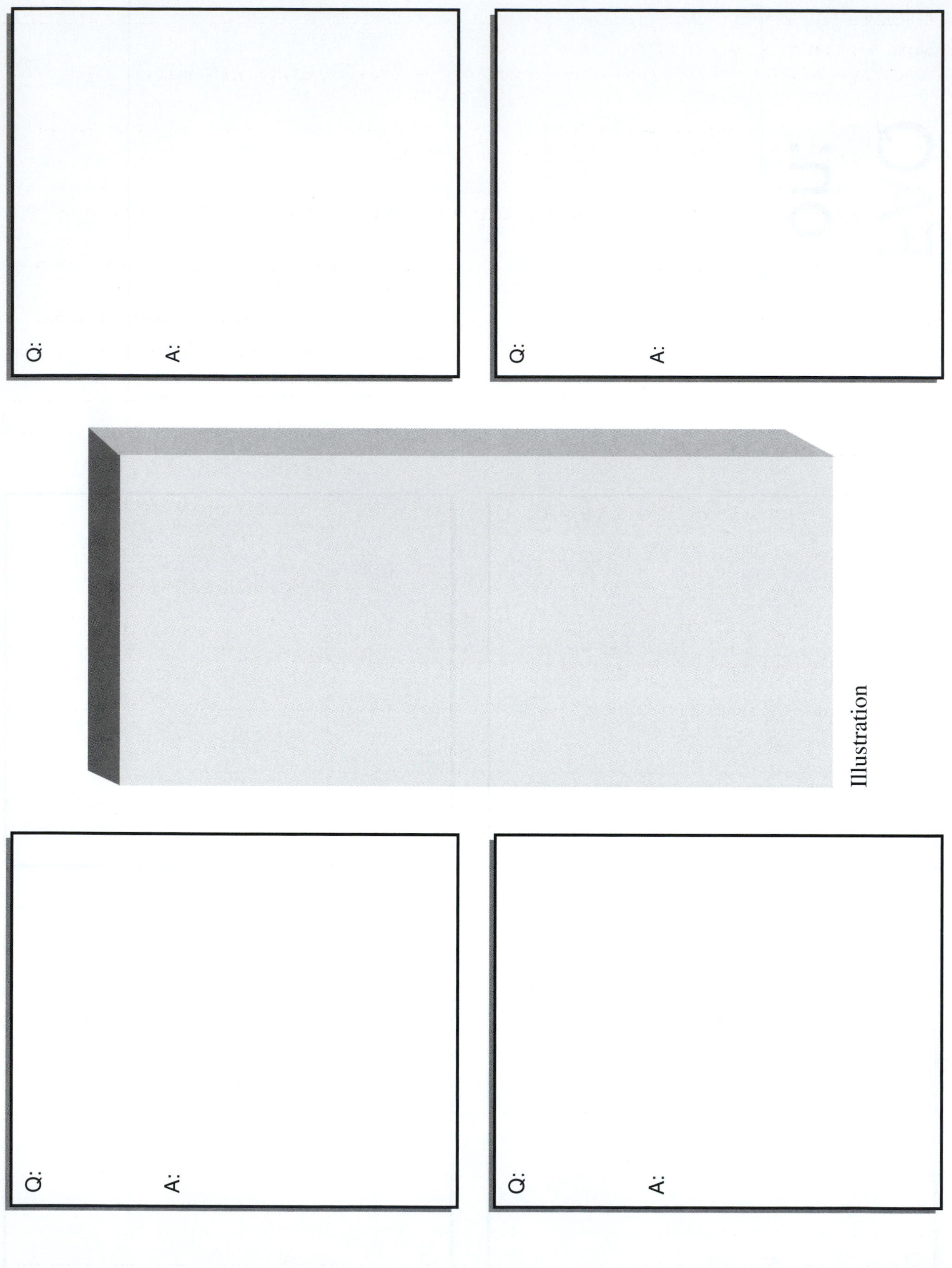
Q:
A:
Q:
A:
Illustration
Q:
A:
Q:
A:

PRACTICE FOR COMPETENCY

Local Application of Heat and Cold

Procedures 22-1, 22-2, and 22-3: Application of Heat. Apply the following heat treatments, and record the procedure in the chart provided: heating pad, hot soak, hot compress, and chemical hot pack.

Procedures 22-4, 22-5, and 22-6: Application of Cold. Apply the following cold treatments, and record the results in the chart provided: ice bag, cold compress, and chemical cold pack.

Ambulatory Aids

Procedure 22-7: Axillary Crutch Measurement. Measure an individual for axillary crutches, and record the procedure in the chart provided.

Procedure 22-8: Crutch Gaits. Instruct an individual in mastering the following crutch gaits: four-point, two-point, three-point, swing-to, and swing-through. Record the procedure in the chart provided.

Procedure 22-9: Cane. Instruct an individual in the use of a cane, and record the procedure in the chart provided.

Procedure 22-10: Walker. Instruct an individual in the use of a walker, and record the procedure in the chart provided.

CHART	
Date	

Chart	
Date	

EVALUATION OF COMPETENCY

Procedure 22-1: Applying a Heating Pad

Name: ______________________ Date: ______________

Evaluated by: ______________________ Score: ______________

Performance Objective

Outcome:	Apply a heating pad.
Conditions:	Given a heating pad with a protective covering.
Standards:	Time: 5 minutes. Student completed procedure in __________ minutes.
	Accuracy: Satisfactory score on the performance evaluation checklist.

Performance Evaluation Checklist

Trial 1	Trial 2	Point Value	Performance Standards
		●	Sanitized hands.
		●	Assembled equipment.
		●	Greeted the patient and introduced yourself.
		●	Identified the patient and explained the procedure.
		●	Placed the heating pad in protective covering.
		●	Connected the plug to electrical outlet and set selector switch to the proper setting.
		●	Placed heating pad on patient's affected body area and asked how the temperature felt.
		●	Instructed patient not to lie on the pad or turn the temperature setting higher.
		▷	Stated why patient should be instructed not to lie on heating pad.
		▷	Explained why patient may want to increase the temperature.
		●	Checked patient's skin periodically.
		●	Administered treatment for the proper length of time as designated by physician.
		●	Sanitized hands.
		●	Charted the procedure correctly.
		●	Properly cared for and returned equipment to its storage place.
		Ⓐ	Incorporated critical thinking skills when performing patient assessment.
		Ⓐ	Incorporated critical thinking skills when performing patient care.
		*	Completed the procedure within 5 minutes.
			TOTALS

Evaluation of Student Performance

EVALUATION CRITERIA			COMMENTS
Symbol	**Category**	**Point Value**	
∗	Critical Step	16 points	
●	Essential Step	6 points	
Ⓐ	Affective Competency	6 points	
▷	Theory Question	2 points	
Score calculation: 100 points – ____ points missed ____ Score Satisfactory score: 85 or above			

2008 CAAHEP Competencies Achieved
Psychomotor (Skills) ☑ IV. 2. Report relevant information to others succinctly and accurately. ☑ IV. 6. Prepare a patient for procedures and/or treatments. ***Affective (Behavior)*** ☑ I. 1. Apply critical thinking skills in performing patient assessment and care.

2015 CAAHEP Competencies Achieved
Psychomotor (Skills) ☑ I. 8. Instruct and prepare a patient for a procedure or a treatment. ☑ V. 11. Report relevant information concisely and accurately. ***Affective (Behavior)*** ☑ I. 1. Incorporate critical thinking skills when performing patient assessment. ☑ I. 2. Incorporate critical thinking skills when performing patient care.

ABHES Competencies Achieved
☑ 2. c. Identify diagnostic and treatment modalities as they relate to each body system. ☑ 8. e. Display professionalism through written and verbal communications. ☑ 9. e. Perform specialty procedures including but not limited to minor surgery, cardiac, respiratory, OB-GYN, neurological, gastroenterology.

EVALUATION OF COMPETENCY

Procedure 22-2: Applying a Hot Soak

Name: ______________________ Date: ______________

Evaluated by: ______________________ Score: ______________

Performance Objective

Outcome:	Apply a hot soak.
Conditions:	Given the following: soaking solution, bath thermometer, basin, and bath towels.
Standards:	Time: 10 minutes. Student completed procedure in ________ minutes.
	Accuracy: Satisfactory score on the performance evaluation checklist.

Performance Evaluation Checklist

Trial 1	Trial 2	Point Value	Performance Standards
		●	Sanitized hands.
		●	Assembled equipment.
		●	Checked the label on the solution container.
		●	Warmed the soaking solution.
		●	Greeted the patient and introduced yourself.
		●	Identified the patient and explained the procedure.
		●	Filled basin one-half to two-thirds full with the warmed soaking solution.
		●	Checked temperature of the solution with a bath thermometer.
		▷	Stated the safe temperature range that should be used for an adult patient (105°F to 110°F).
		●	Assisted patient in a comfortable position and padded side of the basin with towel.
		●	Slowly and gradually immersed affected body part into the solution and asked patient how the temperature felt.
		●	Kept the solution at a constant temperature by removing cooler solution and adding hot solution.
		●	Placed a hand between patient and solution when adding more solution.
		●	Stirred the solution with your hand while pouring it.
		●	Checked patient's skin periodically.
		●	Applied hot soak for the proper length of time as designated by physician.
		●	Completely dried affected part.

Trial 1	Trial 2	Point Value	Performance Standards
		●	Sanitized hands.
		●	Charted the procedure correctly.
		●	Properly cared for and returned equipment to its storage place.
		Ⓐ	Incorporated critical thinking skills when performing patient assessment.
		Ⓐ	Incorporated critical thinking skills when performing patient care.
		*	Completed the procedure within 10 minutes.
			TOTALS

CHART	
Date	

Evaluation of Student Performance

EVALUATION CRITERIA			**COMMENTS**
Symbol	**Category**	**Point Value**	
*	Critical Step	16 points	
●	Essential Step	6 points	
Ⓐ	Affective Competency	6 points	
▷	Theory Question	2 points	
Score calculation: 100 points – ___ points missed ___ Score Satisfactory score: 85 or above			

2008 CAAHEP Competencies Achieved
Psychomotor (Skills) ☑ IV. 2. Report relevant information to others succinctly and accurately. ☑ IV. 6. Prepare a patient for procedures and/or treatments. ***Affective (Behavior)*** ☑ I. 1. Apply critical thinking skills in performing patient assessment and care.

2015 CAAHEP Competencies Achieved
Psychomotor (Skills) ☑ I. 8. Instruct and prepare a patient for a procedure or a treatment. ☑ V. 11. Report relevant information concisely and accurately. ***Affective (Behavior)*** ☑ I. 1. Incorporate critical thinking skills when performing patient assessment. ☑ I. 2. Incorporate critical thinking skills when performing patient care.

ABHES Competencies Achieved
☑ 2. c. Identify diagnostic and treatment modalities as they relate to each body system. ☑ 8. e. Display professionalism through written and verbal communications. ☑ 9. e. Perform specialty procedures including but not limited to minor surgery, cardiac, respiratory, OB-GYN, neurological, gastroenterology.

Notes

EVALUATION OF COMPETENCY

Procedure 22-3: Applying a Hot Compress

Name: ______________________ Date: ______________

Evaluated by: ______________________ Score: ______________

Performance Objective

Outcome:	Apply a hot compress.
Conditions:	Given the following: solution for the compresses, bath thermometer, basin, washcloths, and a towel.
Standards:	Time: 10 minutes. Student completed procedure in __________ minutes.
	Accuracy: Satisfactory score on the Performance Evaluation Checklist.

Performance Evaluation Checklist

Trial 1	Trial 2	Point Value	Performance Standards
		•	Sanitized hands.
		•	Assembled equipment.
		•	Checked the label on the solution container.
		•	Warmed the soaking solution.
		•	Greeted the patient and introduced yourself.
		•	Identified the patient and explained the procedure.
		•	Filled basin half full with the warmed solution.
		•	Checked temperature of the solution with a bath thermometer.
		▷	Stated the safe temperature range that should be used for an adult patient (105°F to 110°F).
		•	Completely immersed the compress in the solution.
		•	Squeezed excess solution from compress.
		•	Applied compress to affected body part and asked patient how the -temperature felt.
		•	Placed additional compresses in the solution.
		•	Repeated the application every 2 to 3 minutes for the duration of time specified by physician.
		•	Checked patient's skin periodically.
		•	Checked temperature of the solution periodically, removed cooler fluid, and added hot fluid if needed.
		•	Administered treatment for proper length of time as designated by a physician.

Trial 1	Trial 2	Point Value	Performance Standards
		●	Thoroughly dried affected part.
		●	Sanitized hands.
		●	Charted the procedure correctly.
		●	Properly cared for and returned equipment to its storage place.
		Ⓐ	Incorporated critical thinking skills when performing patient assessment.
		Ⓐ	Incorporated critical thinking skills when performing patient care.
		✶	Completed the procedure within 10 minutes.
			TOTALS

CHART	
Date	

Evaluation of Student Performance

EVALUATION CRITERIA			**COMMENTS**
Symbol	**Category**	**Point Value**	
✶	Critical Step	16 points	
●	Essential Step	6 points	
Ⓐ	Affective Competency	6 points	
▷	Theory Question	2 points	
Score calculation: 100 points – ___ points missed ___ Score Satisfactory score: 85 or above			

2008 CAAHEP Competencies Achieved
Psychomotor (Skills) ☑ IV. 2. Report relevant information to others succinctly and accurately. ☑ IV. 6. Prepare a patient for procedures and/or treatments. ***Affective (Behavior)*** ☑ I. 1. Apply critical thinking skills in performing patient assessment and care.

2015 CAAHEP Competencies Achieved
Psychomotor (Skills) ☑ I. 8. Instruct and prepare a patient for a procedure or a treatment. ☑ V. 11. Report relevant information concisely and accurately. ***Affective (Behavior)*** ☑ I. 1. Incorporate critical thinking skills when performing patient assessment. ☑ I. 2. Incorporate critical thinking skills when performing patient care.

ABHES Competencies Achieved
☑ 2. c. Identify diagnostic and treatment modalities as they relate to each body system. ☑ 8. e. Display professionalism through written and verbal communications. ☑ 9. e. Perform specialty procedures including but not limited to minor surgery, cardiac, respiratory, OB-GYN, neurological, gastroenterology.

Notes

EVALUATION OF COMPETENCY

Procedure 22-4: Applying an Ice Bag

Name: ______________________ Date: ______________

Evaluated by: ______________________ Score: ______________

Performance Objective

Outcome:	Apply an ice bag.
Conditions:	Given the following: ice bag and protective covering, and small pieces of ice.
Standards:	Time: 10 minutes. Student completed procedure in ________ minutes.
	Accuracy: Satisfactory score on the Performance Evaluation Checklist.

Performance Evaluation Checking

Trial 1	Trial 2	Point Value	Performance Standards
		●	Sanitized hands.
		●	Assembled equipment.
		●	Greeted the patient and introduced yourself.
		●	Identified the patient and explained the procedure.
		●	Checked ice bag for leakage.
		●	Filled bag one-half to two-thirds full with small pieces of ice.
		▷	Explained why small pieces of ice are used.
		●	Expelled air from bag.
		▷	Explained the reason for expelling air from bag.
		●	Placed the bag in protective covering.
		▷	Stated the purpose of placing bag in protective covering.
		●	Placed bag on affected body area and asked patient how the temperature felt.
		●	Checked patient's skin periodically.
		▷	Listed skin changes that would warrant removal of bag.
		●	Refilled bag with ice and changed protective covering when needed.
		●	Administered treatment for the proper length of time as designated by physician.
		●	Sanitized hands.
		●	Charted the procedure correctly.

Trial 1	Trial 2	Point Value	Performance Standards
		●	Properly cared for and returned equipment to its storage place.
		Ⓐ	Incorporated critical thinking skills when performing patient assessment.
		Ⓐ	Incorporated critical thinking skills when performing patient care.
		✶	Completed the procedure within 10 minutes.
			TOTALS

CHART	
Date	

Evaluation of Student Performance

EVALUATION CRITERIA			COMMENTS
Symbol	Category	Point Value	
✶	Critical Step	16 points	
●	Essential Step	6 points	
Ⓐ	Affective Competency	6 points	
▷	Theory Question	2 points	
Score calculation: 100 points – ___ points missed ___ Score Satisfactory score: 85 or above			

2008 CAAHEP Competencies Achieved
Psychomotor (Skills) ☑ IV. 2. Report relevant information to others succinctly and accurately. ☑ IV. 6. Prepare a patient for procedures and/or treatments. ***Affective (Behavior)*** ☑ I. 1. Apply critical thinking skills in performing patient assessment and care.

2015 CAAHEP Competencies Achieved
Psychomotor (Skills) ☑ I. 8. Instruct and prepare a patient for a procedure or a treatment. ☑ V. 11. Report relevant information concisely and accurately. ***Affective (Behavior)*** ☑ I. 1. Incorporate critical thinking skills when performing patient assessment. ☑ I. 2. Incorporate critical thinking skills when performing patient care.

ABHES Competencies Achieved
☑ 2. c. Identify diagnostic and treatment modalities as they relate to each body system. ☑ 8. e. Display professionalism through written and verbal communications. ☑ 9. e. Perform specialty procedures including but not limited to minor surgery, cardiac, respiratory, OB-GYN, neurological, gastroenterology.

Notes

EVALUATION OF COMPETENCY

Procedure 22-5: Applying a Cold Compress

Name: ______________________ Date: ______________

Evaluated by: ______________________ Score: ______________

Performance Objective

Outcome:	Apply a cold compress.
Conditions:	Given the following: ice cubes, a basin, and washcloths.
Standards:	Time: 10 minutes. Student completed procedure in __________ minutes.
	Accuracy: Satisfactory score on the Performance Evaluation Checklist.

Performance Evaluation Checklist

Trial 1	Trial 2	Point Value	Performance Standards
		•	Sanitized hands.
		•	Assembled equipment.
		•	Checked the label on the solution.
		•	Greeted the patient and introduced yourself.
		•	Identified the patient and explained the procedure.
		•	Placed large ice cubes in basin and added the solution until the basin is half full.
		▷	Explained why larger pieces of ice are used.
		•	Completely immersed the compress in the solution.
		•	Squeezed excess solution from compress.
		•	Applied compress to affected body part and asked patient how the temperature felt.
		•	Placed additional compresses in the solution.
		•	Repeated the application every 2 to 3 minutes for the duration of time specified by physician.
		•	Checked patient's skin periodically.
		•	Added ice if needed to keep the solution cold.
		•	Administered treatment for proper length of time as designated by physician.
		•	Thoroughly dried affected part.
		•	Sanitized hands.

Trial 1	Trial 2	Point Value	Performance Standards
		●	Charted the procedure correctly.
		●	Properly cared for and returned equipment to its storage place.
		Ⓐ	Incorporated critical thinking skills when performing patient assessment.
		Ⓐ	Incorporated critical thinking skills when performing patient care.
		✶	Completed the procedure within 10 minutes.
			TOTALS

CHART	
Date	

Evaluation of Student Performance

EVALUATION CRITERIA			COMMENTS
Symbol	**Category**	**Point Value**	
✶	Critical Step	16 points	
●	Essential Step	6 points	
Ⓐ	Affective Competency	6 points	
▷	Theory Question	2 points	
Score calculation: 100 points – ___ points missed ___ Score Satisfactory score: 85 or above			

2008 CAAHEP Competencies Achieved
Psychomotor (Skills) ☑ IV. 2. Report relevant information to others succinctly and accurately. ☑ IV. 6. Prepare a patient for procedures and/or treatments. ***Affective (Behavior)*** ☑ I. 1. Apply critical thinking skills in performing patient assessment and care.

2015 CAAHEP Competencies Achieved
Psychomotor (Skills) ☑ I. 8. Instruct and prepare a patient for a procedure or a treatment. ☑ V. 11. Report relevant information concisely and accurately. ***Affective (Behavior)*** ☑ I. 1. Incorporate critical thinking skills when performing patient assessment. ☑ I. 2. Incorporate critical thinking skills when performing patient care.

ABHES Competencies Achieved
☑ 2. c. Identify diagnostic and treatment modalities as they relate to each body system. ☑ 8. e. Display professionalism through written and verbal communications. ☑ 9. e. Perform specialty procedures including but not limited to minor surgery, cardiac, respiratory, OB-GYN, neurological, gastroenterology.

Notes

EVALUATION OF COMPETENCY

Procedure 22-6: Applying a Chemical Pack

Name: ______________________________ Date: ______________

Evaluated by: ______________________________ Score: ______________

Performance Objective

Outcome:	Apply a chemical cold and hot pack.
Conditions:	Given a chemical cold and hot pack.
Standards:	Time: 5 minutes. Student completed procedure in ________ minutes.
	Accuracy: Satisfactory score on the Performance Evaluation Checklist.

Performance Evaluation Checklist

Trial 1	Trial 2	Point Value	Performance Standards
		•	Sanitized hands.
		•	Assembled equipment.
		•	Greeted the patient and introduced yourself.
		•	Identified the patient and explained the procedure.
		•	Shook the crystals to the bottom of bag.
		•	Squeezed bag firmly to break inner water bag.
		•	Shook bag vigorously to mix the contents.
		•	Covered bag with a protective covering.
		•	Applied bag to affected area.
		•	Checked the patient's skin periodically.
		•	Administered treatment for the proper length of time.
		•	Discarded bag in an appropriate receptacle.
		•	Sanitized hands.
		•	Charted the procedure correctly.
		Ⓐ	Incorporated critical thinking skills when performing patient assessment.
		Ⓐ	Incorporated critical thinking skills when performing patient care.
		*	Completed the procedure within 5 minutes.
			TOTALS

Evaluation of Student Performance

EVALUATION CRITERIA			COMMENTS
Symbol	**Category**	**Point Value**	
∗	Critical Step	16 points	
●	Essential Step	6 points	
Ⓐ	Affective Competency	6 points	
▷	Theory Question	2 points	
Score calculation: 100 points – ___ points missed ___ Score Satisfactory score: 85 or above			

2008 CAAHEP Competencies Achieved
Psychomotor (Skills) ☑ IV. 2. Report relevant information to others succinctly and accurately. ☑ IV. 6. Prepare a patient for procedures and/or treatments. ***Affective (Behavior)*** ☑ I. 1. Apply critical thinking skills in performing patient assessment and care.

2015 CAAHEP Competencies Achieved
Psychomotor (Skills) ☑ I. 8. Instruct and prepare a patient for a procedure or a treatment. ☑ V. 11. Report relevant information concisely and accurately. ***Affective (Behavior)*** ☑ I. 1. Incorporate critical thinking skills when performing patient assessment. ☑ I. 2. Incorporate critical thinking skills when performing patient care.

ABHES Competencies Achieved
☑ 2. c. Identify diagnostic and treatment modalities as they relate to each body system. ☑ 8. e. Display professionalism through written and verbal communications. ☑ 9. e. Perform specialty procedures including but not limited to minor surgery, cardiac, respiratory, OB-GYN, neurological, gastroenterology.

EVALUATION OF COMPETENCY

Procedure 22-7: Measuring for Axillary Crutches

Name: ______________________ Date: ______________

Evaluated by: ______________________ Score: ______________

Performance Objective

Outcome:	Measure an individual for axillary crutches.
Conditions:	Given the following: axillary crutches and a tape measure.
Standards:	Time: 10 minutes. Student completed procedure in __________ minutes.
	Accuracy: Satisfactory score on the Performance Evaluation Checklist.

Performance Evaluation Checklist

Trial 1	Trial 2	Point Value	Performance Standards
		●	Asked patient to stand erect.
		●	Positioned crutches with the tips at a distance of 2 inches in front of, and 4 to 6 inches to the side of, each foot.
		●	Adjusted crutch length so that the shoulder rests were approximately 1½ to 2 inches below the axilla.
		●	Asked the patient to support his or her weight by the handgrips.
		●	Adjusted the handgrips so that patient's elbow was flexed-approximately 30 degrees.
		●	Checked the fit of the crutches by placing two fingers between the top of the crutch and patient's axilla.
		●	Charted the procedure correctly.
		Ⓐ	Incorporated critical thinking skills when performing patient assessment.
		Ⓐ	Incorporated critical thinking skills when performing patient care.
		*	Completed the procedure within 10 minutes.
			TOTALS

CHART	
Date	

Evaluation of Student Performance

EVALUATION CRITERIA			COMMENTS
Symbol	**Category**	**Point Value**	
*	Critical Step	16 points	
●	Essential Step	6 points	
Ⓐ	Affective Competency	6 points	
▷	Theory Question	2 points	
Score calculation: 100 points − ___ points missed ___ Score Satisfactory score: 85 or above			

2008 CAAHEP Competencies Achieved
Psychomotor (Skills) ☑ IV. 6. Prepare a patient for procedures and/or treatments. ***Affective (Behavior)*** ☑ I. 1. Apply critical thinking skills in performing patient assessment and care.

2015 CAAHEP Competencies Achieved
Psychomotor (Skills) ☑ I. 8. Instruct and prepare a patient for a procedure or a treatment. ***Affective (Behavior)*** ☑ I. 1. Incorporate critical thinking skills when performing patient assessment. ☑ I. 2. Incorporate critical thinking skills when performing patient care.

ABHES Competencies Achieved
☑ 8. e. Display professionalism through written and verbal communications. ☑ 9. j. Make adaptations with patients with special needs.

EVALUATION OF COMPETENCY

Procedure 22-8: Instructing a Patient in Crutch Gaits

Name: ______________________ Date: ______________

Evaluated by: ______________________ Score: ______________

Performance Objective

Outcome:	Instruct an individual in the following crutch gaits: four-point, two-point, three-point, -swing-to, and swing-through.
Conditions:	Given axillary crutches.
Standards:	Time: 15 minutes. Student completed procedure in ________ minutes.
	Accuracy: Satisfactory score on the Performance Evaluation Checklist.

Performance Evaluation Checklist

Trial 1	Trial 2	Point Value	Performance Standards
			Tripod Position
			Instructed patient:
		●	Stand erect and face straight ahead.
		●	Place the tips of crutches 4 to 6 inches in front of, and 4 to 6 inches to side of, each foot.
		▷	Stated one use of the tripod position.
			Four-Point Gait
			Instructed patient:
		●	Begin in the tripod position.
		●	Move the right crutch forward.
		●	Move the left foot forward to the level of the left crutch.
		●	Move the left crutch forward.
		●	Move the right foot forward to the level of the right crutch.
		●	Repeat the above sequence.
		▷	Stated one use of the four-point gait.
			Two-Point Gait
			Instructed patient:
		●	Begin in the tripod position.
		●	Move the left crutch and the right foot forward at the same time.
		●	Move the right crutch and left foot forward at the same time.

Trial 1	Trial 2	Point Value	Performance Standards
		●	Repeat the above sequence.
		▷	Stated one use of the two-point gait.
			Three-Point Gait
			Instructed patient:
		●	Begin in the tripod position.
		●	Move both crutches and the affected leg forward.
		●	Move the unaffected leg forward while balancing weight on both crutches.
		●	Repeat the above sequence.
		▷	Stated two uses of the three-point gait.
			Swing-To Gait
			Instructed patient:
		●	Begin in the tripod position.
		●	Move both crutches forward together.
		●	Lift and swing body to the crutches.
		●	Repeat the above sequence.
		▷	Stated one use of the swing-to gait.
			Swing-Through Gait
			Instructed patient:
		●	Begin in the tripod position.
		●	Move both crutches forward together.
		●	Lift and swing body past the crutches.
		●	Repeat the above sequence.
		▷	Stated one use of the swing-through gait.
		Ⓐ	Demonstrated: a. empathy b. active listening c. nonverbal communication.
		✶	Completed the procedure within 15 minutes.
			TOTALS

CHART	
Date	

Evaluation of Student Performance

EVALUATION CRITERIA			COMMENTS
Symbol	**Category**	**Point Value**	
✶	Critical Step	16 points	
●	Essential Step	6 points	
Ⓐ	Affective Competency	6 points	
▷	Theory Question	2 points	
Score calculation: 100 points – ___ points missed ___ Score Satisfactory score: 85 or above			

2008 CAAHEP Competencies Achieved

Psychomotor (Skills)

☑ IV. 5. Instruct patients according to their needs to promote health maintenance and disease prevention.
☑ IV. 6. Prepare a patient for procedures and/or treatments.

Affective (Behavior)

☑ I. 2. Use language/verbal skills that enable patients' understanding.
☑ IV. 6. Demonstrate awareness of how an individual's personal appearance affects anticipated responses.

2015 CAAHEP Competencies Achieved

Psychomotor (Skills)

☑ I. 8. Instruct and prepare a patient for a procedure or a treatment.
☑ V. 4. Coach patients regarding: office policies b. health maintenance c. disease prevention d. treatment plans.

Affective (Behavior)

☑ V. 1. Demonstrate: a. empathy b. active listening c. nonverbal communication.

ABHES Competencies Achieved

☑ 8. e. Display professionalism through written and verbal communications.
☑ 9. j. Make adaptations with patients with special needs.

Notes

EVALUATION OF COMPETENCY

Procedures 22-9 and 22-10: Instructing a Patient in Use of a Cane and Walker

Name: ______________________________ Date: ______________

Evaluated by: ______________________________ Score: ______________

Performance Objective

Outcome:	Instruct an individual in the use of a cane and walker.
Conditions:	Given the following: a cane and a walker.
Standards:	Time: 10 minutes. Student completed procedure in ________ minutes.
	Accuracy: Satisfactory score on the Performance Evaluation Checklist.

Performance Evaluation Checklist

Trial 1	Trial 2	Point Value	Performance Standards
			Cane
			Instructed patient:
		●	Hold the cane on the strong side of body.
		●	Place tip of the cane 4 to 6 inches to the side of foot.
		●	Move the cane forward approximately 12 inches.
		●	Move the affected leg forward to the level of the cane.
		●	Move strong leg forward and ahead of the cane and weak leg.
		●	Repeat the above sequence.
		▷	Stated one condition for which a cane is used.
			Walker
			Instructed patient:
		●	Pick up the walker and move it forward approximately 6 inches.
		●	Move the right foot and then the left foot up to the walker.
		●	Repeat the above sequence.
		▷	Stated one condition for which a walker is used.
		Ⓐ	Demonstrated: a. empathy b. active listening c. nonverbal communication.
		*	Completed the procedure within 10 minutes.
			TOTALS

Chart	
Date	

Evaluation of Student Performance

EVALUATION CRITERIA			COMMENTS
Symbol	**Category**	**Point Value**	
✶	Critical Step	16 points	
●	Essential Step	6 points	
Ⓐ	Affective Competency	6 points	
▷	Theory Question	2 points	
Score calculation: 100 points – ___ points missed ___ Score Satisfactory score: 85 or above			

2008 CAAHEP Competencies Achieved
Psychomotor (Skills) ☑ IV. 5. Instruct patients according to their needs to promote health maintenance and disease prevention. ☑ IV. 6. Prepare a patient for procedures and/or treatments. ***Affective (Behavior)*** ☑ I. 2. Use language/verbal skills that enable patients' understanding. ☑ IV. 6. Demonstrate awareness of how an individual's personal appearance affects anticipated responses.

2015 CAAHEP Competencies Achieved
Psychomotor (Skills) ☑ I. 8. Instruct and prepare a patient for a procedure or a treatment. ☑ V. 4. Coach patients regarding: office policies b. health maintenance c. disease prevention d. treatment plans. ***Affective (Behavior)*** ☑ V. 1. Demonstrate: a. empathy b. active listening c. nonverbal communication.

ABHES Competencies Achieved
☑ 8. e. Display professionalism through written and verbal communications. ☑ 9. j. Make adaptations with patients with special needs.

23 The Gynecologic Examination and Prenatal Care

CHAPTER ASSIGNMENTS

✓ After Completing	Date Due	Study Guide Pages	STUDY GUIDE ASSIGNMENTS (CTA = Critical Thinking Activity)	Possible Points	Points You Earned
		513	Pretest	10	
		514-515 516	Key Term Assessment A. Definitions B. Word Parts (Add 1 point for each key term)	47 22	
		516-522	Evaluation of Learning questions	50	
		523	CTA A: Breast Cancer (5 points per question)	15	
			ⓔ Evolve Site: What's on Your Tray? (Record points earned)		
		524-525	CTA B: Methods of Contraception (3 points per each method)	42	
		526-530	CTA C: Herpesvirus and Human Papillomavirus (40 points per brochure)	80	
		531	CTA D: Signs and Symptoms of Pregnancy	16	
		531	CTA E: Calculation of the Expected Date of Delivery	5	
		532	CTA F: Nutrition During Pregnancy	8	
		533	CTA G: Minor Discomforts of Pregnancy	10	
		534	CTA H: Health Promotion During Pregnancy	7	
		535	CTA I: Breast feeding	8	
		535	CTA J: Prenatal Ultrasound	5	
		536	CTA K: Crossword Puzzle	19	
			ⓔ Evolve Site: Road to Recovery Game OB/GYN Terminology (Record points earned)		

✓ After Completing	Date Due	Study Guide Pages	STUDY GUIDE ASSIGNMENTS (CTA = Critical Thinking Activity)	Possible Points	Points You Earned
			Evolve Site: Apply Your Knowledge questions	12	
			Evolve Site: Video Evaluation	48	
		513	Posttest	10	
			ADDITIONAL ASSIGNMENTS		
			TOTAL POINTS		

✓ When Assigned By Your Instructor	Study Guide Pages	Practices Required	LABORATORY ASSIGNMENTS (Procedure Number and Name)	Score*
	537	5	**Practice for Competency** 23-1: Breast Self-Examination Instructions Textbook reference: pp. 498-500	
	545-548		**Evaluation of Competency** 23-1: Breast Self-Examination Instructions	*
	537-538	5	**Practice for Competency** 23-2: Assisting with a Gynecologic Examination Textbook reference: pp. 501-504	
	549-553		**Evaluation of Competency** 23-2: Assisting with a Gynecologic Examination	*
	539-544	5	**Practice for Competency** 23-3: Assisting with a Return Prenatal Examination Textbook reference: pp. 522-524	
	555-558		**Evaluation of Competency** 23-3: Assisting with a Return Prenatal Examination	*
			ADDITIONAL ASSIGNMENTS	

Notes

Name ______________________________ Date ______________

PRETEST

True or False

_______ 1. A complete gynecologic examination consists of a breast examination and a pelvic examination.

_______ 2. The American College of Obstetricians and Gynecologists recommends that a woman perform a breast self-examination weekly.

_______ 3. The purpose of the Pap test is for the early detection of cervical cancer.

_______ 4. The patient should be instructed to douche before having a Pap test.

_______ 5. Trichomoniasis produces a profuse, frothy vaginal discharge.

_______ 6. Another name for candidiasis is a yeast infection.

_______ 7. Prenatal refers to the care of the pregnant woman before delivery of the infant.

_______ 8. During each return prenatal visit, the mother's urine is tested for glucose and protein.

_______ 9. The normal range for the fetal pulse rate is between 120 and 160 beats per minute.

_______ 10. Amniocentesis can be used to diagnose certain genetically transmitted conditions.

POSTTEST

True or False

_______ 1. The patient position for a breast examination is the lithotomy position.

_______ 2. Most breast lumps are discovered by the physician.

_______ 3. Trichomoniasis is caused by a virus.

_______ 4. Chlamydia often occurs in association with syphilis.

_______ 5. In the absence of complications, the first prenatal visit should be scheduled after a woman misses her first period.

_______ 6. True labor pains are referred to as Braxton Hicks contractions.

_______ 7. The purpose of measuring fundal height is to determine the degree of cervical dilation and effacement.

_______ 8. The fetal heart tones can first be detected between 4 and 6 weeks of gestation using a Doppler fetal pulse detector.

_______ 9. Obstetric ultrasound scanning is used to assess fetal lung maturity.

_______ 10. The perineum is the period of time in which the body systems are returning to their prepregnant state.

Term KEY TERM ASSESSMENT

A. Definitions

Gynecologic Examination

Directions: Match each key term with its definition.

_______ 1. Adnexal
_______ 2. Amenorrhea
_______ 3. Atypical
_______ 4. Cervix
_______ 5. Colposcopy
_______ 6. Cytology
_______ 7. Dysmenorrhea
_______ 8. Dyspareunia
_______ 9. Dysplasia
_______ 10. Endocervix
_______ 11. External os
_______ 12. Gynecology
_______ 13. Menopause
_______ 14. Menorrhagia
_______ 15. Metrorrhagia
_______ 16. Perimenopause
_______ 17. Perineum
_______ 18. Risk factor
_______ 19. Vulva

A. The opening of the cervical canal of the uterus into the vagina
B. The mucous membrane lining the cervical canal
C. Deviation from the normal
D. The external region between the vaginal orifice and the anus in a female and between the scrotum and the anus in a male
E. Adjacent
F. The absence or cessation of the menstrual period
G. The region of the female external genital organs
H. The science that deals with the study of cells, including their origin, structure, function, and pathology
I. The branch of medicine that deals with the diseases of the reproductive organs of women
J. Anything that increases an individual's chance of developing a disease
K. The growth of abnormal cells
L. Before the onset of menopause, the phase during which a woman with regular periods changes to irregular cycles and increased periods of amenorrhea
M. Pain in the vagina or pelvis experienced by a woman during sexual intercourse
N. Examination of the cervix using a lighted instrument with a magnifying lens
O. Bleeding between menstrual periods
P. Excessive bleeding during a menstrual period
Q. The lower narrow end of the uterus that opens into the vagina
R. Pain associated with the menstrual period
S. The permanent cessation of menstruation

Prenatal Care

Directions: Match each medical term with its definition.

_______ 1. Abortion

_______ 2. Braxton Hicks contractions

_______ 3. Dilation (of the cervix)

_______ 4. EDD

_______ 5. Effacement

_______ 6. Embryo

_______ 7. Engagement

_______ 8. Fetal heart rate

_______ 9. Fetal heart tones

_______ 10. Fetus

_______ 11. Fundus

_______ 12. Gestation

_______ 13. Gestational age

_______ 14. Infant

_______ 15. Multigravida

_______ 16. Multipara

_______ 17. Nullipara

_______ 18. Obstetrics

_______ 19. Position

_______ 20. Postpartum

_______ 21. Preeclampsia

_______ 22. Prenatal

_______ 23. Presentation

_______ 24. Primigravida

_______ 25. Primipara

_______ 26. Quickening

_______ 27. Toxemia

_______ 28. Trimester

A. A woman who has completed two or more pregnancies to the age of viability, regardless of whether they ended in live infants or stillbirths

B. The entrance of the fetal head or the presenting part into the pelvic inlet

C. Before birth

D. Three months, or one third, of the gestational period of pregnancy

E. The termination of the pregnancy before the fetus reached the age of viability (20 weeks)

F. The dome-shaped upper portion of the uterus between the fallopian tubes

G. The number of times per minute the fetal heart beats

H. The first movements of the fetus in utero as felt by the mother

I. The child in utero, from the third month after conception to birth

J. A woman who has been pregnant more than once

K. Projected birth date of the infant

L. A woman who has carried a pregnancy to fetal viability for the first time, regardless of whether the infant was stillborn or alive at birth

M. The stretching of the external os from an opening a few millimeters wide to an opening large enough to allow the passage of an infant (approximately 10 cm)

N. The period of intrauterine development from conception to birth

O. The thinning and shortening of the cervical canal from its normal length of 1 to 2 cm to a structure with paper-thin edges in which there is no canal at all

P. A woman who has not carried a pregnancy to the point of viability (20 weeks of gestation)

Q. The branch of medicine concerned with the care of the woman during pregnancy, childbirth, and the postpartal period

R. A woman who is pregnant for the first time

S. Occurring after childbirth

T. Intermittent and irregular painless uterine contractions that occur throughout pregnancy

U. The relation of the presenting part of the fetus to the maternal pelvis

V. The sounds of the heartbeat of the fetus heard through the mother's abdominal wall

W. A child from birth to 12 months of age

X. The child in utero from the time of conception through the first 8 weeks of development

Y. The age of the fetus between conception and birth

Z. A major complication of pregnancy characterized by increasing hypertension, albuminuria, and edema

AA. Indication of the part of the fetus that is closest to the cervix and will be delivered first

BB. A condition occurring in pregnant women that includes preeclampsia and eclampsia

B. Word Parts

Directions: Indicate the meaning of each word part in the space provided. List as many medical terms as possible that incorporate the word part in the space provided.

Word Part	Meaning of Word Part	Medical Terms That Incorporate Word Part
1. a-		
2. men/o		
3. -orrhea		
4. colp/o		
5. -scopy		
6. cyt/o		
7. -ology		
8. dys-		
9. plasia		
10. ecto-		
11. endo-		
12. gynec/o		
13. multi-		
14. par/o		
15. nulli-		
16. peri-		
17. post-		
18. pre-		
19. nat/o		
20. -al		
21. prim/i		
22. tri-		

EVALUATION OF LEARNING

Gynecologic Examination

Directions: Fill in each blank with the correct answer.

1. What is the purpose of the gynecologic examination?

____

____

____

2. What is the purpose of performing a breast examination?

____

____

____

3. How often should a woman perform a breast self-examination at home? When should it be performed in relation to the menstrual cycle and why?

____

____

____

4. What are the components of the pelvic examination?

____

____

5. What position is generally used for the pelvic examination?

____

6. How can the medical assistant help the patient to relax during the pelvic examination?

____

____

7. What is the function of a vaginal speculum?

____

____

8. What is the purpose of performing a visual examination of the vagina and the cervix?

____

____

9. What are three examples of vaginal infections that cause a discharge?

____

10. What is the purpose of performing a Pap test?

____

____

11. What causes most cervical cancers?

____

12. Describe the schedule for having a Pap test as recommended by the American Cancer Society.

____

____

____

13. Why should the medical assistant instruct the patient not to douche or insert vaginal medications for 2 days before coming to the medical office to have a Pap test?

14. What are the three types of specimens that may be obtained for a Pap test? Where is each collected?

15. Why must the slides be fixed immediately after collection of a specimen for the direct-smear Pap test method?

16. What are the advantages of using the liquid-based Pap test method?

17. List three conditions that the maturation index can help to evaluate.

18. Why is the Bethesda System recommended for reporting the results of the Pap test?

19. What is the purpose of performing the bimanual pelvic examination?

20. What is the purpose of the rectal–vaginal examination?

21. Describe the laboratory procedure that can be used to identify Trichomonas vaginalis in the medical office.

22. Describe the laboratory procedure that can be used to identify Candida albicans in the medical office.

23. What are the symptoms of PID? What complications can occur from PID?

24. How are chlamydial and gonorrheal infections usually diagnosed?

25. List the symptoms of each of the following sexually transmitted diseases:

a. Trichomoniasis in the female

b. Candidiasis in the female

c. Chlamydia

Female:

Male:

d. Gonorrhea

Female:

Male:

Prenatal Care

Directions: Fill in each blank with the correct answer.

1. What is the purpose of prenatal care?

2. List the three categories of medical office visits for provision of prenatal and postnatal care to the pregnant woman.

3. List the four components of the first prenatal visit.

4. What is the purpose of the prenatal record?

5. List two types of information included in the past medical history (of the prenatal record).

6. List three types of information included in the present pregnancy history.

7. What are the warning signs of a spontaneous abortion?

8. What are the warning signs of preeclampsia?

9. What is the purpose of the interval prenatal history?

10. Explain the importance of performing a physical examination on the prenatal patient.

11. What is the importance of making sure a pregnant woman does not have gonorrhea before delivery of the infant?

12. Why is a pregnant woman tested for group B streptococcus (GBS)? When is the woman tested for GBS?

13. What is the purpose of performing a hemoglobin and hematocrit evaluation on a prenatal patient?

14. What is the importance of assessing the Rh factor and ABO blood type of a pregnant woman?

15. What is the purpose of performing a glucose challenge test on a pregnant woman?

16. What is the purpose of performing a rubella titer test on a pregnant woman?

17. Why does the Centers for Disease Control and Prevention recommend that pregnant women have a blood test to screen for exposure to the hepatitis B virus?

18. What is the purpose of the return prenatal visit? List the usual schedule for return prenatal visits.

19. What tests are performed on the patient's urine specimen at each return visit and why is each performed?

____

____

____

____

20. List two purposes of measuring the fundal height.

____

____

21. What is the normal range for the fetal heart rate?

____

22. What is the purpose of performing a vaginal examination as the patient nears term?

____

____

23. What is the purpose for performing each of the following special tests and procedures?

a. Multiple marker test ____

____

b. Obstetric ultrasound scan ____

____

c. Amniocentesis ____

____

d. Fetal heart rate monitoring ____

____

24. What conditions might warrant performing an amniocentesis?

____

____

____

25. What conditions might warrant performing a fetal heart rate monitoring test?

____

____

____

CRITICAL THINKING ACTIVITIES

A. Breast Cancer

Select three of the following questions that interest you the most. Using the following Internet sites, answer these questions in the space provided.

National Cancer Institute: www.cancer.gov

American Cancer Society: www.cancer.org

Cancer Center: www.cancercenter.com

1. Can a male develop breast cancer? Elaborate on your answer.
2. How does tamoxifen work in treating breast cancer?
3. What are the pros and cons of being tested for the breast cancer gene?
4. What methods are used to reconstruct the breast after a mastectomy?
5. What new diagnostic methods are being explored to detect breast cancer?
6. What complementary and alternative therapies are being used in the treatment of breast cancer?

Question # ____

____

____

____

____

____

____

Question # ____

____

____

____

____

____

Question # ____

____

____

____

____

____

B. Methods of Contraception

Patients coming to the medical office for gynecologic examinations frequently ask the medical assistant questions regarding methods of contraception. The medical assistant should have knowledge of the various types of contraceptives, how they work to prevent pregnancy, and the advantages and disadvantages of each. A list of common contraceptive methods is provided. List the information requested for each in the spaces provided. The contraceptive Internet sites listed under "On the Web" at the end of Chapter 23 in your textbook can be used to complete this activity.

Contraceptive Method	Mode of Action	Advantages	Disadvantages
Oral contraceptives			
Contraceptive injections			
Contraceptive patch			
Birth control implant			
Male condom			

Contraceptive Method	Mode of Action	Advantages	Disadvantages
Female condom			
Spermicide			
Diaphragm			
Cervical cap			
Vaginal sponge			
Vaginal ring			

Contraceptive Method	Mode of Action	Advantages	Disadvantages
Intrauterine device (IUD)			
Fertility awareness-based method			
Surgical sterilization			
Emergency contraception			

C. Herpesvirus and Human Papillomavirus

You are working for an obstetrics and gynecology (OB/GYN) office. Your physician is concerned about the increase in the number of patients contracting herpesvirus and human papillomairus (HPV) infections. He or she asks you to design a colorful, creative, and informative brochure on herpesvirus and HPV infections using the brochures provided on the following pages. These brochures will be published and placed in the waiting room to educate patients about these sexually transmitted diseases (STDs). The STD Internet sites listed under "On the Web" at the end of Chapter 23 in your textbook can be used to complete this activity.

HERPES

How common is herpes?

How can herpes be prevented?

What is herpes?

How do you get herpes?

How is herpes diagnosed?

What are the symptoms?

What causes herpes to recur?

How is herpes treated?

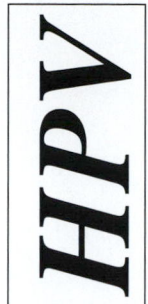

How common is HPV?

What are the complications of HPV?

What is HPV?

How do you get HPV?

How is HPV tested?

What are the symptoms?

How is HPV diagnosed?

How can HPV be prevented?

D. Signs and Symptoms of Pregnancy

Listed here are the common signs and symptoms of pregnancy. Define each of them and, if possible, explain what causes the sign or symptom to occur. The pregnancy and childbirth Internet sites listed under "On the Web" at the end of Chapter 23 in your textbook can be used to obtain information to complete this activity.

1. Amenorrhea

___

___

2. Fatigue

___

___

3. Urinary frequency ___

___

4. Quickening

___

___

5. Goodell's sign ___

___

6. Hegar's sign

___

___

7. Braxton Hicks contractions

___

___

8. Skin changes: striae gravidarum, chloasma, linea nigra

___

___

___

___

E. Calculation of the Expected Date of Delivery

Calculate the expected date of delivery (EDD) for the following patients using the Nägele rule. The first day of each patient's last menstrual period (LMP) is listed.

1. February 10, 2017 ___
2. April 28, 2017 ___
3. July 20, 2017 ___
4. October 2, 2017 ___
5. December 22, 2017 ___

F. Nutrition During Pregnancy

1. Brianna Flint is in your medical office for her first prenatal visit. This is her first pregnancy, and she is concerned about adequate nutrition during her pregnancy. Explain why the following nutrients are of particular importance during pregnancy and provide good food sources of each. The pregnancy and childbirth Internet sites listed in the section "On the Web" at the end of Chapter 23 in your textbook can be used to obtain information to complete this activity.

2. In a classroom situation, select a partner. In a role-playing situation, one student takes the role of the medical assistant, and the other plays the role of the patient. Explain to the patient the importance of these nutrients, and list good food sources of each.

Nutrient	Importance During Pregnancy	Food Sources
Iron		
Calcium		
Protein		
Folic acid		

G. Minor Discomforts of Pregnancy

1. Listed here are the minor discomforts that a prenatal patient may experience during pregnancy. Indicate measures the patient can take to help prevent or relieve each discomfort. The pregnancy and childbirth Internet sites listed in the section "On the Web" at the end of Chapter 23 in your textbook can be used to obtain information to complete this activity.

2. In a classroom situation, select a partner. In a role-playing situation, one student takes the role of the medical assistant, and the other plays the role of the patient. The patient should indicate that she has a problem with each of these discomforts, and the medical assistant should respond by describing measures the patient can take to help prevent or relieve each problem.

   a. Nausea (morning sickness)

   ____

   ____

   b. Heartburn

   ____

   ____

   c. Fatigue

   ____

   ____

   d. Constipation

   ____

   ____

   e. Backache

   ____

   ____

   f. Breathing difficulties

   ____

   ____

   g. Varicose veins

   ____

   ____

   h. Hemorrhoids

   ____

   ____

   i. Leg cramps

   ____

   ____

   j. Swelling of the lower legs and feet

   ____

   ____

H. Health Promotion During Pregnancy

1. Obtain a prenatal guidebook, and list the guidelines the patient should follow with respect to each of the areas provided. The pregnancy and childbirth Internet sites listed under "On the Web" at the end of Chapter 23 in your textbook can be used to obtain information to complete this activity.

2. In a classroom situation, select a partner. In a role-playing situation, one student takes the role of the medical assistant, and the other plays the role of the patient. The patient should ask for guidance regarding each of these areas, and the medical assistant should respond with appropriate information.

   a. Nutrition

   ____

   ____

   b. Employment

   ____

   ____

   c. Exercise

   ____

   ____

   d. Travel

   ____

   ____

   e. Smoking

   ____

   ____

   f. Alcohol

   ____

   ____

   g. Medication

   ____

   ____

I. Breast feeding

1. Lucy Clark asks you for information regarding the advantages and disadvantages of breastfeeding and -bottle–feeding. List these in the following chart. The pregnancy and childbirth Internet sites listed under "On the Web" at the end of Chapter 23 in your textbook can be used to obtain information to complete this activity.
2. In a classroom situation, select a partner. In a role-playing situation, one student takes the role of the medical -assistant, and the other plays the role of the patient. The patient should ask for information regarding the advantages and disadvantages of both methods, and the medical assistant should respond with appropriate information.

Bottle-feeding	
Advantages	*Disadvantages*
Breastfeeding	
Advantages	*Disadvantages*

J. Prenatal Ultrasound

View obstetric ultrasound scans at the following Internet sites:

www.ob-ultrasound.net/frames.htm

www.layyous.com/ultasound/ultrasound_video.htm

The following scans can be viewed at these sites:

1. Gestational sac
2. Fetus at various gestational ages
3. Fetal measurements
4. Fetal organs
5. Three-dimensional (3D) and four-dimensional (4D) images of the fetus

K. Crossword Puzzle: Gynecology and Obstetrics

Directions: Complete the crossword puzzle using the clues provided.

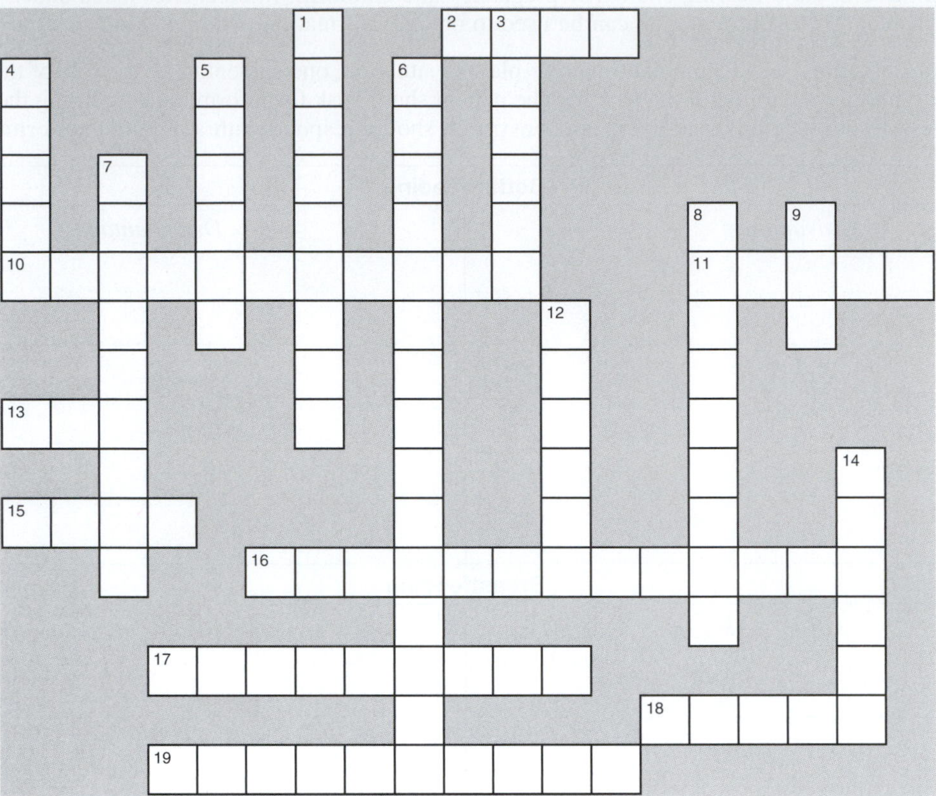

Across

2 Definite minor Pap changes
10 Spread of cancer
11 Slightly abnormal Pap cells
13 Long-term use increases breast cancer risk
15 Warning sign of breast cancer
16 Phase before menopause
17 Growth of abnormal cells
18 Breast cancer increases (age)
19 Examination of the cervix

Down

1 Menstrual cycle ceases
3 Breast examination position
4 Collects both ectocervical and endocervical Pap specimen
5 Determines whether benign or malignant
6 Causes vaginal yeast infection
7 Pelvic examination position
8 Breast radiograph
9 Screening test for GDM
12 What most breast lumps are
14 Age to begin BSE

PRACTICE FOR COMPETENCY

Procedure 23-1: Breast Self-Examination. Instruct an individual about the procedure for performing a breast self-examination and record the procedure in the chart provided.

Procedure 23-2: Gynecologic Examination

1. Complete the cytology request form provided using a female classmate as the patient.
2. Practice the procedure for assisting with a gynecologic examination. Record the vital signs and height and weight in the chart provided.

CHART	
Date	

GYN CYTOLOGY REQUISITION

THOMAS WOODSIDE, MD
501 MAIN ST
ST. LOUIS, MO 63146
(314) 883-0093

PATIENT INFO

Patient's Name (Last)	(First)	(MI)	Date of Birth MO / DAY / YR	Collection Time : AM PM	Collection Date MO / DAY / YR	Patient's ID #

Patient's Address	Phone	
City	State	ZIP

RESP. PARTY

Name of Responsible Party (if different from patient)	
Address of Responsible Party	APT #
City State	ZIP

INSURANCE

Patient's Relationship to Responsible Party ☐ 1. Self ☐ 2. Spouse ☐ 3. Child ☐ 4. Other

Insurance Comany Name	Plan	Carrier Code
Subscriber/Member #	Location	Group #
Insurance Address		Physician's Provider #
City	State	ZIP
Employer's Name or Number		Insured SSN

Diagnosis/Signs/Symptoms in ICD-9 Format (Highest Specificity)

REQUIRED

ICD-9 codes are the internationally accepted method of describing the clinical picture of the patient. All diagnoses should be provided by the ordering physician or his or her authorized designee. The following is a partial list of of common diagnoses in ICD-9 format. Most third party payers require an ICD-9 code to indicate the medical necessity of the test(s) and or profile(s) ordered. For a complete list of all ICD-9 codes, please refer to a current ICD-9 manual.

V76.2	Routine Cervical Pap Smear	616.0	Cervicitis	626.8	Abnormal Bleeding
V15.89	High Risk Cervical Screening	616.10	Vaginitis	627.1	Postmenopausal Bleeding
V22.2	Pregnancy	617.0	Endometriosis, Uterus	627.3	Atrophic Vaginitis
079.4	Human Papillomavirus	622.1	Dysplasia, Cervix	795.0	Abnormal Cervical Pap Smear
180.0	Malignant Neoplasm, Cervix	623.0	Dysplasia, Vagina		

COLLECTION METHOD

Liquid Based Prep

192055 ☐ Thin Prep Pap Test

192039 ☐ Thin Prep Pap Test w/reflex to HPV Hybrid Capture when ASC-US or SIL

192047 ☐ Thin Prep Pap Test w/reflex to high-risk only HPV Hybrid Capture when ASC-US

Pap Smear

009100 ☐ 1 Slide **009191** ☐ 2 Slides

Pap Smear and Maturation Index

009209 ☐ 1 Slide **190074** ☐ 2 Slides

SOURCE OF SPECIMEN

☐ **Cervical**
☐ **Endocervical**
☐ **Vaginal**

Date LMP

____/____/____
Mo Day Year

COLLECTION TECHNIQUE

☐ **Spatula**
☐ **Brush**
☐ **Broom**
☐ **Other** ____________

PATIENT HISTORY

☐ **Pregnant**
☐ **Lactating**
☐ **Oral Contraceptives**
☐ **Postmenopausal**
☐ **Hormone Replacement Therapy**
☐ **PMP Bleeding**
☐ **Postpartum**
☐ **IUD**
☐ **Postcoital Bleeding**
☐ **DES Exposure**
☐ **Previous Abnormal Pap Test**

☐ **Other** ____________

PREVIOUS TREATMENT

PREVIOUS TREATMENT	Date/Results
☐ None	
☐ Colposcopy and Bx	____________
☐ Cryosurgery	____________
☐ LEEP	____________
☐ Laser Vaporization	____________
☐ Conization	____________
☐ Hysterectomy	____________
☐ Radiation	____________
☐ Chemotherapy	____________

Procedure 23-3: Return Prenatal Examination

1. Complete the prenatal health history form provided using a female classmate as the patient.
2. Prepare the patient and assist with a return prenatal examination. Record the results of procedures you performed on the chart provided.

CHART	
Date	

Chart	
Date	

PRENATAL HEALTH HISTORY

PATIENT INFORMATION

Date: ______________________ EDD: ____________________ Referred By: ________________________

Name: ____ Phone (home): ________________________

LAST FIRST MIDDLE

Phone (work): ________________________

Address: ____ Emergency Contact: ________________________

____ Phone: ________________________

CITY STATE ZIP

Date of Birth: ___/___/___ Age: ____ Marital Status: ________________________

Occupation: ____

Education: ☐ High School ☐ College ☐ Post-graduate

PAST MEDICAL HISTORY

	O Neg + Pos	DETAIL POSITIVE REMARKS INCLUDE DATE AND TREATMENT			O Neg + Pos	DETAIL POSITIVE REMARKS INCLUDE DATE AND TREATMENT
1. DIABETES				16. D (Rh) SENSITIZED		
2. HYPERTENSION				17. PULMONARY (TB, ASTHMA)		
3. HEART DISEASE				18. RHEUMATIC FEVER		
4. AUTOIMMUNE DISORDER				19. BLEEDING TENDENCY		
5. KIDNEY DISEASE/UTI				20. GYN SURGERY		
6. NEUROLOGIC/EPILEPSY						
7. PSYCHIATRIC				21. OPERATIONS/HOSPITALIZATIONS (YEAR AND REASON)		
8. HEPATITIS/LIVER DISEASE						
9. VARICOSITIES/PHLEBITIS						
10. THYROID DYSFUNCTION						
11. TRAUMA/DOMESTIC VIOLENCE				22. ANESTHETIC COMPLICATIONS		
12. BLOOD TRANSFUSION				23. HISTORY OF ABNORMAL PAP		
	AMT/DAY PREPREG.	AMT/DAY PREG.	# YEARS USE	24. UTERINE ANOMALY/DES		
				25. INFERTILITY		
13. TOBACCO				26. SEXUALLY TRANSMITTED DISEASE		
14. ALCOHOL						
15. STREET DRUGS				27. OTHER		

IMMUNIZATIONS:

Mark an X next to those you have had.

☐ Influenza ☐ Chickenpox

☐ Hepatitis B ☐ Pneumococcal

☐ Hib ☐ Tuberculin Test

☐ Polio ☐ Tetanus Booster

☐ MMR

ALLERGIES:

List all allergies (foods, drugs, environment). ☐ None

____

____

____

____

____

____

MENSTRUAL HISTORY

Menarche: Age of Onset ____________________

Frequency: Q________Days

Duration: ____________Days

Amount of Flow: ☐ Small ☐ Moderate ☐ Large

GYN Disorders (List): ____________________

____

____

On contraceptive at conception? ☐ Yes ☐ No

OBSTETRIC HISTORY

G ________ (Total Pregnancies) T ________ (Term) P ________ (Preterm) A ________ (Abortions) L ________ (Living Children)

PREVIOUS PREGNANCIES:

DATE MONTH/ YEAR	WEEKS GEST.	LENGTH OF LABOR	BIRTH WEIGHT	SEX M/F	TYPE DELIVERY	ANES.	MATERNAL COMPLICATIONS	INFANT COMPLICATIONS

PRESENT PREGNANCY HISTORY

NAUSEA			ABDOMINAL PAIN		
VOMITING			URINARY COMPLAINTS		
FATIGUE			VAGINAL BLEEDING		
BREAST CHANGES			VAGINAL DISCHARGE		
INDIGESTION			PRURITIS		
CONSTIPATION			ACCIDENTS		
PERSISTENT HEADACHES			SURGERY		
DIZZINESS			X-RAYS		
VISUAL DISTURBANCE			RUBELLA EXPOSURE		
EDEMA (SPECIFY AREA)			OTHER VIRAL INFECTIONS		

LMP ____ / ____ / ____ (Mo / Day / Year) **Amount of Flow:** ☐ **Small** ☐ **Moderate** ☐ **Large**

CURRENT MEDICATIONS: (Include prescription, OTC, herbal, and vitamins). ☐ **None**

Medication **Frequency**

____

____

INITIAL PHYSICAL EXAMINATION

DATE ___/___/___

1. HEENT	☐ NORMAL	☐ ABNORMAL	12. VULVA	☐ NORMAL	☐ CONDYLOMA	☐ LESIONS
2. FUNDI	☐ NORMAL	☐ ABNORMAL	13. VAGINA	☐ NORMAL	☐ INFLAMMATION	☐ DISCHARGE
3. TEETH	☐ NORMAL	☐ ABNORMAL	14. CERVIX	☐ NORMAL	☐ INFLAMMATION	☐ LESIONS
4. THYROID	☐ NORMAL	☐ ABNORMAL	15. UTERUS SIZE	_____ WEEKS		☐ FIBROIDS
5. BREASTS	☐ NORMAL	☐ ABNORMAL	16. ADNEXA	☐ NORMAL	☐ MASS	
6. LUNGS	☐ NORMAL	☐ ABNORMAL	17. RECTUM	☐ NORMAL	☐ ABNORMAL	
7. HEART	☐ NORMAL	☐ ABNORMAL	18. DIAGONAL CONJUGATE	☐ REACHED	☐ NO	_____ CM
8. ABDOMEN	☐ NORMAL	☐ ABNORMAL	19. SPINES	☐ AVERAGE	☐ PROMINENT	☐ BLUNT
9. EXTREMITIES	☐ NORMAL	☐ ABNORMAL	20. SACRUM	☐ CONCAVE	☐ STRAIGHT	☐ ANTERIOR
10. SKIN	☐ NORMAL	☐ ABNORMAL	21. SUBPUBIC ARCH	☐ NORMAL	☐ WIDE	☐ NARROW
11. LYMPH NODES	☐ NORMAL	☐ ABNORMAL	22. GYNECOID PELVIC TYPE	☐ YES	☐ NO	

COMMENTS (Number and explain abnormals): ______________________________

____

____

______________________ **EXAM BY** ______________________

PATIENT'S NAME ____________________

INTERVAL PRENATAL HISTORY

Date 20__	Weeks Gestation	Height of Fundus (cm)	Weight	B/P	Urine Glucose	Urine Protein	FHT	Vaginal Examination	Presentation	Edema	Discharge	Bleeding	Contractions	Fetal Activity	NST	Next Appt.	Initials

PLANS/EDUCATION (COUNSELED ☑)

- ☐ ANESTHESIA PLANS ____________________
- ☐ TOXOPLASMOSIS PRECAUTIONS (CATS/RAW MEAT) ____
- ☐ CHILDBIRTH CLASSES ____________________
- ☐ PHYSICAL/SEXUAL ACTIVITY ____________________
- ☐ LABOR SIGNS ____________________
- ☐ NUTRITION COUNSELING ____________________
- ☐ BREAST OR BOTTLE FEEDING ____________________
- ☐ NEWBORN CAR SEAT ____________________
- ☐ POSTPARTUM BIRTH CONTROL ____________________
- ☐ ENVIRONMENTAL/WORK HAZARDS ____________________
- ☐ TUBAL STERILIZATION ____________________
- ☐ VBAC COUNSELING ____________________
- ☐ CIRCUMCISION ____________________
- ☐ TRAVEL ____________________
- ☐ LIFESTYLE, TOBACCO, ALCOHOL ____________________

REQUESTS ____________________

____

____

TUBAL STERILIZATION DATE INITIALS

CONSENT SIGNED ___/___/___ ____________

LABORATORY		PATIENT'S NAME ______________________________		
INITIAL LABS	**DATE**	**RESULTS**	**REVIEWED**	**COMMENTS**
BLOOD TYPE	/ /	A B AB O		
Rh FACTOR	/ /	☐ Pos ☐ Neg		
Rh ANTIBODY SCREEN	/ /	☐ Pos ☐ Neg		
HCT/HGB	/ /	____% ____ g/dL		
RUBELLA ANTIBODY TITER	/ /	Immune Nonimmune		
VDRL	/ /	☐ NR ☐ R		
HBsAg (HEPATITIS B)	/ /	☐ Pos ☐ Neg		
HIV	/ /	☐ Pos ☐ Neg ☐ Declined		
URINE CULTURE/SCREEN	/ /			
PAP TEST	/ /	☐ Normal ☐ Abnormal		
CHLAMYDIA (DNA PROBE)	/ /	☐ Pos ☐ Neg		
GONORRHEA (DNA PROBE)	/ /	☐ Pos ☐ Neg		
7–20 WEEK LABS (WHEN INDICATED/ELECTED)	**DATE**	**RESULTS**	**REVIEWED**	**COMMENTS**
ULTRASOUND #1 (7–13 WEEKS)	/ /	EDD:		
ULTRASOUND #2 (18–20 WEEKS)	/ /	EFW:		
TRIPLE SCREEN (15–20 WEEKS)	/ /			
CVS	/ /			
AMNIOCENTESIS	/ /			
24–28 WEEK LABS (WHEN INDICATED)	**DATE**	**RESULTS**	**REVIEWED**	**COMMENTS**
HCT/HGB	/ /	____ % ____ g/dL		
GCT (24–28 WKS)	/ /	1 Hour ____________		
GTT (IF SCREEN ABNORMAL)	/ /	____ FBS ____ 1 Hour ____ 2 Hour ____ 3 Hour		
D (Rh) ANTIBODY SCREEN	/ /			
D IMMUNE GLOBULIN (RhIG) GIVEN (28 WKS)	/ /	SIGNATURE		
32–36 WEEK LABS	**DATE**	**RESULTS**	**REVIEWED**	**COMMENTS**
HCT/HGB (32 WKS)	/ /	____ % ____ g/dL		
ULTRASOUND #3 (34 WKS)	/ /	EFW:		
GROUP B STREP (35–37 WKS)	/ /	☐ Pos ☐ Neg		
ADDITIONAL LAB TESTS	**DATE**	**RESULTS**	**REVIEWED**	**COMMENTS**
	/ /			
	/ /			
	/ /			
	/ /			
	/ /			

EVALUATION OF COMPETENCY

Procedure 23-1: Breast Self-Examination Instructions

Name: ______________________ Date: ______________

Evaluated by: ______________________ Score: ______________

Performance Objective

Outcome:	Instruct a patient in the procedure for performing a breast self-examination.
Conditions:	Small pillow.
Standards:	Time: 10 minutes. Student completed procedure in __________ minutes.
	Accuracy: Satisfactory score on the performance evaluation checklist.

Performance Evaluation Checklist

Trial 1	Trial 2	Point Value	Performance Standards
		●	Greeted the patient and introduced yourself.
		●	Identified patient and explained that you will be instructing the patient in a BSE.
		●	Explained the purpose of the exam, when to perform it, and the three methods of examination.
		▷	Explained why three methods are used to examine the breasts.
			Instructed patient:
			1. Before a mirror
		●	Remove clothing from the waist up.
		●	Place arms at sides and inspect the breasts.
		●	Inspect for a change in size or shape; swelling, puckering, or dimpling; change in skin texture; nipple retraction; change in nipple size or position compared with other breast.
		▷	Described what may cause puckering or dimpling of the skin.
		●	Slowly raise arms over head and inspect the breasts.
		▷	Stated what should normally occur when the arms are moved at the same time.
		●	Rest palms on hips, press down firmly, and inspect the breasts.
		▷	Stated the purpose of flexing the chest muscles.
		●	Gently squeeze each nipple and look for a discharge.
			2. Lying down
		●	Place a pillow (or folded towel) under right shoulder.

Trial 1	Trial 2	Point Value	Performance Standards
		●	Place right hand behind head.
		▷	Stated the purpose of the pillow and hand placement.
		●	Use the finger pads of the middle three fingers of the left hand.
		▷	Explained why the finger pads should be used.
		●	Use small rotating motions and continuous firm pressure.
		●	Use one of the following patterns to move around the breast: circular, vertical strip, or wedge.
		▷	Stated why a pattern is used.
			Circular pattern:
		●	Visualize breast as a clock face.
		●	Start at outside edge of breast.
		●	Proceed clockwise until you return to starting point.
		●	Move in 1 inch, and repeat the circle.
		●	Continue until nipple is reached.
			Vertical strip:
		●	Divide breast into strips.
		●	Start at underarm.
		●	Slowly move fingers down until they are below the breast.
		●	Move fingers 1 inch toward middle and move back up.
		●	Repeat until entire breast has been examined.
			Wedge:
		●	Divide breasts into wedges.
		●	Start at outer edge of breast.
		●	Move fingers toward the nipple and back to edge of breast.
		●	Repeat until entire breast has been examined.
			Use the following techniques during the examination:
		●	Press firmly enough to feel the different breast tissues.
		●	Palpate for lumps, hard knots, or thickening.
		▷	Explained how normal breast tissue feels.
		●	Examine the entire chest area from your collarbone to the base of a properly fitted bra and from the breastbone to the underarm.

Trial 1	Trial 2	Point Value	Performance Standards
		●	Pay special attention to the area between the breast and underarm including the underarm itself.
		▷	Explained why the underarm should be examined.
		●	Continue the examination until every part of the right breast has been examined, including the nipple.
		●	Repeat the procedure on the left breast, with a pillow or rolled towel under the left shoulder, the left hand behind the head, and using the right hand to palpate.
			3. In the shower
		●	Gently lather each breast.
		▷	Explained why the breasts should be examined in the shower.
		●	Place right hand behind head.
		●	Use the finger pads of the middle three fingers of the left hand.
		●	Use small, rotating motions and continuous, firm pressure.
		●	Use your preferred pattern to thoroughly examine the right breast and underarm for lumps, hard knots, or thickening.
		●	Repeat the procedure on the left breast using the pads of your right fingers.
		●	Instructed the patient to report any lumps or changes to the physician immediately.
		▷	Explained why it is important to report changes immediately.
		●	Charted the procedure correctly.
		Ⓐ	Showed awareness of a patient's concerns related to the procedure being performed.
		Ⓐ	Explained to a patient the rationale for performance of a procedure.
		*	Completed the procedure within 10 minutes.
			TOTALS

CHART	
Date	

Evaluation of Student Performance

EVALUATION CRITERIA			COMMENTS
Symbol	**Category**	**Point Value**	
∗	Critical Step	16 points	
●	Essential Step	6 points	
Ⓐ	Affective Competency	6 points	
▷	Theory Question	2 points	
Score calculation: 100 points – ____ points missed ____ Score Satisfactory score: 85 or above			

2008 CAAHEP Competencies Achieved
Psychomotor (Skills) ☑ IV. 5. Instruct patients according to their needs to promote health maintenance and disease prevention. ☑ IV. 9. Document patient education. ***Affective (Behavior)*** ☑ I. 2. Use language/verbal skills that enable patients' understanding. ☑ IV. 3. Use appropriate body language and other nonverbal skills in communicating with patients, family, and staff.

2015 CAAHEP Competencies Achieved
Psychomotor (Skills) ☑ V. 4. Coach patients regarding: a. office policies b. health maintenance c. disease prevention d. treatment plan. ☑ X. 3. Document patient care accurately in the medical record. ***Affective (Behavior)*** ☑ I. 3. Show awareness of a patient's concerns related to the procedure being performed. ☑ V. 4. Explain to a patient the rationale for performance of a procedure.

ABHES Competencies Achieved
☑ 4. a. Follow documentation guidelines. ☑ 8. f. Display professionalism through written and verbal communications. ☑ 9. h. Teach self-examination, disease management and health promotion.

EVALUATION OF COMPETENCY

Procedure 23-2: Assisting with a Gynecologic Examination

Name: ______________________________ Date: ______________

Evaluated by: ______________________________ Score: ______________

Performance Objective

Outcome:	Assist with a gynecologic examination.
Conditions:	Using an examining table.
	Given the following: disposable gloves, examining gown and drape, disposable vaginal speculum, lubricant, gauze pads, collection vial, plastic spatula and endocervical brush or cytology broom, Hemoccult slide and developing solution, tissues, biohazard waste container, cytology request form, biohazard specimen transport bag.
Standards:	Time: 15 minutes. Student completed procedure in __________ minutes.
	Accuracy: Satisfactory score on the Performance Evaluation Checklist.

Performance Evaluation Checklist

Trial 1	Trial 2	Point Value	Performance Standards
		•	Sanitized hands.
		•	Assembled equipment.
		•	Completed as much of the cytology request form as possible.
		•	Checked the expiration date and labeled the collection vial.
		•	Greeted the patient and introduced yourself.
		•	Escorted the patient to the examining room.
		•	Identified the patient.
		•	Asked patient if she has any problems or concerns and charted the information.
		•	Completed the cytology request by asking necessary questions.
		•	Measured vital signs and height and weight and charted the results correctly.
			Prepared patient for the examination:
		•	Asked patient if she needs to empty bladder.
		▷	Explained why the bladder should be empty for the examination.
		•	Instructed the patient to undress and put on the examining gown with opening in front.
		•	Informed patient that physician would be in soon.
		•	Left the room to provide patient privacy.

Trial 1	Trial 2	Point Value	Performance Standards
		●	Made medical record available for review by the physician (if using a PPR).
		●	Checked to make sure patient is ready.
		●	Informed physician that the patient was ready.
			Assisted the physician:
		●	Positioned and draped patient in a supine position for the breast examination.
		●	Positioned and draped patient in the lithotomy position for the pelvic examination.
		●	Prepared the vaginal speculum and handed it to the physician.
		●	Prepared the light for physician.
		●	Handed vaginal speculum to physician.
		●	Reassured patient and helped her to relax during the examination.
		▷	Explained why patient should be relaxed during the examination.
			Assisted with Pap specimen collection:
		●	Applied gloves.
			1a. ThinPrep spatula and brush method
		●	Held the vial to receive the collection device from the physician.
		●	Correctly rinsed each collection device in the liquid preservative.
		▷	Explained why the collection device should be swirled vigorously.
		●	Discarded each collection device in a biohazard waste container.
		●	Tightened the cap on the vial.
			1b. ThinPrep broom method
		●	Held the vial to receive the broom from the physician.
		●	Correctly rinsed the broom in the liquid preservative.
		●	Discarded the broom in a biohazard waste container.
		●	Tightened the cap on the vial.
			2. SurePath spatula and brush method
		●	Held the vial to receive each collection device from the physician.
		●	Broke off or disconnected tip of each collection device.
		●	Discarded each handle in a regular waste container.
		●	Tightened cap on the vial.
			Assisted with the remainder of the examination:
		●	Removed light source.

Trial 1	Trial 2	Point Value	Performance Standards
		●	Discarded vaginal speculum in a biohazard waste container.
		●	Provided the physician with lubricant for the bimanual and rectal-vaginal examinations.
		●	Assisted as required with the collection of the fecal occult blood specimen.
		●	Assisted the patient into a sitting position and allowed her to rest.
		▷	Explained why the patient should be allowed to rest.
		●	Offered the patient tissues to remove lubricant from the perineum.
		●	Assisted patient from the examining table.
		●	Instructed patient to get dressed.
		●	Informed patient of the method used by the medical office to relay test results.
		●	Tested the fecal occult blood specimen and charted the results.
		●	Prepared Pap specimen for transport to the laboratory.
		●	Placed specimen in a biohazard specimen bag and sealed the bag.
		●	Inserted the cytology requisition into the outside pocket of bag.
		●	Placed bag in appropriate location for pickup by the laboratory.
		●	Charted the transport of the Pap specimen to an outside laboratory.
		●	Cleaned the examining room.
		Ⓐ	Incorporated critical thinking skills when performing patient assessment.
		Ⓐ	Showed awareness of a patient's concerns related to the procedure being performed.
		Ⓐ	Protected the integrity of the medical record.
		✶	Completed the procedure within 15 minutes.
			TOTALS

CHART	
Date	

Evaluation of Student Performance

EVALUATION CRITERIA			COMMENTS
Symbol	Category	Point Value	
✶	Critical Step	16 points	
●	Essential Step	6 points	
Ⓐ	Affective Competency	6 points	
▷	Theory Question	2 points	
Score calculation: 100 points – ___ points missed ___ Score Satisfactory score: 85 or above			

2008 CAAHEP Competencies Achieved
Psychomotor (Skills) ☑ I. 10. Assist physician with patient care. ☑ IV. 5. Instruct patients according to their needs to promote health maintenance and disease prevention. ☑ IV. 6. Prepare a patient for procedures and/or treatments. ***Affective (Behavior)*** ☑ III. 3. Show awareness of patients' concerns. ☑ IV. 1. Demonstrate empathy in communicating with patients, family, and staff.

2015 CAAHEP Competencies Achieved
Psychomotor (Skills) ☑ I. 3. Perform screening using established protocols. ☑ I. 8. Instruct and prepare a patient for a procedure or a treatment. ☑ I. 9. Assist provider with a patient exam. ☑ V. 1. Use feedback techniques to obtain patient information including: a. reflection b. restatement c. clarification. ☑ V. 4. Coach patients regarding: a. office policies b. health maintenance c. disease prevention d. treatment plan. ☑ X. 2. Apply HIPAA rules in regard to: a. privacy b. release of information. ☑ X. 3. Document patient care accurately in the medical record. ***Affective (Behavior)*** ☑ I. 1. Incorporate critical thinking skills when performing patient assessment. ☑ I. 3. Show awareness of a patient's concerns related to the procedure being performed. ☑ X. 2. Protect the integrity of the medical record.

ABHES Competencies Achieved
☑ 4. a. Follow documentation guidelines. ☑ 8. f. Display professionalism through written and verbal communications. ☑ 9. d. Assist provider with specialty examination including cardiac, respiratory, OB-GYN, neurological, gastroenterology procedures. ☑ 9. e. Perform specialty procedures including but not limited to minor surgery, cardiac, respiratory, OB-GYN, neurological, gastroenterology. ☑ 9. h. Teach self-examination, disease management and health promotion.

GYN CYTOLOGY REQUISITION

THOMAS WOODSIDE, MD
501 MAIN ST
ST. LOUIS, MO 63146
(314) 883–0093

PATIENT INFO

Patient's Name (Last) | (First) | (MI) | Date of Birth MO DAY YR | Collection Time : AM PM | Collection Date MO DAY YR | Patient's ID #

Patient's Address | Phone

City | State | ZIP

RESP. PARTY

Name of Responsible Party (if different from patient)

Address of Responsible Party | APT #

City | State | ZIP

INSURANCE

Patient's Relationship to Responsible Party: 1. Self 2. Spouse 3. Child 4. Other

Insurance Comany Name | Plan | Carrier Code

Subscriber/Member # | Location | Group #

Insurance Address | Physician's Provider #

City | State | ZIP

Employer's Name or Number | Insured SSN

Diagnosis/Signs/Symptoms in ICD-9 Format (Highest Specificity)

REQUIRED

ICD-9 codes are the internationally accepted method of describing the clinical picture of the patient. All diagnoses should be provided by the ordering physician or his or her authorized designee. The following is a partial list of of common diagnoses in ICD-9 format. Most third party payers require an ICD-9 code to indicate the medical necessity of the test(s) and or profile(s) ordered. For a complete list of all ICD-9 codes, please refer to a current ICD-9 manual.

V76.2	Routine Cervical Pap Smear	616.0	Cervicitis	626.8	Abnormal Bleeding
V15.89	High Risk Cervical Screening	616.10	Vaginitis	627.1	Postmenopausal Bleeding
V22.2	Pregnancy	617.0	Endometriosis, Uterus	627.3	Atrophic Vaginitis
079.4	Human Papillomavirus	622.1	Dysplasia, Cervix	795.0	Abnormal Cervical Pap Smear
180.0	Malignant Neoplasm, Cervix	623.0	Dysplasia, Vagina		

COLLECTION METHOD

Liquid Based Prep

192055 ☐ Thin Prep Pap Test

192039 ☐ Thin Prep Pap Test w/reflex to HPV Hybrid Capture when ASC-US or SIL

192047 ☐ Thin Prep Pap Test w/reflex to high-risk only HPV Hybrid Capture when ASC-US

Pap Smear

009100 ☐ 1 Slide 009191 ☐ 2 Slides

Pap Smear and Maturation Index

009209 ☐ 1 Slide 190074 ☐ 2 Slides

SOURCE OF SPECIMEN

☐ Cervical
☐ Endocervical
☐ Vaginal

Date LMP

___/___/___
Mo Day Year

COLLECTION TECHNIQUE

☐ Spatula
☐ Brush
☐ Broom
☐ Other ____________

PATIENT HISTORY

☐ Pregnant
☐ Lactating
☐ Oral Contraceptives
☐ Postmenopausal
☐ Hormone Replacement Therapy
☐ PMP Bleeding
☐ Postpartum
☐ IUD
☐ Postcoital Bleeding
☐ DES Exposure
☐ Previous Abnormal Pap Test
☐ Other ____________

PREVIOUS TREATMENT | Date/Results

☐ None
☐ Colposcopy and Bx ____________
☐ Cryosurgery ____________
☐ LEEP ____________
☐ Laser Vaporization ____________
☐ Conization ____________
☐ Hysterectomy ____________
☐ Radiation ____________
☐ Chemotherapy ____________

Notes

EVALUATION OF COMPETENCY

Procedure 23-3: Assisting with a Return Prenatal Examination

Name: ______________________________ Date: ______________

Evaluated by: ______________________________ Score: ______________

Performance Objective

Outcome:	Prepare the patient and assist with a return prenatal examination.
Conditions:	Using an examining table.
	Given the following: centimeter tape measure, Doppler fetal pulse detector, ultrasound coupling agent, paper towel, disposable vaginal speculum, disposable gloves, lubricant, gauze pads, examining gown and drape, and a biohazard waste container.
Standards:	Time: 15 minutes. Student completed procedure in __________ minutes.
	Accuracy: Satisfactory score on the Performance Evaluation Checklist.

Performance Evaluation Checklist

Trial 1	Trial 2	Point Value	Performance Standards
		•	Sanitized hands.
		•	Set up the tray for the prenatal examination.
		•	Greeted the patient and introduced yourself.
		•	Identified patient and explained the procedure.
		•	Asked the patient to obtain a urine specimen.
		•	Escorted the patient to the examining room and asked her to be seated.
		•	Asked the patient if she has experienced any problems since her last visit and recorded information in the prenatal record.
		•	Measured patient's blood pressure and charted the results correctly.
		•	Weighed the patient and charted the results correctly.
		▷	Stated the importance of weighing the patient.
		•	Instructed and prepared patient for the examination.
		•	Left room to provide patient with privacy.
		•	Made medical record available for review by the physician (if using a PPR).
		•	Tested the urine specimen for glucose and protein, and charted the results correctly.
		•	Checked to make sure the patient is ready to be seen by physician.
		•	Informed physician that patient is ready.
		▷	Stated how the physician can be informed that the patient is ready.

Trial 1	Trial 2	Point Value	Performance Standards
		●	Assisted patient into a supine position and properly draped her.
			Assisted physician during the examination:
		●	Handed physician the tape measure for determination of fundal height.
		●	Applied coupling gel to the patient's abdomen and handed physician Doppler device.
		●	Removed gel from patient's abdomen.
		●	Cleaned the probe head of the Doppler device.
		●	Assisted patient into the lithotomy position if a vaginal specimen is to be obtained or if vaginal examination is to be performed.
			After completion of the examination:
		●	Assisted patient into a sitting position and allowed her to rest.
		●	Assisted patient from examining table.
		●	Provided patient teaching and explanation of physician's instructions as required.
		●	Escorted patient to the reception area.
		●	Cleaned the examining room in preparation for the next patient.
		●	Prepared any specimens collected for transport to an outside laboratory.
		Ⓐ	Incorporated critical thinking skills when performing patient assessment.
		Ⓐ	Showed awareness of a patient's concerns related to the procedure being performed.
		Ⓐ	Protected the integrity of the medical record.
		*	Completed the procedure within 15 minutes.
			TOTALS

CHART	
Date	

Evaluation of Student Performance

EVALUATION CRITERIA			COMMENTS
Symbol	**Category**	**Point Value**	
✶	Critical Step	16 points	
●	Essential Step	6 points	
Ⓐ	Affective Competency	6 points	
▷	Theory Question	2 points	
Score calculation: 100 points – ___ points missed ___ Score Satisfactory score: 85 or above			

2008 CAAHEP Competencies Achieved

Psychomotor (Skills)

☑ I. 10. Assist physician with patient care.
☑ II. 2. Maintain laboratory test results using flow sheets.
☑ IV. 1. Use reflection, restatement, and clarification techniques to obtain a patient history.
☑ IV. 5. Instruct patients according to their needs to promote health maintenance and disease prevention.
☑ IV. 6. Prepare a patient for procedures and/or treatments.
☑ IX. 7. Document accurately in the patient record.

Affective (Behavior)

☑ IV. 2. Apply active listening skills.
☑ IV. 8. Analyze communications in providing appropriate responses or feedback.

2015 CAAHEP Competencies Achieved

Psychomotor (Skills)

☑ I. 3. Perform screening using established protocols.
☑ I. 8. Instruct and prepare a patient for a procedure or a treatment.
☑ I. 9. Assist provider with a patient exam.
☑ II. 3. Maintain lab test results using flow sheets.
☑ V. 1. Use feedback techniques to obtain patient information including: a. reflection b. restatement c. clarification.
☑ V. 4. Coach patients regarding: a. office policies b. health maintenance c. disease prevention d. treatment plan.
☑ V. 5. Coach patients appropriately considering: a. cultural diversity b. developmental life stage c. communication barriers.
☑ X. 2. Apply HIPAA rules in regard to: a. privacy b. release of information.
☑ X. 3. Document patient care accurately in the medical record.

Affective (Behavior)

☑ I. 1. Incorporate critical thinking skills when performing patient assessment.
☑ I. 3. Show awareness of a patient's concerns related to the procedure being performed.
☑ X. 2. Protect the integrity of the medical record.

ABHES Competencies Achieved

☑ 4. a. Follow documentation guidelines.
☑ 5. d. Discuss developmental stages of life.
☑ 8. f. Display professionalism through written and verbal communications.
☑ 9. b. Obtain vital signs, obtain patient history, and formulate chief complaint.
☑ 9. d. Assist provider with specialty examination including cardiac, respiratory, OB-GYN, neurological, gastroenterology procedures.
☑ 9. e. Perform specialty procedures including but not limited to minor surgery, cardiac, respiratory, OB-GYN, neurological, gastroenterology.
☑ 9. h. Teach self-examination, disease management and health promotion.

PATIENT'S NAME ______________________________

INTERVAL PRENATAL HISTORY

Date 20__	Weeks Gestation	Height of Fundus (cm)	Weight	B/P	Urine Glucose	Urine Protein	FHT	Vaginal Examination	Presentation	Edema	Discharge	Bleeding	Contractions	Fetal Activity	NST	Next Appt.	Initials
				/													
				/													
				/													
				/													
				/													
				/													
				/													
				/													
				/													
				/													
				/													
				/													
				/													
				/													

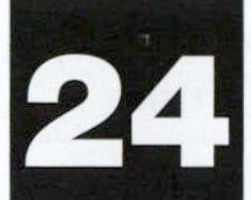

The Pediatric Examination

CHAPTER ASSIGNMENTS

✓ After Completing	Date Due	Study Guide Pages	STUDY GUIDE ASSIGNMENTS (CTA = Critical Thinking Activity)	Possible Points	Points You Earned
		563	Pretest	10	
		564	Term Key Term Assessment	12	
		564-567	Evaluation of Learning questions	35	
		568	CTA A: Pediatric Weight	7	
			Evolve Site: Pounds and Ounces (Record points earned)		
		568	CTA B: Pediatric Length	8	
			Evolve Site: Inch by Inch (Record points earned)		
		568	CTA C: Growth Charts	18	
		569	CTA D: Motor and Social Development (5 points per each category)	65	
		569	CTA E: Intramuscular Injection	15	
		570-571	CTA F: Vaccine Information Statement	11	
		571	CTA G: Locating and Interpreting a Vaccine Information Statement	20	
		571-572	CTA H: Immunization Administration Record	40	
		573	CTA I: Crossword Puzzle	28	
			Evolve Site: Apply Your Knowledge questions (Record points earned)	10	

✓ After Completing	Date Due	Study Guide Pages	STUDY GUIDE ASSIGNMENTS (CTA = Critical Thinking Activity)	Possible Points	Points You Earned
			Evolve Site: Video Evaluation	31	
		563	Posttest	10	
			ADDITIONAL ASSIGNMENTS		
			TOTAL POINTS		

✓ When Assigned By Your Instructor	Study Guide Pages	Practices Required	LABORATORY ASSIGNMENTS (Procedure Number and Name)	Score*
	575	3	**Practice for Competency** 24-A: Carrying an Infant Textbook reference: p. 531	
	579-580		**Evaluation of Competency** 24-A: Carrying an Infant	*
	576	5	**Practice for Competency** 24-1: Measuring the Weight and Length of an Infant Textbook reference: pp. 536-537	
	581-583		**Evaluation of Competency** 24-1: Measuring the Weight and Length of an Infant	*
	577	5	**Practice for Competency** 24-2: Measuring Head and Chest Circumference of an Infant Textbook reference: pp. 537-538	
	585-586		**Evaluation of Competency** 24-2: Measuring Head and Chest Circumference of an Infant	*
	576	5	**Practice for Competency** 24-3: Calculating Growth Percentiles Textbook reference: pp. 539-541	
	587-588		**Evaluation of Competency** 24-3: Calculating Growth Percentiles	*
	577	5	**Practice for Competency** 24-4: Applying a Pediatric Urine Collector Textbook reference: pp. 544-546	
	589-591		**Evaluation of Competency** 24-4: Applying a Pediatric Urine Collector	*
			ADDITIONAL ASSIGNMENTS	

Notes

Name ______________________________ Date ______________

PRETEST

True or False

_______ 1. A pediatrician is a medical doctor who specializes in the diagnosis and treatment of disease in children.

_______ 2. The first well-child visit is usually scheduled 4 weeks after birth of the infant.

_______ 3. Length is measured with the child standing with his or her back to the measuring device.

_______ 4. Blood pressure should be taken for a child starting at 8 years of age.

_______ 5. It is best not to tell a child that an immunization will hurt.

_______ 6. The vastus lateralis muscle site is recommended for administering an injection to an infant.

_______ 7. An MMR injection includes the following immunizations: measles, meningitis, and rubella.

_______ 8. A Vaccine Information Statement explains the benefits and risks of a vaccine in lay terminology.

_______ 9. The hepatitis B vaccine can be given to a newborn.

_______ 10. The blood specimen for a newborn screening test is obtained from the infant's earlobe.

POSTTEST

True or False

_______ 1. A well-child visit is also referred to as a health maintenance visit.

_______ 2. A reason for weighing a child is to determine proper medication dosage.

_______ 3. Growth charts can be used to identify children with growth abnormalities.

_______ 4. Measuring pediatric blood pressure helps to identify children at risk for type 1 diabetes.

_______ 5. Using a blood pressure cuff that is too large for the child can result in a falsely low reading.

_______ 6. The length of the needle used for a pediatric IM injection depends on the amount of medication being administered.

_______ 7. The resistance of the body to pathogenic microorganisms or their toxins is known as inflammation.

_______ 8. The recommended route of administration for an MMR vaccine is subcutaneous.

_______ 9. Before administering a pediatric immunization, the National Childhood Vaccine Injury Act (NCVIA) requires that the parent sign a consent form.

_______ 10. If phenylketonuria (PKU) is left untreated, it can lead to malnutrition.

KEY TERM ASSESSMENT

Directions: Match each key term with its definition.

_______ 1. Immunity
_______ 2. Immunization
_______ 3. Infant
_______ 4. Length
_______ 5. Pediatrician
_______ 6. Pediatrics
_______ 7. Preschooler
_______ 8. School-age child
_______ 9. Toddler
_______ 10. Toxoid
_______ 11. Vaccine
_______ 12. Vertex

A. A physician who specializes in the care and development of children and the diagnosis and treatment of children's diseases
B. A child between 1 and 3 years old
C. The top of the head
D. The resistance of the body to the effects of a harmful agent such as a pathogenic microorganism or its toxins
E. The branch of medicine that deals with the care and development of children and the diagnosis and treatment of children's diseases
F. A suspension of attenuated or killed microorganisms administered to an individual to prevent an infectious disease
G. The process of becoming immune or of rendering an individual immune through the use of a vaccine or toxoid
H. The measurement from the vertex of the head to the heel of the foot in a supine position
I. A toxin that has been treated by heat or chemicals to destroy its harmful properties administered to an individual to prevent an infectious disease
J. A child from birth to 12 months old
K. A child from 3 to 6 years old
L. A child from 6 to 12 years old

EVALUATION OF LEARNING

Directions: Fill in each blank with the correct answer.

1. What are the components of the well-child visit?

____

____

2. What topics are commonly included in anticipatory guidance?

____

____

3. What is the usual schedule for well-child visits?

____

____

____

4. What is the purpose of the sick-child visit?

____

____

5. What procedures are often performed by the medical assistant during pediatric office visits?

____

____

____

6. Why is it important for the medical assistant to develop a rapport with the pediatric patient?

7. List the two positions that can be used to safely carry an infant.

8. Why is it important to measure the growth (weight and height or length) of the child during each office visit?

9. What is the difference between height and length?

10. What is the purpose of measuring head circumference?

11. What is the primary use of growth charts?

12. What is the primary cause of childhood obesity?

13. What problems are associated with childhood obesity?

14. List five guidelines for preventing childhood obesity.

15. According to the American Academy of Pediatrics, at what age and how often should blood pressure be measured in children?

16. What is the importance of measuring blood pressure in children?

17. What criteria must be followed to determine the correct cuff size for a child?

18. What occurs if the blood pressure cuff is too small or too large?

19. What three factors must be taken into consideration when determining if a child has hypertension?

20. List three reasons for collecting a urine specimen from a child.

21. Why should the child's genitalia be cleansed before applying a pediatric urine collector?

22. What gauge and length (range) of needle are recommended for giving an intramuscular injection to a child?

23. Why is the dorsogluteal site not recommended for use as an intramuscular injection site in infants and young children?

24. Why is the vastus lateralis muscle recommended as a good site for giving an intramuscular injection to an infant or young child? How is this site located?

25. At what age can the deltoid site be used to administer an IM injection to a child? Explain the reason for this.

26. What is the recommended subcutaneous injection site for each of the following?

   a. An infant younger than 12 months of age: ______

   b. A child that is 12 months of age or older: ______

27. What is the difference between a vaccine and a toxoid?

28. What immunizations are included in the following?

a. DTaP:

b. MMR:

29. According to the American Academy of Pediatrics, what immunizations are recommended for each of the following pediatric patients?

a. 2-month-old infant:

b. 6-month-old infant:

c. 12-month-old infant:

d. 5-year-old child:

30. What information must be provided to parents as required by the NCVIA?

31. What information is included in a VIS?

32. According to the NCVIA, what information must be recorded in the patient's medical record after a pediatric immunization has been administered?

33. The newborn screening test screens for which metabolic diseases?

34. What are the symptoms of PKU if left untreated?

35. Why can the PKU screening test be performed earlier on infants on formula compared with breast-fed babies?

CRITICAL THINKING ACTIVITIES

A. Pediatric Weight

Locate the following weight values on a pediatric balance scale. Place a check mark next to each one after it has been correctly located.

1. 7 lb, 9 oz ______________
2. 8 lb, 5 oz ______________
3. 12 lb, 10 oz ______________
4. 15 lb, 11 oz ______________
5. 19 lb, 7 oz ______________
6. 23 lb, 6 oz ______________
7. 25 lb, 3 oz ______________

B. Pediatric Length

Locate the following length values on your pediatric measuring device. Place a check mark next to each after it has been correctly located.

1. 20½ inches ______________
2. 22½ inches ______________
3. 24 inches ______________
4. 25¾ inches ______________
5. 28½ inches ______________
6. 31 inches ______________
7. 33¼ inches ______________
8. 36½ inches ______________

C. Growth Charts

Matthew Williams, age 2 years (24 months), has had health maintenance visits at the intervals listed below. His length and weight measurements were taken during each visit and are recorded here. Plot these on the growth chart on page 480 of your textbook. You can also print out a growth chart from your computer by going to the following website: www.cdc.gov/growthcharts. Calculate the percentile for each and record it in the space provided. (Note: His birth weight was 7 lb, 8 oz and his length was 20 inches.)

Well-Child Visit

Age	Weight	Percentile	Length	Percentile
1 month	9 lb, 10 oz		22 in	
2 months	12 lb, 4 oz		23½ in	
4 months	16 lb, 5 oz		25¼ in	
6 months	18 lb, 8 oz		27 in	
9 months	22 lb, 4 oz		29¼ in	
12 months	24 lb, 4 oz		30½ in	
15 months	26 lb, 8 oz		31½ in	
18 months	27 lb		32½ in	
24 months	28 lb		35¾ in	

D. Motor and Social Development

Using a reference source, describe the motor and social development of the age groups listed here. The first one is done for you.

Age	Motor and Social Development
Birth to 3 months	Raises head but not stable, can turn head from side to side, activities are limited to reflexes, cries when hungry, responsive social smile, coos, eyes can focus on an object and follow a moving object 180 degrees.
4 to 6 months	
7 to 9 months	
10 to 12 months	
1 year	
2 years	
3 years	
4 years	
5 years	
6 years	
7 years	
8 to 10 years	
Preadolescent	
Adolescent	

E. Intramuscular Injection

How would you prepare the following children for an intramuscular injection of penicillin to reduce apprehension and fear? Table 24-2, Techniques for Interacting with Children, on page 533 of your textbook can be used as a reference for this activity.

a. Katie Waugh, age 5

____

____

____

b. Patrick Williams, age 8

____

____

____

c. Julie Anderson, age 15

____

____

____

F. Vaccine Information Statement

Refer to the Diphtheria, Tetanus, and Pertussis Vaccine Information Statement (VIS) in your textbook (page 552), and answer the following questions:

1. How does an individual contract tetanus?

___

___

2. What are the symptoms of the following diseases?

   a. Diphtheria ___

   b. Tetanus ___

   c. Pertussis ___

3. Why is DTaP now used instead of DTP?

___

___

4. What is the immunization schedule for DTaP?

___

___

5. Who should not get a DTaP immunization?

___

___

6. What does Td protect against, and what is the recommended immunization schedule for Td?

___

___

7. What mild problems may occur from a DTaP vaccine?

___

___

8. What moderate problems may occur from a DTaP vaccine?

___

___

9. What should be done if the patient develops fever and pain after receiving a DTaP?

___

___

10. What are the symptoms of a serious reaction to DTaP?

___

11. What should be done if a moderate or severe reaction occurs after a DTaP immunization?

____

____

G. Locating and Interpreting a Vaccine Information Statement

Obtain a VIS for a vaccine that you would like to know more about (other than the DTaP vaccine already included in your textbook). List the information that would be important for a parent to know before this immunization is administered to his or her child. The following Internet sites can be used to obtain a VIS:

www.cdc.gov/vaccines/hcp/vis/index.html
www.immunize.org/vis

Name of Immunization: ____

Publication Date: ____

Information to Relay to a Parent:

____

____

____

____

____

____

____

____

____

____

H. Immunization Administration Record

Complete the following immunization record form for an infant at his or her 2-month, 4-month, and 6-month visits using Figure 24-11 (immunization schedule) in the textbook to determine which immunizations are administered during these well-child visits. The website (www.immunize.org/catg.d/p2022.pdf) provides an example of a completed immunization administration form to assist you in completing this form.

IMMUNIZATION ADMINISTRATION RECORD

Name ______________________________
(first) (MI) (last)

DOB ______________________________

Physician ______________________________

Address ______________________________

____

SITE ABBREVIATIONS:
RVL: Right vastus lateralis
LVL: Left vastus lateralis
RD: Right deltoid
LD: Left deltoid
PO: By mouth
IN: Intranasal

Vaccine	Type of Vaccine[1] (generic abbreviation)	Date Given (mo/day/yr)	Dose	Site	Vaccine		Vaccine Information Statement		Signature and Title of Vaccinator
					Lot #	Mfr.	Date on VIS	Date Given	
Hepatitis B[2] (e.g., HepB, Hib-HepB, DTaP-HepB-IPV) Give IM.									
Diphtheria, Tetanus, Pertussis[2] (e.g., DTaP, DTaP-Hib, DTaP-HepB-IPV, DT, DTaP-HiB-IPV, Tdap, DTaP-IPV, Td) Give IM.									
Haemophilus influenzae type b[2] (e.g., Hib, Hib-HepB, DTaP-HiB-IPV, DTaP-Hib) Give IM.									
Polio[2] (e.g., IPV, DTaP-HepB-IPV, DTaP-HiB-IPV, DTaP-IPV) Give IPV SC or IM. Give all others IM.									
Pneumococcal (e.g., PCV, conjugate; PPV, polysaccharide) Give PCV IM. Give PPV SC or IM.									
Rotavirus Give oral.									
Measles, Mumps, Rubella (e.g., MMR, MMRV) Give SC.									
Varicella (e.g., Var, MMRV) Give SC.									
Hepatitis A (HepA) Give IM									
Meningococcal (e.g., MCV4, MPSV4) Give MCV4 IM and MPSV4 SC.									
Human papillomavirus (e.g., HPV) Give IM									
Influenza (e.g., TIV, inactivated; LAIV, live attenuated) Give TIV IM. Give LAIV IN.									
Other									

1. Record the generic abbreviation for the type of vaccine given (e.g., DTaP-Hib, PCV), *not* the trade name.
2. For combination vaccines, fill in a row for each separate antigen in the combination.

I. Crossword Puzzle: The Pediatric Examination

Directions: Complete the crossword puzzle using the clues provided.

Across

1 Right size for child's BP?
3 Title expires at 1 year
6 Child's vaccine act
9 German measles
10 Not for pregnant women
13 Whooping cough
16 PKU puncture site
17 3-in-1 vaccine
20 Do not weigh infant in this
21 Stand up straight
22 Begin at 3
23 First breast milk
24 Baby doctor
25 MMR administration route
26 Can give at birth vaccine
27 Injection site for infants

Down

1 Hold-me position
2 Not a kid reward
4 Common immunization side effect
5 From 1 to 3 years
7 Resistance to microorganisms
8 No phenylalanine enzyme disease
11 Vertex to heel
12 Child's work
14 Childhood obesity can cause this
15 Not caused by chickens
18 Fights with a microorganism
19 Immunization explainer

Notes

PRACTICE FOR COMPETENCY

Procedure 24-A: Carrying an Infant

Practice the procedure for carrying an infant, using a pediatric training mannequin in the following positions: cradle and upright.

Carrying Position	Number Of Practices

Procedures 24-1 and 24-3: Weight, Length, and Growth Charts

1. **Weight and Length.** Measure the weight of an infant using a pediatric training mannequin. Record the results in the chart provided.
2. **Growth Charts**. Calculate growth percentiles on a growth chart using the values presented below. Assume these values were taken from the same (female) child over the course of her first year of life.

Age	Weight	Length
2 months	9 pounds	21 inches
4 months	11 pounds, 8 ounces	23½ inches
6 months	14 pounds, 8 ounces	25¼ inches
9 months	18 pounds, 8 ounces	27¼ inches
12 months	21 pounds, 6 ounces	28¾ inches

Chart	
Date	

Procedure 24-2: Head and Chest Circumference. Measure the head and chest circumference of an infant using a pediatric training mannequin. Record the results in the chart provided.

Procedure 24-4: Pediatric Urine Collector. Practice the procedure for applying a pediatric urine collector, using a pediatric training mannequin. Record the procedure in the chart provided.

Chart	
Date	

Chart

Date	

EVALUATION OF COMPETENCY

Procedure 24-A: Carrying an Infant

Name: ______________________________ Date: ______________

Evaluated by: ______________________________ Score: ______________

Performance Objective

Outcome:	Carry an infant in the following positions: cradle and upright.
Conditions:	Given a pediatric training mannequin.
Standards:	Time: 5 minutes. Student completed procedure in __________ minutes.
	Accuracy: Satisfactory score on the performance evaluation checklist.

Performance Evaluation Checklist

Trial 1	Trial 2	Point Value	Performance Standards
			Cradle position:
		•	Slid the left hand and arm under infant's back.
		•	Grasped infant's upper arm from behind.
		•	Encircled infant's upper arm with the thumb and fingers.
		•	Supported infant's head, shoulders, and back on your arm.
		•	Slipped the right arm up and under the infant's buttocks.
		•	Cradled infant in your arms with the infant's body resting against your chest.
			Upright position:
		•	Slipped the right hand under infant's head and shoulders.
		•	Spread the fingers apart to support infant's head and neck.
		•	Slipped the left forearm under infant's buttocks.
		•	Allowed infant to rest against your chest.
		Ⓐ	Demonstrated: a. empathy b. active listening c. nonverbal communication.
		*	Completed the procedure within 5 minutes.
			TOTALS

CHART	
Date	

Evaluation of Student Performance

EVALUATION CRITERIA			COMMENTS
Symbol	**Category**	**Point Value**	
∗	Critical Step	16 points	
●	Essential Step	6 points	
Ⓐ	Affective Competency	6 points	
▷	Theory Question	2 points	
Score calculation: 100 points – ____ points missed ____ Score Satisfactory score: 85 or above			

2008 CAAHEP Competencies Achieved
Psychomotor (Skills) ☑ IV. 6. Prepare a patient for procedures and/or treatments. ***Affective (Behavior)*** ☑ IV. 1. Demonstrate empathy in communicating with patients, family, and staff.

2015 CAAHEP Competencies Achieved
Psychomotor (Skills) ☑ I. 8. Instruct and prepare a patient for a procedure or a treatment. ***Affective (Behavior)*** ☑ V. 1. Demonstrate: a. empathy b. active listening c. nonverbal communication.

ABHES Competencies Achieved
☑ 9. c. Assist provider with general/physical examination.

EVALUATION OF COMPETENCY

Procedure 24-1: Measuring the Weight and Length of an Infant

Name: ______________________ Date: ______________

Evaluated by: ______________________ Score: ______________

Performance Objective

Outcome:	Measure the weight and length of an infant.
Conditions:	Using a pediatric training mannequin and a pediatric balance scale (table model).
	Given a paper protector.
Standards:	Time: 5 minutes Student completed procedure in ________ minutes.
	Accuracy: Satisfactory score on the performance evaluation checklist.

Performance Evaluation Checklist

Trial 1	Trial 2	Point Value	Performance Standards
			Weight:
		●	Sanitized hands.
		●	Greeted the infant's parent and introduced yourself.
		●	Identified the infant.
		●	Explained the procedure to the child's parent.
		●	Based on the medical office policy asked parent to: a. Remove infant's clothing and put on a dry diaper. b. Remove infant's clothing including the diaper.
		▷	Stated why the infant should not be weighed with a wet diaper.
		●	Unlocked pediatric scale and placed a clean paper protector on it.
		▷	Stated the purpose of the paper protector.
		●	Checked the balance scale for accuracy.
		▷	Stated the purpose for balancing the scale.
		●	Gently placed infant on his or her back on the scale.
		●	Placed one hand slightly above infant.
		●	Balanced scale.
		●	Read results while infant was lying still.
		●	Jotted down value or made a mental note of it.
		*	The reading was identical to the evaluator's reading.
		●	Returned balance to its resting position and locked the scale.

Trial 1	Trial 2	Point Value	Performance Standards
			Length:
		●	Placed the vertex of infant's head against the headboard at the zero mark.
		●	Asked parent to hold infant's head in position.
		●	Straightened infant's knees and placed soles of infant's feet firmly against the upright footboard.
		●	Read infant's length in inches from the measure.
		●	Jotted down value or made a mental note of it.
		*	The reading was identical to the evaluator's reading.
		●	Removed infant from the scale and handed him or her to the parent.
		●	Returned headboard and footboard to their resting positions.
		●	Sanitized hands.
		●	Charted the results correctly.
		Ⓐ	Incorporated critical thinking skills when performing patient assessment.
		Ⓐ	Demonstrated: a. empathy b. active listening c. nonverbal communication.
		*	Completed the procedure within 5 minutes.
			TOTALS

CHART	
Date	

Evaluation of Student Performance

EVALUATION CRITERIA			COMMENTS
Symbol	**Category**	**Point Value**	
*	Critical Step	16 points	
●	Essential Step	6 points	
Ⓐ	Affective Competency	6 points	
▷	Theory Question	2 points	
Score calculation: 100 points – ___ points missed ___Score Satisfactory score: 85 or above			

2008 CAAHEP Competencies Achieved
Psychomotor (Skills) ☑ IV. 6. Prepare a patient for procedures and/or treatments. ***Affective (Behavior)*** ☑ I. 2. Use language/verbal skills that enable patients' understanding. ☑ IV. 7. Demonstrate recognition of the patient's level of understanding in communications.

2015 CAAHEP Competencies Achieved
Psychomotor (Skills) ☑ I. 1. f. Measure and record weight. ☑ I. 1. g. Measure and record length (infant) ☑ V. 5. Coach patients appropriately considering: a. cultural diversity b. developmental life stage c. communication barriers. ***Affective (Behavior)*** ☑ I. 1. Incorporate critical thinking skills when performing patient assessment. ☑ V. 1. Demonstrate: a. empathy b. active listening c. nonverbal communication.

ABHES Competencies Achieved
☑ 4. a. Follow documentation guidelines. ☑ 5. d. Discuss developmental stages of life. ☑ 9. c. Assist provider with general/physical examination.

Notes

EVALUATION OF COMPETENCY

Procedure 24-2: Measuring Head and Chest Circumference of an Infant

Name: ______________________________ Date: ______________

Evaluated by: ______________________________ Score: ______________

Performance Objective

Outcome:	Measure the head and chest circumference of an infant.
Conditions:	Given a flexible, nonstretch tape measure (in centimeters).
Standards:	Time: 5 minutes Student completed procedure in __________ minutes.
	Accuracy: Satisfactory score on the performance evaluation checklist.

Performance Evaluation Checklist

Trial 1	Trial 2	Point Value	Performance Standards
			Measurement of head circumference:
		●	Sanitized hands.
		●	Assembled equipment.
		●	Positioned the infant.
		▷	Stated what positions can be used to measure head circumference.
		●	Positioned the measuring device around the infant's head.
		●	The tape measure was placed slightly above the eyebrows and pinna of the ears, and around the occipital prominence at the back of the skull.
		●	Read the results in centimeters (or inches).
		●	Jotted down value or made a mental note of it.
		*	The reading was identical to the evaluator's reading.
		●	Sanitized hands.
		●	Charted the results correctly.
			Measurement of chest circumference:
		●	Positioned the infant on his or her back on the examining table.
		●	Encircled the measuring device around the infant's chest at the nipple line.
		●	Ensured that the measuring device was snug but not too tight.
		●	Read the results in centimeters (or inches).
		●	Jotted down this value or made a mental note of it.
		*	The reading was identical to the evaluator's reading.
		●	Charted the results correctly.

Trial 1	Trial 2	Point Value	Performance Standards
		Ⓐ	Incorporated critical thinking skills when performing patient assessment.
		✶	Completed the procedure within 5 minutes.
			TOTALS

CHART	
Date	

Evaluation of Student Performance

EVALUATION CRITERIA			COMMENTS
Symbol	**Category**	**Point Value**	
✶	Critical Step	16 points	
●	Essential Step	6 points	
Ⓐ	Affective Competency	6 points	
▷	Theory Question	2 points	
Score calculation: 100 points – ___ points missed ___ Score Satisfactory score: 85 or above			

2008 CAAHEP Competencies Achieved
Psychomotor (Skills) ☑ IV. 6. Prepare a patient for procedures and/or treatments. ***Affective (Behavior)*** ☑ I. 1. Apply critical thinking skills in performing patient assessment and care.

2015 CAAHEP Competencies Achieved
Psychomotor (Skills) ☑ I. 1. h. Measure and record head circumference (infant). ***Affective (Behavior)*** ☑ I. 1. Incorporate critical thinking skills when performing patient assessment.

ABHES Competencies Achieved
☑ 4. a. Follow documentation guidelines. ☑ 9. c. Assist provider with general/physical examination.

EVALUATION OF COMPETENCY

Procedure 24-3: Calculating Growth Percentiles

Name: ______________________________ Date: ______________

Evaluated by: ______________________________ Score: ______________

Performance Objective

Outcome:	Plot a pediatric growth value on a growth chart.
Conditions:	Given a pediatric growth chart.
Standards:	Time: 5 minutes Student completed procedure in ________ minutes.
	Accuracy: Satisfactory score on the performance evaluation checklist.

Performance Evaluation Checklist

Trial 1	Trial 2	Point Value	Performance Standards
		●	Selected the proper growth chart.
		●	Located the child's age in the horizontal column at the bottom of the chart.
		●	Located the growth value in the vertical column under the appropriate category.
		●	Drew a (imaginary) vertical line from the child's age mark and an imaginary horizontal line from the growth mark.
		●	Found the site at which the two lines intersected on the graph.
		●	Placed a dot on this site.
		●	Determined the percentile by following the curved percentile line upward.
		●	Read the value located on the right side of the chart.
		●	Estimated the results if the value did not fall exactly on a percentile line.
		●	Charted the results correctly.
		✶	The value was within ±2 percentage points of the evaluator's determination.
		Ⓐ	Explained to a patient the rationale for performance of a procedure.
		✶	Completed the procedure within 5 minutes.
			TOTALS

CHART	
Date	

Evaluation of Student Performance

EVALUATION CRITERIA			COMMENTS
Symbol	**Category**	**Point Value**	
✶	Critical Step	16 points	
●	Essential Step	6 points	
Ⓐ	Affective Competency	6 points	
▷	Theory Question	2 points	
Score calculation: 100 points – ___ points missed ___ Score Satisfactory score: 85 or above			

2008 CAAHEP Competencies Achieved
Psychomotor (Skills) ☑ II. 3. Maintain growth charts. ***Affective (Behavior)*** ☑ II. 2. Distinguish between normal and abnormal test results.

2015 CAAHEP Competencies Achieved
Psychomotor (Skills) ☑ II. 4. Document on a growth chart. ***Affective (Behavior)*** ☑ V. 4. Explain to a patient the rationale for performance of a procedure.

ABHES Competencies Achieved
☑ 4. a. Follow documentation guidelines. ☑ 5. d. Discuss developmental stages of life.

EVALUATION OF COMPETENCY

Procedure 24-4: Applying a Pediatric Urine Collector

Name: ______________________________ Date: ______________

Evaluated by: ______________________________ Score: ______________

Performance Objective

Outcome:	Apply a pediatric urine collector.
Conditions:	Using a pediatric training mannequin.
	Given the following: disposable gloves, personal antiseptic wipes, pediatric urine collector bag, urine specimen container and label, and a waste container.
Standards:	Time: 10 minutes Student completed procedure in ________ minutes.
	Accuracy: Satisfactory score on the performance evaluation checklist.

Performance Evaluation Checklist

Trial 1	Trial 2	Point Value	Performance Standards
		●	Sanitized hands.
		●	Assembled equipment.
		●	Greeted the child's parent and introduced yourself.
		●	Identified the child and explained the procedure to the parent.
		●	Applied gloves.
		●	Positioned child on his or her back with legs spread apart.
			Cleanse the area and apply the bag:
			Females
		●	Cleansed each side of the meatus with a separate wipe using a front-to-back motion.
		●	Cleansed directly down the middle with a third wipe.
		●	Discarded each wipe after cleansing.
		▷	Stated the reason for cleansing the urinary meatus.
		●	Allowed the area to dry completely.
		▷	Explained why the area should be allowed to dry.
		●	Removed paper backing from urine collector bag.
		●	Placed the bottom of the adhesive ring on the perinuem and work upward.

Trial 1	Trial 2	Point Value	Performance Standards
		●	Firmly pressed the adhesive surface firmly to the skin surrounding the external genitalia.
		●	Made sure there was no puckering.
		●	Opening of the bag was placed directly over the urinary meatus.
		●	Excess length of the bag was positioned toward the feet.
			Males
		●	Retracted the foreskin of the penis if the child is not circumcised.
		●	Cleansed each side of the urethral orifice with a separate wipe.
		●	Cleansed directly over the urethral orifice.
		●	Cleansed the scrotum.
		●	Discarded each wipe after cleansing.
		●	Allowed the area to dry completely.
		●	Removed the paper backing from urine collector bag.
		●	Positioned the bag so that child's penis and scrotum are projected through the opening of the bag.
		●	Firmly pressed the adhesive surface firmly to the skin.
		●	Excess length of the bag was positioned toward the feet.
			Completed the procedure:
		●	Loosely diapered child.
		●	Checked bag every 15 minutes until urine specimen was obtained.
		●	Gently removed collector bag from top to bottom.
		●	Cleansed genital area with a personal antiseptic wipe and rediapered child.
		●	Transferred urine specimen into specimen container and tightly applied the lid.
		●	Applied label to the container.
		●	Disposed of collector bag in a regular waste container.
		●	Tested the specimen or prepared it for transfer to an outside laboratory.
		▷	Explained why the urine specimen should not be allowed to stand at room temperature.
		●	Removed gloves and sanitized hands.
		●	Charted the procedure correctly.
		Ⓐ	Explained to a patient the rationale for performance of a procedure.
		*	Completed the procedure within 5 minutes.
			TOTALS

Chart	
Date	

Evaluation of Student Performance

EVALUATION CRITERIA			COMMENTS
Symbol	**Category**	**Point Value**	
✶	Critical Step	16 points	
●	Essential Step	6 points	
Ⓐ	Affective Competency	6 points	
▷	Theory Question	2 points	
Score calculation: 100 points – ___ points missed ___ Score Satisfactory score: 85 or above			

2008 CAAHEP Competencies Achieved
Psychomotor (Skills) ☑ IV. 6. Prepare a patient for procedures and/or treatments. ***Affective (Behavior)*** ☑ III. 2. Explain the rationale for performance of a procedure to the patient.

2015 CAAHEP Competencies Achieved
Psychomotor (Skills) ☑ I. 11. c. Obtain specimens and perform CLIA waived urinalysis. ***Affective (Behavior)*** ☑ V. 4. Explain to a patient the rationale for performance of a procedure.

ABHES Competencies Achieved
☑ 4. a. Follow documentation guidelines. ☑ 10. d. Collect, label and process specimens.

Notes

25 Minor Office Surgery

CHAPTER ASSIGNMENTS

✓ After Completing	Date Due	Study Guide Pages	STUDY GUIDE ASSIGNMENTS (CTA = Critical Thinking Activity)	Possible Points	Points You Earned
		597	Pretest	10	
		598 599	Term Key Term Assessment A. Definitions B. Word Parts (Add 1 point for each key term)	26 9	
		599-604	Evaluation of Learning questions	51	
		604-605	CTA A: Medical and Surgical Asepsis	10	
		606	CTA B: Violation of Surgical Asepsis	10	
		607-608	CTA C: Surgical Instruments (2 points each)	22	
			Evolve Site: It's Instrumental (Record points earned)		
			Evolve Site: Keep it Sterile (Record points earned)		
		609	CTA D: Pioneers in Surgical Asepsis (5 points each)	15	
		609-610	CTA E: Patient Instruction Sheet	20	
		611	CTA F: Crossword Puzzle	24	
			Evolve Site: Apply Your Knowledge questions	10	
			Evolve Site: Video Evaluation	69	
		597	Posttest	10	
			ADDITIONAL ASSIGNMENTS		
			TOTAL POINTS		

Notes

✓ When Assigned By Your Instructor	Study Guide Pages	Practices Required	Laboratory Assignments (Procedure Number and Name)	Score*
	613-614	5	**Practice for Competency** 25-1: Applying and Removing Sterile Gloves Textbook reference: pp. 568-570	
	615-616		**Evaluation of Competency** 25-1: Applying and Removing Sterile Gloves	*
	613-614	5	**Practice for Competency** 25-2: Opening a Sterile Package Textbook reference: pp. 571-572	
	617-618		**Evaluation of Competency** 25-2: Opening a Sterile Package	*
	613-614	5	**Practice for Competency** Using Commercially Prepared Sterile Packages Textbook reference: p. 568	
	619-620		**Evaluation of Competency** Using Commercially Prepared Sterile Packages	*
	613-614	3	**Practice for Competency** 25-3: Pouring a Sterile Solution Textbook reference: p. 573	
	621-622		**Evaluation of Competency** 25-3: Pouring a Sterile Solution	*
	613-614	5	**Practice for Competency** 25-4: Changing a Sterile Dressing Textbook reference: pp. 576-568	
	623-626		**Evaluation of Competency** 25-4: Changing a Sterile Dressing	*
	613-614	Sutures: 3 Staples: 3	**Practice for Competency** 25-5: Removing Sutures and Staples Textbook reference: pp. 583-585	
	627-629		**Evaluation of Competency** 25-5: Removing Sutures and Staples	*
	613-614	3	**Practice for Competency** 25-6: Applying and Removing Adhesive Skin Closures Textbook reference: pp. 586-589	
	631-634		**Evaluation of Competency** 25-6: Applying and Removing Adhesive Skin Closures	*

✓ When Assigned By Your Instructor	Study Guide Pages	Practices Required	Laboratory Assignments (Procedure Number and Name)	Score*
	613-614	5	**Practice for Competency** 25-7: Assisting with Minor Office Surgery Textbook reference: pp. 594-598	
	635-638		**Evaluation of Competency** 25-7: Assisting with Minor Office Surgery	*
	613-614	Each bandage turn: 3	**Practice for Competency** 25-A: Bandage Turns Textbook reference: pp. 608-609	
	639-641		**Evaluation of Competency** 25-A: Bandage Turns	*
			ADDITIONAL ASSIGNMENTS	

Name ______________________________ Date ______________

PRETEST

True or False

_______ 1. Surgical asepsis refers to practices that keep objects and areas free from all microorganisms.

_______ 2. Something that is sterile is contaminated if it comes in contact with a pathogen.

_______ 3. Reaching over a sterile field is a violation of sterile technique.

_______ 4. An incision is a jagged tearing of the tissues.

_______ 5. The skin is the first line of defense of the body.

_______ 6. One of the local signs of inflammation is fever.

_______ 7. Sutures approximate the edges of a wound until proper healing occurs.

_______ 8. A biopsy is usually performed to determine if an infection is present.

_______ 9. An ingrown toenail can be caused by shoes that are too tight.

_______ 10. One of the functions of a bandage is to hold a dressing in place.

POSTTEST

True or False

_______ 1. Measuring a patient's temperature requires the use of surgical asepsis.

_______ 2. Hemostatic forceps are used to clamp off blood vessels.

_______ 3. An instrument with a ratchet should be kept in a closed position when not in use.

_______ 4. The physician would most likely order a tetanus booster for an abrasion.

_______ 5. Inflammation is the protective response of the body to trauma and the entrance of foreign substances.

_______ 6. A serous exudate is red in color.

_______ 7. Size 4-0 sutures have a smaller diameter than size 3 sutures.

_______ 8. Sebaceous cysts are commonly found on the palm of the hand.

_______ 9. Colposcopy is frequently used to evaluate lesions of the cervix.

_______ 10. Cryosurgery is used in the treatment of cervical cancer.

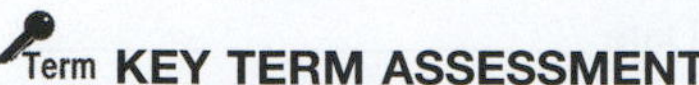

A. Definitions

Directions: Match each key term with its definition.

_______ 1. Abrasion
_______ 2. Abscess
_______ 3. Absorbable suture
_______ 4. Approximation
_______ 5. Bandage
_______ 6. Biopsy
_______ 7. Capillary action
_______ 8. Colposcope
_______ 9. Colposcopy
_______ 10. Contaminate
_______ 11. Contusion
_______ 12. Cryosurgery
_______ 13. Fibroblast
_______ 14. Forceps
_______ 15. Furuncle
_______ 16. Hemostasis
_______ 17. Incision
_______ 18. Infection
_______ 19. Inflammation
_______ 20. Laceration
_______ 21. Nonabsorbable suture
_______ 22. Puncture
_______ 23. Sterile
_______ 24. Surgery
_______ 25. Surgical asepsis
_______ 26. Wound

A. A protective response of the body to trauma and the entrance of foreign matter
B. To cause a sterile object or surface to become unsterile
C. A wound made by a sharp pointed object piercing the skin
D. The condition in which the body is invaded by a pathogen
E. A collection of pus in a cavity surrounded by inflamed tissue
F. The arrest of bleeding by natural or artificial means
G. Free of all living microorganisms and bacterial spores
H. A wound in which the tissues are torn apart, leaving ragged and irregular edges
I. A lighted instrument with a binocular magnifying lens used to examine the vagina and cervix
J. A localized staphylococcal infection that originates deep within a hair follicle; also known as a boil
K. An injury to the tissues under the skin that causes blood vessels to rupture, allowing blood to seep into the tissues
L. The surgical removal and examination of tissue from the living body
M. A wound in which the outer layers of the skin are damaged
N. The action that causes liquid to rise along a wick, a tube, or a gauze dressing
O. A two-pronged instrument for grasping and squeezing
P. Practices that keep objects and areas sterile or free from microorganisms
Q. A break in the continuity of an external or internal surface caused by physical means
R. The therapeutic use of freezing temperatures to destroy abnormal tissue
S. The visual examination of the vagina and cervix using a lighted instrument with a magnifying lens
T. Suture material that is gradually digested and absorbed by the body
U. The process of bringing two parts, such as tissue, together through the use of sutures or other means
V. A strip of woven material used to wrap or cover a part of the body
W. A clean cut caused by a cutting instrument
X. Suture material that is not absorbed by the body
Y. An immature cell from which connective tissue can develop
Z. The branch of medicine that deals with operative and manual procedures for correction of deformities and defects, repair of injuries, and diagnosis and treatment of certain diseases

B. Word Parts

Directions: Indicate the meaning of each word part in the space provided. List as many medical terms as possible that incorporate the word part in the space provided.

Word Part	Meaning of Word Part	Medical Terms That Incorporate Word Part
1. bi/o		
2. -opsy		
3. colp/o		
4. -scope		
5. -scopy		
6. cry/o		
7. fibr/o		
8. hem/o		
9. stasis		

EVALUATION OF LEARNING

Directions: Fill in each blank with the correct answer.

1. List the characteristics of a minor surgical procedure.

2. List the responsibilities of the medical assistant during a minor surgical operation.

3. What is the purpose of serrations found on some instruments?

4. What is the difference in function between mosquito hemostatic forceps and standard hemostatic forceps?

5. List five guidelines that should be followed in caring for instruments.

6. What is the difference between a closed and an open wound?

7. Why does a puncture wound encourage the growth of tetanus bacteria?

8. What is the purpose of inflammation?

9. List the four local signs that occur during inflammation.

10. What occurs during the inflammatory phase of wound healing?

11. What occurs during the granulation phase of wound healing?

12. What occurs during the maturation phase of wound healing?

13. What is an exudate?

14. Describe the appearance of the following types of exudates:

    a. Serous

    b. Sanguineous

    c. Purulent

    d. Serosanguineous

    e. Purosanguineous

15. List two functions of a sterile dressing.

16. The names and sizes of sutures are listed. In each set, circle the suture that has the smaller diameter:
    a. 4-0 silk
       2-0 silk
    b. 0 chromic surgical gut
       3-0 chromic surgical gut
    c. 2-0 polypropylene
       2 polypropylene

17. List five examples of materials used for nonabsorbable sutures.

18. What is a swaged needle? List advantages of using a swaged needle.

19. Why are sutures inserted in the head and neck generally removed sooner than other sutures?

20. List two advantages of using surgical skin staples to approximate a wound.

21. List three advantages of adhesive skin closures.

22. What is the purpose of preparing the patient's skin before minor office surgery?

23. What is the purpose of a fenestrated drape?

24. What are the characteristics of a local anesthetic?

25. What is the purpose of adding epinephrine to a local anesthetic?

26. What is the name of the local anesthetic most frequently used in the medical office during minor office surgery.

27. Explain how an instrument should be handed to the physician during minor office surgery.

28. What is a sebaceous cyst, and what causes it to form?

29. What is the purpose of using gauze packing or a rubber Penrose drain after incising a localized infection?

30. What is the difference between congenital nevi and acquired nevi?

31. What are the characteristics of benign moles?

32. What are skin tags? Where are they most frequently found on the body?

33. Describe the appearance of dysplastic nevi. What concern exists with dysplastic nevi?

34. List the characteristics of melanoma.

35. What are the postoperative instructions for toenail removal?

36. What are the most common methods used to remove moles?

37. What is the purpose of a biopsy?

38. What is an ingrown toenail?

39. List three causes of an ingrown toenail.

40. List two reasons for performing a colposcopy.

41. What is the purpose of performing a cervical punch biopsy?

42. List the postoperative instructions that must be relayed to the patient after a cervical punch biopsy.

43. List two uses of cryosurgery.

44. List the postoperative instructions that must be relayed to the patient after cervical cryosurgery.

45. List three functions of a bandage.

46. List four guidelines to follow when applying a bandage.

47. List four signs that may indicate a bandage is too tight.

48. Why should the medical assistant be careful when applying an elastic bandage?

49. What is the purpose of reversing the spiral during a spiral-reverse turn?

50. List two uses of the figure-eight bandage turn.

51. What type of bandage turn is used to anchor a bandage?

CRITICAL THINKING ACTIVITIES

A. Medical and Surgical Asepsis

Refer to Chapter 17, and describe the difference between medical asepsis and surgical asepsis.

Which technique (medical asepsis or surgical asepsis) would be employed during the following procedures? For procedures requiring surgical asepsis, indicate which of the following reasons necessitate the use of surgical asepsis: caring for broken skin, penetrating a skin surface, or entering a body cavity that is normally sterile.

1. Administering oral medication

____

____

2. Inserting sutures

____

____

3. Measuring oral temperature

____

____

4. Applying a bandage to the forearm

____

____

5. Performing a needle biopsy

____

____

6. Removing a sebaceous cyst

____

____

7. Obtaining a Pap specimen

____

____

8. Inserting a urinary catheter

____

____

9. Incision and drainage of an abscess

____

____

10. Applying a dressing to an open wound

____

____

B. Violation of Surgical Asepsis

In the situations that follow, the principles of surgical asepsis have been violated. In the space provided, explain why the techniques should not be performed in this manner.

1. Placing a sterile 4 × 4 gauze pad within the 1-inch border around the sterile field

2. Wearing rings during the application of sterile gloves

3. Talking over a sterile field

4. Reaching over a sterile field

5. Holding sterile gauze below waist level

6. Not palming the label when pouring an antiseptic solution

7. Spilling an antiseptic solution on the sterile field

8. Passing a soiled dressing over the sterile field

9. Placing a vial of Xylocaine on the sterile field

10. Using bare hands to arrange articles on the sterile field

C. Surgical Instruments

In the space provided, state the name and use of each of the following types of surgical instruments. Identify any of the following parts present on each instrument by labeling the instrument: box lock, spring handle, ratchets, serrations, cutting edge, and teeth.

(Courtesy of Elmed Incorporated, Addison, IL.)

1. Name: ____________________
   Use ____________________
   ____

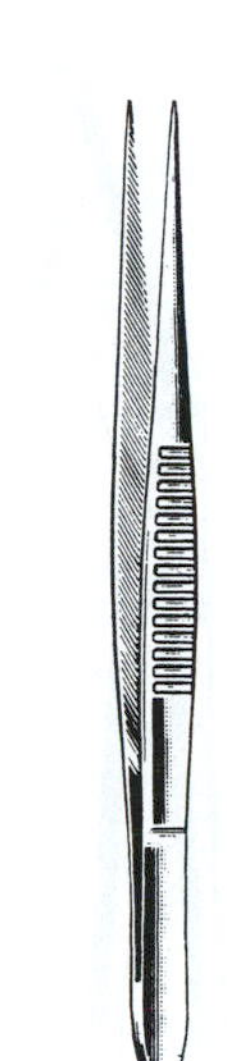

2. Name: ____________________
   Use ____________________
   ____

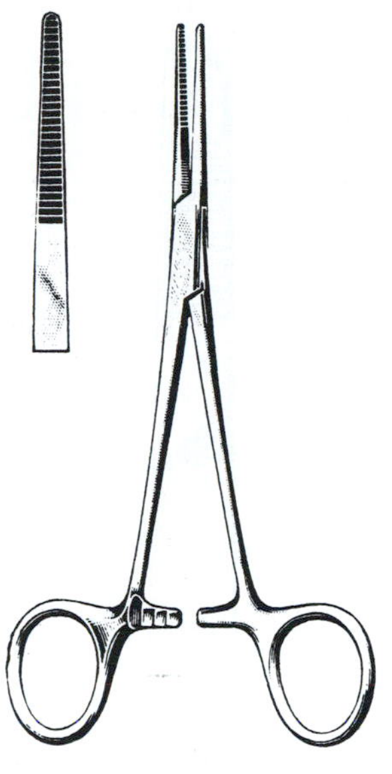

3. Name: ____________________
   Use ____________________
   ____

(Courtesy of Elmed Incorporated, Addison, IL.)

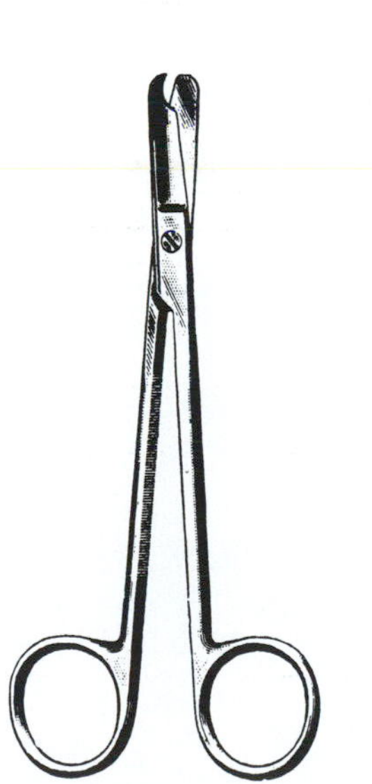

4. Name: ____________________
   Use ____________________
   ____

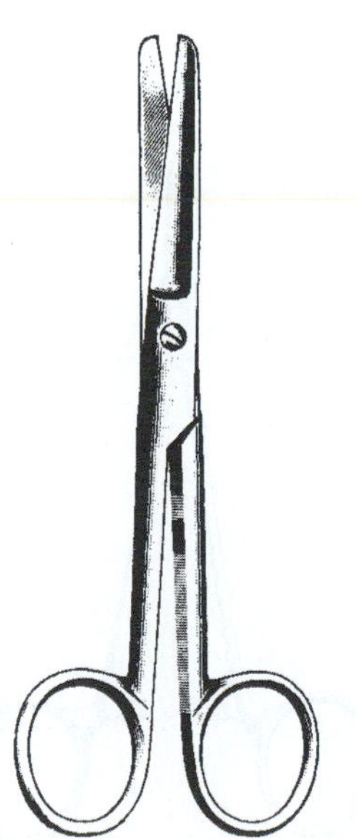

5. Name: ____________________
   Use ____________________
   ____

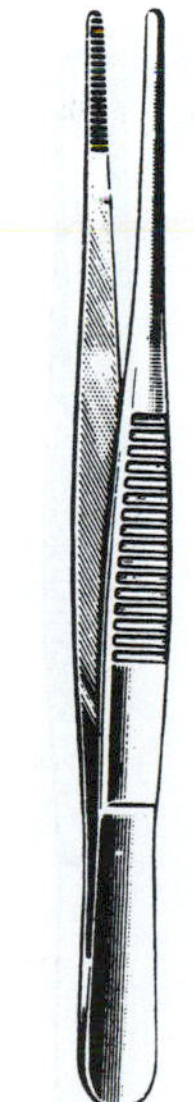

6. Name: ____________________
   Use ____________________
   ____

(Courtesy of Elmed Incorporated, Addison, IL.)

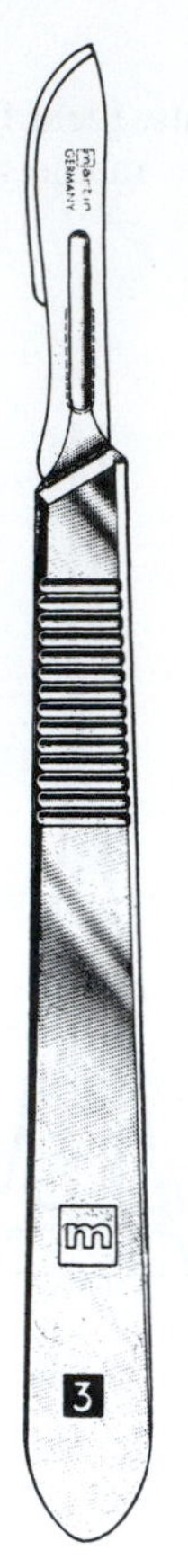

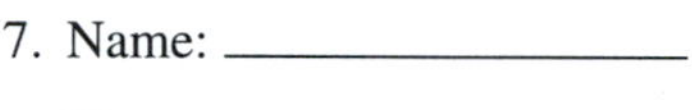

7. Name: ____________________

Use ____________________

____

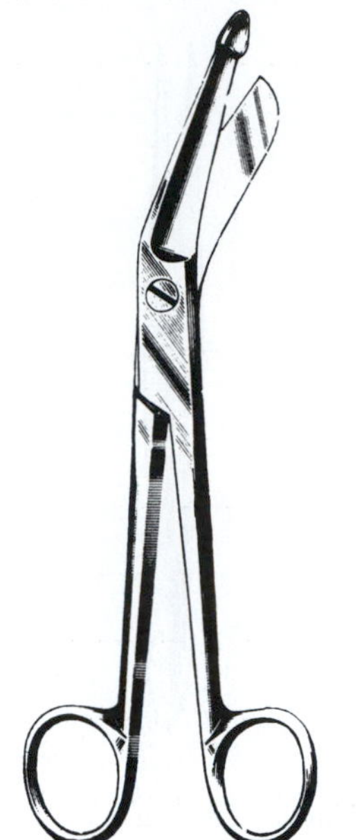

8. Name: ____________________

Use ____________________

____

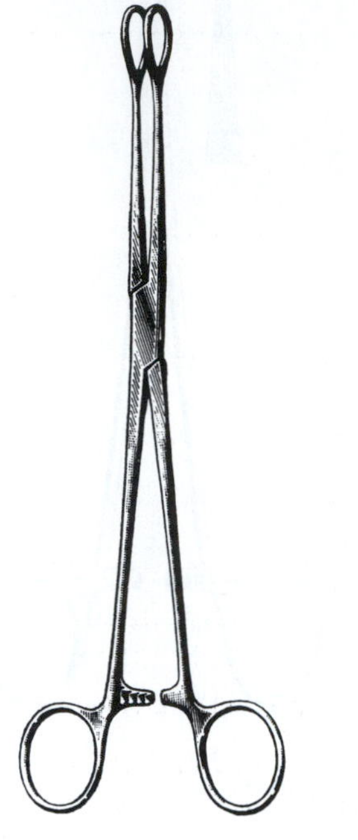

9. Name: ____________________

Use ____________________

____

(Courtesy of Elmed Incorporated, Addison, IL.)

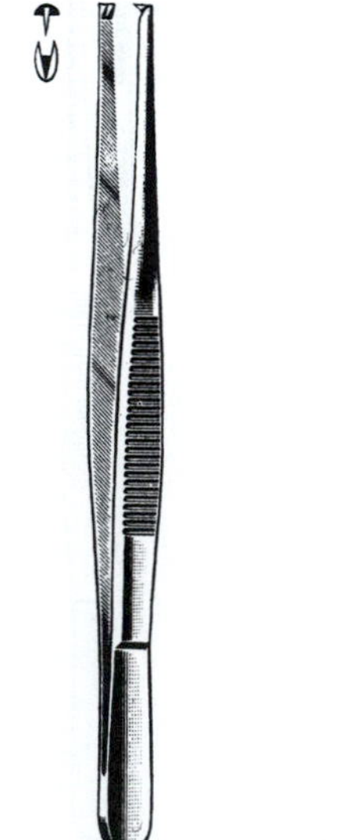

10. Name: ____________________

Use ____________________

____

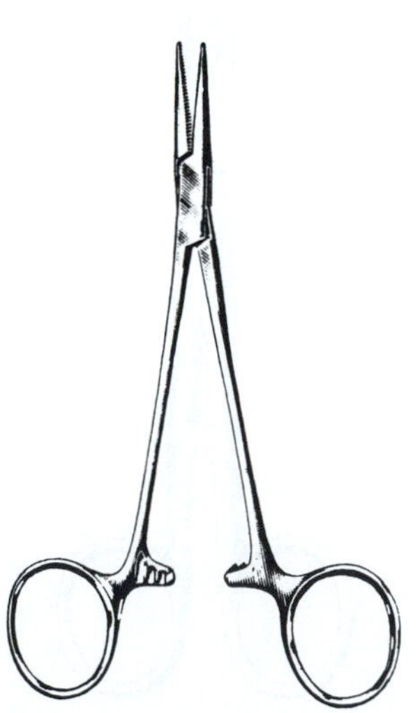

11. Name: ____________________

Use ____________________

____

D. Pioneers In Surgical Asepsis

Using a reference source, describe the contributions the following men made to medicine, especially regarding surgical asepsis:

1. Ignaz Semmelweis

____

____

____

2. Louis Pasteur

____

____

____

3. Joseph Lister

____

____

____

E. Patient Instruction Sheet

1. You are working for a surgeon who would like you to develop a patient instruction sheet for minor surgery. Select one of the minor operations provided. Using the following instruction sheet, develop a sheet that would be informative and visually appealing to a patient. Be as creative as possible in designing your sheet.
2. Select a partner. Have your partner play the role of a patient who is going to have the minor surgery performed, and explain the information on the sheet. Ask the patient to sign the sheet, and witness the patient's signature.

Minor Office Operations

a. Sebaceous cyst removal
b. Mole removal
c. Needle biopsy
d. Ingrown toenail removal
e. Colposcopy and biopsy
f. Cervical cryosurgery

PATIENT INSTRUCTION SHEET

NAME OF THE PROCEDURE:

DESCRIPTION OF PROCEDURE:

PURPOSE OF THE PROCEDURE:

HOW TO PREPARE FOR THE PROCEDURE:

WHAT TO DO FOLLOWING THE PROCEDURE:

I have received and understand the above instructions:

Patient's Signature ____

Witness: ____ Date: ____________

F. Crossword Puzzle: Minor Office Surgery

Directions: Complete the crossword puzzle using the clues presented below.

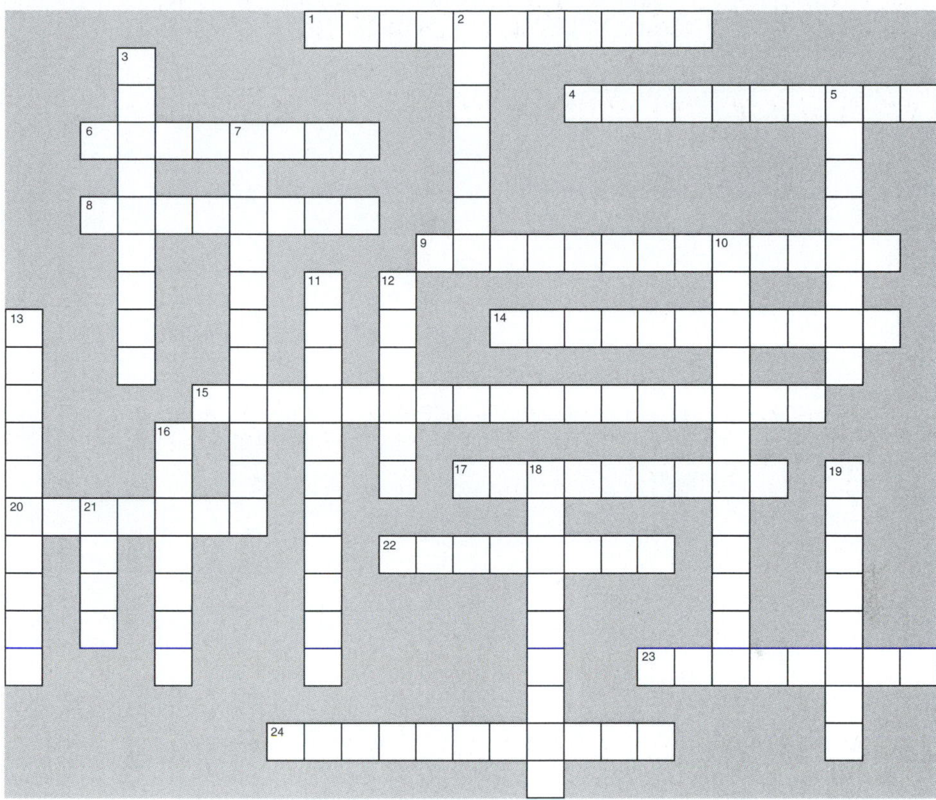

Across

1 Drape with a hole
4 Produces collagen
6 Clean, smooth cut
8 Boil
9 Sac containing oil secretions
14 Pus formation
15 Clamps off blood vessels
17 Local anesthetic brand name
20 Pus in a cavity
22 Tetanus may grow here
23 A local sign of inflammation
24 Bring together

Down

2 Free of all MOs and spores
3 Bruise
5 Scrape
7 Exudate containing blood
10 Suture/needle combination
11 Tx for chronic cervicitis
12 Father of modern surgery
13 Ragged and irregular wound
16 Discovered penicillin
18 Position for colposcopy
19 Antiseptic brand name
21 Nonabsorbable suture material

Notes

PRACTICE FOR COMPETENCY

Sterile Technique

Procedure 25-1: Applying and Removing Sterile Gloves. Apply and remove sterile gloves.

Procedure 25-2: Sterile Package. Open a sterile package. Add a sterile article to a sterile field using a commercially prepared peel-apart package. Practice each of the methods used to transfer articles to a sterile field as shown in Figure 25-4 of your textbook.

Procedure 25-3: Sterile Solution. Pour a sterile solution into a container on a sterile field.

Minor Surgical Procedures

Procedure 25-4: Sterile Dressing. Change a sterile dressing and record the procedure in the chart provided.

Procedure 25-5: Suture and Staple Removal. Practice the procedure for removing sutures and staples, and record the procedure in the chart provided.

Procedure 25-6: Adhesive Skin Closures. Practice the procedure for applying and removing adhesive skin closures, and record the procedure in the chart provided.

Procedure 25-7: Assisting with Minor Office Surgery. Obtain eight index cards. For each of the following minor office surgeries, indicate (on one side of the card) the equipment and supplies required for the side table. On the other side of the card, indicate the equipment and supplies required for the sterile tray setup. Set up a surgical tray for the procedures listed using your index cards. In the chart provided, record the instructions relayed to the patient following the surgery.

a. Suture insertion
b. Sebaceous cyst removal
c. Incision and drainage of a localized infection
d. Mole removal
e. Needle biopsy
f. Ingrown toenail removal
g. Colposcopy
h. Cervical punch biopsy
i. Cervical cryosurgery

Procedure 25-A: Bandage Turns. Practice the following bandage turns:

a. Circular turn
b. Spiral turn
c. Spiral-reverse turn
d. Figure-eight turn
e. Recurrent turn

CHART	
Date	

Chart	
Date	

EVALUATION OF COMPETENCY

Procedure 25-1: Applying and Removing Sterile Gloves

Name: ______________________________ Date: ______________________

Evaluated by: ______________________________ Score: ______________________

Performance Objective

Outcome:	Apply and remove sterile gloves.
Conditions:	Given the appropriate-sized sterile gloves.
	Using a clean flat surface.
Standards:	Time: 5 minutes. Student completed procedure in __________ minutes.
	Accuracy: Satisfactory score on the Performance Evaluation Checklist.

Performance Evaluation Checklist

Trial 1	Trial 2	Point Value	Performance Standards
			Application of gloves:
		•	Removed rings and washed hands with an antimicrobial soap.
		▷	Explained why the hands should be washed.
		•	Selected the appropriate-sized gloves.
		▷	Explained what may occur if the gloves are too small or too large.
		•	Placed the glove package on a clean flat surface.
		•	Opened the sterile glove package without touching the inside of the wrapper.
		•	Picked up the first glove on the inside of the cuff without contaminating.
		•	Did not touch the outside of the glove with the bare hand.
		•	Stepped back and pulled on glove and allowed the cuff to remain turned back on itself.
		•	Picked up the second glove by slipping sterile gloved fingers under its cuff and grasping the opposite side with the thumb.
		•	Pulled the glove on and turned back the cuff.
		•	Turned back the cuff of the first glove without contaminating it.
		•	Adjusted the gloves to a comfortable position.
		•	Inspected the gloves for tears.
		▷	Explained what should be done if a glove is torn.
			Removal of gloves:
		•	Grasped the outside of the right glove 1 to 2 inches from the top with the gloved left hand.
		•	Slowly pulled right glove off the hand.

Trial 1	Trial 2	Point Value	Performance Standards
		●	Pulled the right glove free and scrunched it into a ball with the gloved left hand.
		●	Placed index and middle fingers of the right hand on the inside of left glove.
		●	Did not allow the clean hand to touch the outside of the glove.
		●	Pulled the glove off the left hand, enclosing the balled-up right glove.
		●	Discarded both gloves in an appropriate waste container.
		▷	Stated how to discard gloves if they are visibly contaminated with blood.
		●	Sanitized hands.
		Ⓐ	Recognized the implications for failure to comply with Center for Disease (CDC) regulations in healthcare settings.
		✶	Completed the procedure within 5 minutes.
			TOTALS

Evaluation of Student Performance

EVALUATION CRITERIA			COMMENTS
Symbol	**Category**	**Point Value**	
✶	Critical Step	16 points	
●	Essential Step	6 points	
Ⓐ	Affective Competency	6 points	
▷	Theory Question	2 points	
Score calculation: 100 points – ____ points missed ____Score Satisfactory score: 85 or above			

2008 CAAHEP Competencies Achieved

Psychomotor (Skills)

☑ III. 3. Select appropriate barrier/personal protective equipment (PPE) for potentially infectious situations.

2015 CAAHEP Competencies Achieved

Psychomotor (Skills)

☑ III. 2. Select appropriate barrier/personal protective equipment (PPE).

Affective (Behavior)

☑ III. 1. Recognize the implications for failure to comply with Center for Disease (CDC) regulations in healthcare settings.

ABHES Competencies Achieved

☑ 4. f. Comply with federal, state and local health laws as they relate to healthcare settings.
☑ 9. a. Practice standard precautions and perform disinfection/sterilization techniques.

EVALUATION OF COMPETENCY

Procedure 25-2: Opening a Sterile Package

Name: ______________________ Date: ______________

Evaluated by: ______________________ Score: ______________

Performance Objective

Outcome:	Open a sterile package.
Conditions:	Given a sterile package.
	Using a clean flat surface.
Standards:	Time: 5 minutes. Student completed procedure in ________ minutes.
	Accuracy: Satisfactory score on the Performance Evaluation Checklist.

Performance Evaluation Checklist

Trial 1	Trial 2	Point Value	Performance Standards
		•	Sanitized hands.
		•	Assembled equipment.
		•	Checked pack to make sure it is not wet, torn, or opened.
		•	Checked the autoclave tape on the pack.
		▷	Stated the purpose of autoclave tape.
		•	Positioned the pack on the table so that the top flap of wrapper will open away from the body.
		•	Removed the fastener on wrapped package and discarded it.
		•	Opened the first flap away from the body.
		•	Opened the left and right flaps without contaminating contents.
		•	Opened the flap closest to the body.
		•	In all cases, touched only the outside of the wrapper.
		•	In all cases, did not reach over the sterile contents of the package.
		▷	Stated why the medical assistant should not reach over the contents of the package.
		•	Adjusted the sterile wrapper by the corners as needed.
		•	Checked the sterilization indicator on the inside of the pack.
		▷	Stated the reason for checking the sterilization indicator.
		*	Completed the procedure within 5 minutes.
			TOTALS

Evaluation of Student Performance

EVALUATION CRITERIA			COMMENTS
Symbol	Category	Point Value	
∗	Critical Step	16 points	
●	Essential Step	6 points	
Ⓐ	Affective Competency	6 points	
▷	Theory Question	2 points	
Score calculation: 100 points – ___ points missed ___Score Satisfactory score: 85 or above			

2008 CAAHEP Competencies Achieved
Psychomotor (Skills) ☑ I. 10. Assist physician with patient care.

2015 CAAHEP Competencies Achieved
Psychomotor (Skills) ☑ III. 6. Prepare a sterile field. ☑ III. 7. Perform within a sterile field.

ABHES Competencies Achieved
☑ 9. e. Perform specialty procedures including but not limited to minor surgery, cardiac, respiratory, OB-GYN, neurological, gastroenterology.

EVALUATION OF COMPETENCY

Using Commercially Prepared Sterile Packages

Name: ______________________________ Date: ______________

Evaluated by: ______________________________ Score: ______________

Performance Objective

Outcome:	Add a sterile article to a sterile field from a peel-apart package by ejecting its contents onto the field.
Conditions:	Given the following: peel-apart package and a sterile field.
Standards:	Time: 3 minutes. Student completed procedure in __________ minutes.
	Accuracy: Satisfactory score on the Performance Evaluation Checklist.

Performance Evaluation Checklist

Trial 1	Trial 2	Point Value	Performance Standards
		•	Sanitized hands.
		•	Grasped the two unsterile flaps of the peel-pack between thumbs.
		•	Pulled the package apart using a rolling-outward motion.
		▷	Stated what parts of the peel-pack must remain sterile.
		•	Stepped back slightly from the sterile field.
		▷	Explained the reason for stepping back.
		•	Gently ejected contents of the peel-pack onto the center of the sterile field.
		*	Completed the procedure within 3 minutes.
			TOTALS

Evaluation of Student Performance

EVALUATION CRITERIA			COMMENTS
Symbol	**Category**	**Point Value**	
∗	Critical Step	16 points	
●	Essential Step	6 points	
Ⓐ	Affective Competency	6 points	
▷	Theory Question	2 points	
Score calculation: 100 points – ___ points missed ___ Score Satisfactory score: 85 or above			

2008 CAAHEP Competencies Achieved
Psychomotor (Skills) ☑ I. 10. Assist physician with patient care.

2015 CAAHEP Competencies Achieved
Psychomotor (Skills) ☑ III. 7. Perform within a sterile field.

ABHES Competencies Achieved
☑ 9. e. Perform specialty procedures including but not limited to minor surgery, cardiac, respiratory, OB-GYN, neurological, gastroenterology.

EVALUATION OF COMPETENCY

Procedure 25-3: Pouring a Sterile Solution

Name: ______________________________ Date: ________________

Evaluated by: ______________________________ Score: ________________

Performance Objective

Outcome:	Pour a sterile solution.
Conditions:	Given the following: sterile solution, sterile container, and a sterile towel.
Standards:	Time: 5 minutes. Student completed procedure in __________ minutes.
	Accuracy: Satisfactory score on the Performance Evaluation Checklist.

Performance Evaluation Checklist

Trial 1	Trial 2	Point Value	Performance Standards
		●	Checked the label of the solution.
		●	Checked expiration date on the solution.
		▷	Explained why an outdated solution should not be used.
		●	Checked solution label a second time.
		●	Palmed the label of the bottle.
		▷	Explained why the label should be palmed.
		●	Removed cap and placed it on a flat surface with the open end up.
		▷	Stated why cap should be placed with the open end up.
		●	Rinsed the lip of the bottle.
		▷	Explained why the lip of the bottle should be rinsed.
		●	Poured the proper amount of solution into a sterile container at a height of 6 inches.
		●	Did not allow the neck of the bottle to come in contact with container.
		●	Did not allow any of the solution to splash onto the sterile field.
		▷	Explained why the sterile solution should not be allowed to splash onto the sterile field.
		●	Replaced cap on container without contaminating.
		●	Checked the label a third time.
		*	Completed the procedure within 5 minutes.
			TOTALS

Evaluation of Student Performance

EVALUATION CRITERIA			COMMENTS
Symbol	**Category**	**Point Value**	
✶	Critical Step	16 points	
●	Essential Step	6 points	
Ⓐ	Affective Competency	6 points	
▷	Theory Question	2 points	
Score calculation: 100 points – ____ points missed ____ Score Satisfactory score: 85 or above			

2008 CAAHEP Competencies Achieved
Psychomotor (Skills) ☑ I. 10. Assist physician with patient care.

2015 CAAHEP Competencies Achieved
Psychomotor (Skills) ☑ III. 7. Perform within a sterile field.

ABHES Competencies Achieved
☑ 9. e. Perform specialty procedures including but not limited to minor surgery, cardiac, respiratory, OB-GYN, neurological, gastroenterology.

EVALUATION OF COMPETENCY

Procedure 25-4: Changing a Sterile Dressing

Name: ______________________ Date: ______________

Evaluated by: ______________________ Score: ______________

Performance Objective

Outcome:	Change a sterile dressing.
Conditions:	Given the following: Mayo stand, biohazard waste container, clean and disposable gloves, antiseptic swabs, sterile gloves, plastic waste bag, adhesive tape and scissors, sterile dressing, and thumb forceps.
Standards:	Time: 10 minutes. Student completed procedure in __________ minutes.
	Accuracy: Satisfactory score on the Performance Evaluation Checklist.

Performance Evaluation Checklist

Trial 1	Trial 2	Point Value	Performance Standards
		•	Washed hands with an antimicrobial soap.
		•	Assembled equipment.
		•	Set up nonsterile items on a side table or counter.
		•	Positioned the plastic waste bag in a convenient location.
		•	Greeted the patient and introduced yourself.
		•	Identified patient and explained the procedure.
		•	Instructed patient not to move during procedure.
		•	Adjusted the light.
		•	Applied clean gloves.
		•	Loosened the tape and carefully removed soiled dressing by pulling it upward.
		•	Did not touch inside of dressing next to the wound.
		▷	Explained why the inside of the dressing should not be touched.
		▷	Described what should be done if the dressing is stuck to the wound.
		•	Placed soiled dressing in the waste bag without touching outside of bag.
		•	Inspected the wound.
		▷	Stated what type of inspection should be performed.
		•	Opened the antiseptic swabs and placed the pouch in a convenient location or held the pouch in your hand.
		•	Applied the antiseptic to the wound.

Trial 1	Trial 2	Point Value	Performance Standards
		●	Used a new swab for each motion.
		●	Discarded each contaminated swab in the waste bag after use.
		●	Removed gloves and discarded them without contaminating.
		●	Sanitized hands and prepared the sterile field.
		●	Instructed patient not to talk, laugh, sneeze, or cough over the sterile field.
		●	Opened sterile glove package and applied sterile gloves.
		●	Picked up sterile dressing from the tray using sterile gloves or sterile forceps.
		●	Placed sterile dressing over the wound by lightly dropping it in place.
		●	Did not move dressing after dropping it in place.
		▷	Explained why the dressing should be dropped onto the wound and then not moved.
		●	Discarded gloves (and forceps) in the waste bag.
		●	Applied hypoallergenic tape to hold sterile dressing in place.
		●	Provided the patient with written wound care instructions.
		●	Instructed patient in wound care.
		▷	Described the wound care that should be relayed to the patient.
		●	Asked patient to sign instruction sheet.
		●	Witnessed the patient's signature.
		●	Gave a signed copy to the patient.
		●	Filed original in the patient's medical record.
		▷	Stated the purpose of filing original in patient's chart.
		●	Returned equipment.
		●	Disposed of plastic bag in a biohazard waste container.
		●	Sanitized hands.
		●	Charted the procedure correctly.
		Ⓐ	Incorporated critical thinking skills when performing patient care.
		Ⓐ	Showed awareness of a patient's concerns related to the procedure being performed.
		Ⓐ	Explained to a patient the rationale for performance of a procedure.
		*	Completed the procedure within 10 minutes.
			TOTALS

Chart	
Date	

Evaluation of Student Performance

EVALUATION CRITERIA			COMMENTS
Symbol	Category	Point Value	
*	Critical Step	16 points	
●	Essential Step	6 points	
Ⓐ	Affective Competency	6 points	
▷	Theory Question	2 points	
Score calculation: 100 points – ___ points missed ___ Score Satisfactory score: 85 or above			

2008 CAAHEP Competencies Achieved
Psychomotor (Skills) ☑ IV. 5. Instruct patients according to their needs to promote health maintenance and disease prevention. ☑ IV. 6. Prepare a patient for procedures and/or treatments. ☑ IV. 8. Document patient care. ☑ IV. 9. Document patient education. ***Affective (Behavior)*** ☑ III. 2. Explain the rationale for performance of a procedure to the patient. ☑ III. 3. Show awareness of patients' concerns regarding their perceptions related to the procedure being performed.

2015 CAAHEP Competencies Achieved
Psychomotor (Skills) ☑ I. 8. Instruct and prepare a patient for a procedure or a treatment. ☑ III. 6. Prepare a sterile field. ☑ III. 7. Perform within a sterile field. ☑ III. 8. Perform wound care. ☑ III. 9. Perform dressing change. ☑ III. 10. Demonstrate proper disposal of biohazardous material: regulated wastes: a. sharps b. regulates wastes. ☑ V. 4. Coach patient regarding: office policies b. health maintenance c. disease prevention d. treatment plan. ☑ X. 3. Document patient care accurately in the medical record. ***Affective (Behavior)*** ☑ I. 2. Incorporate critical thinking skills when performing patient care. ☑ I. 3. Show awareness of a patient's concerns related to the procedure being performed. ☑ V. 4. Explain to a patient the rationale for performance of a procedure.

ABHES Competencies Achieved
☑ 4. a. Follow documentation guidelines. ☑ 8. f. Display professionalism through written and verbal communications. ☑ 9. e. Perform specialty procedures including but not limited to minor surgery, cardiac, respiratory, OB-GYN, neurological, gastroenterology. ☑ 9. h. Teach self-examination, disease management and health promotion. ☑ 10. c. Dispose of biohazardous materials.

EVALUATION OF COMPETENCY

Procedure 25-5: Removing Sutures and Staples

Name: ______________________ Date: ______________

Evaluated by: ______________________ Score: ______________

Performance Objective

Outcome:	Remove sutures and staples.
Conditions:	Given the following: Mayo stand, antiseptic swabs, clean and disposable gloves, sterile 4 × 4 gauze, surgical tape, biohazard waste container, suture removal kit, and staple removal kit.
Standards:	Time: 10 minutes. Student completed procedure in __________ minutes.
	Accuracy: Satisfactory score on the Performance Evaluation Checklist.

Performance Evaluation Checklist

Trial 1	Trial 2	Point Value	Performance Standards
		•	Washed hands with an antimicrobial soap.
		•	Assembled equipment.
		•	Greeted the patient and introduced yourself.
		•	Identified patient and explained the procedure.
		•	Positioned the patient as required.
		•	Adjusted the light.
		•	Checked to make sure the sutures (or staples) were intact.
		•	Checked to make sure the incision line was approximated and free from infection.
		▷	Explained what to do if the incision line is not approximated.
		•	Opened the suture or staple removal kit.
		•	Applied clean gloves.
		•	Cleaned the incision line with antiseptic swabs using a new swab for each motion.
		•	Allowed the skin to dry.
		•	Informed the patient that he or she would feel a pulling sensation as each suture (or staple) is removed.
			Removed sutures as follows:
		•	Picked up the knot of suture with thumb forceps.
		•	Placed curved tip of suture scissors under the suture.
		•	Cut suture below the knot on the side of suture closest to the skin.

Trial 1	Trial 2	Point Value	Performance Standards
		●	Gently pulled suture out of the skin, using a smooth, continuous motion.
		●	Did not allow any portion of suture previously on the outside to be pulled through the tissue lying beneath the incision line.
		●	Placed the suture on the gauze.
		●	Repeated above sequence until all sutures were removed.
			Removed staples as follows:
		●	Gently placed the jaws of the staple remover under the staple.
		●	Squeezed the staple handles until they were fully closed.
		●	Lifted the staple remover upward to remove the staple.
		●	Placed staple on gauze.
		●	Continued until all the staples were removed.
		●	Counted number of sutures or staples and checked number with chart.
		●	Cleansed the site with an antiseptic swab.
		●	Applied adhesive skin closures if directed by physician.
		●	Applied DSD, directed to do so by physician.
		●	Disposed of sutures or staples and gauze in biohazard waste container.
		●	Removed gloves and sanitized hands.
		●	Charted the procedure correctly.
		Ⓐ	Incorporated critical thinking skills when performing patient care.
		Ⓐ	Showed awareness of a patient's concerns related to the procedure being performed.
		Ⓐ	Demonstrated: a. empathy b. active listening c. nonverbal communication.
		*	Completed the procedure within 10 minutes.
			TOTALS

Chart	
Date	

Evaluation of Student Performance

EVALUATION CRITERIA			COMMENTS
Symbol	**Category**	**Point Value**	
∗	Critical Step	16 points	
●	Essential Step	6 points	
Ⓐ	Affective Competency	6 points	
▷	Theory Question	2 points	
Score calculation: 100 points − ___ points missed ___ Score Satisfactory score: 85 or above			

2008 CAAHEP Competencies Achieved

Psychomotor (Skills)

☑ IV. 5. Instruct patients according to their needs to promote health maintenance and disease prevention.
☑ IV. 6. Prepare a patient for procedures and/or treatments.
☑ IV. 8. Document patient care.

Affective (Behavior)

☑ III. 3. Show awareness of patients' concerns regarding their perceptions related to the procedure being performed.
☑ IV. 1. Demonstrate empathy in communicating with patients, family, and staff.

2015 CAAHEP Competencies Achieved

Psychomotor (Skills)

☑ I. 8. Instruct and prepare a patient for a procedure or a treatment.
☑ III. 8. Perform wound care.
☑ III. 10. Demonstrate proper disposal of biohazardous material: regulated wastes: a. sharps b. regulates wastes.
☑ V. 4. Coach patient regarding: office policies b. health maintenance c. disease prevention d. treatment plan.
☑ X. 3. Document patient care accurately in the medical record.

Affective (Behavior)

☑ I. 2. Incorporate critical thinking skills when performing patient care.
☑ I. 3. Show awareness of a patient's concerns related to the procedure being performed.
☑ V. 1. Demonstrate: a. empathy b. active listening c. nonverbal communication.

ABHES Competencies Achieved

☑ 4. a. Follow documentation guidelines.
☑ 8. f. Display professionalism through written and verbal communications.
☑ 9. e. Perform specialty procedures including but not limited to minor surgery, cardiac, respiratory, OB-GYN, neurological, gastroenterology.
☑ 9. h. Teach self-examination, disease management and health promotion.
☑ 10. c. Dispose of biohazardous materials.

Notes

EVALUATION OF COMPETENCY

Procedure 25-6: Applying and Removing Adhesive Skin Closures

Name: ______________________ Date: ______________

Evaluated by: ______________________ Score: ______________

Performance Objective

Outcome:	Apply and remove adhesive skin closures.
Conditions:	Given the following: clean and disposable gloves, sterile gloves, antiseptic solution, surgical scrub brush, antiseptic swabs, tincture of benzoin, sterile cotton-tipped applicator, adhesive skin closure strips, sterile 4 × 4 gauze pads, surgical tape, and a biohazard waste container.
Standards:	Time: 10 minutes. Student completed procedure in __________ minutes.
	Accuracy: Satisfactory score on the Performance Evaluation Checklist.

Performance Evaluation Checklist

Trial 1	Trial 2	Point Value	Performance Standards
			Application of adhesive skin closures:
		•	Washed hands with an antimicrobial soap.
		•	Assembled equipment.
		•	Checked expiration date on the adhesive skin closures.
		•	Greeted patient and introduced yourself.
		•	Identified patient and explained the procedure.
		•	Positioned the patient as required.
		•	Adjusted the light.
		•	Applied clean gloves.
		•	Inspected the wound for redness, swelling, and drainage.
		•	Scrubbed the wound with an antiseptic solution.
		•	Allowed the skin to dry or patted dry with gauze pads.
		•	Applied antiseptic using a new swab for each motion.
		•	Allowed the skin to dry.
		▷	Explained why the skin must be completely dry.
		•	Applied tincture of benzoin without letting it touch the wound.
		▷	Stated the purpose of tincture of benzoin.
		•	Allowed the skin to dry.

Trial 1	Trial 2	Point Value	Performance Standards
		●	Removed gloves and washed hands.
		●	Opened the package of adhesive strips and laid them on a flat surface.
		●	Applied sterile gloves and tore the tab off the card of strips.
		●	Peeled a strip of tape off the card.
		●	Checked to make sure the skin surface was dry.
		●	Positioned the first strip over the center of the wound.
		●	Secured one end of the strip to the skin by pressing down firmly on the tape.
		●	Stretched the strip across the incision until the edges of the wound were approximated.
		●	Secured the strip to the skin on the other side of the wound.
		●	Applied the second strip on one side of center strip at an 18-inch interval.
		●	Applied a third strip at a 18-inch interval on the other side of the center strip.
		●	Continued applying the strips at 18-inch intervals until the edges of the wound were approximated.
		▷	Explained why the strips should be spaced at 18-inch intervals.
		●	Applied two closures approximately ½ -inch from the ends of the strips.
		▷	Stated the purpose of applying a strip along each edge.
		●	Applied a sterile dressing over the strips if indicated by the physician.
		●	Removed gloves and sanitized hands.
		●	Provided patient with written wound care instructions.
		●	Explained the wound care instructions to the patient.
		●	Asked patient to sign instruction sheet and witnessed patient's signature.
		●	Gave a signed copy to the patient and filed original in the patient's medical record.
		●	Charted the procedure correctly.
			Removal of adhesive skin closures:
		●	Sanitized hands.
		●	Greeted patient and introduced yourself.
		●	Identified patient and explained the procedure.
		●	Positioned the patient as required.
		●	Adjusted the light.
		●	Checked to make sure the incision line was approximated and free from infection.
		●	Positioned a 4 × 4 gauze pad in a convenient location.

Trial 1	Trial 2	Point Value	Performance Standards
		●	Applied clean gloves.
		●	Peeled off each half of the strip from the outside toward the wound margin.
		●	Stabilized the skin with one finger.
		●	Gently lifted the strip up and away from the wound and placed it on the gauze.
		●	Continued until all closures were removed.
		●	Cleansed the site with an antiseptic swab.
		●	Applied a sterile dressing if indicated by the physician.
		●	Disposed of strips and gauze in a biohazard waste container.
		●	Removed gloves and sanitized hands.
		●	Charted the procedure correctly.
		Ⓐ	Incorporated critical thinking skills when performing patient care.
		Ⓐ	Showed awareness of a patient's concerns related to the procedure being performed.
		Ⓐ	Explained to a patient the rationale for performance of a procedure.
		✶	Completed the procedure within 10 minutes.
			TOTALS

CHART	
Date	

Evaluation of Student Performance

EVALUATION CRITERIA			COMMENTS
Symbol	**Category**	**Point Value**	
✶	Critical Step	16 points	
●	Essential Step	6 points	
Ⓐ	Affective Competency	6 points	
▷	Theory Question	2 points	
Score calculation: 100 points – ___ points missed ___ Score Satisfactory score: 85 or above			

2008 CAAHEP Competencies Achieved
Psychomotor (Skills) ☑ IV. 5. Instruct patients according to their needs to promote health maintenance and disease prevention. ☑ IV. 6. Prepare a patient for procedures and/or treatments. ☑ IV. 8. Document patient care ***Affective (Behavior)*** ☑ III. 2. Explain the rationale for performance of a procedure to the patient. ☑ III. 3. Show awareness of patients' concerns regarding their perceptions about the procedure being performed.

2015 CAAHEP Competencies Achieved
Psychomotor (Skills) ☑ I. 8. Instruct and prepare a patient for a procedure or a treatment. ☑ III. 8. Perform wound care. ☑ V. 4. Coach patient regarding: office policies b. health maintenance c. disease prevention d. treatment plan. ☑ X. 3. Document patient care accurately in the medical record. ***Affective (Behavior)*** ☑ I. 2. Incorporate critical thinking skills when performing patient care. ☑ I. 3. Show awareness of a patient's concerns related to the procedure being performed. ☑ V. 4. Explained to a patient the rationale for performance of a procedure.

ABHES Competencies Achieved
☑ 4. a. Follow documentation guidelines. ☑ 8. f. Display professionalism through written and verbal communications. ☑ 9. e. Perform specialty procedures including but not limited to minor surgery, cardiac, respiratory, OB-GYN, neurological, gastroenterology. ☑ 9. h. Teach self-examination, disease management and health promotion. ☑ 10. c. Dispose of biohazardous materials.

EVALUATION OF COMPETENCY

Procedure 25-7: Assisting with Minor Office Surgery

Name: ______________________ Date: ______________

Evaluated by: ______________________ Score: ______________

Performance Objective

Outcome:	Set up the surgical tray and assist with minor office surgery.
Conditions:	Given a Mayo stand, biohazard waste container, and the instruments and supplies required for a specific minor office surgery as designed by the instructor.
Standards:	Time: 15 minutes. Student completed procedure in ________ minutes.
	Accuracy: Satisfactory score on the Performance Evaluation Checklist.

Performance Evaluation Checklist

Trial 1	Trial 2	Point Value	Performance Standards
		•	Determined the type of minor office surgery to be performed.
		•	Prepared examining room.
		•	Sanitized hands.
		•	Set up articles required that are not sterile on a side table or counter.
		•	Labeled the specimen container (if included in the setup).
		•	Washed hands with an antimicrobial soap.
		•	Set up the minor office surgery tray on a clean, dry, flat surface, using the principles of surgical asepsis.
			Prepackaged sterile setup
		•	Selected the appropriate package from supply shelf and placed it on a flat surface.
		•	Opened the setup using the inside of wrapper as the sterile field.
		•	Checked the sterilization indicator on inside of pack.
		•	Added any additional articles required for the surgery and covered tray setup with a sterile towel.
			Transferring articles to a sterile field:
		•	Placed sterile towel on a flat surface by two corner ends, making sure not to contaminate it.
		•	Transferred sterile articles to the field from wrapped or peel-apart packages.
		•	Applied sterile glove.
		•	Arranged articles neatly on the sterile field with sterile glove.

Trial 1	Trial 2	Point Value	Performance Standards
		●	Checked to make sure all articles were available on the sterile field.
		●	Covered the tray setup with a sterile towel without allowing arms to pass over the sterile field.
			Prepared the patient:
		●	Greeted the patient and introduced yourself.
		●	Identified patient, explained the procedure, and reassured the patient.
		●	Asked patient if he or she needs to void before the surgery.
		●	Instructed patient on clothing removal.
		●	Instructed patient not to move during procedure or to talk, laugh, sneeze, or cough over the sterile field.
		●	Positioned patient as required for the type of surgery to be performed.
		●	Adjusted the light so that it was focused on the operative site.
			Prepared the patient's skin:
		●	Applied clean disposable gloves.
		●	Shaved skin (if required).
		●	Cleansed skin with an antiseptic solution.
		●	Rinsed and dried the area.
		●	Applied antiseptic using antiseptic swabs.
		●	Allowed the skin to dry.
		●	Removed gloves and sanitized hands.
		●	Checked to make sure that everything was ready and informed physician.
			Assisted the physician:
		●	Uncovered the tray setup.
		●	Opened the outer glove wrapper for physician.
		●	Held the vial while physician withdrew the local anesthetic.
		●	Adjusted the light as required.
		●	Restrained patient (e.g., child).
		●	Relaxed and reassured patient.
		●	Handed instruments and supplies to physician. Sterile gloves required.
		●	Kept the sterile field neat and orderly. Sterile gloves required.
		●	Held basin for physician to deposit soiled instruments and supplies. Clean gloves required.
		●	Retracted tissue. Sterile gloves required.

Trial 1	Trial 2	Point Value	Performance Standards
		●	Sponged blood from operative site. Sterile gloves required.
		●	Added instruments and supplies as necessary to the sterile field.
		●	Held specimen container to accept specimen. Clean gloves required.
		●	Cut ends of suture material after insertion by physician. Sterile gloves required.
			After surgery:
		●	Applied sterile dressing to the surgical wound if ordered by physician.
		●	Stayed with patient as a safety precaution.
		●	Assisted and instructed patient as required.
		●	Verified that patient understood postoperative instructions.
		●	Provided patient with verbal and written wound care instructions.
		▷	Stated the patient instructions that should be relayed for wound and suture care.
		●	Asked patient to sign instruction sheet and witnessed the patient's signature.
		●	Gave a signed copy to the patient and filed original in patient's medical record.
		●	Relayed information regarding the return visit
		●	Assisted patient off table.
		●	Instructed patient to get dressed.
		●	Prepared any specimens collected for transfer to the laboratory with a completed biopsy request.
		●	Charted correctly.
		●	Cleaned examining room.
		●	Discarded disposable contaminated articles in a biohazard waste container.
		●	Sanitized and sterilized instruments.
		Ⓐ	Showed awareness of a patient's concerns related to the procedure being performed.
		Ⓐ	Demonstrated: a. empathy b. active listening c. nonverbal communication.
		Ⓐ	Explained to a patient the rationale for performance of a procedure.
		*	Completed the procedure within 15 minutes.
			TOTALS

Chart	
Date	

Evaluation of Student Performance

EVALUATION CRITERIA			COMMENTS
Symbol	**Category**	**Point Value**	
∗	Critical Step	16 points	
●	Essential Step	6 points	
Ⓐ	Affective Competency	6 points	
▷	Theory Question	2 points	
Score calculation: 100 points – ___ points missed ___ Score Satisfactory score: 85 or above			

2008 CAAHEP Competencies Achieved

Psychomotor (Skills)

☑ I. 10. Assist physician with patient care.
☑ IV. 5. Instruct patients according to their needs to promote health maintenance and disease prevention.
☑ IV. 6. Prepare a patient for procedures and/or treatments.
☑ IV. 8. Document patient care.
☑ IX. 1. Respond to issues of confidentiality.

Affective (Behavior)

☑ III. 2. Explain the rationale for performance of a procedure to the patient.
☑ III. 3. Show awareness of patients' concerns regarding their perceptions related to the procedure being performed.
☑ IV. 6. Demonstrate awareness of how an individual's personal appearance affects anticipated responses.
☑ IX. 3. Recognize the importance of local, state, and federal legislation and regulations in the practice setting.

2015 CAAHEP Competencies Achieved

Psychomotor (Skills)

☑ I. 8. Instruct and prepare a patient for a procedure or a treatment.
☑ III. 6. Prepare a sterile field.
☑ III. 7. Perform within a sterile field.
☑ III. 10. Demonstrate proper disposal of biohazardous material: regulated wastes: a. sharps b. regulates wastes.
☑ V. 4. Coach patient regarding: office policies b. health maintenance c. disease prevention d. treatment plan.
☑ X. 3. Document patient care accurately in the medical record.
☑ X. 4. Apply the Patient's Bill of Rights as it relates to: a. choice of treatment b. consent for treatment c. refusal of treatment.

Affective (Behavior)

☑ I. 3. Show awareness of a patient's concerns related to the procedure being performed.
☑ V. 1. Demonstrate: a. empathy b. active listening c. nonverbal communication.
☑ V. 4. Explain to a patient the rationale for performance of a procedure.

ABHES Competencies Achieved

☑ 4. a. Follow documentation guidelines.
☑ 8. f. Display professionalism through written and verbal communications.
☑ 9. d. Assist provider with specialty examination including cardiac, respiratory, OB-GYN, neurological, gastroenterology procedures.
☑ 9. e. Perform specialty procedures including but not limited to minor surgery, cardiac, respiratory, OB-GYN, neurological, gastroenterology.
☑ 9. g. Recognize and respond to medical office emergencies.
☑ 9. h. Teach self-examination, disease management and health promotion.
☑ 9. j. Make adaptations with patients with special needs.
☑ 10. c. Dispose of biohazardous materials.

EVALUATION OF COMPETENCY

Procedure 25-A: Bandage Turns

Name: ______________________ Date: ______________

Evaluated by: ______________________ Score: ______________

Performance Objective

Outcome:	Apply the following bandage turns: circular, spiral, spiral-reverse, figure-eight, and recurrent.
Conditions:	Given the following: a roller bandage and an elastic bandage.
Standards:	Time: 15 minutes. Student completed procedure in __________ minutes.
	Accuracy: Satisfactory score on the Performance Evaluation Checklist.

Performance Evaluation Checklist

Trial 1	Trial 2	Point Value	Performance Standards
			Circular turn:
		●	Placed the end of a bandage on a slant.
		●	Encircled the body part while allowing the corner of the bandage to extend.
		●	Turned down corner of bandage.
		●	Made another circular turn around the body part.
		▷	Stated a use of the circular turn.
			Spiral turn:
		●	Anchored bandage using a circular turn.
		●	Encircled the body part while keeping bandage at a slant.
		●	Carried each spiral turn upward at a slight angle.
		●	Overlapped each previous turn by one half to two thirds of the width of the bandage.
		▷	Stated a use of the spiral turn.
			Spiral-reverse turn:
		●	Anchored bandage using a circular turn.
		●	Encircled the body part while keeping bandage at a slant.
		●	Reversed the spiral turn using the thumb or index finger.
		●	Directed bandage downward and folded it on itself.
		●	Kept bandage parallel to the lower edge of the previous turn.
		●	Overlapped each previous turn by two thirds the width of the bandage.

Trial 1	Trial 2	Point Value	Performance Standards
		▷	Stated a use of the spiral-reverse turn.
			Figure-eight turn:
		●	Anchored bandage using a circular turn.
		●	Slanted bandage turns to alternately ascend and descend around the body part.
		●	Crossed the turns over one another in the middle to resemble a figure eight
		●	Overlapped each previous turn by two thirds of the width of the bandage.
		▷	Stated a use of the figure-eight turn.
			Recurrent turn:
		●	Anchored bandage using two circular turns.
		●	Passed bandage back and forth over the tip of the body part being bandaged.
		●	Overlapped each previous turn by two thirds of the width of the bandage.
		▷	Stated a use of the recurrent turn.
		Ⓐ	Incorporated critical thinking skills when performing patient care.
		✶	Completed the procedure within 15 minutes.
			TOTALS

CHART	
Date	

Evaluation of Student Performance

EVALUATION CRITERIA			COMMENTS
Symbol	Category	Point Value	
✶	Critical Step	16 points	
●	Essential Step	6 points	
Ⓐ	Affective Competency	6 points	
▷	Theory Question	2 points	
Score calculation:	100 points – ___ points missed ___ Score		
Satisfactory score: 85 or above			

2008 CAAHEP Competencies Achieved
Psychomotor (Skills) ☑ IV. 5. Instruct patients according to their needs to promote health maintenance and disease prevention. ☑ IV. 6. Prepare a patient for procedures and/or treatments. ***Affective (Behavior)*** ☑ I. 1. Apply critical thinking skills in performing patient assessment and care.

2015 CAAHEP Competencies Achieved
Psychomotor (Skills) ☑ I. 8. Instruct and prepare a patient for a procedure or a treatment. ☑ V. 4. Coach patient regarding: office policies b. health maintenance c. disease prevention d. treatment plan. ***Affective (Behavior)*** ☑ I. 2. Incorporate critical thinking skills when performing patient care.

ABHES Competencies Achieved
☑ 9. h. Teach self-examination, disease management and health promotion. ☑ 9. j. Make adaptations with patients with special needs.

Notes

26 Administration of Medication and Intravenous Therapy

CHAPTER ASSIGNMENTS

✓ After Completing	Date Due	Study Guide Pages	STUDY GUIDE ASSIGNMENTS (CTA = Critical Thinking Activity)	Possible Points	Points You Earned
		649	Pretest	10	
		 650 651	Key Term Assessment A. Definitions B. Word Parts (Add 1 point for each key term)	 26 13	
		651-657	Evaluation of Learning questions	65	
		657-660	CTA A: Using the PDR	38	
		660-661	CTA B: Locating Information in a Drug Insert	15	
		662	CTA C: Drug Classifications (3 points each)	30	
			Evolve Site: Road to Recovery: Drug Categories		
		662	CTA D: Medication Record	20	
		663	CTA E: Seven Rights of Medication Administration	35	
			Evolve Site: Script It! (Record points earned)		
		664	CTA F: Liquid Measurement	11	
		664	CTA G: Parts of a Needle and Syringe	11	
			Evolve Site: Take the Plunge (Record points earned)		
		664-665	CTA H: Hypodermic Syringe Calibrations	10	
			Evolve Site: Which Needle? (Record points earned)		

✓ After Completing	Date Due	Study Guide Pages	STUDY GUIDE ASSIGNMENTS (CTA = Critical Thinking Activity)	Possible Points	Points You Earned
		665	CTA I: Insulin Syringe Calibrations	20	
		665-666	CTA J: Tuberculin Syringe Calibrations	30	
			Evolve Site: Draw It Up! (Record points earned)		
		666	CTA K: Syringe and Needle Labels (3 points each)	12	
		666	CTA L: Angle of Insertion for Injections	3	
		666-667	CTA M: Preparing and Administering Parenteral Medication	18	
		668	CTA N: Measuring Mantoux Test Reactions	5	
		669	CTA O: Interpreting Mantoux Skin Test Reactions	11	
		669	CTA P: Anaphylactic Reaction	20	
		670-685	CTA Q: Researching Drugs (5 points per drug researched)	200	
		686	CTA R: Crossword Puzzle	37	
			Evolve Site: Math Review (Record points earned)		
			Evolve Site: Apply Your Knowledge questions	10	
			Evolve Site: Video Evaluation	60	
		649	Posttest	10	
			ADDITIONAL ASSIGNMENTS		
			TOTAL POINTS		

✓ After Completing	Date Due	Study Guide Pages	STUDY GUIDE ASSIGNMENTS Drug Dose Calculation: Supplemental Education for Chapter 26	Possible Points	Points You Earned
		725	Unit 1: The Metric System A. Units of Measurement	10	
		726	Unit 1: The Metric System B. Metric Abbreviations	6	
		726	Unit 1: The Metric System C. Metric Notation	15	
		727	Unit 2: The Household System A. Units of Measurements	4	
		727	Unit 3: Medication Orders A. Medical Abbreviations	25	
		728-729	Unit 3: Medication Orders B. Interpreting Medication Orders (3 points each)	30	
		729-730	Unit 4: Converting Units of Measurement A. Using Conversion Tables (2 points each)	40	
		730-732	Unit 4: Converting Units of Measurement B. Converting Units within the Metric System (2 points each)	40	
		732-734	Unit 4: Converting Units of Measurement C. Converting Units Within the Household System (2 points each)	20	
		734-736	Unit 5: Ratio and Proportion A. Ratio and Proportion Guidelines (6 points each)	48	
		736-738	Unit 5: Ratio and Proportion B. Converting Units Using Ratio and Proportion (2 points each)	20	
		738-744	Unit 6: Determining Drug Dose A. Oral Administration (2 points each)	30	

✓ After Completing	Date Due	Study Guide Pages	STUDY GUIDE ASSIGNMENTS Drug Dose Calculation: Supplemental Education for Chapter 26	Possible Points	Points You Earned
		745-749	Unit 6: Determining Drug Dose B. Parenteral Administration (2 points each)	20	
			ADDITIONAL ASSIGNMENTS		
			TOTAL POINTS		

✓ When Assigned By Your Instructor	Study Guide Pages	Practices Required	LABORATORY ASSIGNMENTS (Procedure Number and Name)	Score*
	687	5	**Practice for Competency** 26-1: Administering Oral Medication Textbook reference: pp. 646-647	
	693-695		**Evaluation of Competency** 26-1: Administering Oral Medication	*
	687	Vial: 5 Ampule: 5	**Practice for Competency** 26-2: Preparing an Injection Textbook reference: pp. 657-660	
	697-700		**Evaluation of Competency** 26-2: Preparing an Injection	*
	687	3	**Practice for Competency** 26-3: Reconstituting Powdered Drugs Textbook reference: p. 661	
	701-703		**Evaluation of Competency** 26-3: Reconstituting Powdered Drugs	*
	687	5	**Practice for Competency** 26-4: Administering a Subcutaneous Injection Textbook reference: pp. 662-664	
	705-707		**Evaluation of Competency** 26-4: Administering a Subcutaneous Injection	*
	688-691	5	**Practice for Competency** 26-A: Locating Intramuscular Injection Sites Textbook reference: pp. 654-656	
	709-712		**Evaluation of Competency** 26-A: Locating Intramuscular Injection Sites	*
	688-691	5	**Practice for Competency** 26-5: Administering an Intramuscular Injection Textbook reference: pp. 664-666	
	713-715		**Evaluation of Competency** 26-5: Administering an Intramuscular Injection	*
	688-691	5	**Practice for Competency** 26-6: Z-Track Intramuscular Injection Technique Textbook reference: p. 667	
	717-719		**Evaluation of Competency** 26-6: Z-Track Intramuscular Injection Technique	*

✓ When Assigned By Your Instructor	Study Guide Pages	Practices Required	LABORATORY ASSIGNMENTS (Procedure Number and Name)	Score*
	688-691	5	**Practice for Competency** 26-7: Administering an Intradermal Injection Textbook reference: pp. 668-671	
	721-724		**Evaluation of Competency** 26-7: Administering an Intradermal Injection	*
			ADDITIONAL ASSIGNMENTS	

Name ____ Date ____________________

PRETEST

True or False

_______ 1. A drug is a chemical that is used for treatment, prevention, or diagnosis of disease.

_______ 2. The generic name of a drug is assigned by the pharmaceutical manufacturer who develops the drug.

_______ 3. The Rx symbol comes from the Latin word recipe and means "take."

_______ 4. An anaphylactic reaction can be life threatening.

_______ 5. The dorsogluteal site is the most common site for administering injections in infants.

_______ 6. A subcutaneous injection is given into muscle tissue.

_______ 7. The purpose of aspirating when administering an injection is to make sure the needle is not in a blood vessel.

_______ 8. The Mantoux tuberculin skin test is administered through a subcutaneous injection.

_______ 9. The peripheral veins of the arm and hand are used most often for administering IV therapy.

_______ 10. Chemotherapy is the use of chemicals to treat disease.

POSTTEST

True or False

_______ 1. OSHA is responsible for determining whether drugs are safe before release for human use.

_______ 2. An enteric-coated tablet does not dissolve until it reaches the intestines.

_______ 3. The apothecary system is most often used to administer medication in the medical office.

_______ 4. The parenteral route of administering medications is used when the patient is allergic to the oral form of the drug.

_______ 5. Hypodermic syringes are calibrated in milliliters.

_______ 6. The maximum amount of medication that can be administered through the subcutaneous route is 2 mL.

_______ 7. A patient with latent tuberculosis infection has a negative reaction to a TB test.

_______ 8. A tuberculin skin test result should be read 15 to 20 minutes after administration.

_______ 9. The administration of fluids, medications, or nutrients through the IV route is known as an infusion.

_______ 10. The administration of blood through the IV route is known as an IV push.

KEY TERM ASSESSMENT

A. Definitions

Directions: Match each key term with its definition.

_______ 1. Adverse reaction
_______ 2. Allergen
_______ 3. Allergy
_______ 4. Ampule
_______ 5. Anaphylactic reaction
_______ 6. Chemotherapy
_______ 7. Controlled drug
_______ 8. Dose
_______ 9. Drug
_______ 10. Gauge
_______ 11. Induration
_______ 12. Infusion
_______ 13. Inhalation administration
_______ 14. Intradermal injection
_______ 15. Intramuscular injection
_______ 16. Intravenous therapy
_______ 17. Oral administration
_______ 18. Parenteral
_______ 19. Pharmacology
_______ 20. Prescription
_______ 21. Subcutaneous injection
_______ 22. Sublingual administration
_______ 23. Topical administration
_______ 24. Transfusion
_______ 25. Vial
_______ 26. Wheal

A. Application of a drug to a particular spot, usually for a local action
B. Introduction of medication into the dermal layer of the skin
C. A small, sealed glass container that holds a single dose of medication
D. A physician's order authorizing the dispensing of a drug by a pharmacist
E. An unintended and undesirable effect produced by a drug
F. An abnormal hypersensitivity of the body to substances that are ordinarily harmless
G. The administration of a liquid agent directly into a patient's vein, where it is distributed throughout the body by way of the circulatory system
H. A tense, pale raised area of the skin
I. Introduction of medication beneath the skin, into the subcutaneous or fatty layer of the body
J. An abnormally raised hardened area of the skin with clearly defined margins
K. A closed glass container with a rubber stopper that holds medication
L. The administration of medication by way of air or other vapor being drawn into the lungs
M. A serious allergic reaction that requires immediate treatment
N. Administration of medication by mouth
O. A drug that has restrictions placed on it by the federal government because of its potential for abuse
P. Introduction of medication into the muscular layer of the body
Q. Administration of medication by placing it under the tongue
R. The quantity of a drug to be administered at one time
S. A substance that is capable of causing an allergic reaction
T. A chemical used for the treatment, prevention, or diagnosis of disease
U. The diameter of the lumen of a needle used to administer medication
V. Administration of medication by injection
W. The study of drugs
X. The use of chemicals to treat disease; most often refers to the treatment of cancer using antineoplastic medications
Y. The administration of fluids, medications, or nutrients into a vein
Z. The administration of whole blood or blood products through the intravenous route

B. Word Parts

Directions: Indicate the meaning of each word part in the space provided. List as many medical terms as possible that incorporate the word part in the space provided.

Word Part	Meaning of Word Part	Medical Terms That Incorporate Word Part
1. chem/o		
2. -therapy		
3. intra-		
4. derm/o		
5. muscul/o		
6. -ar		
7. ven/o		
8. -ous		
9. pharmac/o		
10. sub-		
11. cutane/o		
12. lingu/o		
13. trans-		

EVALUATION OF LEARNING

Directions: Fill in each blank with the correct answer.

Administration of Medication

1. What is the difference between administering, prescribing, and dispensing medication at the medical office?

____

____

____

____

2. What is the difference between the generic name and the brand name of a drug?

____

____

____

____

3. What is a liniment?

____

____

4. What is a spray?

5. What is a syrup?

6. What is a tablet?

7. What is the purpose of scoring a tablet?

8. List two drugs that come in the form of chewable tablets.

9. List two reasons for enterically coating a tablet.

10. What is a capsule?

11. Why must a suppository have a cylindrical or conical shape?

12. What is a transdermal patch?

13. Why is the metric system used most often to administer medication?

14. Define the term *volume.*

15. Describe the use of the household system of measurement.

16. When is conversion required?

17. What is a controlled drug?

18. In what forms can a prescription be authorized?

19. What requirements must be followed when issuing a prescription for a schedule II drug?

20. List five brand names of schedule II analgesics.

21. What requirements must be followed when issuing a prescription for a schedule III drug?

22. What is a schedule IV drug?

23. List two brand names of schedule IV analgesics.

24. List three brand names of schedule IV antianxiety agents.

25. What is included in each of the following parts of a prescription?

    a. Superscription: ______

    b. Inscription: ______

    c. Subscription: ______

    d. Signatura: ______

26. Why is it important for the patient's age to be indicated on a prescription?

27. What functions can be performed by an EMR prescription program?

28. What types of medications should be recorded on a medication record form?

29. List and describe three factors that affect the action of drugs in the body.

30. What are the symptoms and treatment of an anaphylactic reaction?

31. What are the advantages and disadvantages of using the parenteral route of administration?

32. How do safety-engineered syringes reduce the risk of a needlestick injury?

33. What is the purpose of using a filter needle when withdrawing medication from an ampule?

34. What sites are used most frequently to administer a subcutaneous injection?

35. List three medications commonly administered through a subcutaneous injection.

36. Why is medication absorbed faster through the intramuscular route than through the subcutaneous route?

____

____

37. List the four intramuscular (IM) injection sites, and explain why these sites must be used to administer an IM injection.

____

____

____

____

38. What types of medication are given using the Z-track technique?

____

____

39. What sites are used most frequently to administer an intradermal injection?

____

40. What is the most frequent use of an intradermal injection?

____

41. What are the symptoms of active pulmonary tuberculosis?

____

42. What is latent tuberculosis infection?

____

43. What are examples of categories of individuals who should have a tuberculin test?

____

____

____

44. Why might a person who was recently infected with tuberculosis have a negative tuberculin skin test result?

____

____

45. What is induration, and what causes it?

____

____

46. What procedures are performed if a patient has a positive reaction to a tuberculin skin test?

____

____

47. Who should have a two-step tuberculin skin test?

48. What does it mean if the first test of a two-step tuberculin skin test is negative and the second test is positive? What does it mean if both tests are negative?

49. What is the name of the blood test for tuberculosis?

50. What are 10 examples of common allergens?

51. What is the general treatment for allergies?

52. What is the purpose of patch testing?

53. How long does it take for a reaction to occur with a skin-prick test?

54. Explain what is meant by each of the following intradermal skin test reactions.

a. ±1

b. +2

c. +3

55. What are the advantages of in vitro blood testing over direct skin testing?

Intravenous Therapy

1. What is intravenous therapy?

2. Which veins are most often used for IV therapy?

3. What types of liquid agents are administered through IV therapy?

4. List examples of outpatient sites in which IV therapy may be administered.

5. List five reasons for administering IV therapy in an outpatient setting?

6. What are the advantages of outpatient IV therapy?

7. What requirements must be met before an entry level medical assistant (MA) can perform IV therapy at a medical office?

8. What must be determined by the physician before prescribing IV therapy?

9. What are the responsibilities of the physician in prescribing IV therapy?

10. What instructions should the MA relay to a patient scheduled for outpatient IV therapy?

CRITICAL THINKING ACTIVITIES

A. Using the PDR

This activity assists you in learning how to use the *Physicians' Desk Reference* (PDR). Refer to Figure 26-1 in your textbook to answer the following questions.

Manufacturer's Index

1. What information is included in the Manufacturer's Index?

2. What company manufactures the drugs listed in the Manufacturer's Index?

3. What number would you call if you had an emergency on the weekend regarding one of these drugs?

4. What page would you turn to in the PDR for product information on Nitrostat tablets?

5. Is a photograph included in the PDR for Accupril Tablets?

6. What page would you turn to in the PDR to find a color photograph of Nardil tablets?

Brand and Generic Name Index

1. What information is included in the Brand and Generic Name Index?

2. To what page in the current PDR edition would you turn to find product information on Lipitor tablets manufactured by Parke-Davis?

3. What is the generic name of Prinivil tablets?

4. What company manufactures Prinivil tablets?

5. What page would you turn to in the PDR to find product information on Prinivil tablets?

6. What page would you turn to in the PDR to find product identification information on Prinivil tablets?

7. Who manufactures Lisinopril Tablets?

8. Does the PDR contain full product information on Lisinopril Tablets?

Product Category Index

1. What information is included in the Product Category Index?

2. What is the drug category for Flexeril Tablets?

3. Who manufactures Soma Tablets?

4. What page would you turn to in the current PDR edition to find product information on Skelaxin Tablets?

5. Who manufactures Valium Tablets?

Product Identification Guide

1. What is included in the Product Identification Guide?

2. How can this section assist the user?

Product Information

Under which heading would you look in this section to find information on the following subjects?

1. Conditions the drug is approved by the FDA to treat

2. Information to relay to the patient to ensure safe and effective use of the drug

3. Route of administration

4. Symptoms associated with an overdose of the drug

5. Diseased states or situations that require special consideration when the drug is being taken.

6. Generic name of the drug

7. How the drug functions in the body to produce its therapeutic effect

8. Situations in which the drug should not be used

9. Recommended adult dose and duration of treatment

____

10. How to pronounce the brand name of the drug

____

11. Handling and storage conditions

____

12. Serious adverse reactions that may occur with the drug

____

13. The dosage forms in which the drug is available.

____

14. Unintended and undesirable effects that may occur with the use of the drug

____

15. Modification of dose needed for children

____

16. Laboratory tests that may be affected when taking the drug

____

17. Interactions of the drug that may occur with other drugs

____

B. Locating Information in a Drug Insert

Obtain a drug insert for a prescription drug, and answer the following questions:

1. What is the brand name of the drug?

____

2. What is the generic name of the drug?

____

3. What is the drug category of this drug?

____

4. What are the dose forms for this drug?

____

5. What is the route of administration of this drug?

____

6. What are the indications and usage for this drug?

7. What are the contraindications for this drug?

8. List the warnings for this drug.

9. What are the general precautions for this drug?

10. What information should be relayed to patients regarding this drug?

11. What laboratory tests may be affected when taking this drug?

12. What are the adverse reactions for this drug?

13. What are the symptoms associated with an overdose of this drug?

14. What is the dosage and administration for this medication?

15. How should this drug be stored?

C. Drug Classifications

Inspect the package labels of 10 drugs (or use other means) to assess the classification of each drug based on preparation and action. List the name of each drug along with its appropriate category in the spaces provided. Compare results. Example: drug: Tylenol elixir; classification based on preparation: elixir; classification based on action: analgesic, antipyretic.

	Drug	Classification Based On: Preparation	Classification Based On: Action
1.			
2.			
3.			
4.			
5.			
6.			
7.			
8.			
9.			
10.			

D. Medication Record

Complete the following medication record form using yourself as the patient. Make sure to include all prescription medications and OTC medications, including vitamin supplements and herbal products. Use Figure 26-5 in your textbook as a guide in completing this form.

MEDICATION RECORD

Patient ______________________

Birthdate ______________________

ALLERGY

DATE	MEDICATION AND DOSAGE	FREQUENCY	RX	OTC	REFILLS			STOP

E. Seven Rights of Medication Administration

You are the office manager at a large clinic. Six new MAs were just hired. Your physician asks you to design an illustrated poster portraying the seven rights of medication administration to remind the new employees of the importance of following these guidelines. Use the diagram below to design your poster.

Follow the Seven Rights	
Right Drug	Right Dose
Right Time	Right Patient
Right Route	Right Technique
Right Documentation	

F. Liquid Measurement

Obtain a medicine cup that is graduated into the metric (milliliters), apothecary (drams and ounces), and household (teaspoons and tablespoons) systems. Complete the following:

1. What is its capacity? ______________________ ounces

   ______________________ milliliters

   ______________________ tablespoons

   ______________________ drams

2. Practice pouring oral liquid medication by pouring the following amounts of water into the medicine cup. Place a check mark by each amount after it has been properly poured.

   20 mL ______________________

   4 drams ______________________

   1 ounce ______________________

   10 mL ______________________

   1/2 ounce ______________________

   1 tablespoon ______________________

   2 drams ______________________

G. Parts of a Needle and Syringe

Obtain a needle and syringe. Locate the following parts of each and explain their function.

Needle **Function**

1. Hub ______________________
2. Shaft ______________________
3. Lumen ______________________
4. Point ______________________
5. Bevel ______________________
6. What is the gauge of the needle? ______________________
7. What is the length of the needle? ______________________

Syringe **Function**

8. Barrel ______________________
9. Flange ______________________
10. Plunger ______________________
11. What is the capacity of the syringe? ______________________

H. Hypodermic Syringe Calibrations

1. Obtain a 3-mL syringe that is divided into tenths of a milliliter. Locate the following calibrations on the syringe. Place a check mark in the blank next to each calibration after it has been correctly located.

   Calibration (mL)

   0.5 mL ______________________

   1.0 mL ______________________

   1.2 mL ______________________

   2.5 mL ______________________

   2.7 mL ______________________

2. Locate each calibration (listed in the previous question) on the illustration of the hypodermic syringe by placing an arrow on the correct calibration line and labeling it with the calibration.

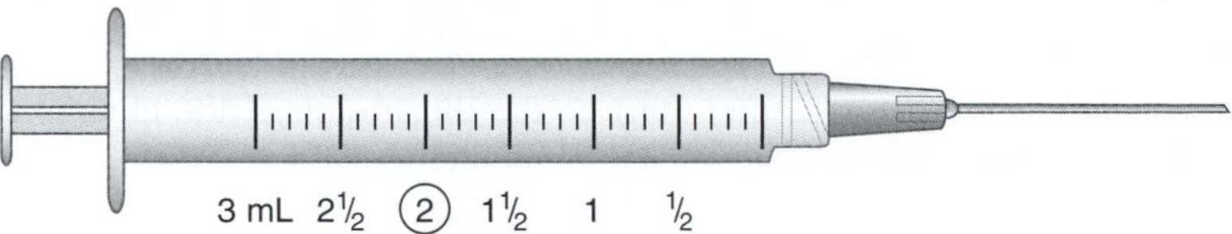

I. Insulin Syringe Calibrations

1. Obtain a U-100 insulin syringe. Locate the following calibrations (units) on the syringe, and place a check mark in the blank next to each calibration after it has been correctly located.

Calibration (units)

10 ____________________

16 ____________________

20 ____________________

44 ____________________

60 ____________________

68 ____________________

70 ____________________

86 ____________________

90 ____________________

100 ____________________

2. Locate each calibration (listed in the previous question) on the illustration of the insulin syringe by placing an arrow on the correct calibration line and labeling it with the calibration.

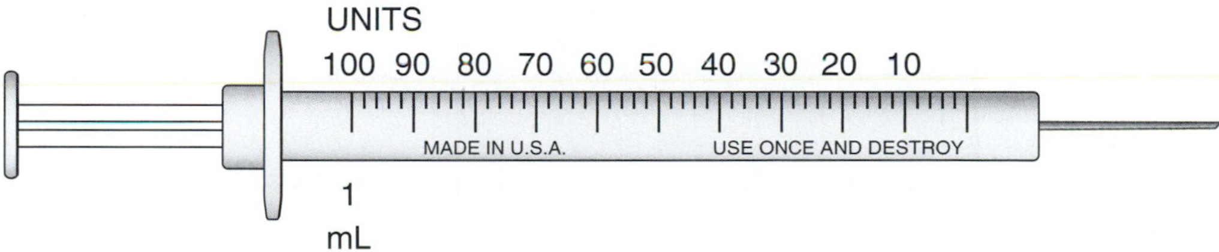

J. Tuberculin Syringe Calibrations

1. Obtain a 1-mL tuberculin syringe that is divided into tenths and hundredths of a milliliter. Locate the following calibrations on the syringe. Place a check mark in the blank next to each calibration after it has been correctly located.

Calibration (mL)

0.05 mL ____________________

0.10 mL ____________________

0.15 mL ____________________

0.34 mL ____________________

0.52 mL ____________________

0.75 mL ____________________

0.92 mL ____________________

2. Locate each calibration (listed in the previous question) on the illustration of the tuberculin syringe by placing an arrow on the correct calibration line and labeling it with the calibration.

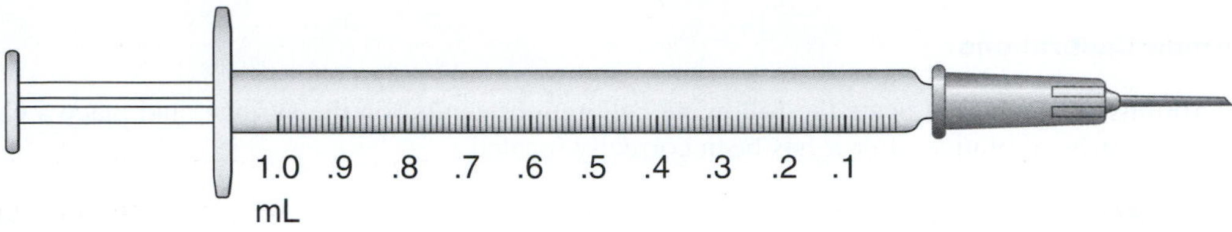

K. Syringe and Needle Labels

Refer to Figure 26-8 in your textbook, and indicate the following information for each syringe and needle: the syringe capacity and the gauge and length of the needle.

a. ____________________

b. ____________________

c. ____________________

d. ____________________

L. Angle of Insertion for Injections

In the diagram that follows, draw three lines indicating the angle of insertion into the correct body tissue for an intradermal, a subcutaneous, and an intramuscular injection. Label the lines.

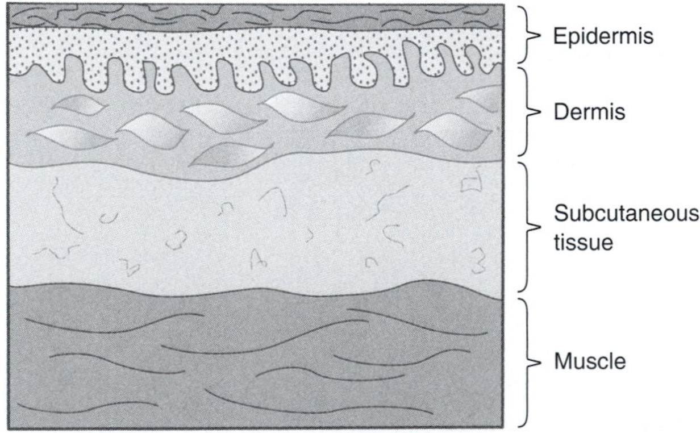

M. Preparing and Administering Parenteral Medication

For each of the following situations involving the preparation and administration of medication, write C if the technique is correct and I if it is incorrect. If the technique is correct, state the principle underlying the technique. If the technique is incorrect, explain what might happen if it were performed.

_______ 1. The expiration date of the medication is checked before administering the medication.

____

_______ 2. The MA is unfamiliar with the drug to be administered, so he or she looks it up in a drug reference.

____

_______ 3. The MA compares the medication label with the physician's instructions three times: as it is taken from the shelf, before preparing the medication, and after preparing the medication.

____

_______ 4. The rubber stopper of the multidose vial is cleansed with an antiseptic wipe before withdrawing the medication.

____

_______ 5. Air is not injected into the multidose vial before withdrawing the medication.

____

_______ 6. Air bubbles are present in the medication in the syringe that has been withdrawn from an ampule.

____

_______ 7. The injection sites are not rotated when repeated injections are given.

____

_______ 8. The antiseptic is not allowed to dry before administering an injection.

____

_______ 9. The skin is stretched taut before an intramuscular injection is given.

____

_______ 10. The needle is inserted slowly and steadily for an IM injection.

____

_______ 11. An IM injection is given in the deltoid site to a patient who has a tight sleeve.

____

_______ 12. An IM injection is given into the dorsogluteal site when the site is not fully exposed.

____

_______ 13. The MA does not aspirate when giving an intramuscular injection.

____

_______ 14. The medication is injected quickly for an IM injection.

____

_______ 15. The needle is withdrawn at the same angle as for insertion.

____

_______ 16. The intradermal needle is inserted with the bevel facing downward.

____

_______ 17. The MA does not aspirate when giving an intradermal injection.

____

_______ 18. Pressure is applied to the injection site after an intradermal injection is given.

____

N. Measuring Mantoux Test Reactions

Measure the diameter of the following circles, which represent induration from a Mantoux tuberculin skin test. A millimeter ruler is provided below. Cut it out and use it to measure the tuberculin reactions. Record results in the chart provided.

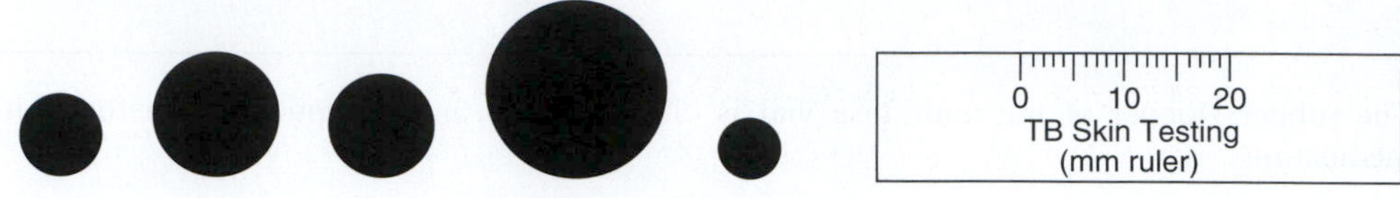

CHART	
Date	

O. Interpreting Mantoux Skin Test Reactions

Tuberculin skin test reactions are listed for various individuals. Using Table 26-7 in your textbook as a reference, determine if the individual's test results are positive or negative, and indicate your answer in the space provided.

_______ a. 2 mm of induration; an individual who is caring for a parent with active TB

_______ b. 7 mm of induration; a student attending college

_______ c. 12 mm of induration; an individual who is 12% below ideal body weight

_______ d. 8 mm of induration; an HIV-infected individual

_______ e. Erythema that is 6 mm wide (no induration); an individual with rheumatoid arthritis on Enbrel

_______ f. 16 mm of induration; a dietitian working in a nursing home

_______ g. 12 mm of induration; an individual who recently traveled to Canada

_______ h. 5 mm of induration; a child living with a parent who has active TB

_______ i. 6 mm of induration; an individual with diabetes mellitus

_______ j. 11 mm of induration; a recent immigrant from Africa

_______ k. 9 mm of induration; an individual working in a home and garden center

P. Anaphylactic Reaction

Create a profile of an individual who is experiencing an anaphylactic reaction following these guidelines:

1. Using a blank piece of paper, colored pencils, crayons, or markers, draw a figure of an individual exhibiting the symptoms of an anaphylactic reaction. Be as creative as possible.
2. Do not use any text on your drawing other than to label items you have drawn in your picture. (A picture is worth a thousand words!)
3. Try to include as many of the symptoms of an anaphylactic reaction as possible.
4. In the classroom, find a partner, and trade drawings. Identify the symptoms in your partner's drawing. With your partner, discuss what causes an anaphylactic reaction and how to prevent it. Also discuss the method of treatment for an anaphylactic reaction.

Q. Researching Drugs

Obtain a drug reference book, and look up the following information for each of the drugs listed on the Pharmacology Drug Sheets: generic name and drug classification, indications, and patient teaching. Record this information in the appropriate space on the Pharmacology Drug Sheets.

Pharmacology Drug Sheet

Name: ______________________________

Generic Name and Drug Classification	Indications	Patient Teaching
Accupril		
Abilify		
Adderall		
Adrenalin		

Pharmacology Drug Sheet

Name: ______________________________

Generic Name and Drug Classification	Indications	Patient Teaching
Advair Diskus		
Ambien		
Amoxil		
Aricept		

Pharmacology Drug Sheet

Name: ______________________________

Generic Name and Drug Classification	Indications	Patient Teaching
Ativan		
Bentyl		
Cardizem		
Catapres		

Pharmacology Drug Sheet

Name: ______________________

Generic Name and Drug Classification	Indications	Patient Teaching
Celebrex		
Cipro		
Coumadin		
Cozaar		

Pharmacology Drug Sheet

Name: ____________________

Generic Name and Drug Classification	Indications	Patient Teaching
Crestor		
Cymbalta		
Depo-Medrol		
Depo-Provera		

Pharmacology Drug Sheet

Name: ______________________________

Generic Name and Drug Classification	Indications	Patient Teaching
Detrol		
Diflucan		
Dilantin		
Flagyl		

Pharmacology Drug Sheet

Name: ______________________________

Generic Name and Drug Classification	Indications	Patient Teaching
Flexeril		
Flonase		
Fosamax		
Glucotrol XL		

Pharmacology Drug Sheet

Name: ______________________________

Generic Name and Drug Classification	Indications	Patient Teaching
Humulin		
Imitrex		
InFed		
Keflex		

Pharmacology Drug Sheet

Name: ____________________

Generic Name and Drug Classification	Indications	Patient Teaching
Lamisil		
Lanoxin		
Lasix		
Lipitor		

Pharmacology Drug Sheet

Name: ______________________________

Generic Name and Drug Classification	Indications	Patient Teaching
Loestrin Fe		
Lomotil		
Lyrica		
Macrobid		

Pharmacology Drug Sheet

Name: ______________________________

Generic Name and Drug Classification	Indications	Patient Teaching
Mexate		
Nitro-Bid		
Norvasc		
Percocet		

Pharmacology Drug Sheet

Name: ____________________

Generic Name and Drug Classification	Indications	Patient Teaching
Phenergan		
Plavix		
Premarin		
Prevacid		

Pharmacology Drug Sheet

Name: ____________________

Generic Name and Drug Classification	Indications	Patient Teaching
Prinivil		
Prozac		
Requip		
Rocephin		

Pharmacology Drug Sheet

Name: ______________________________

Generic Name and Drug Classification	Indications	Patient Teaching
Singulair		
Synthroid		
Tessalon		
Toprol XL		

Pharmacology Drug Sheet

Name: ____________________

Generic Name and Drug Classification	Indications	Patient Teaching
Valium		
Valtrex		
Viagra		
Vicodin		

Pharmacology Drug Sheet

Name: ____________________

Generic Name and Drug Classification	Indications	Patient Teaching
Xanax		
Zithromax		
Zyban		
Zyloprim		
Zyrtec		

R. Crossword Puzzle: Administration of Medication

Directions: Complete the crossword puzzle using the clues provided.

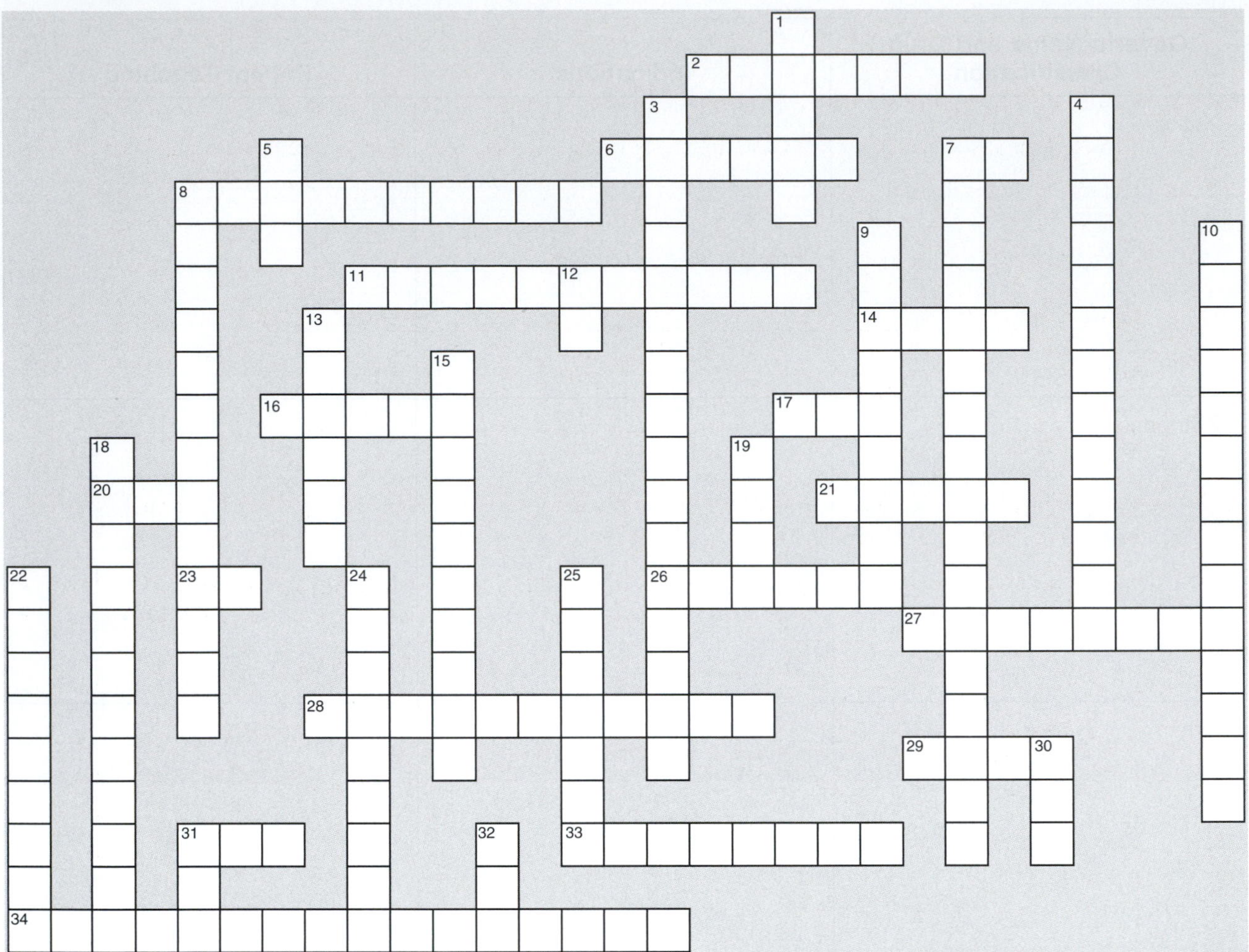

Across

2 Discovered penicillin
6 Most aggressive Hymenoptera
7 1 mL = 1 _______
8 Present with a + Mantoux
11 Used to treat anaphylactic reaction
14 Metric weight unit
16 Ranges between 18 and 27
17 Aspirin
20 Available w/o a Rx
21 Needle opening
23 Before meals
26 Sym: wheezing and dyspnea
27 Allergy to molds and pollen
28 Conditions a drug is approved to treat
29 Immediately!
31 Tuberculin is made of this
33 Causes house dust allergy
34 Runny and inflamed allergic nose

Down

1 Slant of the needle
3 Do not use this drug!
4 Drug to d/c before allergy testing
5 Approves drugs
7 Symptoms include itching, erythema, vesiculation
8 Abnormal or peculiar reaction
9 Medication label info
10 Calibrated in units
12 By mouth
13 Prevents syringe from rolling
15 This drug may cause an allergic reaction
18 Do not use this IM site for children
19 Blood test for allergies
22 Hives
24 Rx requirement for controlled drug
25 Max of 1 mL at this site
30 Three times per day
31 Drug reference (ex)
32 As needed

PRACTICE FOR COMPETENCY

Prerequisite. Complete the Drug Dose Calculation: Supplemental Education for Chapter 26 (pp. 725-749 in this manual).

Procedure 26-1: Oral Medication. Administer oral solid and liquid medication, and record the procedure in the chart provided.

Procedure 26-2: Preparing the Injection. Prepare an injection from an ampule and a vial.

Procedure 26-3: Reconstituting Powdered Drugs. Reconstitute a powdered drug for parenteral administration.

Procedure 26-4: Subcutaneous Injection. Administer an allergy injection, and record the procedure in the allergy injection form provided.

ALLERGY INJECTION (IMMUNOTHERAPY) RECORD

Name____

Date of Birth____________________________________

ADMINISTRATION GUIDELINES:

Allergy injections are administered weekly. The allergy extract should be increased by 0.05 mL per week until symptomatic improvement is achieved or until a maximum dosage of 0.5 mL is reached.

The patient should remain in the office for 20 minutes following the injection and the reaction noted. If no reaction occurs, the abbreviation NR should be recorded. If a reaction occurs, it should be recorded in mm.

Do not administer the allergy injection in the following situations:

a. The patient is ill with a temperature that is greater than 101° F
b. The patient is having an acute asthma attack
c. The patient is experiencing shortness of breath

Vial Number: **Vial Expiration Date:** ________________________

____1
____2
____3
____4

DATE	DOSAGE (mL)	Left Arm	Right Arm	REACTION (mm)	ADMINISTERED BY:

Procedure 26-A: Intramuscular Injection Sites. Locate the following intramuscular injection sites: dorsogluteal, deltoid, vastus lateralis, and ventrogluteal.

Procedure 26-5: Intramuscular Injection. Administer an intramuscular injection, and record the procedure in the chart provided.

Procedure 26-6: Z-track Method. Administer an intramuscular injection using the Z-track method. Record the procedure in the chart provided.

Procedure 26-7: Intradermal Injection. Administer an intradermal injection, and record the procedure in the chart provided. Read and interpret the test results, and record them in the chart. . Complete three TB test record cards located on the following page.

Chart	
Date	

Chart	
Date	

Chart	
Date	

TUBERCULOSIS TEST RECORD

Name	Date Admin: / /
	Date Read: / /
MANTOUX TEST	**RESULT**
	____ mm

Logan Family Practice
401 St. George St.
St. Augustine, FL 32084
(904) 555-3933

Performed by ______________________________

TUBERCULOSIS TEST RECORD

Name	Date Admin: / /
	Date Read: / /
MANTOUX TEST	**RESULT**
	____ mm

Logan Family Practice
401 St. George St.
St. Augustine, FL 32084
(904) 555-3933

Performed by ______________________________

TUBERCULOSIS TEST RECORD

Name	Date Admin: / /
	Date Read: / /
MANTOUX TEST	**RESULT**
	____ mm

Logan Family Practice
401 St. George St.
St. Augustine, FL 32084
(904) 555-3933

Performed by ______________________________

Notes

EVALUATION OF COMPETENCY

Procedure 26-1: Administering Oral Medication

Name: ______________________ Date: ______________

Evaluated by: ______________________ Score: ______________

Performance Objective

Outcome:	Administer oral solid and liquid medication.
Conditions:	Given the following: appropriate medication, medicine cup, and a medication tray.
Standards:	Time: 5 minutes. Student completed procedure in ________ minutes.
	Accuracy: Satisfactory score on the Performance Evaluation Checklist.

Performance Evaluation Checklist

Trial 1	Trial 2	Point Value	Performance Standards
		•	Sanitized hands.
		•	Assembled equipment.
		•	Worked in a quiet, well-lit atmosphere.
		•	Selected the correct medication from the shelf.
		•	Compared the medication with the physician's instructions.
		•	Checked the drug label.
		•	Checked the expiration date.
		•	Calculated the correct dose to be given, if needed.
		•	Removed the bottle cap.
		•	Checked the drug label and poured the medication.
			Solid medication
		*	Poured the correct number of capsules or tablets into the bottle cap.
		▷	Explained why the medication is poured into the bottle cap.
		•	Transferred the medication to a medicine cup.
			Liquid medication
		•	Placed lid of bottle on a flat surface with the open end facing up.
		•	Palmed the surface of the drug label.
		▷	Explained why the surface of the drug label should be palmed.
		•	Placed thumbnail at the proper calibration on medicine cup.
		•	Held medicine cup at eye level.

Trial 1	Trial 2	Point Value	Performance Standards
		✶	Poured the correct amount of medication and read the dose at the lowest level of the meniscus.
		●	Replaced the bottle cap.
		●	Checked the drug label and returned the medication to its storage location.
		●	Greeted the patient and introduced yourself.
		●	Identified the patient and explained the procedure.
		●	Handed the medicine cup to the patient.
		●	Offered water to patient.
		▷	Stated one instance when water should not be offered.
		●	Remained with patient until the medication was swallowed.
		●	Sanitized hands.
		●	Charted the procedure correctly.
		Ⓐ	Incorporated critical thinking skills when performing patient care.
		Ⓐ	Showed awareness of a patient's concerns related to the procedure being performed.
		✶	Completed the procedure within 10 minutes.
			TOTALS

CHART	
Date	

Evaluation of Student Performance

EVALUATION CRITERIA			COMMENTS
Symbol	**Category**	**Point Value**	
✶	Critical Step	16 points	
●	Essential Step	6 points	
Ⓐ	Affective Competency	6 points	
▷	Theory Question	2 points	
Score calculation: 100 points – ___ points missed ___ Score Satisfactory score: 85 or above			

2008 CAAHEP Competencies Achieved

Psychomotor (Skills)

☑ I. 8. Administer oral medications.
☑ II. 1. Prepare proper dosages of medication for administration.
☑ IX. 7. Document accurately in the patient record.

Affective (Behavior)

☑ II. 1. Verify ordered doses or dosages before administration.
☑ IX. 2. Demonstrate awareness of the consequences of not working within the legal scope of practice.

2015 CAAHEP Competencies Achieved

Psychomotor (Skills)

☑ I. 4. Verify the rules of medication administration: a. right patient b. right medication c. right dose d. right route e. right time f. right documentation.
☑ I. 6. Administer oral medication.
☑ II. 1. Calculate proper dosages of medication for administration.
☑ X. 3. Document patient care accurately in the medical record.

Affective (Behavior)

☑ I. 2. Incorporate critical thinking skills when performing patient care.
☑ I. 3. Show awareness of a patient's concerns related to the procedure being performed.

ABHES Competencies Achieved

☑ 4. a. Follow documentation guidelines.
☑ 6. b. Demonstrate accurate occupational math and metric conversion for proper medication administration.
☑ 9. f. Prepare and administer oral and parenteral medications and monitor intravenous (IV) infusions.

Notes

EVALUATION OF COMPETENCY

Procedure 26-2: Preparing an Injection

Name: ______________________________ Date: ______________

Evaluated by: ______________________________ Score: ______________

Performance Objective

Outcome:	Prepare an injection from an ampule and a vial.
Conditions:	Given the following: medication ordered by the physician, needle and syringe, antiseptic wipe, and medication tray.
Standards:	Time: 10 minutes. Student completed procedure in __________ minutes.
	Accuracy: Satisfactory score on the Performance Evaluation Checklist.

Performance Evaluation Checklist

Trial 1	Trial 2	Point Value	Performance Standards
		•	Sanitized hands.
		•	Assembled equipment.
		•	Worked in a quiet, well-lit atmosphere.
		*	Selected the proper medication from its storage location.
		•	Checked the drug label.
		•	Compared the medication with the physician's instructions.
		•	Checked the expiration date.
		*	Calculated the correct dose to be given, if needed.
		•	Opened syringe and needle packages.
		•	Assembled needle and syringe if necessary.
		•	Made sure that needle is attached firmly to syringe and moved the plunger back and forth.
		•	Checked the drug label a second time.
		•	If required, mixed the medication.
			Withdrew medication from a vial
		•	Removed metal or plastic cap if vial is new.
		•	Cleansed the rubber stopper of the vial with an antiseptic wipe and allowed it to dry.
		•	Placed vial in an upright position on a flat surface.
		•	Removed the needle guard.

Trial 1	Trial 2	Point Value	Performance Standards
		●	Drew air into syringe equal to the amount of medication to be withdrawn.
		●	Inserted needle through rubber stopper until it reached the empty space between stopper and the fluid level.
		●	Pushed down on plunger to inject air into the vial.
		●	Kept needle above the fluid level.
		▷	Explained why air must be injected into the vial.
		●	Inverted the vial while holding onto syringe and plunger.
		*	Held syringe at eye level and withdrew the proper amount of medication.
		●	Kept the needle opening below the fluid level.
		▷	Explained why the needle opening must be kept below the fluid level.
		●	Removed any air bubbles in syringe by tapping barrel with the fingertips.
		▷	Explained why air bubbles should be removed from the syringe.
		●	Removed any air remaining at the top of syringe by pushing the plunger forward.
		●	Held the syringe at eye level and checked to make sure the proper amount of medication had been drawn up.
		●	Removed the needle from rubber stopper and replaced the needle guard.
		●	If required, removed the needle and replaced it with a new needle.
		●	Checked the drug label for a third time and returned the medication to its storage location.
			Withdrew medication from an ampule
		●	Removed regular needle from syringe and attached a filter needle.
		▷	Stated the purpose of a filter needle.
		●	Cleansed the neck of the vial with an antiseptic wipe.
		●	Tapped the stem of the ampule lightly to remove any medication in the neck of ampule.
		●	Checked the medication label a second time.
		●	Placed piece of gauze around the neck of ampule.
		●	Broke off the stem by snapping it quickly and firmly away from the body.
		●	Discarded the stem and gauze in a biohazard sharps container.
		●	Placed the ampule on a flat surface.
		●	Removed the needle guard.
		●	Inserted needle opening below the fluid level.
		*	Withdrew the proper amount of medication.

Trial 1	Trial 2	Point Value	Performance Standards
		●	Kept needle opening below the fluid level.
		▷	Explained why needle opening must be kept below the fluid level.
		●	Held the syringe at eye level and checked to make sure the proper amout of medication had been drawn up.
		●	Removed needle from ampule and replaced needle guard.
		●	Checked drug label for a third time.
		●	Discarded the ampule in a biohazard sharps container.
		●	Removed the filter needle and reapplied the regular needle (and guard) to the syringe.
		●	Tapped the syringe to remove air bubbles.
		●	Removed needle guard and expelled air remaining at the top of syringe.
		●	Replaced the needle guard.
		Ⓐ	Incorporated critical thinking skills when performing patient care.
		✶	Completed the procedure within 10 minutes.
			TOTALS

Evaluation of Student Performance

EVALUATION CRITERIA			COMMENTS
Symbol	**Category**	**Point Value**	
✶	Critical Step	16 points	
●	Essential Step	6 points	
Ⓐ	Affective Competency	6 points	
▷	Theory Question	2 points	
Score calculation: 100 points – ____ points missed ____ Score Satisfactory score: 85 or above			

2008 CAAHEP Competencies Achieved
Psychomotor (Skills) ☑ II. 1. Prepare proper dosages of medication for administration. ***Affective (Behavior)*** ☑ II. 1. Verify ordered doses or dosages before administration.

2015 CAAHEP Competencies Achieved
Psychomotor (Skills)
☑ I. 4. Verify the rules of medication administration: a. right patient b. right medication c. right dose d. right route e. right time f. right documentation.
☑ II. 1. Calculate proper dosages of medication for administration.
Affective (Behavior)
☑ I. 2. Incorporate critical thinking skills when performing patient care.

ABHES Competencies Achieved
☑ 6. b. Demonstrate accurate occupational math and metric conversion for proper medication administration.
☑ 9. f. Prepare and administer oral and parenteral medications and monitor intravenous (IV) infusions.

EVALUATION OF COMPETENCY

Procedure 26-3: Reconstituting Powdered Drugs

Name: ______________________ Date: ______________

Evaluated by: ______________________ Score: ______________

Performance Objective

Outcome:	Reconstitute a powdered drug for parenteral administration.
Conditions:	Given the following: vial containing the powdered drug, reconstituting liquid, and a needle and syringe.
Standards:	Time: 5 minutes. Student completed procedure in __________ minutes.
	Accuracy: Satisfactory score on the Performance Evaluation Checklist.

Performance Evaluation Checklist

Trial 1	Trial 2	Point Value	Performance Standards
		•	Sanitized hands.
		•	Assembled equipment.
		*	Selected the proper medication from its storage location.
		•	Checked the drug label.
		•	Compared the medication with the physician's instructions.
		•	Checked the expiration date.
		*	Calculated the correct dose to be given, if needed.
		•	Opened syringe and needle packages.
		•	Assembled needle and syringe, if necessary.
		•	Made sure that the needle is attached firmly to syringe and moved the plunger back and forth.
		•	Checked the drug label a second time.
		•	Withdrew an amount of air equal to the amount of liquid to be injected into the vial from the vial containing the powdered drug.
		•	Injected the air into the vial of diluent.
		*	Inverted the diluent vial and withdrew the proper amount of liquid into the syringe.
		•	Removed air bubbles from the syringe.
		•	Held the syringe at eye level and checked to make sure the proper amount of diluent had been drawn up.
		•	Removed the needle from the vial.

Trial 1	Trial 2	Point Value	Performance Standards
		●	Inserted the needle into the powdered drug vial.
		●	Injected the diluent into the vial.
		●	Removed the needle from the vial and discarded the syringe and needle in a biohazard sharps container.
		●	Rolled the vial between hands to mix it.
		●	Labeled multiple-dose vials with the date of preparation and your initials.
		●	Prepared the injection and administered the medication.
		●	Stored multiple-dose vials as indicated in the manufacturer's instructions.
		▷	Explained the importance of checking the date of preparation of a reconstituted multiple-dose vial before administering it.
		Ⓐ	Incorporated critical thinking skills when performing patient care.
		✶	Completed the procedure within 5 minutes.
			TOTALS

Evaluation of Student Performance

EVALUATION CRITERIA			COMMENTS
Symbol	Category	Point Value	
✶	Critical Step	16 points	
●	Essential Step	6 points	
Ⓐ	Affective Competency	6 points	
▷	Theory Question	2 points	
Score calculation: 100 points – ___ points missed ___Score Satisfactory score: 85 or above			

2008 CAAHEP Competencies Achieved
Psychomotor (Skills) ☑ II. 1. Prepare proper dosages of medication for administration. ***Affective (Behavior)*** ☑ II. 1. Verify ordered doses/dosages prior to administration.

2015 CAAHEP Competencies Achieved
Psychomotor (Skills) ☑ I. 4. Verify the rules of medication administration: a. right patient b. right medication c. right dose d. right route e. right time f. right documentation. ☑ II. 1. Calculate proper dosages of medication for administration. ***Affective (Behavior)*** ☑ I. 2. Incorporate critical thinking skills when performing patient care.

ABHES Competencies Achieved
☑ 6. b. Demonstrate accurate occupational math and metric conversion for proper medication administration. ☑ 9. f. Prepare and administer oral and parenteral medications and monitor intravenous (IV) infusions.

Notes

EVALUATION OF COMPETENCY

Procedure 26-4: Administering a Subcutaneous Injection

Name: ______________________ Date: ______________

Evaluated by: ______________________ Score: ______________

Performance Objective

Outcome:	Administer a subcutaneous injection.
Conditions:	Given the following: appropriate medication, appropriate needle and syringe, antiseptic wipe, 2 × 2 gauze pad, disposable gloves, and a biohazard sharps container.
Standards:	Time: 5 minutes. Student completed procedure in ________ minutes.
	Accuracy: Satisfactory score on the Performance Evaluation Checklist.

Performance Evaluation Checklist

Trial 1	Trial 2	Point Value	Performance Standards
		●	Sanitized hands.
		●	Prepared the injection.
		●	Greeted the patient and introduced yourself.
		●	Identified the patient and explained the procedure and purpose of the injection.
		●	Selected an appropriate subcutaneous injection site.
		▷	Stated the sites that can be used to administer a subcutaneous injection.
		●	Cleansed area with an antiseptic wipe and allowed it to dry completely.
		▷	Explained why the site should be allowed to dry.
		●	Applied gloves.
		●	Removed needle guard.
		●	Properly positioned the hand on area surrounding the injection site.
		▷	Explained when the area should be grasped and when it should be held taut.
		●	Inserted needle to the hub at a 45-degree or 90-degree angle (depending on the length of the needle) with a quick, smooth motion.
		▷	Explained how needle length determines the angle of insertion for a subcutaneous injection.
		●	Removed the hand from the skin.
		▷	Explained why the hand should be removed from the skin.
		▷	Explained why aspiration of a subcutaneous injection is not necessary.
		●	Injected the medication slowly and steadily while holding the syringe steady.
		▷	Described what would happen if the medication were injected rapidly.

Trial 1	Trial 2	Point Value	Performance Standards
		●	Placed a gauze pad gently over the injection site and removed needle quickly at the same angle as insertion.
		▷	Explained why the needle should be removed at the angle of insertion.
		●	Applied gentle pressure to the injection site.
		▷	Stated why the site should not be vigorously massaged.
		●	Activated the safety shield on the needle.
		●	Properly disposed of needle and syringe.
		●	Removed gloves and sanitized hands.
		●	Charted the procedure correctly.
		●	Remained with patient to make sure there were no unusual reactions.
		▷	Stated the steps to follow if the patient has been given an allergy injection.
		Ⓐ	Incorporated critical thinking skills when performing patient care.
		Ⓐ	Showed awareness of a patient's concerns related to the procedure being performed.
		Ⓐ	Explained to a patient the rationale for performance of a procedure.
		✶	Completed the procedure within 5 minutes.
			TOTALS

CHART	
Date	

Evaluation of Student Performance

EVALUATION CRITERIA			COMMENTS
Symbol	Category	Point Value	
✶	Critical Step	16 points	
●	Essential Step	6 points	
Ⓐ	Affective Competency	6 points	
▷	Theory Question	2 points	
Score calculation: 100 points − points missed ___Score Satisfactory score: 85 or above			

2008 AAHEP Competencies Achieved
Psychomotor (Skills) ☑ I. 7. Select proper sites for administering parenteral medication. ☑ I. 9. Administer parenteral (excluding IV) medications. ☑ IX. 7. Document accurately in the patient record. ☑ XI. 5. Demonstrate proper use of the following equipment: c. Sharps disposal containers. ***Affective (Behavior)*** ☑ III. 3. Show awareness of patients' concerns regarding their perceptions related to the procedure being performed.

2015 AAHEP Competencies Achieved
Psychomotor (Skills) ☑ I. 4. Verify the rules of medication administration: a. right patient b. right medication c. right dose d. right route e. right time f. right documentation. ☑ I. 5. Select proper sites for administering parenteral medication. ☑ I. 7. Administer parenteral (excluding IV) medications. ☑ III. 10. Demonstrate proper disposal of biohazardous material: a. sharps b. regulated waste ☑ V. 2. Respond to nonverbal communication. ☑ X. 3. Document patient care accurately in the medical record. ☑ XII. 2. c. Demonstrate proper use of sharps disposal containers. ***Affective (Behavior)*** ☑ I. 2. Incorporate critical thinking skills when performing patient care. ☑ I. 3. Show awareness of a patient's concerns related to the procedure being performed. ☑ V. 4. Explain to a patient the rationale for performance of a procedure.

ABHES Competencies Achieved
☑ 4. a. Follow documentation guidelines. ☑ 9. f. Prepare and administer oral and parenteral medications and monitor intravenous (IV) infusions. ☑ 10. c. Dispose of biohazardous materials.

Notes

EVALUATION OF COMPETENCY

Procedure 26-A: Locating Intramuscular Injection Sites

Name: ______________________ Date: ______________

Evaluated by: ______________________ Score: ______________

Performance Objective

Outcome:	Locate intramuscular injection sites.
Conditions:	None required.
Standards:	Time: 5 minutes. Student completed procedure in ________ minutes.
	Accuracy: Satisfactory score on the Performance Evaluation Checklist.

Performance Evaluation Checklist

Trial 1	Trial 2	Point Value	Performance Standards
			DORSOGLUTEAL SITE
			Method 1:
		•	Asked the patient to lie on the abdomen with the toes pointed inward.
		•	Made sure the injection site was fully exposed.
		▷	Stated why the injection site should be fully exposed.
		•	Located the greater trochanter through palpation.
		•	Located the posterior superior iliac spine through palpation.
		•	Drew an imaginary line between these two points.
		•	Stated that the injection is administered above and outside this area.
			Method 2:
		•	Asked the patient to lie on the abdomen with the toes pointed inward.
		•	Made sure the injection area was fully exposed.
		•	Divided the buttocks into quadrants.
		•	Stated that the injection is administered into the upper outer quadrant approximately 2 to 3 inches below the iliac crest.
		▷	Explained why it is important to maintain proper boundary lines.
			DELTOID SITE
		•	Placed the patient in a sitting position.
		•	Pulled up the patient's sleeve or removed the sleeve from the arm.
		▷	Explained why a tight sleeve should be avoided.

Trial 1	Trial 2	Point Value	Performance Standards
		●	Ensured that the entire arm was exposed.
		●	Palpated the lower edge of the acromion process.
		●	Placed 4 fingers horizontally across the deltoid muscle with the top finger along the acromion process.
		●	Explained that the injection site is located 2 to 3 finger-widths below the acromion process (approximately 1 to 2 inches below the acromion process).
		▷	Identified the maximum amount of medication that can be administered into this site.
			VASTUS LATERALIS SITE
			Adult:
		●	Placed the patient in a supine or sitting position.
		●	Located the midanterior thigh (on the front of the leg).
		●	Located the midlateral thigh (on the side of the leg).
		●	Located the proximal boundary by coming down a hand's breadth from the greater trochanter.
		●	Located the distal boundary by coming up a hand's breadth from the knee.
		●	Stated that the injection is administered within the boundaries identified above.
			Infants and Children:
		●	Placed the infant or child in a supine position or have the parent hold the infant in a sitting position on his or her lap.
		●	Located the midanterior thigh (on the front of the leg).
		●	Located the midlateral thigh (on the side of the leg).
		●	Located the greater trochanter through palpation.
		●	Located the knee joint through palpation.
		●	Divided the area between the greater trochanter and knee joint into thirds and made a mental note of the middle third of the divided area.
		●	Stated that the injection is administered within the boundaries identified above.
		▷	Explained why this site is commonly used with children younger than 3 years of age.
			VENTROGLUTEAL SITE
		●	Placed the patient in a prone position or lying on one side.
		●	Located the greater trochanter through palpation.
		●	Located the anterior superior iliac spine and the iliac crest through palpation.
			For an injection being administered into the left side:

Trial 1	Trial 2	Point Value	Performance Standards
		●	Placed the palm of the right hand on the greater trochanter.
		●	Placed the index finger on the anterior superior iliac spine.
		●	Spread the middle finger posteriorly as far as possible away from the index finger to touch the iliac crest.
		●	Stated that the injection is administered into the triangle formed by the fingers.
			For an injection being administered into the right side:
		●	Placed the palm of the left hand on the greater trochanter.
		●	Placed the index finger on the anterior superior iliac spine.
		●	Spread the middle finger posteriorly as far as possible away from the index finger to touch the iliac crest.
		●	Stated that the injection is administered into the triangle formed by the fingers.
		Ⓐ	Incorporated critical thinking skills when performing patient care.
		✶	Completed the procedure within 5 minutes.
			Totals

Evaluation of Student Performance

EVALUATION CRITERIA			COMMENTS
Symbol	**Category**	**Point Value**	
✶	Critical Step	16 points	
●	Essential Step	6 points	
Ⓐ	Affective Competency	6 points	
▷	Theory Question	2 points	
Score calculation: 100 points – ____ points missed ____ Score Satisfactory score: 85 or above			

2008 CAAHEP Competencies Achieved
Psychomotor (Skills) ☑ II. 1. Prepare proper dosages of medication for administration. ***Affective (Behavior)*** ☑ II. 1. Verify ordered doses or dosages before administration.

2015 CAAHEP Competencies Achieved
Psychomotor (Skills) ☑ I. 4. Verify the rules of medication administration: a. right patient b. right medication c. right dose d. right route e. right time f. right documentation. ☑ I. 5. Select proper sites for administering parenteral medication. ***Affective (Behavior)*** ☑ I. 2. Incorporate critical thinking skills when performing patient care.

ABHES Competencies Achieved
☑ 9. f. Prepare and administer oral and parenteral medications and monitor intravenous (IV) infusions.

EVALUATION OF COMPETENCY

Procedure 26-5: Administering an Intramuscular Injection

Name: ______________________________ Date: ______________

Evaluated by: ______________________________ Score: ______________

Performance Objective

Outcome:	Administer an intramuscular injection.
Conditions:	Given the following: appropriate medication, appropriate needle and syringe, antiseptic wipe, 2 × 2 gauze pad, disposable gloves, and a biohazard sharps container.
Standards:	Time: 5 minutes. Student completed procedure in __________ minutes.
	Accuracy: Satisfactory score on the Performance Evaluation Checklist.

Performance Evaluation Checklist

Trial 1	Trial 2	Point Value	Performance Standards
		•	Sanitized hands.
		•	Prepared the injection.
		•	Greeted the patient and introduced yourself.
		•	Identified the patient and explained the procedure and purpose of the injection.
		*	Located the appropriate intramuscular injection site.
		▷	Stated what tissue layer of the body the medication will be injected into.
		•	Cleansed area with an antiseptic wipe and allowed it to dry completely.
		•	Applied gloves.
		•	Removed needle guard.
		•	Stretched the skin taut over the injection site.
		▷	Explained why the skin should be stretched taut.
		•	Held the barrel of syringe like a dart and inserted needle quickly at a 90-degree angle to the patient's skin with a firm motion.
		•	Inserted the needle to the hub.
		▷	Explained why the needle should be inserted at a 90-degree angle and to the hub.
		*	Aspirated to make sure that the needle was not in a blood vessel.
		▷	Described what would happen if the medication was injected into a blood vessel.
		•	Injected the medication slowly and steadily.
		▷	Described what would happen if the medication was injected rapidly.

Trial 1	Trial 2	Point Value	Performance Standards
		●	Placed a gauze pad gently over the injection site and removed needle quickly at the same angle as insertion.
		▷	Applied gentle pressure to the injection site.
		▷	Stated the reason for applying pressure to the injection site.
		●	Activated the safety shield on the needle.
		●	Properly disposed of needle and syringe.
		●	Removed gloves and sanitized hands.
		●	Charted the procedure correctly.
		▷	Stated the purpose of the lot number on the medication vial.
		●	Remained with patient to make sure there were no unusual reactions.
		Ⓐ	Incorporated critical thinking skills when performing patient care.
		Ⓐ	Showed awareness of a patient's concerns related to the procedure being performed.
		Ⓐ	Explained to a patient the rationale for performance of a procedure.
		✶	Completed the procedure within 5 minutes.
			TOTALS

CHART	
Date	

Evaluation of Student Performance

EVALUATION CRITERIA			COMMENTS
Symbol	**Category**	**Point Value**	
✶	Critical Step	16 points	
●	Essential Step	6 points	
Ⓐ	Affective Competency	6 points	
▷	Theory Question	2 points	
Score calculation: 100 points – points missed Score Satisfactory score: 85 or above			

2008 CAAHEP Competencies Achieved
Psychomotor (Skills) ☑ I. 7. Select proper sites for administering parenteral medication. ☑ I. 9. Administer parenteral (excluding IV) medications. ☑ IX. 7. Document accurately in the patient record. ☑ XI. 5. Demonstrate proper use of the following equipment: c. Sharps disposal containers. ***Affective (Behavior)*** ☑ III. 3. Show awareness of patients' concerns regarding their perceptions related to the procedure being performed.

2015 CAAHEP Competencies Achieved
Psychomotor (Skills) ☑ I. 4. Verify the rules of medication administration: a. right patient b. right medication c. right dose d. right route e. right time f. right documentation. ☑ I. 5. Select proper sites for administering parenteral medication. ☑ I. 7. Administer parenteral (excluding IV) medications. ☑ III. 10. Demonstrate proper disposal of biohazardous material: a. sharps b. regulated waste ☑ V. 2. Respond to nonverbal communication. ☑ X. 3. Document patient care accurately in the medical record. ☑ XII. 2. c. Demonstrate proper use of sharps disposal containers. ***Affective (Behavior)*** ☑ I. 2. Incorporate critical thinking skills when performing patient care. ☑ I. 3. Show awareness of a patient's concerns related to the procedure being performed. ☑ V. 4. Explain to a patient the rationale for performance of a procedure.

ABHES Competencies Achieved
☑ 4. a. Follow documentation guidelines. ☑ 9. f. Prepare and administer oral and parenteral medications and monitor intravenous (IV) infusions. ☑ 10. c. Dispose of biohazardous materials.

Notes

EVALUATION OF COMPETENCY

Procedure 26-6: Z-Track Intramuscular Injection Technique

Name: ______________________________ Date: ______________

Evaluated by: ______________________________ Score: ______________

Performance Objective

Outcome:	Administer an intramuscular injection using the Z-track method.
Conditions:	Given the following: appropriate medication, appropriate needle and syringe, antiseptic wipe, disposable gloves, and a biohazard sharps container.
Standards:	Time: 5 minutes. Student completed procedure in __________ minutes.
	Accuracy: Satisfactory score on the Performance Evaluation Checklist.

Performance Evaluation Checklist

Trial 1	Trial 2	Point Value	Performance Standards
		•	Sanitized hands.
		•	Prepared the injection.
		•	Greeted the patient and introduced yourself.
		•	Identified the patient and explained the procedure and purpose of the injection.
		•	Selected and properly located the intramuscular injection site.
		•	Cleansed area with an antiseptic wipe and allowed it to dry completely.
		•	Applied gloves.
		•	Removed needle guard.
		•	Pulled the skin away laterally from the injection site with the nondominant hand approximately 1 to 1½ inches.
		•	Inserted needle quickly and smoothly at a 90-degree angle.
		*	Aspirated to make sure that the needle was not in a blood vessel.
		•	Injected the medication slowly and steadily.
		•	Waited 10 seconds before withdrawing the needle.
		▷	Explained why there should be a 10-second waiting period.
		•	Withdrew needle quickly at the same angle as that of insertion.
		•	Released the traction on the skin.
		▷	Described what occurs when the skin traction is released.
		•	Did not apply pressure to the injection site.

Trial 1	Trial 2	Point Value	Performance Standards
		▷	Stated why pressure should not be applied to the injection site.
		●	Activated the safety shield on the needle.
		●	Properly disposed of needle and syringe.
		●	Removed gloves and sanitized hands.
		●	Charted the procedure correctly.
		●	Remained with patient to make sure there were no unusual reactions.
		Ⓐ	Incorporated critical thinking skills when performing patient care.
		Ⓐ	Showed awareness of a patient's concerns related to the procedure being performed.
		Ⓐ	Explained to a patient the rationale for performance of a procedure.
		*	Completed the procedure within 5 minutes.
			TOTALS

CHART	
Date	

Evaluation of Student Performance

EVALUATION CRITERIA			COMMENTS
Symbol	Category	Point Value	
*	Critical Step	16 points	
●	Essential Step	6 points	
Ⓐ	Affective Competency	6 points	
▷	Theory Question	2 points	
Score calculation: 100 points – ___ points missed ___ Score Satisfactory score: 85 or above			

2008 CAAHEP Competencies Achieved

Psychomotor (Skills)

☑ I. 7. Select proper sites for administering parenteral medication.
☑ I. 9. Administer parenteral (excluding IV) medications.
☑ IX. 7. Document accurately in the patient record.
☑ XI. 5. Demonstrate proper use of the following equipment: c. Sharps disposal containers.

Affective (Behavior)

☑ III. 3. Show awareness of patients' concerns regarding their perceptions related to the procedure being performed.

2015 CAAHEP Competencies Achieved

Psychomotor (Skills)

☑ I. 4. Verify the rules of medication administration: a. right patient b. right medication c. right dose d. right route e. right time f. right documentation.
☑ I. 5. Select proper sites for administering parenteral medication.
☑ I. 7. Administer parenteral (excluding IV) medications.
☑ III. 10. Demonstrate proper disposal of biohazardous material: a. sharps b. regulated waste
☑ V. 2. Respond to nonverbal communication.
☑ X. 3. Document patient care accurately in the medical record.
☑ XII. 2. c. Demonstrate proper use of sharps disposal containers.

Affective (Behavior)

☑ I. 2. Incorporate critical thinking skills when performing patient care.
☑ I. 3. Show awareness of a patient's concerns related to the procedure being performed.
☑ V. 4. Explain to a patient the rationale for performance of a procedure.

ABHES Competencies Achieved

☑ 4. a. Follow documentation guidelines.
☑ 9. f. Prepare and administer oral and parenteral medications and monitor intravenous (IV) infusions.
☑ 10. c. Dispose of biohazardous materials.

Notes

EVALUATION OF COMPETENCY

Procedure 26-7: Administering an Intradermal Injection

Name: ______________________________ Date: ____________________

Evaluated by: ______________________________ Score: ____________________

Performance Objective

Outcome:	Administer an intradermal injection and read the test results.
Conditions:	Given the following: skin testing solution, appropriate needle and syringe, antiseptic wipe, 2 × 2 gauze pad, disposable gloves, millimeter ruler, TB skin test record card, and a biohazard sharps container.
Standards:	Time: 5 minutes. Student completed procedure in __________ minutes.
	Accuracy: Satisfactory score on the Performance Evaluation Checklist.

Performance Evaluation Checklist

Trial 1	Trial 2	Point Value	Performance Standards
		•	Sanitized hands.
		•	Prepared the injection.
		•	Greeted the patient and introduced yourself.
		•	Identified the patient and explained the procedure and purpose of the injection.
		•	Selected an appropriate intradermal injection site.
		▷	Stated the recommended sites for an intradermal injection.
		•	Cleansed area with an antiseptic wipe and allowed it to dry completely.
		•	Applied gloves.
		•	Removed needle guard.
		•	Stretched the skin taut at the site of administration.
		▷	Explained why the skin is held taut.
		•	Inserted needle at an angle of 10 to 15 degrees and with the bevel upward.
		•	The bevel of the needle just penetrated the skin.
		▷	Stated why the bevel should face upward.
		•	Injected the medication slowly and steadily, ensuring that a wheal formed (approximately 6 to 10 mm in diameter).
		▷	Explained what to do if a wheal does not form.
		•	Placed a gauze pad gently over the injection site and removed the needle quickly at the same angle as that of insertion.

Trial 1	Trial 2	Point Value	Performance Standards
		•	Did not apply pressure to the injection site.
		▷	Explained why pressure should not be applied to the site.
		•	Activated the safety shield on the needle.
		•	Properly disposed of needle and syringe.
		•	Removed gloves and sanitized hands.
		•	Remained with patient to make sure that there were no unusual reactions.
			Allergy skin tests
		•	Read the test results within 20 to 30 minutes.
		•	Inspected and palpated the site of the skin tests.
		•	Interpreted the skin test results.
		•	Charted the procedure correctly.
			Mantoux tuberculin test
		•	Informed the patient to return in 48 to 72 hours to have the results read.
		▷	Stated what must be done if the patient does not return to have the results read.
		•	Instructed the patient in the care of the test site.
		▷	Stated the instructions that must be relayed to the patient.
		•	Charted the procedure correctly.
			Reading Mantoux test results
		•	Greeted the patient and introduced yourself.
		•	Identified the patient and explained the procedure.
		•	Worked in a quiet, well-lit atmosphere.
		•	Checked the patient's chart to determine the site of administration of the test.
		•	Sanitized hands and applied gloves.
		•	Positioned patient's arm on a firm surface with the arm flexed at the elbow.
		•	Located the application site.
		•	Gently rubbed the fingertip over the test site.
		•	If induration is present, rubbed the area lightly, going from the area of normal skin to the indurated area to assess the size of the indurated area.
		•	Measured the diameter of the induration with a millimeter ruler.
		*	The measurement was recorded in millimeters and was identical to the evaluator's measurement.
		•	Removed gloves and sanitized hands.

Trial 1	Trial 2	Point Value	Performance Standards
		●	Charted the results correctly.
		●	Completed a TB test record card and gave it to the patient.
		Ⓐ	Incorporated critical thinking skills when performing patient care.
		Ⓐ	Showed awareness of a patient's concerns related to the procedure being performed.
		Ⓐ	Explained to a patient the rationale for performance of a procedure.
		*	Completed the procedure within 10 minutes.
			TOTALS

CHART	
Date	

TUBERCULOSIS TEST RECORD

Name	Date Admin: / /
	Date Read: / /
MANTOUX TEST	**RESULT**
	____ mm

Logan Family Practice
401 St. George St.
St. Augustine, FL 32084
(904) 555-3933

Performed by ____________________

Evaluation of Student Performance

EVALUATION CRITERIA			COMMENTS
Symbol	Category	Point Value	
*	Critical Step	16 points	
●	Essential Step	6 points	
Ⓐ	Affective Competency	6 points	
▷	Theory Question	2 points	
Score calculation: 100 points – ____ points missed ____ Score Satisfactory score: 85 or above			

2008 CAAHEP Competencies Achieved
Psychomotor (Skills) ☑ I. 7. Select proper sites for administering parenteral medication. ☑ I. 9. Administer parenteral (excluding IV) medications. ☑ IX. 7. Document accurately in the patient record. ☑ XI. 5. Demonstrate proper use of the following equipment: c. Sharps disposal containers. ***Affective (Behavior)*** ☑ III. 3. Show awareness of patients' concerns regarding their perceptions related to the procedure being performed.

2015 CAAHEP Competencies Achieved
Psychomotor (Skills) ☑ I. 4. Verify the rules of medication administration: a. right patient b. right medication c. right dose d. right route e. right time f. right documentation. ☑ I. 5. Select proper sites for administering parenteral medication. ☑ I. 7. Administer parenteral (excluding IV) medications. ☑ III. 10. Demonstrate proper disposal of biohazardous material: a. sharps b. regulated waste ☑ V. 2. Respond to nonverbal communication. ☑ X. 3. Document patient care accurately in the medical record. ☑ XII. 2. c. Demonstrate proper use of sharps disposal containers. ***Affective (Behavior)*** ☑ I. 2. Incorporate critical thinking skills when performing patient care. ☑ I. 3. Show awareness of a patient's concerns related to the procedure being performed. ☑ V. 4. Explain to a patient the rationale for performance of a procedure.

ABHES Competencies Achieved
☑ 4. a. Follow documentation guidelines. ☑ 9. f. Prepare and administer oral and parenteral medications and monitor intravenous (IV) infusions. ☑ 10. c. Dispose of biohazardous materials.

DRUG DOSE CALCULATION: SUPPLEMENTAL EDUCATION FOR CHAPTER 26

This section is designed as supplemental education for Chapter 26 (Administration of Medication) in your textbook. Completion of these exercises will enable you to calculate drug dose effectively and accurately, which is essential for administering the proper amount of medication to patients and preventing medication errors. Because each unit builds on the next one; therefore, you should become completely familiar with each step before proceeding to the next.

Learning Objectives

After completing this chapter, you should be able to:

1. Identify metric abbreviations
2. Indicate dose quantity using metric notation guidelines
3. Identify common medical abbreviations used in writing medication orders
4. Interpret medication orders
5. Convert units of measurement within the following systems: metric and household
6. Convert units of measurement using ratio and proportion
7. Convert units of measurement between the metric and household systems
8. Determine oral drug dose
9. Determine parenteral drug dose

UNIT 1: THE METRIC SYSTEM

A. Units of Measurement: Practice Problems

The basic units of measurement in the metric system are the gram, liter, and meter. The gram is a unit of weight used to measure solids, the liter is a unit volume used to measure liquids, and the meter is a unit of length used to measure distance. In the space provided, indicate whether each of the following metric units of measurement is a unit of weight (W), volume (V), or length (L).

_______ 1. milligram

_______ 2. cubic centimeter

_______ 3. meter

_______ 4. kilogram

_______ 5. liter

_______ 6. milliliter

_______ 7. kiloliter

_______ 8. millimeter

_______ 9. microgram

_______ 10. gram

B. Metric Abbreviations: Practice Problems

Review the metric abbreviations in your textbook before completing these problems. In the space provided, indicate the correct abbreviation for each of the metric units of measurement.

_______ 1. milligram

_______ 2. gram

_______ 3. kilogram

_______ 4. liter

_______ 5. microgram

_______ 6. milliliter

C. Metric Notations: Practice Problems

To read prescriptions and medication orders, to record medication administration, and to avoid medication errors, the MA must be able to use metric notation guidelines. Review the Metric Notation Guidelines on page 633 of your textbook before completing the following practice problems. In the space provided, use metric notation guidelines to indicate the dose quantities.

_______ 1. 25 milligrams

_______ 2. 5 grams

_______ 3. 1½ liters

_______ 4. 10 milliliters

_______ 5. ½ gram

_______ 6. 50 milligrams

_______ 7. 4 milliliters

_______ 8. 2 kilograms

_______ 9. 120 milliliters

_______ 10. ½ gram

_______ 11. 250 milligrams

_______ 12. ½ liter

_______ 13. 500 milliliters

_______ 14. 5 kilograms

_______ 15. 2½ grams

UNIT 2: THE HOUSEHOLD SYSTEM

The household system is a more complicated and less accurate method for administering medication than the metric system. However, most individuals are familiar with this system because of its frequent use in the United States. This system of measurement may be the only one the patient can fully relate to and therefore may safely use to administer liquid medication at home.

A. Units of Measurement: Practice Problems

Volume is the only household unit of measurement used to administer medication. The basic unit of liquid volume is the drop. The remaining units, in order of increasing volume, are the teaspoon, tablespoon, ounce, cup, and glass. In the space provided, indicate the correct abbreviation for each of the household units of measurement listed.

_______ 1. drop

_______ 2. teaspoon

_______ 3. tablespoon

_______ 4. ounce

UNIT 3: MEDICATION ORDERS

A. Medical Abbreviations: Practice Problems

To safely administer medication, the MA must be completely familiar with common medical abbreviations. Review Table 26-5 in your textbook before completing the following practice problems. In the space provided, write the meaning of the following medical abbreviations.

_______ 1. NPO

_______ 2. prn

_______ 3. tab

_______ 4. ac

_______ 5. DAW

_______ 6. pc

_______ 7. qid

_______ 8. $\bar{c}$

_______ 9. $\bar{s}$

_______ 10. bid

_______ 11. tid

_______ 12. qh

_______ 13. gtts

_______ 14. q4h

_______ 15. qs

_______ 16. IM

_______ 17. caps

_______ 18. po

_______ 19. ad lib

_______ 20. $\overline{aa}$

_______ 21. OTC

_______ 22. subcut

_______ 23. per

_______ 24. SL

_______ 25. STAT

B. Interpreting Medication Orders: Practice Problems

To safely administer medication and instruct patients on administering medication at home, the medical assistant must be able to interpret medication orders. Interpret the following medication orders, and using a drug reference, indicate the drug category based on action and a brand name for each medication.

1. Tetracycline 250 mg po qid × 10 days

 ____

 Drug category: ______________________________

 Brand name: ______________________________

2. Lansoprazole 30 mg po every day ac

 ____

 Drug category: ______________________________

 Brand name: ______________________________

3. Alprazolam 0.25 mg po tid

 ____

 Drug category: ______________________________

 Brand name: ______________________________

4. Diltiazem 50 mg po q4h

 ____

 Drug category: ______________________________

 Brand name: ______________________________

5. Ciprofloxacin 500 mg q12h

 ____

 Drug category: ______________________________

 Brand name: ______________________________

6. Hydrocodone/acetaminophen 5 mg q4h prn

 ____

 Drug category: ______________________________

 Brand name: ______________________________

7. Furosemide 40 mg po q AM

 ____

 Drug category: ______________________________

 Brand name: ______________________________

8. Paroxetine 20 mg po every day in AM

 ____

 Drug category: ______________________________

 Brand name: ______________________________

9. Cetirizine 5 mg po every day

____

Drug category: ______________________________

Brand name: ________________________________

10. Cyclobenzaprine 10 mg po tid × 1 wk

____

Drug category: ______________________________

Brand name: ________________________________

UNIT 4: CONVERTING UNITS OF MEASUREMENT

A. Using Conversion Tables

Changing from one unit of measurement to another is known as conversion. Conversion is required when medication is ordered in one unit of measurement and the medication label expresses the drug strength in a different unit. The dose quantity must be mathematically translated or converted to the unit of measurement of the medication on hand. For example, if the physician orders 5 grams of an oral solid medication and the medication label expresses the drug strength in milligrams, the medical assistant must convert the grams into milligrams to know how much medication to administer. Converting units of measurement can be classified as follows:

1. Conversion of units within a measurement system
2. Conversion of units from one measurement system to another

Converting units within a measurement system allows a quantity to be expressed in a different but equal unit of measurement within the same system. An example of converting between units of weight within the metric system is as follows: 1 gram is equal to 1000 milligrams.

Converting from one measurement system to another allows a quantity to be expressed in a unit of measurement of another system. An example of a conversion between the household and metric systems is as follows: 1 ounce (household system) is equivalent to 30 milliliters (metric system). Methods used to convert units of measurement are presented in this unit and in Unit 5.

Conversion requires the use of a conversion table to indicate the equivalent values between units of measurement. The practice problems that follow can assist you in attaining competency in using conversion tables.

Conversion Tables: Practice Problems

Refer to the conversion tables at the end of this chapter. Locate and record the equivalent value for each of the units of measurement listed.

		ANSWER
1. 1 g	=	_______ mg
2. 1 ounce	=	_______ mL
3. 1 tablespoon	=	_______ teaspoons
4. 1 mg	=	_______ mcg
5. 1 liter	=	_______ mL
6. 1 kiloliter	=	_______ liters
7. 1 teacup	=	_______ ounces
8. 1 teaspoon	=	_______ drops
9. 1 mL	=	_______ cc
10. 1 cup	=	_______ ounces
11. 1 drop	=	_______ mL

		ANSWER	
12. 1 kg	=	______	g
13. 1 mL	=	______	drops
14. 1 teaspoon	=	______	mL
15. 1 ounce	=	______	tablespoons
16. 1 tablespoon	=	______	mL
17. 1 ounce	=	______	teaspoons
18. 1 glass	=	______	mL
19. 1 teaspoon	=	______	mL
20. 1 glass	=	______	ounces

B. Converting Units within the Metric System

Drug administration often requires conversion within the metric system to prepare the correct dose. Metric conversion involves converting a larger unit to a smaller unit (e.g., grams to milligrams) or converting a smaller unit to a larger unit (e.g., milliliters to liters). Methods used to convert one metric unit to another are described in the next sections.

Converting a Larger Unit to a Smaller Unit

Converting a larger unit to a smaller unit within the metric system can be accomplished using one of three methods. The method chosen is based on personal preference and the level of difficulty of the conversion problem. For example, more difficult problems require the use of ratio and proportion as the method of conversion. Examples of converting a larger unit to a smaller unit are as follows:

1. grams to milligrams
2. liters to milliliters
3. kilograms to grams

METHODS OF CONVERSION: To convert a larger unit to a smaller unit within the metric system, use one of the following:

Method 1: Multiply the unit to be changed by 1000.
Method 2: Move the decimal point of the unit to be changed three places to the right.
Method 3: Ratio and proportion (see Unit 5).

GUIDELINE: When converting a larger unit to a smaller unit, expect the quantity to become larger. Use this guideline to assist in making accurate conversions. The problems illustrate this guideline.

EXAMPLES

PROBLEM 2 L = ______ mL

Method 1: Multiply the unit to be changed by 1000.
$2 \times 1000 = 2000$ mL

Method 2: Move the decimal point of the unit to be changed three places to the right.
2.0 0 0. = 2000 mL

Answer 2 L = 2000 mL

PROBLEM $4\ g =$ ______ mg

Method 1: Multiply the unit to be changed by 1000.

$4 \times 1000 = 4000$ mg

Method 2: Move the decimal point of the unit to be changed three places to the right.

4.0 0 0. = 4000 mg

Answer	4 g = 4000 mg

Converting a Smaller Unit to a Larger Unit

Converting a smaller unit to a larger unit within the metric system can be accomplished using one of three methods of conversion as outlined below. Examples of converting a smaller unit to a larger unit are as follows:

1. milligrams to grams
2. milliliters to liters
3. grams to kilograms

> METHOD OF CONVERSION: To convert a smaller unit to a larger unit within the metric system, use one of the following:
>
> *Method 1*: Divide the unit to be changed by 1000.
> *Method 2*: Move the decimal point of the unit to be changed three places to the left.
> *Method 3*: Ratio and proportion (see Unit 5).
>
> GUIDELINE: When converting a smaller unit to a larger unit, expect the quantity to become smaller. The problems illustrate this guideline.

EXAMPLES

PROBLEM 250 mg = ______ g

Method 1: Divide the unit to be changed by 1000.

$250 \div 1000 = 0.25$ g

Method 2: Move the decimal point of the unit to be changed three places to the left.

.2 5 0. = 0.25 g

Answer	250 mg = 0.25 g

PROBLEM 1500 mL = ______ L

Method 1: Divide the unit to be changed by 1000.

$1500 \div 1000 = 1.5$ L

Method 2: Move the decimal point of the unit to be changed three places to the left.

1.5 0 0. = 1.5 L

Answer	1500 mL = 1.5 L

Converting Units within the Metric System: Practice Problems

Directions: Convert the following metric units of measurement using Method 1 or Method 2. In the space provided, indicate if the conversion is going from a larger to smaller unit (L→S) or smaller to larger unit (S→L).

		ANSWER	CONVERSION
1. 1 g	=	______ mg	____________
2. 750 mg	=	______ g	____________
3. 2 kg	=	______ g	____________

		ANSWER	CONVERSION
4. 1000 g	=	______ kg	______
5. 1.5 L	=	______ mL	______
6. 250 mL	=	______ L	______
7. 5 g	=	______ mg	______
8. 0.25 kg	=	______ g	______
9. 1000 mg	=	______ g	______
10. 2.5 g	=	______ mg	______
11. 475 mL	=	______ L	______
12. 0.05 g	=	______ mg	______
13. 0.5 L	=	______ mL	______
14. 1000 mL	=	______ L	______
15. 500 g	=	______ kg	______
16. 50 mg	=	______ g	______
17. 1 L	=	______ mL	______
18. 40 g	=	______ mg	______
19. 50 mL	=	______ L	______
20. 1 kg	=	______ g	______

C. Converting Units Within the Household System

Household system conversion involves converting a larger unit to a smaller unit (e.g., tablespoons to teaspoons) or converting a smaller unit to a larger unit (e.g., tablespoons to ounces). Methods used to convert one unit to another are described.

Converting a Larger Unit to a Smaller Unit

Converting a larger unit to a smaller unit within the household system is accomplished using the equivalent value method or the ratio and proportion method. The method chosen is based on personal preference and on the level of difficulty of the conversion problem. Examples of converting a larger unit to a smaller unit follow:

Volume:
teaspoons to drops
tablespoons to teaspoons
ounces to teaspoons
ounces to tablespoons
teacup to ounces
glass to ounces

METHOD OF CONVERSION: To convert a larger unit to a smaller unit within the household system, use one of the following:

Method 1:

a. Look at Table 26-2 (Household Conversion) at the end of this chapter to determine the equivalent value between the two units of measurement.
b. Multiply the equivalent value by the number next to the larger unit of measurement.

Method 2: Ratio and proportion (see Unit 5)

EXAMPLES

PROBLEM 2 tablespoons = _____ teaspoons

Method 1:

a. Look at the conversion table to determine the equivalent value:

1 tablespoon = 3 teaspoons

3 = the equivalent value

b. Multiply the equivalent value by the number next to the larger unit of measurement:

$2 \times 3 = 6$ teaspoons

Answer	2 tablespoons = 6 teaspoons

PROBLEM ½ teaspoon = _____ drops

Method 1:

a. Look at the conversion table to determine the equivalent value:

1 teaspoon = 60 drops

60 = the equivalent value

b. Multiply the equivalent value by the number next to the larger unit of measurement:

$\frac{1}{2} \times 60 = 30$ drops

Answer	½ tablespoon = 30 drops

Converting a Smaller Unit to a Larger Unit

Converting a smaller unit to a larger unit within the household system is accomplished using the equivalent value method or the ratio and proportion method. Examples of converting from a smaller unit to a larger unit follow:

Volume
drops to teaspoons
teaspoons to tablespoons
teaspoons to ounces
tablespoons to ounces
ounces to teacups
ounces to glasses

METHOD OF CONVERSION: To convert a smaller unit to a larger unit within the household system, use one of the following:

Method 1:

a. Look at Table 26-2 (Household Conversion) at the end of this chapter to determine the equivalent value between the two units of measurement.
b. Divide the equivalent value into the number next to the smaller unit of measurement.

Method 2: Ratio and proportion (see Unit 5).

EXAMPLES

PROBLEM 4 tablespoons = _____ ounces

Method 1:

a. Look at the conversion table to determine the equivalent value:

1 ounce = 2 tablespoons

2 = the equivalent value

b. Divide the equivalent value into the number next to the smaller unit of measurement:

$4 \div 2 = 2$ ounces

Answer	4 tablespoon = 2 ounces

PROBLEM 24 ounces = _____ glasses

Method 1:

a. Look at the conversion table to determine the equivalent value:

1 glass = 8 ounces

8 = the equivalent value

b. Divide the equivalent value into the number next to the smaller unit of measurement:

24 ÷ 8 = 3 glasses

Answer	24 ounces = 3 glasses

Converting Units within the Household System: Practice Problems

Directions: Convert the following household units of measurement using the equivalent value method of conversion. In the space provided, indicate the equivalent value for each problem.

		ANSWER	EQUIVALENT VALUE
1. 12 teaspoons	=	_______ ounces	_______________
2. 4 ounces	=	_______ glasses	_______________
3. 90 drops	=	_______ teaspoons	_______________
4. ½ ounce	=	_______ tablespoons	_______________
5. 6 teaspoons	=	_______ tablespoons	_______________
6. 3 tablespoons	=	_______ ounces	_______________
7. 18 ounces	=	_______ teacups	_______________
8. ½ ounce	=	_______ teaspoons	_______________
9. 3 tablespoons	=	_______ teaspoons	_______________
10. ½ teaspoon	=	_______ drops	_______________

UNIT 5: RATIO AND PROPORTION

Ratio and proportion are used to convert units of measurement. This method of conversion has the advantage of clarifying the mathematical rationale for the methods of conversion previously presented. It is also useful in converting units of measurement that are more difficult to calculate, such as converting between systems, such as when converting a metric unit of measurement to a household unit of measurement.

A. Ratio and Proportion Guidelines

Some guidelines must be followed when using ratio and proportion:

1. A ratio is composed of two related numbers separated by a colon. It indicates the relationship between two quantities or numbers. The ratio example shows a relationship between milligrams and grams (i.e., 1000 mg = 1 g).

   EXAMPLE 1000 mg : 1 g

2. A proportion shows the relationship between two equal ratios. The proportion consists of two ratios separated by an equal sign (=), which indicates that the two ratios are equal. This proportion example shows the relationship between two equal ratios of milligrams and grams.

   EXAMPLE 1000 mg : 1 g = 2000 mg : 2 g

3. The units of measurement in the two ratios of a proportion must be expressed in the same sequence. The correct sequencing in the proportion example is mg : g = mg : g, not mg : g = g : mg.

   EXAMPLE *Correct:* 1000 mg : 1 g = 2000 mg : 2 g
   Incorrect: 1000 mg : 1 g = 2 g : 2000 mg

4. The numbers on the ends of a proportion are called the extremes, and the numbers in the middle of the proportion are known as the means. In this example, the means consist of 1 g and 2000 mg, and the extremes are 1000 mg and 2 g.

EXAMPLE 1000 mg : 1 g = 2000 mg : 2 g
(means: 1 g and 2000 mg; extremes: 1000 mg and 2 g)

5. The product of the means equals the product of the extremes. The calculation of the product of the means in the example is $1 \times 2000 = 2000$. The calculation of the product of the extremes is $1000 \times 2 = 2000$. The product of the means equals the product of the extremes or $2000 = 2000$.

EXAMPLE 1000 mg : 1 g = 2000 mg : 2 g

$$1 \times 2000 = 1000 \times 2$$

$$2000 = 2000$$

6. In setting up a proportion, one side of the equation consists of the known quantities, and the other side of the equation consists of the unknown quantity. The letter x is commonly used to express the unknown quantity. To be consistent, the known quantities are indicated on the left side of the equation, and the unknown quantity is indicated on the right side of the equation. Using the previous proportion example, but inserting an unknown quantity, or x, the equation is set up as follows:

EXAMPLE 1000 mg : 1 g = x mg : 2 g
(known quantities) (unknown quantity)

Ratio and Proportion: Practice Problems

Answer the following questions.

1. What is a ratio?

____

2. In the space provided, place a check mark next to each correct example of a ratio.

_______ a. 1000 mg x 10 grams

_______ b. 1000 mL = 1 L

_______ c. 1 mg : 1000 mcg

_______ d. 1000mg/1 gram

_______ e. 1 tablespoons : 1 ounce

_______ f. 1 mL : 1 cc

3. What is a proportion?

____

____

____

4. In the space provided, place a check mark next to each correct example of a proportion.

_______ a. 1 mL : 1 cc

_______ b. 2 tablespoons : 1 ounce 4 tablespoons : 2 ounces

_______ c. 2x = 60 mg

_______ d. 1000 mL : 1 L = 500 mL : 0.5 L

_______ e. 1000 mg : 1 gram = 1000 mL : 1 L

5. In the space provided, place a check mark next to each proportion that has correct sequencing for the units of measurement.

_______ a. 1000 g : 1 kg = 1500 g : 1.5 kg

_______ b. 3 teaspoons : 1 tablespoon = 2 tablespoons : 6 teaspoonsc.1000 mg : 1 g = 2000 mg : *x* g

6. Circle the means and underline the extremes in each of the following proportions:

a. 1000 mg : 1 g = 500 mg : 0.5 g

b. 8 ounces : 1 glass = 16 ounces : 2 glassesc.1 mL : 1 cc = 2 mL : 2cc

7. In each of the following proportions, what is the product of the means, and what is the product of the extremes?

a. 1000 g : 1 kg = 1500 g : 1.5 kg

_______ product of the means

_______ product of the extremes

b. 60 drops : 1 teaspoon = 120 drops : 2 teaspoons

_______ product of the means

_______ product of the extremes

c. 1 ounce : 30 mL = 4 ounces : 120 mL _______ product of the means

_______ product of the extremes

8. In each of the following proportions, circle the known quantities and underline the unknown quantity.

a. 1000 mg : 1 g = 500 mg : *x* g

b. 2 tablespoons : 1 ounce = 6 tablespoons : *x* ouncesc.1000 mL : 1 L = *x* mL : 2 L

B. Converting Units Using Ratio and Proportion

Units can be converted using ratio and proportion.

METHOD OF CONVERSION: To convert a unit of measurement using ratio and proportion, use the following steps:

a. Look at the appropriate conversion table at the end of this chapter to determine what is known about the two units of measurement (equivalent value).
b. State the known quantities as a ratio.
c. Determine the unknown quantity.
d. State the unknown quantity as a ratio.
e. Set up the proportion with the known quantities on the left side and the unknown quantity on the right side of the equation.
f. To solve the equation, multiply the product of the means and the product of the extremes. Divide the equation by the numbers before the x.
g. Include the unit of measure corresponding to x in the original equation with the answer.

EXAMPLES

PROBLEM $2\ g =$ ________ mg

a. Look at Table 26-1 (Metric Conversion) to determine what is known about the two units of measurement:

   $1000\ mg = 1\ g$

b. State the known quantities as a ratio:

   $1000\ mg : 1\ g$

c. Determine the unknown quantity:

   $2\ g = x\ mg$

d. State the unknown quantity as a ratio using the correct unit of measurement sequencing:

   $x\ mg : 2\ g$

e. Set up the proportion with the known quantities on the left side and the unknown quantity on the right side of the equation:

   $1000\ mg : 1\ g = x\ mg : 2\ g$

f. Solve the equation by multiplying the product of the means and the product of the extremes and dividing the equation by the number before the x:

   $1000\ mg : 1\ g = x\ mg : 2\ g$

   $1 \times x = 1000 \times 2$

   $1x = 2000$

   $x = 2000$

g. Include the unit of measure corresponding to x in the original equation with the answer:

   $x = 2000\ mg$

Answer	2 g = 2000 mg

PROBLEM

4 ounces = ________ mL

The steps previously outlined are followed here. However, they are combined as they would be in working an actual conversion problem.

$1\ ounce : 30\ mL = 4\ ounces : x\ mL$

$30 \times 4 = 1 \times x$

$120 = 1\ x$

$x = 120\ mL$

Answer	4 ounces = 120 mL

Converting Units Using Ratio and Proportion: Practice Problems

Directions: Use ratio and proportion to convert between the metric, and household systems by completing the problems below. In the space at the right, indicate what is known regarding the two units of measurement.

			ANSWER	KNOWN QUANTITIES
1.	30 drops	=	_______ mL	____________
2.	2 ounces	=	_______ mL	____________
3.	90 mL	=	_______ ounces	____________
4.	2 glasses	=	_______ mL	____________
5.	360 mL	=	_______ teacups	____________
6.	10 mL	=	_______ teaspoons	____________
7.	60 drops	=	_______ mL	____________
8.	60 mL	=	_______ tablespoons	____________
9.	3 teaspoons	=	_______ mL	____________
10.	5 mL	=	_______ drops	____________

UNIT 6: DETERMINING DRUG DOSE

A. Oral Administration

Dose refers to the amount of medication to be administered to the patient. Each medication has a certain dose range or range of quantities that produce therapeutic effects. It is important to administer the exact drug dose. If the dose is too small, it will not produce a therapeutic effect, whereas too large a dose could harm or even kill the patient. The steps to follow in determining drug dose depend on the unit of measurement in which the drug is ordered and the unit of measurement of the drug you have available, or the dose on hand.

1. If the dose on hand is the same as that ordered, no calculation is required. In this example, the dose ordered and the dose on hand are in the same unit of measurement, and one tablet is administered to the patient.

   EXAMPLE The physician orders 50 mg of a medication po.
   The drug label reads 50 mg/tablet.

2. If the dose ordered is in the same unit of measurement as that indicated on the medication label, only one calculation step is required. In this example, the dose ordered and the dose on hand are in the same unit of measurement, or milligrams. The calculation determines the number of tablets to administer to the patient.

   EXAMPLE The physician orders 500 mg of a medication po.
   The drug label reads 250 mg/tablet.

3. If the dose ordered is in a different unit of measurement than indicated on the drug label, two calculation steps are required to determine the amount of medication to administer to the patient. In this example, the dose ordered and the dose on hand are stated in different units of measurement, or in grams and milligrams. The first step requires conversion of the dose ordered to the unit of measurement of the dose on hand; in this example, grams must be converted to milligrams. The second step is to determine the number of tablets to administer to the patient.

   EXAMPLE The physician orders 1 g of a medication po.
   The drug label reads 500 mg/tablet.

A detailed discussion of determining drug dose for administration of oral medication follows. The method used to calculate drug dose when the units of measurement are the same is presented first, followed by the method used when the units of measurement are different.

Determining Drug Dose with the Same Units of Measurement

Determining the correct drug dose to be administered when the units of measurement are the same requires the use of a drug dose formula.

> DRUG DOSE FORMULA
>
> D (*dose ordered*) / H (on hand) × V (vehicle) = x (Amount of medication to be administered)
>
> D (*dose ordered*): This is the amount of medication ordered by the physician.
>
> H (*drug strength on hand*): This is the dose strength available as indicated on the medication label or the dose on hand.
>
> V (*vehicle*): The vehicle refers to the type of preparation containing the dose on hand (e.g., tablet, capsule, liquid).
>
> x: The letter x is used to express the unknown quantity or the amount of medication to be administered.
>
> GUIDELINES
>
> 1. The units of measurement must be included when setting up the problem.
> 2. The values for D and H must be in the same unit of measurement.
> 3. The value of x is expressed in the same unit as V.
> 4. When determining the drug dose for oral liquid medication, the vehicle must also include the amount of liquid in which the available drug is contained. For example, if the medication label reads 250 mg/5 mL, the value of V is 5 mL.

The method to follow to determine drug dose using this formula is outlined in the following examples. The first problem illustrates determining dose for solid medication taken orally.

EXAMPLES

PROBLEM *Oral* solid medication:
The physician orders 50 mg of a medication po.
The medication label reads 25 mg/tablet.
How much medication should be administered to the patient?

Drug dose formula:

$D/H \times V = x$

a. Identify the dose ordered.
$D = 50$ mg

b. Identify the strength of the drug on hand.
$H = 25$ mg

c. Determine the vehicle containing the dose on hand.
$V = 1$ tablet

d. Calculate the amount of medication to administer to the patient. The units of measurement must be included when setting up the problem, and the values for D and H must be in the same unit of measurement. The value of x is expressed in the same unit as V; in this problem V = 1 tablet.

$50 \text{ mg}/25 \text{ mg} \times 1 \text{ tablet} = x$

$(50 \div 25 = 2) \times 1 \text{ tablet} = x$

$2 \times 1 \text{ tablet} = x$

$x = 2$ tablets

> ***Answer*** 2 tablets administered to the patient

The next problem illustrates the determination of drug dose for liquid medication taken orally. The steps previously outlined are followed; however, they are combined as should be done when working out drug dose problems. Remember, with oral liquid medication, the vehicle must also include the amount of liquid in which the available drug is contained; in the following problem, V = 5 mL.

PROBLEM *Oral liquid medication:*
The physician orders 500 mg of a medication.
The medication label reads 250 mg/5 mL.
How much medication should be administered to the patient?

$D/H \times 1 \text{ tablet} = x$

$500 \text{ mg}/250 \text{ mg} \times 1 \text{ tablet} = x$

$(500 \div 250 = 2) \times 5 \text{ mL} = x$

$2 \times 5 \text{ mL} = x$

$x = 10 \text{ mL}$

Answer	A dose of 10 mL of medication is administered to the patient.

Determining Drug Dose with Different Units of Measurement

Sometimes, the medication ordered is in a different unit of measurement than indicated on the drug label. In this case, the desired dose quantity must be converted to the unit of measurement of the dose on hand before the drug dose is determined. The method chosen to convert a unit of measurement is based on personal preference. Refer to Units 4 and 5 to review methods of conversion before completing this section.

> The following steps are required to determine drug dose when the units of measurement are different:
>
> *Step 1:* Convert the dose quantities to the same unit of measurement. For consistency, it is best to convert to the unit of measurement of the drug on hand.
>
> *Step 2:* Determine the amount of medication to administer to the patient, using the drug dose formula.

EXAMPLES

PROBLEM *Oral solid medication:*
The physician orders .5 gram of medication po.
The medication label reads 250 mg/tablet.
How much medication should be administered to the patient?

Step 1: The dose ordered must be converted to the unit of measurement of the medication on hand. In this problem, .5 gram must be converted to milligrams. The ratio and proportion method of conversion is used to make the conversion.

1 gram = _____ mg

$1 \text{ gram} : 1000 \text{ mg} = .5 \text{ gram} : x \text{ mg}$

$500 = 1\,x$

$x = 500 \text{ mg}$

Answer	.5 gram = 500 mg

The medication ordered is in the same unit of measurement as the medication on hand.
Step 2: Determine the amount of medication to administer to the patient using the drug dose formula.

$D/H \times V = x$

$500\ mg/250\ mg \times 1$ tablet

$(500 \div 250 = 2) \times 1$ tablet $= x$

2×1 tablet $= x$

$x = 2$ tablets

Answer	A dose of 2 tablets is administered to the patient.

PROBLEM *Oral liquid medication:*
The physician orders .5 gram of a medication po.
The medication label reads 125 mg/5mL
How much medication should be administered to the patient?

Step 1: Convert .5 gram to milligrams using ratio and proportion:

.5 gram = _____ mg

1 gram : 1000 mg = .5 gram : x mg

$1\ x = 500$ mg

$x = 500$ mg

Answer	.5 gram = 500 mg

Step 2: Determine the amount of medication to administer to the patient using the drug dose formula.

$D/H \times V = x$

$500\ mg/125\ mg \times 5\ mL = x$

$(500 \div 125 = 4) \times 5\ mL = x$

$4 \times 5\ mL = x$

$x = 20\ mL$

Answer	A dose of 20 mL of medication is administered to the patient.

Oral Administration: Practice Problems

Directions: Determine the drug dose to be administered for each of the following oral medication orders, and record your answer below. In the space provided, indicate the drug category based on action for each medication using a drug reference.

Oral Solid Medications

1. The physician orders Inderal 160 mg po.
   Medication label:

Inderal propranolol 80 mg/capsule

   How much medication should be administered? ______________________

   Drug category: ______________________

2. The physician orders Tagamet 600 mg po.
   Medication label:

Tagamet cimetidine 300 mg/tablet

   How much medication should be administered? ______________________

   Drug category: ______________________

3. The physician orders Amoxil 0.5 g po.
   Medication label:

Amoxil amoxicillin 250 mg/capsule

   How much medication should be administered? ______________________

   Drug category: ______________________

4. The physician orders Lasix 80 mg po.
   Medication label:

Lasix furosemide 40 mg/tablet

   How much medication should be administered? ______________________

   Drug category: ______________________

5. The physician orders Lomotil 5 mg po.
   Medication label:

Lomotil diphenoxylate/atropine 2.5 mg/tablet

   How much medication should be administered? ______________________

   Drug category: ______________________

6. The physician orders Zithromax 0.5 g po.
Medication label:

Zithromax azithromycin 250 mg/tablet

How much medication should be administered? ______________________________

Drug category: ______________________________

7. The physician orders Calan 120 mg po.
Medication label:

Calan verapamil 40 mg/tablet

How much medication should be administered? ______________________________

Drug category: ______________________________

8. The physician orders Xanax 0.5 mg po.
Medication label:

Xanax alprazolam 0.25 mg/tablet

How much medication should be administered? ______________________________

Drug category: ______________________________

9. The physician orders Phenergan 25 mg po.
Medication label:

Phenergan promethazine 12.5 mg/tablet

How much medication should be administered? ______________________________

Drug category: ______________________________

10. The physician orders Procardia XL 30 mg po.
Medication label:

Procardia nifedipine 10 mg/tablet

How much medication should be administered? ______________________________

Drug category: ______________________________

Oral Liquid Medications

1. The physician orders Sumycin Suspension 250 mg po.
Medication label:

Sumycin Suspension tetracycline 125 mg/5 mL

How much medication should be administered? ______________________________

Drug category: ______________________________

2. The physician orders Tagamet liquid 300 mg po.
Medication label:

Tagamet Cimetidine liquid 300 mg/5 mL

How much medication should be administered? ______________________________

Drug category: ______________________________

3. The physician orders Tylenol Elixir 60 mg po.
Medication label:

Tylenol Elixir acetaminophen 120 mg/5 mL

How much medication should be administered? ______________________________

Drug category: ______________________________

4. The physician orders Amoxil Suspension 0.5 g po.
Medication label:

Amoxil Suspension amoxicillin 125 mg/5 mL

How much medication should be administered? ______________________________

Drug category: ______________________________

5. The physician orders Gantanol Suspension 1 g po.
Medication label:

Gantanol Suspension sulfamethoxazole 500 mg/5 mL

How much medication should be administered? ______________________________

Drug category: ______________________________

B. Parenteral Administration

Medications for parenteral administration must be suspended in solution. The medication label indicates the amount of the drug contained in each milliliter of solution. For example, if a medication label reads 10 mg/mL, there are 10 mg of medication for each 1 mL of liquid volume. Some medications, such as penicillin, insulin, and heparin, are ordered and measured in units (e.g., 300,000 units/mL). This refers to their biologic activity in animal tests or the amount of the drug that is required to produce a particular response.

Parenteral medication is available in several dispensing forms, including ampules, single-dose vials, and multiple-dose vials. After the proper drug dose has been determined, the medication is drawn into a syringe from the dispensing unit. Most syringes are calibrated in milliliters (mL).

Determining drug dose for parenteral administration is calculated in a similar manner as that for oral liquid medication. The first problem illustrates the determination of drug dose when the medication is ordered in a different unit of measurement from the dose on hand, requiring two calculation steps.

EXAMPLES

PROBLEM The physician orders 0.5 g of a medication IM.
The medication label reads 250 mg/2 mL.
How much medication should be administered?

Step 1: Convert 0.5 gram to milligrams.

$0.5\ \text{g} = \text{mg}$

$1000\ \text{mg} : 1\ \text{g} = x\ \text{mg} : 0.5\ \text{g}$

$1\,x = 500$

$x = 500\ \text{mg}$

Answer	0.5 mg = 500 mg

Step 2: Determine the amount of medication to administer to the patient:

$\text{D/H} \times \text{V} = \text{x}$

$500\ \text{mg}/250\ \text{mg} \times 2\ \text{mL} = x$

$(500 \div 250 = 2) \times 2\ \text{mL} = x$

$2 \times 2\ \text{mL} = x$

$x = 4\ \text{mL}$

Answer	A dose of 4 mL of medication is administered to the patient

The next problem illustrates the determination of drug dose with a medication ordered in units. Notice that the dose ordered and the dose on hand are in the same unit of measurement; therefore, conversion of units of measurement is not necessary.

PROBLEM The physician orders 600,000 units of a medication IM.
The medication label reads 300,000 units/mL.
How much medication should be administered?

$\text{D/H} \times \text{V} = \text{x}$

$6000{,}000\ \text{units}/300{,}000\ \text{units} \times 1\ \text{mL} = x$

$(600{,}000, 300{,}000 = 2) \times 1\ \text{mL} = x$

$x = 2\ \text{mL}$

Answer	A dose of 2 mL of medication is administered to the patient.

Parenteral Administration: Practice Problems

Determine the drug dose to be administered for each of the following parenteral medication orders, and record your answer. In the space provided, indicate the drug category based on action using a drug reference.

1. The physician orders Vistaril 75 mg IM.
   Medication label:

Vistaril hydroxyzine injection 50 mg/mL

   How much medication should be administered? ____________________

   Drug category: ____________________

2. The physician orders Cobex (vitamin B_{12}) 200 mcg IM.
   Medication label:

Cobex cyanocobalamin injection 100 mcg/mL

   How much medication should be administered? ____________________

   Drug category: ____________________

3. The physician orders Depo-Medrol 40 mg IM.
   Medication label:

Depo-Medrol methylprednisolone injection 80 mg/mL

   How much medication should be administered? ____________________

   Drug category: ____________________

4. The physician orders Wycillin 600,000 units IM.
   Medication label:

Wycillin porcine penicillin G injection 300,000 units/mL

   How much medication should be administered? ____________________

   Drug category: ____________________

5. The physician orders Rocephin 1000 mg IM.
Medication label:

Rocephin ceftriaxone injection 1 g/mL

How much medication should be administered? ______________________

Drug category: ______________________

6. The physician orders INFeD 100 mg IM.
Medication label:

INFeD iron dextran injection 50 mg/mL

How much medication should be administered? ______________________

Drug category: ______________________

7. The physician orders Bicillin 1.2 million units IM.
Medication label:

Bicillin benzathine penicillin G injection 600,000 units/mL

How much medication should be administered? ______________________

Drug category: ______________________

8. The physician orders Depo-Provera 150 mg IM.
Medication label:

Depo-Provera medroxyprogesterone 150 mg/mL

How much medication should be administered? ______________________

Drug category: ______________________

9. The physician orders Pronestyl 0.25 g IM.
Medication label:

Pronestyl procainamide injection 500 mg/mL

How much medication should be administered? ______________________

Drug category: ______________________

10. The physician orders Compazine 7 mg IM.
Medication label:

Compazine prochlorperazine injection 5 mg/mL

How much medication should be administered? ______________________________

Drug category: ______________________________

Table 26-1. Metric System Conversion of Equivalent Values
WEIGHT
1000 micrograms = 1 milligram
1000 milligrams = 1 gram
1000 grams = 1 kilogram
VOLUME
1000 milliliters = 1 liter
1000 liters = 1 kiloliter
1 milliliter = 1 cubic centimeter

Table 26-2. Household System: Conversion of Equivalent Values
ABBREVIATIONS
drop : gtt
teaspoon : tsp
tablespoon : T
ounce : oz
cup : c
VOLUME
60 drops = 1 teaspoon
3 teaspoons = 1 tablespoon
6 teaspoons = 1 ounce
2 tablespoons = 1 ounce
6 ounces = 1 teacup
8 ounces = 1 glass
8 ounces = 1 cup

Table 26-3. Conversion Chart for Household and Metric Equivalents (Volume)

Household	Metric
1 drop	= 0.06 mL
15 drops	= 1 mL (cc)
1 teaspoon	= 5 (4) mL
1 tablespoon	= 15 mL
2 tablespoons	= 30 mL
1 ounce	= 30 mL
1 teacup	= 180 mL
1 glass	= 240 mL

Notes

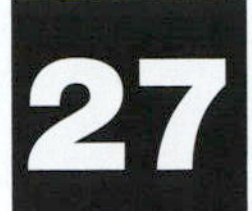

27 Cardiopulmonary Procedures

CHAPTER ASSIGNMENTS

✓ After Completing	Date Due	Study Guide Pages	STUDY GUIDE ASSIGNMENTS (CTA = Critical Thinking Activity)	Possible Points	Points You Earned
		755	Pretest	10	
		756 756-757	Term Key Term Assessment A. Definitions B. Word Parts (Add 1 point for each key term)	21 15	
		757-764	Evaluation of Learning questions	54	
		764	CTA A: Chest Leads	5	
			Evolve Activity: Find That Lead (Record points earned)		
		764	CTA B: ECG Cycle	10	
			Evolve Site: It's a Cycle (Record points earned)		
			Evolve Site: It's an Artifact (Record points earned)		
		765-768	CTA C: Myocardial Infarction	20	
		769	CTA D: Crossword Puzzle	22	
			Evolve Site: Apply Your Knowledge questions	10	
			Evolve Site: Video Evaluation	33	
		755	Posttest	10	
			ADDITIONAL ASSIGNMENTS		
			TOTAL POINTS		

Notes

✓ When Assigned By Your Instructor	Study Guide Pages	Practices Required	LABORATORY ASSIGNMENTS (Procedure Number and Name)	Score*
	771-772	3	**Practice for Competency** 27-1: Running a 12-Lead, Three-Channel Electrocardiogram Textbook reference: pp. 701-704	
	773-775		**Evaluation of Competency** 27-1: Running a 12-Lead, Three-Channel Electrocardiogram	*
	771-772	3	**Practice for Competency** 27-A: Spirometry Testing Textbook reference: p. 706	
	777-779		**Evaluation of Competency** 27-A: Spirometry Testing	*
	771-772	3	**Practice for Competency** 27-2: Measuring Peak Flow Rate Textbook reference: pp. 711-713	
	781-783		**Evaluation of Competency** 27-2: Measuring Peak Flow Rate	*
			ADDITIONAL ASSIGNMENTS	

Notes

Name ______________________________ Date ______________

PRETEST

True or False

_______ 1. The cardiac cycle represents one complete heartbeat.

_______ 2. The portion of the ECG between two waves is known as a segment.

_______ 3. A standard electrocardiogram consists of 10 leads.

_______ 4. An electrolyte facilitates the transmission of electrical impulses.

_______ 5. Leads V_1 through V_6 are known as the augmented leads.

_______ 6. Electrodes that are too loose can cause a 60-cycle interference artifact.

_______ 7. When running an ECG, the medical assistant should work on the left side of the patient.

_______ 8. An electrocardiographic (ECG) result that is within normal limits is said to indicate a normal sinus rhythm.

_______ 9. The purpose of a pulmonary function test is to assess cardiac functioning.

_______ 10. During an asthma attack, the bronchial tubes constrict, swell, and become clogged with mucus.

POSTTEST

True or False

_______ 1. An electrocardiogram is a recording of the electrical activity of the heart.

_______ 2. The amplifier is a device placed on the skin that picks up electrical impulses released by the heart.

_______ 3. The P wave represents the contraction of the ventricles.

_______ 4. If the electrocardiograph is standardized, the standardization mark will be 20 mm high.

_______ 5. A muscle artifact can be identified by its fuzzy, irregular baseline.

_______ 6. A spirometer measures how much air is exhaled from the lungs and how fast it is exhaled.

_______ 7. Spirometry can be used to assess a patient with emphysema.

_______ 8. Quick-relief asthma medication is used to prevent asthma symptoms.

_______ 9. The amount of supplemental oxygen prescribed for a patient is known as the flow rate.

_______ 10. A nasal cannula interferes with a patient's ability to talk, eat, and drink.

Term KEY TERM ASSESSMENT

A. Definitions

Directions: Match each key term with its definition.

_______ 1. Artifact
_______ 2. Atherosclerosis
_______ 3. Baseline
_______ 4. Cardiac cycle
_______ 5. Dysrhythmia
_______ 6. ECG cycle
_______ 7. Electrocardiogram
_______ 8. Electrocardiograph
_______ 9. Flow rate
_______ 10. Electrode
_______ 11. Electrolyte
_______ 12. Hypoxemia
_______ 13. Hypoxia
_______ 14. Interval
_______ 15. Ischemia
_______ 16. Normal sinus rhythm
_______ 17. Oxygen therapy
_______ 18. Peak flow rate
_______ 19. Segment
_______ 20. Spirometer
_______ 21. Wheezing

A. A chemical substance that promotes conduction of an electrical current
B. The flat, horizontal line that separates the various waves of the ECG cycle
C. The instrument used to record the electrical activity of the heart
D. Additional electrical activity picked up by the electrocardiograph that interferes with the normal appearance of the ECG cycles
E. Refers to an electrocardiogram that is within normal limits
F. One complete heartbeat
G. The graphic representation of the electrical activity of the heart
H. The length of a wave or the length of a wave with a segment
I. The graphic representation of a heartbeat
J. A conductor of electricity, which is used to promote contact between the body and the electrocardiograph
K. The portion of the ECG between two waves
L. Deficiency of blood in a body part
M. An instrument for measuring air taken into and expelled from the lungs
N. Buildup of fibrous plaques of fatty deposits and cholesterol on the inner walls of an artery that causes narrowing, obstruction, and hardening of the artery
O. An irregular heart rate or rhythm
P. The number of liters of oxygen per minute that come out of an oxygen delivery system
Q. A decrease in the oxygen saturation of the blood
R. A reduction in the oxygen supply to the tissues of the body
S. The administration of supplemental oxygen at concentrations greater than room air to treat or prevent hypoxemia
T. The maximum volume of air that can be exhaled when a patient blows into a peak flow meter as forcefully and as rapidly as possible
U. A continuous, high-pitched whistling musical sound heard particularly during exhalation and sometimes during inhalation

B. Word Parts

Directions: Indicate the meaning of each word part in the space provided. List as many medical terms as possible that incorporate the word part in the space provided.

Word Part	Meaning of Word Part	Medical Terms That Incorporate Word Part
1. ather/o		
2. -sclerosis		
3. cardi/o		
4. electr/o		
5. cardi/o		
6. -gram		
7. -graph		
8. hypo-		

Word Part	Meaning of Word Part	Medical Terms That Incorporate Word Part
9. ox/i		
10. -emia		
11. -ia		
12. isch/o		
13. spir/o		
14. -meter		
15. -metry		

EVALUATION OF LEARNING

Directions: Fill in each blank with the correct answer.

1. What is the purpose of electrocardiography?

____

____

____

2. What is the cardiac cycle?

____

3. Label the following on the ECG cycle:

P wave   P–R segment

QRS complex   ST segment

T wave   P–R interval

Q–T interval

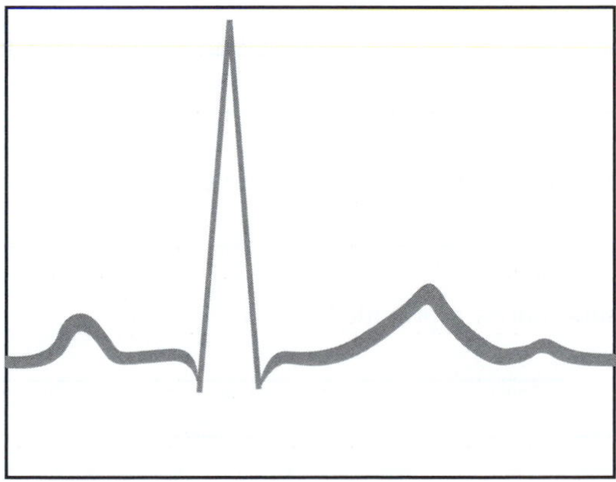

4. Explain what each component of the ECG cycle represents.

P wave ______

QRS complex ______

T wave ______

P–R segment ______

ST segment ______

P–R interval ______

Q–T interval ______

5. Why is the R wave taller than the P wave on the ECG graph cycle?

______

______

6. Why does atrial repolarization not appear as a separate wave on the ECG cycle?

______

______

7. Why is the baseline flat following the U wave?

______

______

8. What changes can occur on an ECG due to the following?

a. Coronary artery disease: ______

b. Myocardial infarction: ______

9. What is the purpose of standardizing the electrocardiograph?

______

______

______

10. How high should the standardization mark be when the electrocardiograph is standardized?

______

11. What is a lead, and what information does it provide?

______

______

12. What is the function of an electrode?

______

______

13. What is the function of each of the following?

    a. Amplifier: ______________________________

    b. Galvanometer: ______________________________

    c. Thermal print head: ______________________________

14. Which electrode is used as a ground reference? ______________________________

15. Why must an electrolyte be used when recording an electrocardiogram?

    ____

    ____

    ____

16. Why should the expiration date on an electrode pouch be checked?

    ____

17. How should electrodes be stored?

    ____

    ____

18. Diagram the bipolar leads on the following illustration:

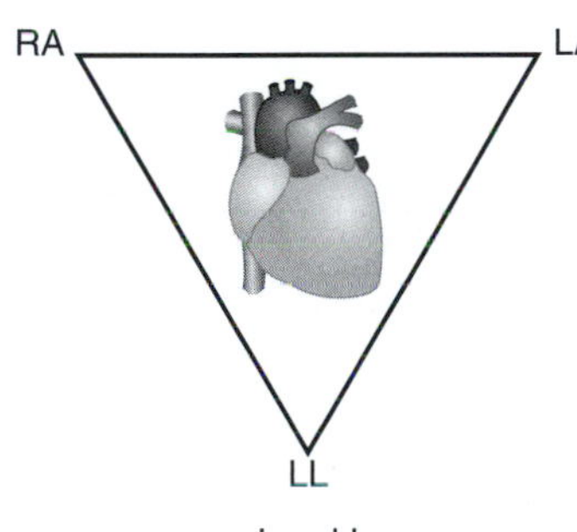

RA LA

LL

Lead II

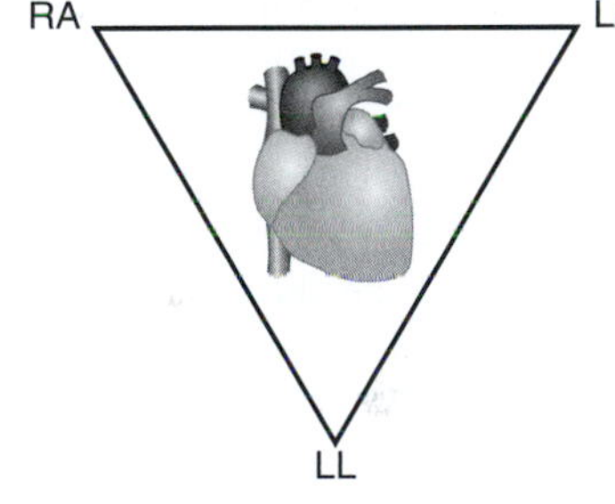

19. Locate and label the locations of the chest electrodes on the following illustration:

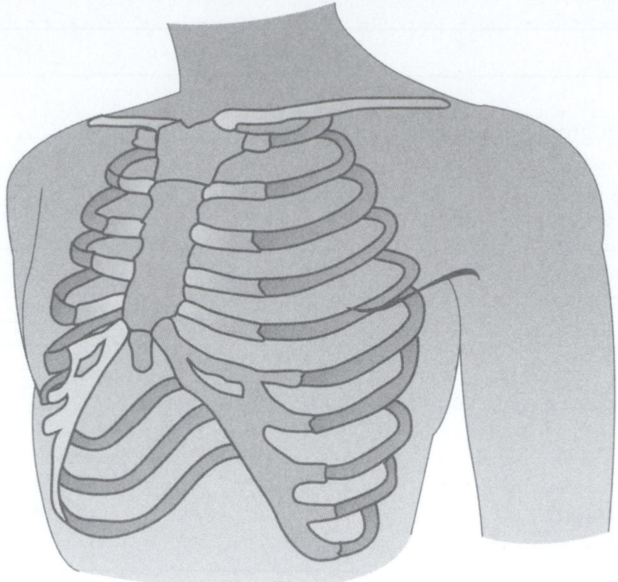

20. What patient preparation is required for an ECG?

____

____

21. What maintenance should be performed on an ECG machine?

____

____

22. At what speed does the paper move while recording a normal electrocardiogram?

____

23. What is the difference between a three-channel and a single-channel electrocardiograph?

____

____

____

24. What is the purpose of each of the following electrocardiograph capabilities?

a. Interpretive capability

____

____

b. EMR connectivity

c. Teletransmission

25. Why should artifacts be eliminated if they occur in an ECG recording?

26. What is the function of an artifact filter?

27. List three possible causes of muscle artifacts.

28. List three possible causes of wandering baseline.

29. List three possible causes of 60-cycle interference artifacts.

30. List four uses of Holter monitor electrocardiography.

31. List examples of cardiac dysrhythmias.

32. What is the purpose of a pulmonary function test?

33. What are the indications for performing spirometry?

34. What patient preparation is required for spirometry?

35. What is the purpose of postbronchodilator spirometry?

36. What are the characteristics of asthma?

37. What are five examples of allergens that may trigger an asthma attack?

38. What are five examples of environmental irritants, activities, or events that may trigger an asthma attack?

39. What happens to the bronchial tubes during an asthma attack?

40. What is the purpose of long-term-control asthma medication?

41. What is the purpose of quick-relief asthma medication?

42. What is the purpose of a peak flow meter?

43. What is the difference between a low-range and full-range peak flow meter?

44. What is the purpose of peak flow measurements?

45. Why is oxygen needed by the body?

46. What occurs when the body cannot maintain an adequate oxygen level?

47. What conditions may require home oxygen therapy?

48. What is the purpose of the regulator and flow meter on an oxygen cylinder?

49. What is liquid oxygen?

50. What is an oxygen concentrator?

51. What is the primary advantage of using a nasal cannula to administer oxygen?

52. List two reasons for using a face mask to administer oxygen therapy.

53. What occurs if oxygen comes in contact with a fire?

54. How should oxygen be stored?

CRITICAL THINKING ACTIVITIES

A. Chest Leads

Practice locating the six chest leads on five individuals. Select individuals of both genders and of varying ages and body contours. Record each person's name here after you have successfully located the chest leads. Record any problems you encountered locating the leads.

1.
2.
3.
4.
5.

B. ECG Cycle

Attach part of an ECG from a recording. Identify and label the various waves, intervals, and segments making up an ECG cycle on two of the leads.

C. Myocardial Infarction

You are working for a cardiologist. Your physician is concerned about the increase in the numbers of patients having heart attacks. He asks you to design a colorful, creative, and informative brochure on heart attacks using the brochure provided on the following page. This brochure will be published and placed in the waiting room to provide patients with education about heart attacks. The heart disease Internet sites listed under "On the Web" at the end of Chapter 27 in your textbook can be used to complete this activity.

Notes

FAQ on:

Q:

A:

Q:

A:

Q:

A:

Q:

A:

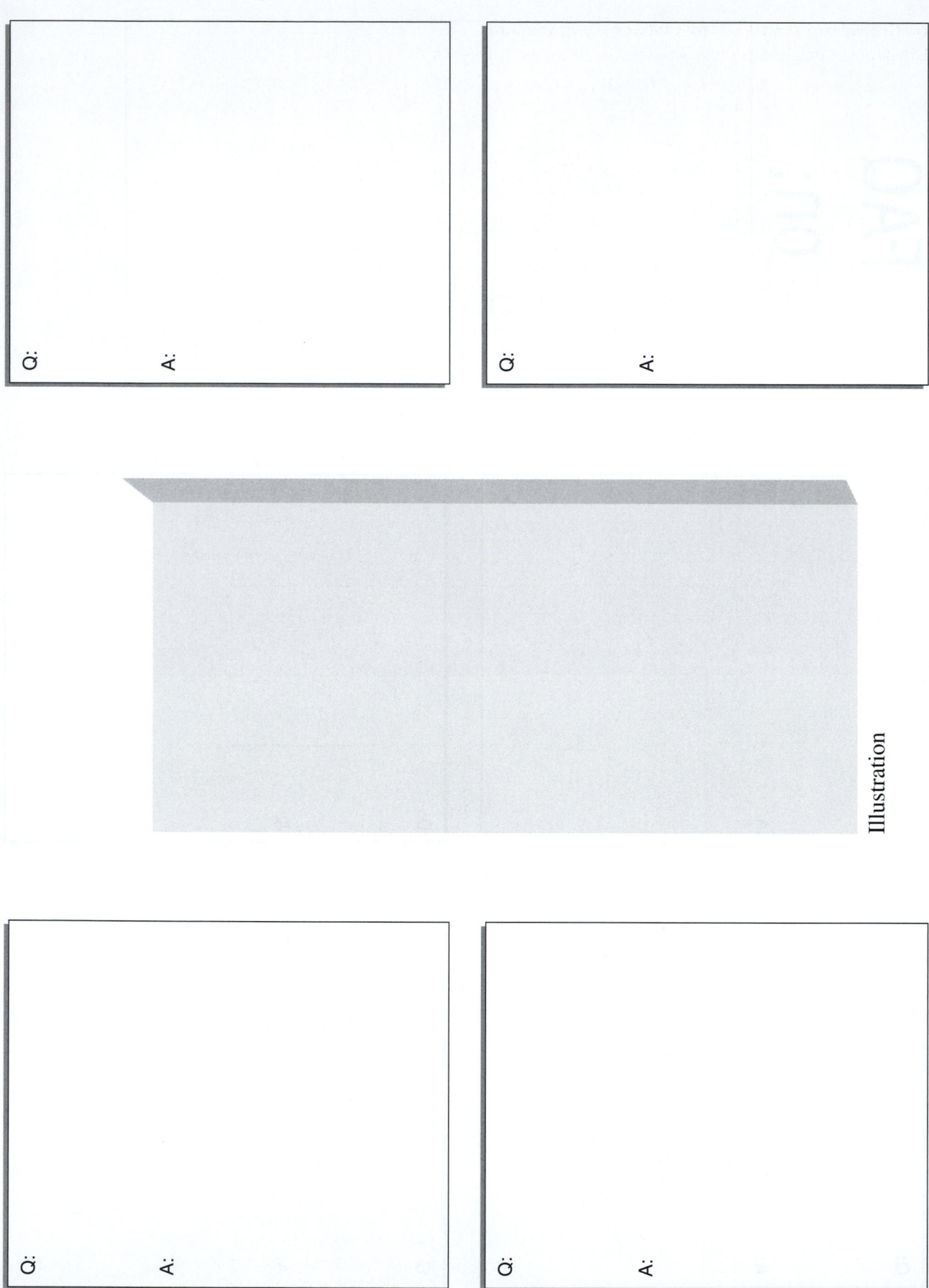

Q:
A:
Q:
A:
Illustration
Q:
A:
Q:
A:

D. Crossword Puzzle: Cardiopulmonary Procedures

Directions: Complete the crossword puzzle using the clues provided.

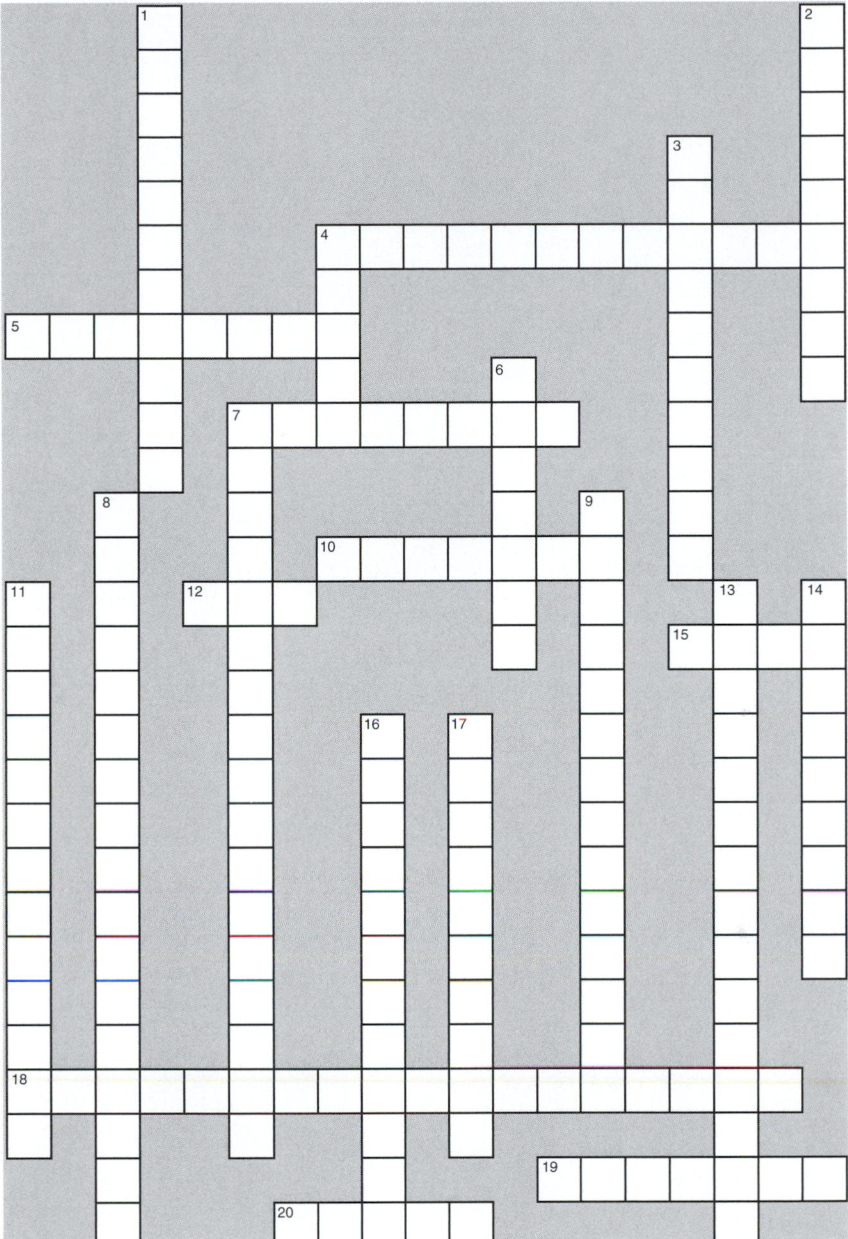

Across

4 Inflammation of heart's lining
5 Not enough blood to a body part
7 High-pitched whistling sound
10 Leads I, II, III
12 ECG std mark in mm
15 Fourth intercostals to the left
18 Separates oxygen out of air
19 Primary cause of COPD
20 The ventricles are recovering

Down

1 Rhythm not normal
2 Damaged alveoli disease
3 "How well can you breathe" test
4 Atria contract
6 Delivers asthma med
7 "Too loose" electrodes causes this
8 ECG within normal limits
9 Drug that opens air passages
11 Ambulatory ECG
13 Coronary artery plaque condition
14 Asthma allergen trigger
16 Oxygen administration device
17 Contraction of the ventricles

Notes

PRACTICE FOR COMPETENCY

Procedure 27-1: 12-Lead Electrocardiogram. Practice the procedure for running a 12-lead electrocardiogram and record the procedure in the chart provided.

Procedure 27-A: Spirometry. Practice the procedure for performing a spirometry test, and record the procedure in the chart provided.

Procedure 27-2: Peak Flow Rate Measurement. Practice the procedure for measuring peak flow rate, and record the procedure in the chart provided.

CHART	
Date	

Chart	
Date	

EVALUATION OF COMPETENCY

Procedure 27-1: Running a 12-Lead, Three-Channel Electrocardiogram

Name: ______________________________ Date: ______________

Evaluated by: ______________________________ Score: ______________

Performance Objective

Outcome:	Record a 12-lead electrocardiogram.
Conditions:	Using a three-channel electrocardiograph.
Standards:	Given ECG paper and disposable electrodes.
	Time: 15 minutes. Student completed procedure in __________ minutes.
	Accuracy: Satisfactory score on the Performance Evaluation Checklist.

Performance Evaluation Checklist

Trial 1	Trial 2	Point Value	Performance Standards
		•	Worked in a quiet atmosphere away from sources of electrical interference.
		•	Sanitized hands.
		•	Checked the expiration date of the electrodes.
		▷	Explained what may occur if the electrodes are outdated.
		•	Greeted the patient and introduced yourself.
		•	Identified the patient and explained the procedure.
		•	Instructed patient that he or she will need to lie still, breathe normally, and not talk during the procedure.
		▷	Explained why the patient should lie still and not talk.
		•	Asked patient to remove appropriate clothing.
		•	Assisted patient into a supine position on the table.
		•	Made sure that patient's arms and legs were adquately supported on the table.
		•	Draped patient properly.
		•	Positioned the electrocardiograph with the power cord pointing away from patient and not passing under the table.
		•	Worked on the left side of the patient.
		•	Prepared the patient's skin for application of the disposable electrodes.
		▷	Explained why the patient's skin must be prepared properly.
		•	Applied the limb electrodes.
		•	Properly located each chest position and applied the chest electrodes.

Trial 1	Trial 2	Point Value	Performance Standards
		▷	Explained why the tabs of the electrodes should be positioned correctly.
		●	Connected the lead wires to the electrodes.
		●	Arranged lead wires to follow body contour.
		▷	Explained why the lead wires should follow body contour.
		●	Plugged the patient's cable into machine and properly supported the cable.
		●	Turned on the electrocardiograph.
		●	Entered patient's data using the soft-touch keypad.
		▷	Stated the purpose of entering patient's data.
		●	Reminded patient to lie still, and pressed the AUTO -button to run the recording.
		●	Checked to make sure the standardization mark is 10 mm high.
		●	Checked to make sure the R wave has a positive deflection.
		▷	Stated what would cause the R wave to have a negative deflection.
		●	Checked the recording for artifacts and corrected them if they occurred.
		●	Informed the patient he or she can move and talk.
		●	Turned off the electrocardiograph.
		●	Disconnected the lead wires.
		●	Removed and discarded the disposable electrodes.
		●	Assisted patient from the table.
		●	Sanitized hands.
		●	Charted the procedure correctly.
		●	Placed the recording in the appropriate place to be reviewed by physician.
		●	Returned equipment to proper place.
		Ⓐ	Incorporated critical thinking skills when performing patient assessment.
		Ⓐ	Showed awareness of a patient's concerns related to the procedure being performed.
		Ⓐ	Explained to a patient the rationale for performance of a procedure.
		*	Completed the procedure within 15 minutes.
			TOTALS

CHART	
Date	

Evaluation of Student Performance

EVALUATION CRITERIA			COMMENTS
Symbol	**Category**	**Point Value**	
∗	Critical Step	16 points	
●	Essential Step	6 points	
Ⓐ	Affective Competency	6 points	
▷	Theory Question	2 points	
Score calculation: 100 points – ___ points missed ____ Score Satisfactory score: 85 or above			

2008 CAAHEP Competencies Achieved
Psychomotor (Skills) ☑ I. 5. Perform electrocardiography. ***Affective (Behavior)*** ☑ I. 2. Use language/verbal skills that enable patients' understanding. ☑ XI. 1. Recognize the effects of stress on all persons involved in -emergency situations.

2015 CAAHEP Competencies Achieved
Psychomotor (Skills) ☑ I. 2. a. Perform electrocardiography. ☑ I. 8. Instruct and prepare a patient for a procedure or a treatment. ☑ V. 3. Use medical terminology correctly and pronounced accurately to communicate information to providers and patients. ☑ VI. 8. Perform routine maintenance of administrative or clinical equipment. ***Affective (Behavior)*** ☑ I. 1. Incorporate critical thinking skills when performing patient assessment. ☑ I. 3. Show awareness of a patient's concerns related to the procedure being performed. ☑ V. 4. Explain to a patient the rationale for performance of a procedure.

ABHES Competencies Achieved
☑ 2. c. Identify diagnostic and treatment modalities as they related to each body system. ☑ 8. f. Display professionalism through written and verbal communications. ☑ 9. e. Perform specialty procedures including but not limited to minor surgery, cardiac, respiratory, OB-GYN, neurological, gastroenterology.

Notes

EVALUATION OF COMPETENCY

Procedure 27-A: Spirometry Testing

Name: ______________________ Date: ______________

Evaluated by: ______________________ Score: ______________

Performance Objective

Outcome:	Perform a spirometry test.
Conditions:	Using a spirometer.
Standards:	Given the following: disposable tubing, disposable mouthpiece, disposable nose clips, waste container.
	Time: 20 minutes. Student completed procedure in __________ minutes.
	Accuracy: Satisfactory score on the Performance Evaluation Checklist.

Performance Evaluation Checklist

Trial 1	Trial 2	Point Value	Performance Standards
		●	Sanitized hands.
		●	Assembled and prepared equipment.
		●	Calibrated the spirometer.
		▷	Stated the reason for calibrating the spirometer.
		●	Applied a disposable mouthpiece to the mouthpiece holder.
		●	Greeted the patient and introduced yourself.
		●	Identified the patient and explained the procedure.
		●	Asked the patient if he or she prepared properly.
		●	Asked the patient to remove heavy or restrictive clothing, to loosen tight clothing, and to discard gum.
		▷	Explained why tight clothing should be loosened.
		●	Measured the patient's weight and height.
		▷	Explained the reason for measuring weight and height.
		●	Asked the patient to sit near the machine.
		●	Entered patient's data into the computer database of the spirometer.
			Described and demonstrated the breathing maneuver:
		●	Relax and take the deepest breath possible.
		●	Place the mouthpiece in your mouth and seal your lips tightly around it.

Trial 1	Trial 2	Point Value	Performance Standards
		●	Blow out as hard as you can for as long as possible.
		●	Do not block the opening of the mouthpiece with your tongue.
		●	Remove the mouthpiece from your mouth.
		▷	Explained why the lips should be tightly sealed around the mouthpiece.
		●	Told the patient the instructions would be repeated during the test.
		●	Encouraged the patient to remain calm.
		●	Gently applied the nose clips.
		▷	Stated the purpose of the nose clips.
		●	Handed mouthpiece to patient.
		●	Began the test and actively coached the patient.
		●	Informed patient of modifications needed if breathing maneuver was not performed correctly.
		●	Continued the test until three acceptable efforts were obtained.
		●	Gently removed the nose clips from patient's nose.
		●	Removed the mouthpiece from its holder.
		●	Disposed of nose clips and mouthpiece in a waste -container.
		●	Allowed the patient to remain seated for a few minutes.
		●	Sanitized your hands.
		●	Printed the report and labeled it.
		●	Charted the procedure correctly.
		●	Placed the spirometry report in appropriate location for review by the physician.
		●	Cleaned the spirometer according to the manufacturer's instructions.
		Ⓐ	Incorporated critical thinking skills when performing patient assessment.
		Ⓐ	Showed awareness of a patient's concerns related to the procedure being performed.
		Ⓐ	Explained to a patient the rationale for performance of a procedure.
		*	Completed the procedure within 20 minutes.
			TOTALS

Chart	
Date	

Evaluation of Student Performance

EVALUATION CRITERIA			COMMENTS
Symbol	**Category**	**Point Value**	
✶	Critical Step	16 points	
●	Essential Step	6 points	
Ⓐ	Affective Competency	6 points	
▷	Theory Question	2 points	
Score calculation: 100 points – ___ points missed ___ Score Satisfactory score: 85 or above			

2008 CAAHEP Competencies Achieved

Psychomotor (Skills)

☑ I. 4. Perform pulmonary function testing.
☑ I. 11. Perform quality control measures.

Affective (Behavior)

☑ I. 2. Use language/verbal skills that enable patients' understanding.

2015 CAAHEP Competencies Achieved

Psychomotor (Skills)

☑ I. 2. d. Perform pulmonary function testing.
☑ I. 8. Instruct and prepare a patient for a procedure or a treatment.
☑ I. 10. Perform a quality control measure.
☑ V. 3. Use medical terminology correctly and pronounced accurately to communicate information to providers and patients.
☑ VI. 8. Perform routine maintenance of administrative or clinical equipment.

Affective (Behavior)

☑ I. 1. Incorporate critical thinking skills when performing patient assessment.
☑ I. 3. Show awareness of a patient's concerns related to the procedure being performed.
☑ V. 4. Explain to a patient the rationale for performance of a procedure.

ABHES Competencies Achieved

☑ 2. c. Identify diagnostic and treatment modalities as they related to each body system.
☑ 8. f. Display professionalism through written and verbal communications.
☑ 9. e. Perform specialty procedures including but not limited to minor surgery, cardiac, respiratory, OB-GYN, neurological, gastroenterology.
☑ 10. a. Practice quality control.

Notes

EVALUATION OF COMPETENCY

Procedure 27-2: Measuring Peak Flow Rate

Name: ______________________ Date: ______________

Evaluated by: ______________________ Score: ______________

Performance Objective

Outcome:	Measure a patient's peak flow rate.
Conditions:	Using a spirometer.
Standards:	Given the following: disposable mouthpiece, waste container.
	Time: 15 minutes. Student completed procedure in __________ minutes.
	Accuracy: Satisfactory score on the Performance Evaluation Checklist.

Performance Evaluation Checklist

Trial 1	Trial 2	Point Value	Performance Standards
		•	Sanitized hands.
		•	Assembled and prepared equipment.
		•	Moved the sliding indicator to the bottom of the scale.
		▷	Stated why the indicator must be moved to the bottom of the scale.
		•	Applied a disposable mouthpiece to the mouthpiece holder.
		▷	Stated the purpose of the disposable mouthpiece.
		•	Greeted the patient and introduced yourself.
		•	Identified the patient and explained the procedure.
		•	Asked the patient to remove heavy or restrictive clothing, to loosen tight clothing, and to discard any gum.
			Described and demonstrated the breathing maneuver:
		•	Relax and take the deepest breath possible.
		•	Place the mouthpiece in your mouth and seal your lips tightly around it.
		•	Blow out as hard and fast as you can.
		•	Try to move the marker as high as you can on the scale.
		•	Do not block the opening of the mouthpiece with your tongue.
		•	Remove the mouthpiece from your mouth.
		•	Told the patient the instructions would be repeated -during the test.
		•	Encouraged the patient to remain calm during the -procedure.

Trial 1	Trial 2	Point Value	Performance Standards
		▷	Explained why the patient should remain calm.
		●	Placed a new disposable mouthpiece on the peak flow meter.
		●	Slid the marker to the bottom of the numbered scale.
		●	Handed the peak flow meter to patient.
		●	Instructed patient to stand up straight and look straight ahead.
		●	Began the test and actively coached the patient.
		●	Noted the number where the indicator stopped on the scale and jotted it down on a piece of paper.
		●	Informed patient of modifications needed if breathing maneuver was not performed correctly.
		●	Continued the test until three acceptable efforts were obtained.
		▷	Explained why three acceptable efforts must be obtained.
		●	The numbers from the three tests were about the same.
		▷	Stated the significance of the three numbers being about the same.
		●	Took the peak flow meter from the patient.
		●	Removed the mouthpiece from its holder and discarded it in a waste container.
		●	Sanitized your hands.
		●	Noted the highest of the three peak flow measurements.
		●	Charted the procedure correctly.
		●	Cleaned the peak flow meter.
		▷	Explained how to clean the peak flow meter.
		Ⓐ	Incorporated critical thinking skills when performing patient assessment.
		Ⓐ	Showed awareness of a patient's concerns related to the procedure being performed.
		Ⓐ	Explained to a patient the rationale for performance of a procedure.
		*	Completed the procedure within 15 minutes.
			TOTALS

CHART	
Date	

Evaluation of Student Performance

EVALUATION CRITERIA			COMMENTS
Symbol	**Category**	**Point Value**	
✶	Critical Step	16 points	
●	Essential Step	6 points	
Ⓐ	Affective Competency	6 points	
▷	Theory Question	2 points	
Score calculation: 100 points – ____ points missed ____ Score Satisfactory score: 85 or above			

2008 CAAHEP Competencies Achieved
Psychomotor (Skills) ☑ I. 4. Perform pulmonary function testing. ***Affective (Behavior)*** ☑ I. 2. Use language/verbal skills that enable patients' understanding.

2015 CAAHEP Competencies Achieved
Psychomotor (Skills) ☑ I. 2. d. Perform pulmonary function testing. ☑ I. 8. Instruct and prepare a patient for a procedure or a treatment. ☑ V. 3. Use medical terminology correctly and pronounced accurately to communicate information to providers and patients. ☑ VI. 8. Perform routine maintenance of administrative or clinical equipment. ***Affective (Behavior)*** ☑ I. 1. Incorporate critical thinking skills when performing patient assessment. ☑ I. 3. Show awareness of a patient's concerns related to the procedure being performed. ☑ V. 4. Explain to a patient the rationale for performance of a procedure.

ABHES Competencies Achieved
☑ 2. c. Identify diagnostic and treatment modalities as they relate to each body system. ☑ 8. f. Display professionalism through written and verbal communications. ☑ 9. e. Perform specialty procedures including but not limited to minor surgery, cardiac, respiratory, OB-GYN, neurological, gastroenterology.

Notes

28 Specialty Examinations and Procedures: Colon Procedures, Male Reproductive Health, and Radiology and Diagnostic Imaging

CHAPTER ASSIGNMENTS

✓ After Completing	Date Due	Study Guide Pages	STUDY GUIDE ASSIGNMENTS (CTA = Critical Thinking Activity)	Possible Points	Points You Earned
		789	Pretest	10	
		790 791	Term Key Term Assessment A. Definitions B. Word Parts (Add 1 point for each key term)	23 23	
		791-800	Evaluation of Learning questions	77	
		800	CTA A: FOBT Patient Preparation	10	
		800-801	CTA B: Capsule Endoscopy	25	
		801	CTA C: Dear Gabby	10	
		801	CTA D: Lower Gastrointestinal Tract	5	
		802	CTA E: Intravenous Pyelogram	5	
		802-803	CTA F: Magnetic Resonance Imaging	7	
		804	CTA G: Crossword Puzzle	27	
			Evolve Site: Apply Your Knowledge questions	12	
			Evolve Site: Video Evaluation	18	
		789	Posttest	10	
			ADDITIONAL ASSIGNMENTS		
			TOTAL POINTS		

Notes

✓ When Assigned By Your Instructor	Study Guide Pages	Practices Required	LABORATORY ASSIGNMENTS (Procedure Number and Name)	Score*
	805	5	**Practice for Competency** 28-1 and 28-2: Fecal Occult Blood Testing: Guaiac Slide Test Method and Developing the Hemoccult Slide Test Textbook reference: pp. 725-727 and 728-729	
	807-810		**Evaluation of Competency** 28-1 and 28-2: Fecal Occult Blood Testing: Guaiac Slide Test Method and Developing the Hemoccult Slide Test	*
	805	5	**Practice for Competency** 28-A: Testicular Self-Examination Instructions Textbook reference: p. 736	
	811-813		**Evaluation of Competency** 28-A: Testicular Self-Examination Instructions	*
	806	3	**Practice for Competency** 28-B: Preparation for Radiology Examinations Textbook reference: pp. 736-742	
	815-816		**Evaluation of Competency** 28-B: Preparation for Radiology Examinations	*
	806	3	**Practice for Competency** 28-C: Preparation for Diagnostic Imaging Procedures Textbook reference: pp. 742-746	
	817-818		**Evaluation of Competency** 28-C: Preparation for Diagnostic Imaging Procedures	*
			ADDITIONAL ASSIGNMENTS	

Notes

Name ______________________________ Date ______________

PRETEST

True or False

_______ 1. Nonvisible blood in the stool is termed *occult blood.*

_______ 2. Colorectal cancer is a common form of cancer in individuals older than 50 years.

_______ 3. If a Hemoccult test result is positive, the physician may order a colonoscopy.

_______ 4. Most prostate cancers are slow growing.

_______ 5. The most common sign of testicular cancer is a small, hard, painless lump on the testicle.

_______ 6. The permanent record of the picture produced on x-ray film is a sonogram.

_______ 7. Mammography can be used to detect breast calcifications.

_______ 8. An IVP is a radiograph of the kidneys, ureters, and bladder.

_______ 9. Ultrasonography allows for continuous viewing of a structure.

_______ 10. A patient must remove all metal before undergoing MRI.

POSTTEST

True or False

_______ 1. Consuming red meat may cause a false-positive result on a fecal occult guaiac slide test.

_______ 2. The Hemoccult test should be stored at room temperature after applying a stool specimen to it.

_______ 3. Patient preparation for a sigmoidoscopy includes partial bowel preparation.

_______ 4. There are often no symptoms in the early stages of prostate cancer.

_______ 5. A prostate-specific antigen (PSA) level of 20 is within normal range.

_______ 6. Bone is an example of a radiolucent structure.

_______ 7. The patient should be instructed not to move during a radiographic examination to prevent confusing shadows on the film.

_______ 8. The breasts are compressed during mammography to prevent radiation burns.

_______ 9. Computed tomography produces a series of cross-sectional images.

_______ 10. A radioactive material is introduced into the body before a nuclear medicine imaging procedure is performed.

Term KEY TERM ASSESSMENT

A. Definitions

Directions: Match each key term with its definition.

_______ 1. Biopsy
_______ 2. Colonoscope
_______ 3. Colonoscopy
_______ 4. Contrast medium
_______ 5. Echocardiogram
_______ 6. Endoscope
_______ 7. Enema
_______ 8. Fluoroscope
_______ 9. Fluoroscopy
_______ 10. Insufflate
_______ 11. Melena
_______ 12. Occult blood
_______ 13. Peroxidase
_______ 14. Radiograph
_______ 15. Radiography
_______ 16. Radiologist
_______ 17. Radiology
_______ 18. Radiolucent
_______ 19. Radiopaque
_______ 20. Sigmoidoscope
_______ 21. Sigmoidoscopy
_______ 22. Sonogram
_______ 23. Ultrasonography

A. A permanent record of a picture of an internal body organ or structure produced on radiographic film
B. The visualization of the rectum and the entire colon using a colonoscope
C. A physician who specializes in the diagnosis and treatment of disease using radiation and other imaging techniques
D. Blood occurring in such a small amount that it is not visually detectable by the unaided eye
E. A substance used to make a particular structure visible on a radiograph
F. The surgical removal and examination of tissue from the living body
G. The record obtained with ultrasonography
H. The visual examination of the rectum and sigmoid colon using a sigmoidoscope
I. An injection of fluid into the rectum to aid in the elimination of feces from the colon
J. The darkening of the stool caused by the presence of blood in an amount of 50 mL or more
K. An instrument that consists of a tube and an optical system that is used for direct visual inspection of organs or cavities
L. A substance that is able to transfer oxygen from hydrogen peroxide to oxidize guaiac, causing the guaiac to turn blue
M. An endoscope that is specially designed for passage through the anus to permit visualization of the rectum and sigmoid colon
N. To blow a powder, vapor, or gas (such as air) into a body cavity
O. An endoscope that is specially designed for passage through the anus to permit visualization of the rectum and the entire length of the colon
P. The branch of medicine that deals with the use of radiation and other imaging techniques in diagnosis and treatment
Q. An instrument used to view internal organs and structures directly
R. Describing a structure that obstructs the passage of x-rays
S. The taking of permanent records of internal body organs and structures by passing x-rays through the body to act on a specially sensitized film
T. Describing a structure that permits the passage of x-rays
U. Examination of a patient with a fluoroscope
V. An ultrasound examination of the heart
W. The use of high-frequency sound waves to produce an image of an organ or tissue

B. Word Parts

Directions: Indicate the meaning of each word part in the space provided. List as many medical terms as possible that incorporate the word part in the space provided.

Word Part	Meaning of Word Part	Medical Terms That Incorporate Word Part
1. bi/o		
2. -opsy		
3. colon/o		
4. -scopy		
5. -scope		
6. endo-		
7. -oxia		
8. -ase		
9. ox/i		
10. sigmoid/o		
11. ech/o		
12. cardi/o		
13. -gram		
14. fluor/o		
15. radi/o		
16. -graph		
17. -graphy		
18. -ologist		
19. -ology		
20. lucent		
21. opaque		
22. son/o		
23. ultra-		

EVALUATION OF LEARNING

Colon Procedures and Male Reproductive Health

Fill in each blank with the correct answer.

1. List five causes of blood in the stool.

____

____

____

____

____

2. Define the term melena, and explain what causes it.

3. What is the primary reason for screening patients for the presence of fecal occult blood?

4. What are the symptoms of colorectal cancer

5. Why must three stool specimens be obtained for the fecal occult guaiac slide test?

6. List two reasons for placing the patient on a high-fiber diet when testing for fecal occult blood.

7. What medications and vitamin supplements must be discontinued before guaiac slide testing?

8. List two factors that could cause false-positive test results on a guaiac slide test.

9. List three examples of diagnostic tests that may be performed if the guaiac slide test result is positive.

10. Why is it important to perform quality control methods when developing the guaiac slide test?

11. How should the guaiac slide test be stored?

12. What factors can cause a failure of the expected control results to occur on a guaiac slide test?

13. List the advantages of the fecal immunochemical test (FIT) compared with the guaiac slide test.

14. How does a fecal DNA test function to detect colorectal cancer?

15. What is the purpose of performing a sigmoidoscopy?

16. Describe the following patient preparation required for a sigmoidoscopy:
    a. The day before the procedure and continuing until the examination is completed:
    b. The evening before the procedure:
    c. The day of the procedure:

17. What is the purpose of performing a digital rectal examination (DRE) before a sigmoidoscopy?

18. What is the purpose of insufflating air into the colon during a sigmoidoscopy?

19. What is the purpose of suctioning during sigmoidoscopy?

20. What is the recommended position of the patient during flexible fiberoptic sigmoidoscopy?

____

21. What parts of the colon are viewed during a colonoscopy?

____

____

22. What is the purpose of a full bowel preparation before a colonoscopy?

____

____

23. How should a patient consume the liquid laxative solution when preparing the bowel for a colonoscopy?

____

____

24. Where is the prostate gland located?

____

____

25. What are the symptoms of prostate cancer?

____

____

____

26. How is the digital rectal examination used for the early detection of prostate cancer?

____

____

27. What conditions can cause an elevated PSA level?

____

____

28. What is the PSA level for each of the following:

    a. Normal range _______________________________
    b. Slightly elevated range _______________________________
    c. Moderately elevated range _______________________________
    d. Highly elevated _______________________________

29. What patient preparation is required for a PSA test?

____

____

30. What tests may be ordered by the physician if the patient has positive prostate screening results?

31. What is the definition of the term screening?

32. What is the American Cancer Society's recommendation for the PSA test and the DRE?

33. When does testicular cancer most commonly occur?

34. When is the best time for a male to perform a testicular self-examination (TSE) and why?

35. What are the risk factors for testicular cancer?

36. What is the most common sign of testicular cancer?

Radiology and Diagnostic Imaging

1. Who discovered x-rays?

2. What is the function of x-rays?

3. What are the two ways in which radiographs can be taken?

4. Why is it important for a patient to prepare properly for a radiographic examination?

5. What is the function of a radiopaque contrast medium?

____

____

6. What are the various ways in which contrast medium can be administered to a patient?

____

____

7. What is the purpose of mammography?

____

____

____

8. Why should the patient be instructed not to apply lotions, powders, or deodorants when having a mammogram?

____

____

9. Why must the breasts be compressed during mammography?

____

____

10. What is the purpose of a bone density scan?

____

____

11. What is osteoporosis?

____

____

12. Who is at particular risk for osteoporosis?

____

13. What patient preparation is required for a bone density scan?

____

____

14. What information is provided by DXA bone density measurements?

____

____

____

____

15. What is the purpose of the upper GI radiographic examination?

16. Why must the GI tract be free of food and fluid before an upper GI radiographic examination is performed?

17. How can the patient prevent constipation after an upper GI examination?

18. A lower GI radiographic examination assists in the diagnosis of what conditions?

19. Why is it important to remove gas and fecal material from the colon before a lower GI radiographic examination is performed?

20. What is the advantage of the air used with a double-contrast barium enema?

21. What is an intravenous pyelogram (IVP)?

22. An IVP assists in the diagnosis of what conditions?

23. What may the patient experience during an IVP when the iodine enters the bloodstream?

24. Define the following:

    a. Angiocardiogram

b. Bronchogram

c. Cerebral angiogram

d. Coronary angiogram

e. Cystogram

25. What are the primary uses of ultrasonography?

26. What are the advantages of ultrasonography?

27. What can be determined during an echocardiogram?

28. What is the purpose of the gel used with ultrasonography?

29. What is the purpose of performing an obstetric ultrasound?

30. Doppler ultrasound assists in the diagnosis of what conditions?

31. What type of image is produced by computed tomography?

32. What are the primary uses of computed tomography?

33. What type of patient preparation is required for computed tomography?

34. What are the primary uses of magnetic resonance imaging?

35. What items must the patient remove before having an MRI scan?

36. What material is used with a nuclear medicine diagnostic imaging procedure?

37. What is the function of a gamma camera used in nuclear medicine?

38. What is the purpose of a bone scan?

39. A nuclear cardiac stress test assists in the evaluation of what heart condition?

40. A PET scan is used to assist in the diagnosis of what conditions?

41. What are the advantages of digital imaging technology?

CRITICAL THINKING ACTIVITIES

A. FOBT Patient Preparation

Frank Morrison has been given a Hemoccult slide kit for fecal occult blood testing (FOBT). In the space provided, plan breakfast, lunch, and dinner for him following the FOBT patient preparation guidelines on page 655 of your textbook.

B. Capsule Endoscopy

Perform an Internet search for capsule endoscopy. Search for textual information and videos of this procedure. Based on your research, answer the following questions regarding this procedure:

1. What is capsule endoscopy?

2. What conditions can be diagnosed using capsule endoscopy?

3. What patient preparation is required for this procedure?

4. What are the advantages of capsule endoscopy?

5. What are the disadvantages of capsule endoscopy?

C. Dear Gabby

Gabby broke her wrist while ice skating and wants you to fill in for her. In the space provided, respond to the following letter using the knowledge you have acquired in this chapter.

Dear Gabby:

I am 15 years old, and my mom just took me to a new doctor for a sports physical examination. I am going to play football this fall at my high school. Before this, I had always gone to the doctor I had since I was little, but I had to switch because I am getting older. After the doctor did my physical, he told me that I needed to examine my testicles every month and that the medical assistant would be in to explain how this is done.

Gabby, I was totally shocked, and you can bet I got out of that office before she had a chance to do that. I am too embarrassed to ask my parents about this. Gabby, what is going on? I am only 15 years old. Are my parents taking me to a quack, and should I report this to someone?

Signed,

Don't Know What to Do

D. Lower Gastrointestinal Tract

Trent Douglas has been having pain in his lower abdomen and occult blood in his stool. Dr. Hartman tells you to schedule him for a lower GI radiographic examination at Grant Hospital. In the space provided, explain how you would instruct Mr. Douglas to prepare for this examination. Include the patient preparation and the reason for each of the measures.

E. Intravenous Pyelogram

Dr. Tristen instructs you to schedule Ellie Ray for an IVP at Grant Hospital. After you have explained to Ms. Ray the instructions for preparing for the examination, she asks you the following questions. Respond to them in the space provided.

1. What body structures will be "x-rayed" during the examination?

____

____

____

2. Why must gas and fecal material be removed from the intestines?

____

____

____

3. Why will iodine be injected into my veins?

____

____

____

4. Will I feel anything when the iodine is injected?

____

____

____

5. What is done if an individual is allergic to iodine?

____

____

F. Magnetic Resonance Imaging

Jason Zindra, a college baseball player, has been experiencing pain in his left shoulder joint. Dr. Baker schedules him for magnetic resonance imaging (MRI) of the left shoulder. Jason asks you the following questions regarding this procedure. Respond to them in the space provided.

1. Is this a safe procedure?

____

____

2. Will there be any pain involved with this procedure?

____

____

3. Will I be exposed to x-rays?

4. What should I wear to the test?

5. May I wear my watch during the procedure to keep track of the time?

6. Does the MRI machine make any noise?

7. Will the technician be in the room with me?

G. Crossword Puzzle: Specialty Examinations and Procedures

Directions: Complete the crossword puzzle using the clues provided.

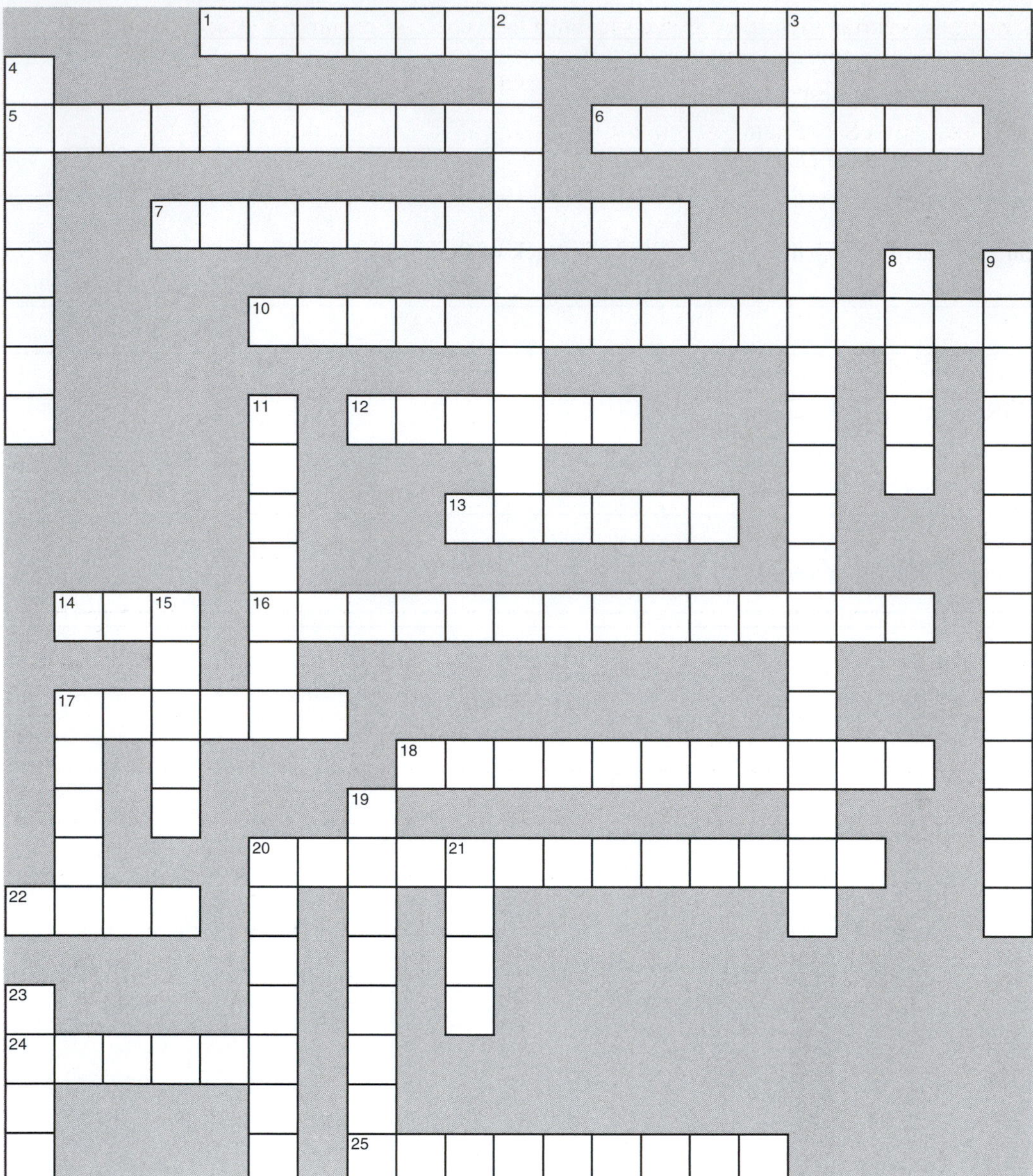

Across

1 Radiograph of coronary arteries
5 Hidden blood
6 Detects a stress fracture
7 Can cause blood in the stool
10 Normally increases PSA level
12 Lower GI contrast medium
13 Produces cross-sectional images
14 Used to diagnose kidney stones
16 US of heart
17 Black and tarlike stool
18 Visualization of colon
20 Secretes fluid that transports sperm
22 Color of positive Hemoccult
24 IVP contrast medium
25 Breast radiograph

Down

2 X-ray doctor
3 Can tell if it's twins
4 Discovered x-rays
8 CRC increases after this age
9 Symptom of CRC
11 Age to start TSE
15 CRC often starts from this
17 Remove during an MRI
19 US recording
20 Prostate CA screening test
21 May be done after elevated PSA
23 Pt position for sigmoidoscopy

PRACTICE FOR COMPETENCY

Procedure 28-1 and 28-2: Hemoccult Slide Test

1. Patient instructions. Instruct the patient in the specimen collection procedure for a fecal occult blood test (e.g.; Hemoccult) . Record these instructions in the chart provided.
2. Developing the test. Develop a fecal occult blood test, and record the results in the chart provided.

Procedure 28-A: Testicular Self-Examination. Instruct an individual about the procedure for testicular self-examination, and record the procedure in the chart provided.

CHART	
Date	

PRACTICE FOR COMPETENCY

Procedure 28-B: Radiology Examinations. Instruct a patient in the proper preparation required for each of the following types of radiographic examinations: mammogram, bone density scan, upper GI, lower GI, and intravenous pyelogram. Record the procedure in the chart provided.

Procedure 28-C: Diagnostic Imaging Procedures. Instruct a patient in the proper preparation required for each of the following types of diagnostic imaging procedures: ultrasonography, computed tomography, magnetic resonance -imaging, and nuclear medicine. Record the procedure in the chart provided.

CHART	
Date	

EVALUATION OF COMPETENCY

Procedures 28-1 and 28-2: Fecal Occult Blood Testing: Guaiac Slide Test Method and Developing the Fecal Occult Blood Test

Name: ______________________ Date: ______________

Evaluated by: ______________________ Score: ______________

Performance Objective

Outcome:	Instruct an individual in the specimen collection procedure for a Hemoccult slide test and develop the test.
Conditions:	Given the following: Hemoccult slide testing kit, disposable gloves, developing solution, reference card, and a waste container.
Standards:	Time: 15 minutes. Student completed procedures in _______ minutes.
	Accuracy: Satisfactory score in the Performance Evaluation Checklist.

Performance Evaluation Checklist

Trial 1	Trial 2	Point Value	Performance Standards
			Instructions for the Hemoccult slide test
		•	Obtained the Hemoccult slide testing kit.
		•	Checked expiration date on the slides.
		▷	Described what may occur if the slides are outdated.
		•	Greeted the patient and introduced yourself.
		•	Identified the patient and explained purpose of the test.
		•	Informed patient when the test should not be performed.
		•	Instructed patient in the proper preparation required for the test.
		•	Encouraged patient to adhere to the diet modifications.
		▷	Explained why the patient should follow the diet -modifications.
		•	Provided patient with the Hemoccult slide test kit.
		•	Instructed patient in completion of the information on the front flap of each card.
		•	Provided instructions on the proper care and storage of the slides.
		▷	Explained why the slides must be stored properly.
			Instructed the patient in the initiation of the test
		•	Began the diet modifications.
		•	Collected a stool specimen from the first bowel movement after the 3-day preparatory period.

Trial 1	Trial 2	Point Value	Performance Standards
			Instructed the patient in the collection of the stool specimen
		•	Filled in the collection date on the front flap.
		•	Used a clean dry container to collect the stool specimen.
		•	Collected the stool sample before it came in contact with toilet bowl water.
		•	Used the wooden applicator to obtain specimen from one part of the stool.
		•	Opened the front flap of the first cardboard slide.
		•	Spread a thin smear of the specimen over the filter paper in the square labeled A.
		•	Obtained another specimen from a different area of the stool, using the other end of the applicator.
		•	Spread a thin smear of the specimen over the filter paper in the square labeled B.
		•	Closed the front flap of the cardboard slide and filled in the date.
		•	Discarded the applicator in a waste container.
		▷	Explained why a sample is collected from two different parts of the stool.
		•	Instructed patient to place slides in a regular envelope to air-dry overnight.
		•	Instructed the patient to continue the testing period on 3 different days until all three specimens have been obtained.
		•	Instructed patient to place the cardboard slides in the foil envelope and return them to the medical office.
		•	Provided patient with an opportunity to ask questions.
		•	Made sure the patient understood the instructions.
		•	Charted the procedure correctly.
			Developing the Hemoccult slide test
		•	Assembled equipment.
		•	Checked expiration date on the developing solution bottle.
		▷	Explained how the solution should be stored.
		•	Sanitized hands and applied gloves.
		•	Opened the back flap of the cardboard slides.
		•	Applied 2 drops of the developing solution to the guaiac test paper underlying the back of each smear.
		•	Did not allow the developing solution to come in contact with skin or eyes.
		•	Read results within 60 seconds.
		*	Results were identical to the evaluator's results.
		▷	Explained why the slides should be read within 60 seconds.
		•	Performed the quality control procedure on each slide.
		•	Read the quality control results after 10 seconds.

Trial 1	Trial 2	Point Value	Performance Standards
		▷	Described what is observed during a normal positive and negative control reaction.
		▷	Stated the purpose of the quality control procedure.
		●	Properly disposed of the slides in a regular waste container.
		●	Removed gloves and sanitized hands.
		●	Charted the results correctly.
		Ⓐ	Explained to a patient the rationale for performance of a procedure.
		Ⓐ	Showed awareness of a patient's concerns related to the procedure being performed.
		Ⓐ	Showed awareness of patient's concerns regarding a dietary change.
		✶	Completed the procedure within 15 minutes.
			TOTALS

Chart	
Date	

Evaluation of Student Performance

EVALUATION CRITERIA			COMMENTS
Symbol	**Category**	**Point Value**	
✶	Critical Step	16 points	
●	Essential Step	6 points	
Ⓐ	Affective Competency	6 points	
▷	Theory Question	2 points	
Score calculation: 100 points – ____ points missed ____ Score Satisfactory score: 85 or above			

2008 CAAHEP Competencies Achieved
Psychomotor (Skills) ☑ I. 11. Perform quality control measures. ☑ IV. 5. Instruct patients according to their needs to promote health -maintenance and disease prevention. ***Affective (Behavior)*** ☑ III. 1. Display sensitivity to patient rights and feelings in collecting -specimens.

2015 CAAHEP Competencies Achieved
Psychomotor (Skills)
☑ i. 10. Perform a quality control measure.
☑ II. 2. Differentiate between normal and abnormal test results.
☑ IV. 1. Instruct a patient according to patient's special dietary needs.
☑ V. 4. Coach patients regarding: a. office policies, b. health maintenance c. disease prevention d. treatment plan.
Affective (Behavior)
☑ I. 3. Show awareness of a patient's concerns related to the procedure being performed.
☑ IV. 1. Show awareness of patient's concerns regarding a dietary change.
☑ V. 4. Explain to a patient the rationale for performance of a procedure.

ABHES Competencies Achieved
☑ 8. f. Display professionalism through written and verbal communication.
☑ 9. e. Perform specialty procedures including but not limited to minor surgery, cardiac, respiratory, OB-GYN, neurological, gastroenterology.
☑ 10. a. Practice quality control.
☑ 10. e. (2). Instruct patients in the collection of fecal specimens.

EVALUATION OF COMPETENCY

Procedure 28-A: Testicular Self-Examination Instructions

Name: ______________________________ Date: ______________

Evaluated by: ______________________________ Score: ______________

Performance Objective

Outcome:	Instruct an individual in the procedure for performing a testicular self-examination (TSE).
Conditions:	None.
Standards:	Time: 10 minutes. Student completed procedure in __________ minutes.
	Accuracy: Satisfactory score on the Performance Evaluation Checklist.

Performance Evaluation Checklist

Trial 1	Trial 2	Point Value	Performance Standards
		●	Greeted the patient and introduced yourself.
		●	Identified patient and explained that you will be instructing the patient in a TSE.
		●	Explained purpose of the examination and when to perform it.
			Instructed the patient as follows:
		●	Take a warm bath or shower.
		●	Stand in front of a mirror.
		●	Inspect for any swelling of the skin of the scrotum.
		●	Place the index and middle fingers of both hands on the underside of one testicle and the thumbs on top of the testicle.
		●	Apply a small amount of pressure, and gently roll the -testicle between the thumb and fingers of both hands.
		●	Palpate for lumps, swelling, or any change in the size, shape, or consistency of the testicle.
		▷	Stated the normal characteristics of a testicle.
		●	Locate the epididymis so that you do not confuse it with a lump.
		▷	Stated the characteristics and function of the epididymis.
		●	Repeatthe examination on the other testicle.
		●	Report any abnormalities to the physician.
		▷	Stated examples of abnormalities that should be reported.

Trial 1	Trial 2	Point Value	Performance Standards
		●	Charted the procedure correctly.
		Ⓐ	Explained to a patient the rationale for performance of a procedure.
		Ⓐ	Demonstrated a. empathy b. active listening c. nonverbal communication.
		Ⓐ	Demonstrated respect for individual diversity including: a gender b. race c. religion d. age e. economic status f. appearance.
		✶	Completed the procedure within 10 minutes.
			TOTALS

Chart	
Date	

Evaluation of Student Performance

EVALUATION CRITERIA			COMMENTS
Symbol	**Category**	**Point Value**	
✶	Critical Step	16 points	
●	Essential Step	6 points	
Ⓐ	Affective Competency	6 points	
▷	Theory Question	2 points	
Score calculation: 100 points – ___ points missed ___Score Satisfactory score: 85 or above			

2008 CAAHEP Competencies Achieved
Psychomotor (Skills) ☑ IV. 5. Instruct patients according to their needs to promote health -main-tenance and disease prevention. ☑ IV. 9. Document patient education. ***Affective (Behavior)*** ☑ I. 2. Use language/verbal skills that enable patients' understanding. ☑ IV. 3. Use appropriate body language and other nonverbal skills in -communicating with patients, family, and staff.

2015 CAAHEP Competencies Achieved
Psychomotor (Skills) ☑ V. 4. Coach patients regarding: a. office policies, b. health maintenance c. disease prevention d. treatment plan. ***Affective (Behavior)*** ☑ V. 1. Demonstrate a. empathy b. active listening c. nonverbal communication. ☑ V. 3. Demonstrate respect for individual diversity including: a gender b. race c. religion d. age e. economic status f. appearance. ☑ V. 4. Explain to a patient the rationale for performance of a procedure.

ABHES Competencies Achieved
☑ 8. f. Display professionalism through written and verbal communication. ☑ 9. h. Teach self-examination, disease management and health promotion.

Notes

EVALUATION OF COMPETENCY

Procedure 28-B: Preparation for Radiology Examinations

Name: ______________________________ Date: ______________

Evaluated by: ______________________________ Score: ______________

Performance Objective

Outcome:	Instruct a patient in the proper preparation required for each of the following radiographic examinations: mammogram, upper GI, lower GI, and intravenous pyelogram.
Conditions:	Given the following: a patient instruction sheet for each radiographic examination.
Standards:	Time: 15 minutes. Student completed procedure in __________ minutes.
	Accuracy: Satisfactory score in the Performance Evaluation Checklist.

Performance Evaluation Checklist

Trial 1	Trial 2	Point Value	Performance Standards
		•	Greeted and identified patient.
		•	Introduced yourself.
			Instructed patient in the proper preparation for each of the following radiographic examinations:
		•	Mammogram
		•	Bone density scan
		•	Upper GI
		•	Lower GI
		•	Intravenous pyelogram
		•	Charted the procedure correctly.
		Ⓐ	Explained to a patient the rationale for performance of a procedure.
		Ⓐ	Showed awareness of a patient's concerns related to the procedure being performed.
		*	Completed the procedure within 15 minutes.
			TOTALS

CHART	
Date	

Evaluation of Student Performance

EVALUATION CRITERIA			COMMENTS
Symbol	**Category**	**Point Value**	
∗	Critical Step	16 points	
●	Essential Step	6 points	
Ⓐ	Affective Competency	6 points	
▷	Theory Question	2 points	
Score calculation: 100 points – ___ points missed ___ Score Satisfactory score: 85 or above			

2008 CAAHEP Competencies Achieved
Psychomotor (Skills) ☑ IV. 6. Prepare a patient for procedures and/or treatments. ***Affective (Behavior)*** ☑ I. 2. Use language/verbal skills that enable patient's understanding.

2015 CAAHEP Competencies Achieved
Psychomotor (Skills) ☑ I. 8. Instruct and prepare a patient for a procedure or a treatment. ☑ IV. 1. Instruct a patient according to patient's special dietary needs. ☑ V. 11. Report relevant information concisely and accurately. ***Affective (Behavior)*** ☑ I. 3. Show awareness of a patient's concerns related to the procedure being performed. ☑ V. 4. Explain to a patient the rationale for performance of a procedure.

ABHES Competencies Achieved
☑ 2. c. Identify diagnostic and treatment modalities as they related to each body system. ☑ 8. f. Display professionalism through written and verbal communication.

EVALUATION OF COMPETENCY

Procedure 28-C: Preparation for Diagnostic Imaging Procedures

Name: ______________________ Date: ______________

Evaluated by: ______________________ Score: ______________

Performance Objective

Outcome:	Instruct a patient in the proper preparation required for each of the following diagnostic imaging procedures: ultrasonography, computed tomography, magnetic resonance imaging, and nuclear medicine.
Conditions:	Given the following: a patient instruction sheet for each diagnostic imaging procedure.
Standards:	Time: 15 minutes. Student completed procedure in ________ minutes.
	Accuracy: Satisfactory score in the Performance Evaluation Checklist.

Performance Evaluation Checklist

Trial 1	Trial 2	Point Value	Performance Standards
		•	Greeted and identified patient.
		•	Introduced yourself.
			Instructed patient in the proper preparation for each of the following diagnostic imaging procedures:
		•	Ultrasonography
		•	Computed tomography
		•	Magnetic resonance imaging
		•	Nuclear medicine
		•	Charted the procedure correctly.
		Ⓐ	Explained to a patient the rationale for performance of a procedure.
		Ⓐ	Showed awareness of a patient's concerns related to the procedure being performed.
		*	Completed the procedure within 15 minutes.
			TOTALS

CHART	
Date	

Evaluation of Student Performance

EVALUATION CRITERIA			COMMENTS
Symbol	**Category**	**Point Value**	
∗	Critical Step	16 points	
●	Essential Step	6 points	
Ⓐ	Affective Competency	6 points	
▷	Theory Question	2 points	
Score calculation: 100 points – ___ points missed ___ Score Satisfactory score: 85 or above			

2008 CAAHEP Competencies Achieved
Psychomotor (Skills) ☑ IV. 6. Prepare a patient for procedures and/or treatments. ***Affective (Behavior)*** ☑ I. 2. Use language/verbal skills that enable patient's understanding.

2015 CAAHEP Competencies Achieved
Psychomotor (Skills) ☑ I. 8. Instruct and prepare a patient for a procedure or a treatment. ☑ V. 11. Report relevant information concisely and accurately. ***Affective (Behavior)*** ☑ I. 3. Show awareness of a patient's concerns related to the procedure being performed. ☑ V. 4. Explain to a patient the rationale for performance of a procedure.

ABHES Competencies Achieved
☑ 2. c. Identify diagnostic and treatment modalities as they related to each body system. ☑ 8. f. Display professionalism through written and verbal communication.

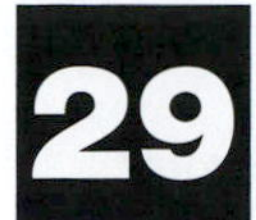

Introduction to the Clinical Laboratory

CHAPTER ASSIGNMENTS

✓ After Completing	Date Due	Study Guide Pages	STUDY GUIDE ASSIGNMENTS (CTA = Critical Thinking Activity)	Possible Points	Points You Earned
		821	Pretest	10	
		822	Term Key Term Assessment	22	
		823-828	Evaluation of Learning questions	44	
		828	CTA A: Laboratory Directory Information	10	
		828-829	CTA B: Specimen Requirements	15	
		829	CTA C: Identifying Abnormal Values	10	
		829-830	CTA D: Laboratory Report	25	
		830-831	CTA E: Laboratory Directory	9	
		831-832	CTA F: Testing Kit Product Insert (3 points for each section)	42	
		833	CTA G: Crossword Puzzle	29	
			Evolve Site: Apply Your Knowledge questions	10	
		821	Posttest	10	
			ADDITIONAL ASSIGNMENTS		
			TOTAL POINTS		

✓ When Assigned By Your Instructor	Study Guide Page	Practices Required	LABORATORY ASSIGNMENTS (Procedure Number and Name)	Score*
	835	2	**Practice for Competency** 29-A: Operate an Emergency Eyewash Station Textbook reference: pp. 756-757	
	837-839		**Evaluation of Competency** 29-A: Operate an Emergency Eyewash Station	*
	836	1	**Practice for Competency** 29-B: Complete a Laboratory Requisition Form Textbook reference: pp. 760-764	

Name ______________________________ Date ______________

PRETEST

True or False

_______ 1. When the body is in homeostasis, an imbalance exists in the body.

_______ 2. A routine test is performed to assist in the early detection of disease.

_______ 3. The laboratory request form provides the outside laboratory with information needed to test the specimen.

_______ 4. The clinical diagnosis is indicated on a laboratory request to correlate laboratory data with the needs of the physician.

_______ 5. The purpose of a laboratory report is to indicate the patient's diagnosis.

_______ 6. A patient who is fasting in preparation for a laboratory test is permitted to drink diet soda.

_______ 7. A small sample taken from the body to represent the nature of the whole is known as a *specimen*.

_______ 8. A laboratory report marked QNS means that the patient did not prepare properly.

_______ 9. Fecal occult blood testing is an example of a CLIA-waived test.

_______ 10. The purpose of quality control is to prevent accidents in the laboratory.

POSTTEST

True or False

_______ 1. Laboratory tests are most frequently ordered by the physician to assist in the diagnosis of pathologic conditions.

_______ 2. A laboratory directory indicates the patient preparation required for laboratory tests.

_______ 3. Laboratory tests called *profiles* contain a number of different tests.

_______ 4. A lipid profile includes a test for glucose.

_______ 5. The purpose of patient preparation for a laboratory test is to ensure the test results fall within the reference range.

_______ 6. A comprehensive metabolic profile requires that the patient fast.

_______ 7. Antibiotics taken by the patient before the collection of a throat specimen for culture may produce a false-positive result.

_______ 8. The purpose of CLIA is to prevent exposure of employees to bloodborne pathogens.

_______ 9. If a POL is performing moderate-complexity tests, CLIA requires that two levels of controls be run daily.

_______ 10. *In vitro* means occurring in the living body.

Term KEY TERM ASSESSMENT

Directions: Match each key term with its definition.

_______ 1. Analyte
_______ 2. Calibration
_______ 3. Clinical diagnosis
_______ 4. Control
_______ 5. Fasting
_______ 6. Homeostasis
_______ 7. In vivo
_______ 8. Laboratory test
_______ 9. Nonwaived test
_______ 10. Plasma
_______ 11. Product insert
_______ 12. Profile
_______ 13. Qualitative test
_______ 14. Quality control
_______ 15. Quantitative test
_______ 16. Reagent
_______ 17. Reference range
_______ 18. Routine test
_______ 19. Serum
_______ 20. Specimen
_______ 21. Test system
_______ 22. Waived test

A. Liquid part of the blood, consisting of a clear, yellowish fluid that comprises approximately 55% of the total blood volume
B. State in which body systems are functioning normally and the internal environment of the body is in equilibrium; the body is in a healthy state
C. Array of laboratory tests for identifying a disease state or evaluating a particular organ or organ system
D. Printed document supplied by the manufacturer with a laboratory test product that contains information on the proper storage and use of the product
E. Solution that is used to monitor a test system to ensure the reliability and accuracy of the test results
F. Test that indicates whether a substance is present in the specimen being tested and provides an approximate indication of the amount of the substance present
G. Application of methods to ensure that test results are reliable and valid and that errors are detected and eliminated
H. Occurring in the living body or organism
I. Test that indicates the exact amount of a chemical substance that is present in the body, with the results being reported in measurable units
J. Substance that is being identified or measured in a laboratory test
K. Substance that produces a reaction with a patient specimen that allows detection or measurement of the substance by the test system
L. A certain established and acceptable parameter of reference range within which the laboratory test results of a healthy individual are expected to fall
M. Tentative diagnosis of a patient's condition obtained through the evaluation of the health history and the physical examination, without the benefit of laboratory or diagnostic tests
N. Abstaining from food or fluids (except water) for a specified amount of time before the collection of a specimen
O. Laboratory test that meets the CLIA criteria for being a simple procedure that is easy to perform and has a low risk of erroneous test results
P. Laboratory test performed routinely on apparently healthy patients to assist in the early detection of disease
Q. Clear, straw-colored part of the blood (plasma) that remains after the solid elements and the clotting factor fibrinogen have been separated from it
R. Mechanism to check the precision and accuracy of a test system, such as an automated analyzer
S. Small sample of something taken to show the nature of the whole
T. Clinical analysis and study of materials, fluids, or tissues obtained from patients to assist in diagnosis and treatment of disease
U. Setup that includes all of the test components required to perform a laboratory test such as testing devices, controls, and testing reagents
V. Complex laboratory test that does not meet the CLIA criteria for waiver and is subject to the CLIA regulations

EVALUATION OF LEARNING

Directions: Fill in each blank with the correct answer.

1. What is the general purpose of a laboratory test?

2. List five specific uses of laboratory test results.

3. What is the purpose of performing a routine test?

4. What is the purpose of CLIA?

5. What requirements must be followed regarding a refrigerator used to store specimens and testing components?

6. What is the purpose of an emergency eyewash station?

7. Why is it important to flush the eyes immediately after they have been exposed to a hazardous substance?

8. What temperature range is usually required for storing testing materials and performing laboratory tests?

9. What information is included in a laboratory directory?

10. What is the purpose of a laboratory request?

11. What is the reason for indicating the following information on the laboratory request form?

   a. Patient's age and gender:

   b. Date and time of collection of the specimen:

   c. Source of the specimen:

   d. Physician's clinical diagnosis:

   e. Medications the patient is taking:

12. How does a laboratory report the results when a laboratory request is marked STAT?

13. What tests are included in the following profiles?

   a. Comprehensive metabolic profile:

   b. Hepatic function profile:

   c. Prenatal profile:

14. What information is included on laboratory reports?

15. Why must the test results of specimens tested by an outside laboratory be compared with the reference ranges supplied by the laboratory?

16. How are laboratory reports delivered to the medical office?

17. If a laboratory request form is completed on a computer, how is it transmitted to the laboratory?

18. Why do some laboratory tests require advance patient preparation?

19. Why is it important to explain the reason for the advance preparation to the patient?

20. Why are fasting specimens usually collected in the morning?

21. What is a specimen?

22. List 10 examples of specimens.

23. What reference source should be used to locate the specimen collection and handling requirements for the following?

    a. Specimen transported to an outside laboratory:

    ____

    b. Specimen tested in the medical office:

    ____

24. Why must the appropriate container be used to collect a specimen?

____

____

25. What is a unique identifier?

____

____

26. What two methods can be used to label a specimen?

____

____

27. Why is it important to properly identify a patient?

____

28. Why must a specimen be properly handled and stored?

____

____

29. List the CLIA-waived tests that are most frequently performed in the medical office.

____

____

____

____

30. What is included in a laboratory testing kit?

____

____

31. What may occur if a testing kit is outdated?

____

____

32. What is a unitized testing device?

____

____

33. Describe a CLIA-waived automated analyzer.

____

____

34. What is the purpose of quality control?

____

____

35. What are the storage requirements for most testing systems?

____

____

36. What should be written on the label of a control that is stable only for a certain period of time after opening it?

____

____

37. What is an internal control?

____

38. An internal control checks for what conditions?

____

____

39. What is the purpose of an external control?

____

____

40. What types of results are produced by the following controls?

    a. Low-level control:

    ____

    b. High-level control:

    ____

41. What may cause a control to fail to produce expected results?

____

____

42. What may cause invalid test results to occur when testing a specimen with a testing kit?

____

____

43. What is the difference between qualitative test results and quantitative test results?

44. List 10 laboratory safety guidelines that should be followed in the medical office to prevent accidents from occurring.

CRITICAL THINKING ACTIVITIES

A. Laboratory Directory Information

Look at a laboratory directory (from an outside medical laboratory), and list the categories of information included in it (e.g., normal range of laboratory tests).

B. Specimen Requirements

Refer to Table 29-1 in your textbook, and list the specimen requirements for each of the following tests:

1. ALT
2. Bilirubin, total
3. Blood group (ABO) and Rh Type
4. BUN, serum
5. Calcium
6. CBC (with differential)
7. CRP
8. Glucose, plasma
9. LD
10. PT/INR
11. RPR

12. Sedimentation rate (ESR) ___

13. Thyroxine (T_4) ___

14. Triglycerides ___

15. Urinalysis ___

C. Identifying Abnormal Values

Refer to the laboratory report in your textbook (Figure 29-7), and circle any abnormal values using a red pen.

D. Laboratory Report

Refer to the laboratory report in your textbook (Figure 29-7). Using the normal values listed on this report, determine whether the following tests fall within normal ranges or whether they are high or low. Mark each test according to the following: **N** = normal, **H** = high, **L** = low. Your patient is an adult female.

1. Glucose: 140 mg/dL ___
2. BUN: 15 mg/dL ___
3. Creatinine: 1.7 mg/dL ___
4. Calcium: 10.2 mg/dL ___
5. Magnesium: 0.4 mmol/L ___
6. Sodium: 156 mmol/L ___
7. Potassium: 5.5 mmol/L ___
8. Chloride: 84 mmol/L ___
9. Carbon dioxide: 18 mmol/L ___
10. Uric acid: 5.2 mg/dL ___
11. Total protein: 4.0 g/dL ___
12. Albumin: 3.5 g/dL ___
13. Total bilirubin: 0.8 mg/dL ___
14. Alkaline phosphatase: 80 U/L ___
15. LD: 132 U/L ___
16. AST: 24 U/L ___
17. ALT: 44 U/L ___
18. Total cholesterol: 260 mg/dL ___
19. HDL cholesterol: 57 mg/dL ___
20. LDL cholesterol: 165 mg/dL ___

21. WBC: 15.5 ($\times 10^3/mm^3$) __________

22. Hemoglobin: 10.4 g/dL __________

23. Hematocrit: 34% __________

24. Prothrombin time: 10 seconds __________

25. Neutrophils: 84% __________

E. Laboratory Directory

Your physician has ordered a triglyceride test on a patient that will be analyzed at an outside laboratory. You are required to collect the specimen and prepare it for transport to the outside laboratory. Using Figure 29-9 in your textbook as a reference, respond to the following questions in the space provided.

1. What is the amount and type of specimen required for this test?

2. What patient preparation is required for this test?

3. What collection supplies are required for this test?

4. What collection techniques must be performed after collecting the specimen?

5. How should you store the specimen while awaiting pickup by the laboratory?

6. What would cause the laboratory to reject the specimen?

7. What are the limitations of this test?

8. When would be the best time to collect this specimen (am or pm)? Explain the reason for your answer.

9. When the laboratory report is returned, the triglyceride test results are 250 mg/dL. How is this interpreted: desirable, borderline high, high, or very high?

____

F. Testing Kit Product Insert

Obtain a product insert from a CLIA-waived testing kit. The product insert can be obtained from an actual testing kit or from a Google search on the Internet. Provide a brief description of the information included in each section of the product insert in the space provided. Examples of brand names of CLIA-waived testing kits include the following:

Hemoccult fecal occult blood test

ColoScreen fecal occult blood test

Seracult fecal occult blood test

Hemoccult ICT test

QuickVue iFOB test

OSOM Mono test

Clearview Mono Test

QuickVue hCG pregnancy test

OSOM hCG urine pregnancy test

ICON hCG urine pregnancy test

QuickVue In-Line Strep A test

OSOM Ultra Strep A test

ICON DS Strep A test

Acceava Strep A test

Name of Testing Kit: ______________________________

Section	Brief description of information included in this section of the product insert
Intended use	
Summary and explanation	
Principles of the procedure	
Precautions and warnings	
Reagents and materials provided	
Materials not provided	
Storage and stability	
Specimen collection and handling	
Test procedure	
Interpretation and reading results	
Quality control	
Limitations of the procedure	
Expected values	
Performance characteristics	

G. Crossword Puzzle: Introduction to the Clinical Laboratory

Directions: Complete the crossword puzzle using the clues provided.

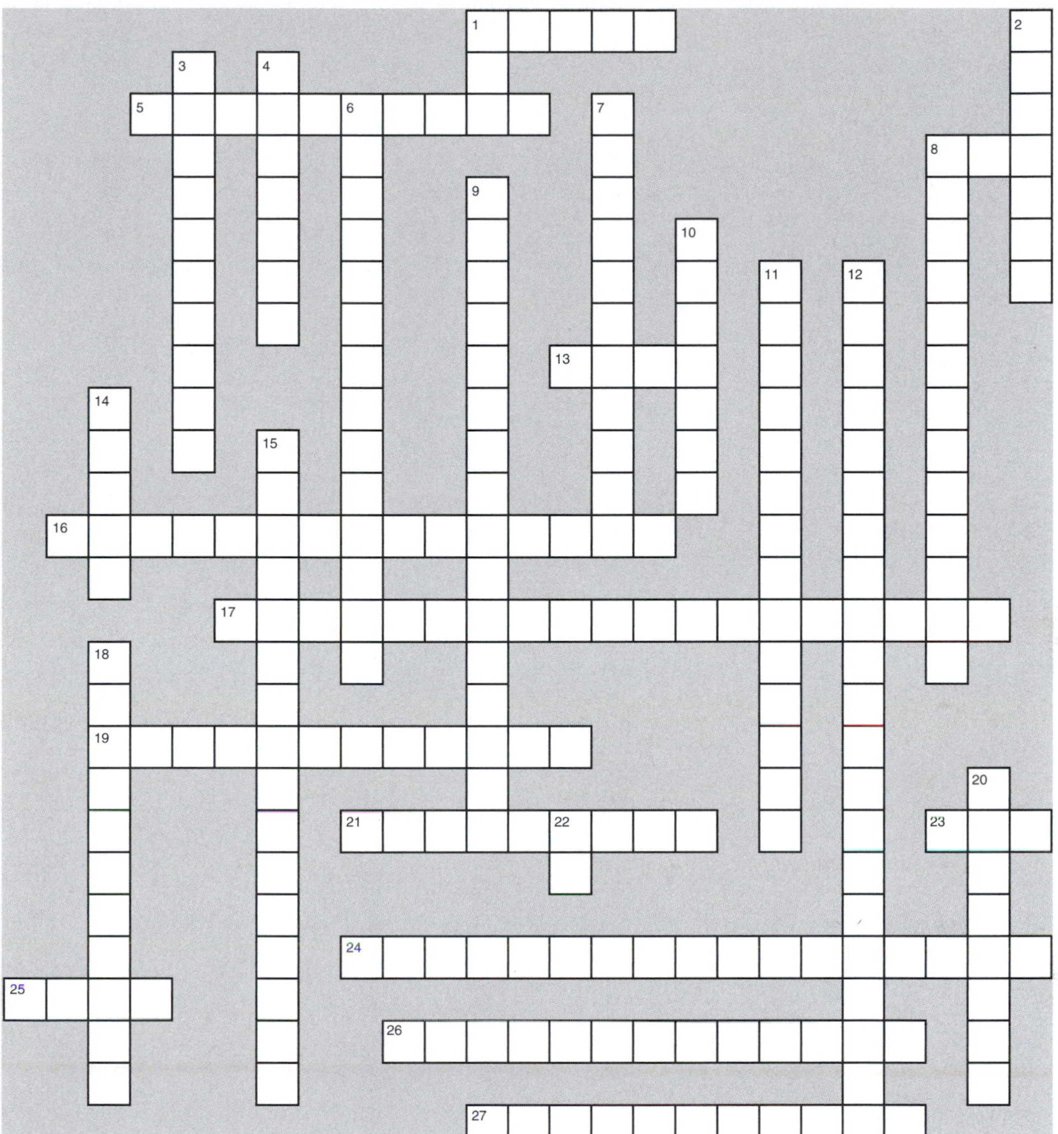

Across

1 For documenting control results
5 Order a laboratory test
8 In-house laboratory
13 As soon as possible
16 Approximate amount of substance present
17 Outside lab reference source
19 Determines CAD risk
21 What are the results?
23 Microscopic analysis of urine (ex)
24 Tentative diagnosis
25 To improve quality of lab testing
26 Complex lab test
27 Detects disease early

Down

1 Not enough specimen?
2 A substance being identified
3 Has a low risk of erroneous test results
4 More than one lab test
6 Accurate and reliable test results
7 Healthy body
8 Provides info on performing lab test
9 Is that you?
10 No food or fluid
11 Where healthy test results should fall
12 Which disease is it?
14 Plasma minus fibrinogen
15 A cause of abnormal control results
18 Test system working ok?
20 Sample of the body
22 CLIA requires 3 times per year

Notes

PRACTICE FOR COMPETENCY

Procedure 29-A: Operate and Inspect an Emergency Eyewash Station. Operate and inspect an emergency eyewash station. Document the inspection on the eyewash inspection tag presented below.

EMERGENCY EYEWASH STATION INSPECTION

INSPECT UNIT CAREFULLY BEFORE SIGNING

DATE	BY	DATE	BY

DO NOT REMOVE THIS TAG

Procedure 29-B: Laboratory Requisition Form. Complete the Laboratory Request form below using a classmate as a patient. The tests that have been ordered by the physician include the following: Basic Metabolic Profile, Lipid Profile, CBC (with Diff), and Rheumatoid Arthritis Factor.

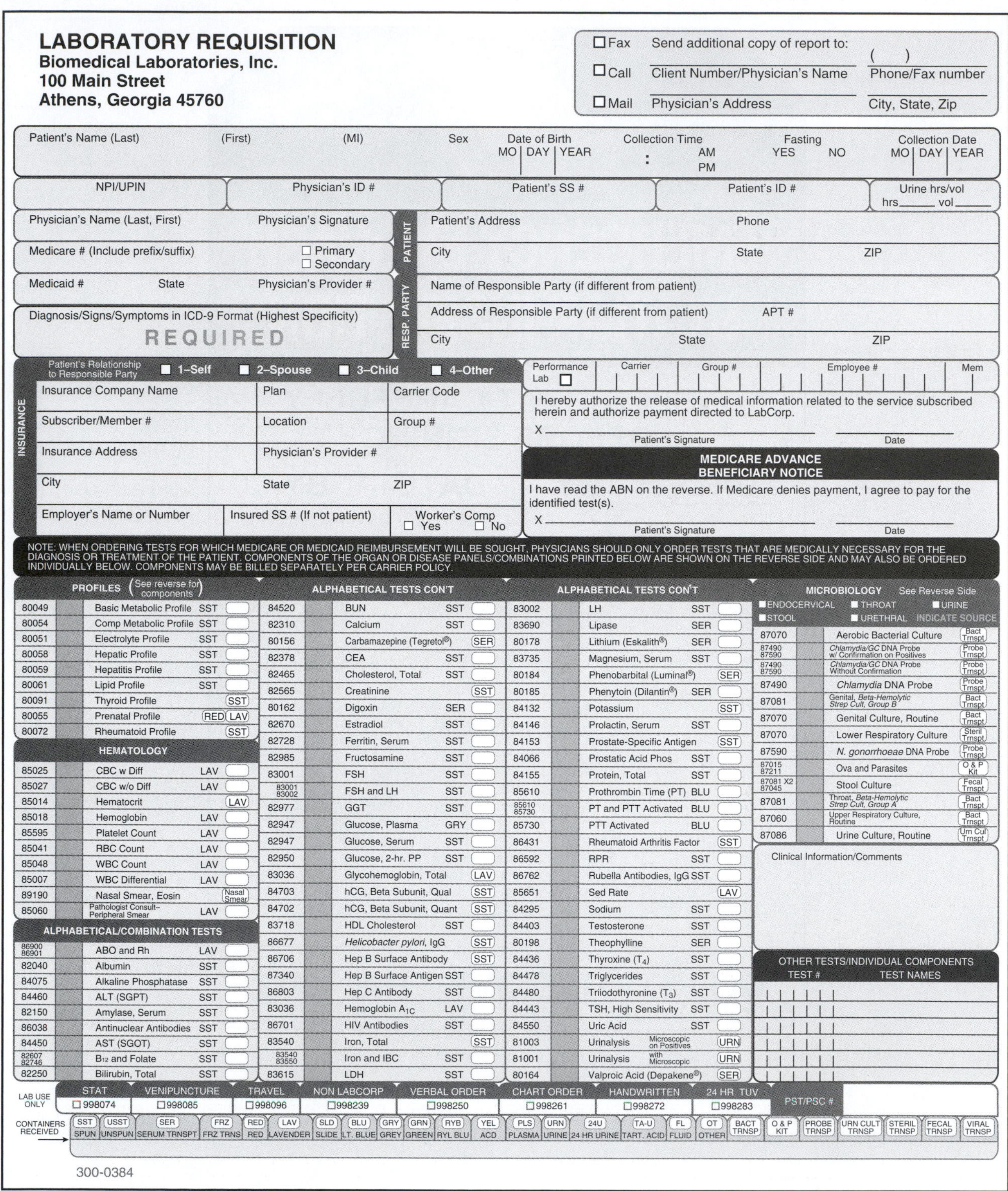

LABORATORY REQUISITION
Biomedical Laboratories, Inc.
100 Main Street
Athens, Georgia 45760

☐ Fax Send additional copy of report to:
☐ Call Client Number/Physician's Name ( ) Phone/Fax number
☐ Mail Physician's Address City, State, Zip

Patient's Name (Last) (First) (MI) Sex Date of Birth MO | DAY | YEAR Collection Time : AM PM Fasting YES NO Collection Date MO | DAY | YEAR

NPI/UPIN | Physician's ID # | Patient's SS # | Patient's ID # | Urine hrs/vol hrs_____ vol_____

Physician's Name (Last, First) Physician's Signature

Medicare # (Include prefix/suffix) ☐ Primary ☐ Secondary

Medicaid # State Physician's Provider #

Diagnosis/Signs/Symptoms in ICD-9 Format (Highest Specificity) REQUIRED

PATIENT: Patient's Address Phone / City State ZIP

RESP. PARTY: Name of Responsible Party (if different from patient) / Address of Responsible Party (if different from patient) APT # / City State ZIP

INSURANCE: Patient's Relationship to Responsible Party ■ 1–Self ■ 2–Spouse ■ 3–Child ■ 4–Other

Insurance Company Name | Plan | Carrier Code
Subscriber/Member # | Location | Group #
Insurance Address | Physician's Provider #
City | State | ZIP
Employer's Name or Number | Insured SS # (If not patient) | Worker's Comp ☐ Yes ☐ No

Performance Lab ☐ | Carrier | Group # | Employee # | Mem

I hereby authorize the release of medical information related to the service subscribed herein and authorize payment directed to LabCorp.
X ______ Patient's Signature ______ Date

MEDICARE ADVANCE BENEFICIARY NOTICE
I have read the ABN on the reverse. If Medicare denies payment, I agree to pay for the identified test(s).
X ______ Patient's Signature ______ Date

NOTE: WHEN ORDERING TESTS FOR WHICH MEDICARE OR MEDICAID REIMBURSEMENT WILL BE SOUGHT, PHYSICIANS SHOULD ONLY ORDER TESTS THAT ARE MEDICALLY NECESSARY FOR THE DIAGNOSIS OR TREATMENT OF THE PATIENT. COMPONENTS OF THE ORGAN OR DISEASE PANELS/COMBINATIONS PRINTED BELOW ARE SHOWN ON THE REVERSE SIDE AND MAY ALSO BE ORDERED INDIVIDUALLY BELOW. COMPONENTS MAY BE BILLED SEPARATELY PER CARRIER POLICY.

PROFILES (See reverse for components)

Code	Test	Container
80049	Basic Metabolic Profile	SST
80054	Comp Metabolic Profile	SST
80051	Electrolyte Profile	SST
80058	Hepatic Profile	SST
80059	Hepatitis Profile	SST
80061	Lipid Profile	SST
80091	Thyroid Profile	SST
80055	Prenatal Profile	RED LAV
80072	Rheumatoid Profile	SST

HEMATOLOGY

Code	Test	Container
85025	CBC w Diff	LAV
85027	CBC w/o Diff	LAV
85014	Hematocrit	LAV
85018	Hemoglobin	LAV
85595	Platelet Count	LAV
85041	RBC Count	LAV
85048	WBC Count	LAV
85007	WBC Differential	LAV
89190	Nasal Smear, Eosin	Nasal Smear
85060	Pathologist Consult–Peripheral Smear	LAV

ALPHABETICAL/COMBINATION TESTS

Code	Test	Container
86900 86901	ABO and Rh	LAV
82040	Albumin	SST
84075	Alkaline Phosphatase	SST
84460	ALT (SGPT)	SST
82150	Amylase, Serum	SST
86038	Antinuclear Antibodies	SST
84450	AST (SGOT)	SST
82607 82746	B_{12} and Folate	SST
82250	Bilirubin, Total	SST

ALPHABETICAL TESTS CON'T

Code	Test	Container
84520	BUN	SST
82310	Calcium	SST
80156	Carbamazepine (Tegretol®)	SER
82378	CEA	SST
82465	Cholesterol, Total	SST
82565	Creatinine	SST
80162	Digoxin	SER
82670	Estradiol	SST
82728	Ferritin, Serum	SST
82985	Fructosamine	SST
83001	FSH	SST
83001 83002	FSH and LH	SST
82977	GGT	SST
82947	Glucose, Plasma	GRY
82947	Glucose, Serum	SST
82950	Glucose, 2-hr. PP	SST
83036	Glycohemoglobin, Total	LAV
84703	hCG, Beta Subunit, Qual	SST
84702	hCG, Beta Subunit, Quant	SST
83718	HDL Cholesterol	SST
86677	*Helicobacter pylori*, IgG	SST
86706	Hep B Surface Antibody	SST
87340	Hep B Surface Antigen	SST
86803	Hep C Antibody	SST
83036	Hemoglobin A_{1C}	LAV
86701	HIV Antibodies	SST
83540	Iron, Total	SST
83540 83550	Iron and IBC	SST
83615	LDH	SST

ALPHABETICAL TESTS CON'T

Code	Test	Container
83002	LH	SST
83690	Lipase	SER
80178	Lithium (Eskalith®)	SER
83735	Magnesium, Serum	SST
80184	Phenobarbital (Luminal®)	SER
80185	Phenytoin (Dilantin®)	SER
84132	Potassium	SST
84146	Prolactin, Serum	SST
84153	Prostate-Specific Antigen	SST
84066	Prostatic Acid Phos	SST
84155	Protein, Total	SST
85610	Prothrombin Time (PT)	BLU
85610 85730	PT and PTT Activated	BLU
85730	PTT Activated	BLU
86431	Rheumatoid Arthritis Factor	SST
86592	RPR	SST
86762	Rubella Antibodies, IgG	SST
85651	Sed Rate	LAV
84295	Sodium	SST
84403	Testosterone	SST
80198	Theophylline	SER
84436	Thyroxine (T_4)	SST
84478	Triglycerides	SST
84480	Triiodothyronine (T_3)	SST
84443	TSH, High Sensitivity	SST
84550	Uric Acid	SST
81003	Urinalysis Microscopic on Positives	URN
81001	Urinalysis with Microscopic	URN
80164	Valproic Acid (Depakene®)	SER

MICROBIOLOGY See Reverse Side
■ ENDOCERVICAL ■ THROAT ■ URINE ■ STOOL ■ URETHRAL INDICATE SOURCE

Code	Test	Container
87070	Aerobic Bacterial Culture	Bact Trnspt
87490 87590	*Chlamydia/GC* DNA Probe w/ Confirmation on Positives	Probe Trnspt
87490 87590	*Chlamydia/GC* DNA Probe Without Confirmation	Probe Trnspt
87490	*Chlamydia* DNA Probe	Probe Trnspt
87081	Genital, *Beta-Hemolytic Strep Cult, Group B*	Bact Trnspt
87070	Genital Culture, Routine	Bact Trnspt
87070	Lower Respiratory Culture	Steril Trnspt
87590	*N. gonorrhoeae* DNA Probe	Probe Trnspt
87015 87211	Ova and Parasites	O & P Kit
87081 X2 87045	Stool Culture	Fecal Trnspt
87081	Throat, *Beta-Hemolytic Strep Cult, Group A*	Bact Trnspt
87060	Upper Respiratory Culture, Routine	Bact Trnspt
87086	Urine Culture, Routine	Urn Cul Trnspt

Clinical Information/Comments

OTHER TESTS/INDIVIDUAL COMPONENTS
TEST # TEST NAMES

LAB USE ONLY: STAT ☐998074 | VENIPUNCTURE ☐998085 | TRAVEL ☐998096 | NON LABCORP ☐998239 | VERBAL ORDER ☐998250 | CHART ORDER ☐998261 | HANDWRITTEN ☐998272 | 24 HR TUV ☐998283 | PST/PSC #

CONTAINERS RECEIVED: SST SPUN | USST UNSPUN | SER SERUM TRNSPT | FRZ FRZ TRNS | RED RED | LAV LAVENDER | SLD SLIDE | BLU LT. BLUE | GRY GREY | GRN GREEN | RYB RYL BLU | YEL ACD | PLS PLASMA | URN URINE | 24U 24 HR URINE | TA-U TART. ACID | FL FLUID | OT OTHER | BACT TRNSP | O & P KIT | PROBE TRNSP | URN CULT TRNSP | STERIL TRNSP | FECAL TRNSP | VIRAL TRNSP

300-0384

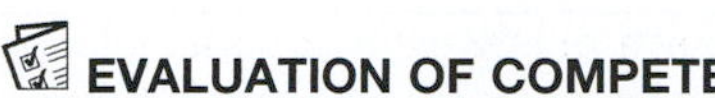

EVALUATION OF COMPETENCY

Procedure 29-A: Operating an Emergency Eyewash Station

Name: ______________________ Date: ______________

Evaluated by: ______________________ Score: ______________

Performance Objective

Outcome:	Operate and inspect an emergency eyewash station.
Conditions:	Using an emergency eyewash station.
	Given a disinfectant.
Standards:	Time: 5 minutes. Student completed procedure in __________ minutes.
	Accuracy: Satisfactory score on the performance evaluation checklist.

Performance Evaluation Checklist

Trial 1	Trial 2	Point Value	Performance Standards
			Operate the Emergency Eyewash Station
		●	Immediately proceeded to the emergency eyewash station after the eye(s) come in contact with a hazardous substance.
		●	Asked for assistance, if needed.
		●	Activated the eyewash station using the activation lever or paddle.
		●	Held both eyelids apart with your thumbs and forefingers.
		▷	Stated why the eyelids must be held apart.
		●	Directed the flow of water at an angle to the eyes from the outside edge of the lower eyes towards the inside of the eyes.
		▷	Stated why the water should not be aimed directly onto the eyes.
		●	If necessary, removed contact lenses.
		▷	Stated why contact lenses should be removed.
		●	Continued to hold the eyelids apart and gently rolled your eyeballs from left to right and up and down.
		▷	Stated why the eyeballs should be gently rolled.
		●	Continued flushing for a full 15 minutes.
		●	Returned the activation lever or paddle to its resting position.
		●	Sought medical attention to determine if further treatment is required.
		●	Cleaned, disinfected, rinsed, and completely dried the eyewash device.

Trial 1	Trial 2	Point Value	Performance Standards
			Inspect the Emergency Eyewash Station
		●	Made sure the access route to the eyewash station is well-lit and free of obstructions.
		▷	Stated what may occur if there is a delay in reaching the eyewash station.
		●	Made sure the eyewash station is well-lit and the area around the eyewash station is free of clutter.
		▷	Stated why the area around the station should be free of clutter.
		●	Made sure the nozzle covers are in place and in good condition.
		▷	Stated the purpose of the nozzle covers.
		●	Made sure the eyewash bowl is clean and free of debris
		●	Activated the eyewash device using the activation lever or paddle.
		●	Made sure the water flow from the nozzles occurred in one second or less following activation of the eyewash.
		●	Made sure the nozzle covers come off automatically when the eyewash device is activated.
		●	Activated the eyewash station for approximately three minutes to flush out the water supply lines.
		▷	Stated the purpose of flushing the water lines.
		●	Made sure that water flows continuously without the use of the hands.
		●	Made sure the nozzle heads are not clogged and that water flows equally from both nozzle heads.
		●	Cleaned, disinfected, rinsed, and completely dried the eyewash device.
		●	Replaced the nozzle covers on the nozzle heads.
		●	Reported any problems to the appropriate personnel.
		●	Documented the inspection date and your initials on the eyewash inspection tag.
		▷	Stated how often the eyewash station should be inspected.
		Ⓐ	Recognized the physical and emotional effects of persons involved in an emergency situation.
		Ⓐ	Demonstrated self-awareness in responding to emergency situations.
		*	Completed the procedure within 20 minutes.
			TOTALS

Evaluation of Student Performance

EVALUATION CRITERIA			COMMENTS
Symbol	**Category**	**Point Value**	
∗	Critical Step	16 points	
●	Essential Step	6 points	
Ⓐ	Affective Competency	6 points	
▷	Theory Question	2 points	
Score calculation: 100 Points – Points missed ____Score Satisfactory score: 85 or above			

2008 CAAHEP Competencies Achieved
☑ III. 1. Participate in training on Standard Precautions. ☑ III. 2. Practice Standard Precautions. ☑ IX. 8. Apply local, state, and federal health care legislation and regulation appropriate to the medical assisting practice setting. ☑ XI. 5. Demonstrate proper use of the following equipment: a. Eyewash b. Fire extinguishers c. Sharps disposal containers ***Affective (Behavior)*** ☑ XI. 1. Recognize the effects of stress on all persons involved in emergency situations. ☑ XI. 2. Demonstrate self-awareness in responding to emergency situations.

2015 CAAHEP Competencies Achieved
Psychomotor (Skills) ☑ III. 1. Participate in bloodborne pathogen training. ☑ VI. 8. Perform routine maintenance of administrative or clinical equipment. ☑ XII. 2. a. Demonstrate proper use of eyewash equipment. ***Affective (Behavior)*** ☑ XII. 1. Recognize the physical and emotional effects of persons involved in an emergency situation. ☑ XII. 2. Demonstrate self-awareness in responding to emergency situations.

ABHES Competencies Achieved
☑ 9. a. Practice standard precautions and perform disinfection/sterilization techniques. ☑ 9. g. Recognize and respond to medical office emergencies.

Notes

30 Urinalysis

CHAPTER ASSIGNMENTS

✓ After Completing	Date Due	Study Guide Pages	STUDY GUIDE ASSIGNMENTS (CTA = Critical Thinking Activity)	Possible Points	Points You Earned
		845	Pretest	10	
		846 846-847	Term Key Term Assessment A. Definitions B. Word Parts (Add 1 point for each key term)	23 16	
		847-850	Evaluation of Learning questions	31	
		850	CTA A: First-Voided Specimen	2	
		850-851	CTA B: Clean-Catch Specimen	4	
		851	CTA C: Urine Testing Kit Instructions	6	
			Evolve Site: Chemical Testing of Urine (Record points earned)		
		852	CTA D: Crossword Puzzle	20	
			Evolve Site: Road to Recovery: Urinalysis Terminology (Record points earned)		
			Evolve Site: Apply Your Knowledge questions	10	
			Evolve Site: Video Evaluation	25	
		845	Posttest	10	
			ADDITIONAL ASSIGNMENTS		
			TOTAL POINTS		

Notes

✓ When Assigned By Your Instructor	Study Guide Pages	Practices Required	LABORATORY ASSIGNMENTS (Procedure Number and Name)	Score*
	853-856	3	**Practice for Competency** 30-1: Clean-Catch Midstream Specimen Collection Instructions Textbook reference: pp. 790-791	
	857-859		**Evaluation of Competency** 30-1: Clean-Catch Midstream Specimen Collection Instructions	*
	853-856	5	**Practice for Competency** 30-A: Assessing Color and Appearance of a Urine Specimen Textbook reference: pp. 791-793	
	861-862		**Evaluation of Competency** 30-A: Assessing Color and Appearance of a Urine Specimen	*
	853-856	5	**Practice for Competency** 30-2: Chemical Testing of Urine with the Multistix 10 SG Reagent Strip Textbook reference: pp. 797-799	
	863-866		**Evaluation of Competency** 30-2: Chemical Testing of Urine with the Multistix 10 SG Reagent Strip	*
	853-856	2	**Practice for Competency** 30-3: Prepare a Urine Specimen for Microscopic Examination: Kova Method Textbook reference: pp. 804-807	
	867-869		**Evaluation of Competency** 30-3: Prepare a Urine Specimen for Microscopic Examination: Kova Method	*
	853-856	2	**Practice for Competency** 30-4: Performing a Urine Pregnancy Test Textbook reference: pp. 810-811	
	871-872		**Evaluation of Competency** 30-4: Performing a Urine Pregnancy Test	*
			ADDITIONAL ASSIGNMENTS	

Notes

Name ______________________________ Date ______________

PRETEST

True or False

_______ 1. Approximately 95% of urine consists of water.

_______ 2. Frequency is the condition of having to urinate often.

_______ 3. An excessive increase in urine output is called *polyuria*.

_______ 4. A clean-catch midstream urine specimen is required for a urine culture.

_______ 5. Urinalysis consists of a physical, chemical, and microscopic examination of urine.

_______ 6. A urine specimen that is light yellow indicates that bacteria are present in the specimen.

_______ 7. The pH of most urine specimens is neutral.

_______ 8. Blood may normally be present in the urine due to menstruation.

_______ 9. Hematuria refers to the presence of blood in the urine.

_______ 10. HCG is a hormone that is present in the urine and blood of a pregnant woman.

POSTTEST

True or False

_______ 1. Urea is a waste product derived from the breakdown of water.

_______ 2. A normal adult excretes approximately 250 mL of urine each day.

_______ 3. Vomiting can result in oliguria.

_______ 4. The distal urethra normally contains microorganisms.

_______ 5. A 24-hour urine specimen may be collected to assist in the diagnosis of a UTI.

_______ 6. If a urine specimen is allowed to stand for more than 1 hour at room temperature, the pH becomes more acidic.

_______ 7. If a freshly voided specimen is cloudy, the patient may have a urinary tract infection.

_______ 8. The normal specific gravity of urine ranges from 1.003 to 1.030.

_______ 9. Dysuria is the inability to control urination at night.

_______ 10. Casts are formed in the urinary bladder.

Term KEY TERM ASSESSMENT

A. Definitions

Directions: Match each key term with its definition.

_______ 1. Anuria
_______ 2. Bilirubinuria
_______ 3. Dysuria
_______ 4. Frequency
_______ 5. Glycosuria
_______ 6. Hematuria
_______ 7. Ketonuria
_______ 8. Ketosis
_______ 9. Micturition
_______ 10. Nephron
_______ 11. Nocturia
_______ 12. Nocturnal enuresis
_______ 13. Oliguria
_______ 14. pH
_______ 15. Polyuria
_______ 16. Proteinuria
_______ 17. Pyuria
_______ 18. Retention
_______ 19. Specific gravity
_______ 20. Urgency
_______ 21. Urinalysis
_______ 22. Urinary incontinence
_______ 23. Void

A. Decreased or scanty output of urine
B. The presence of protein in the urine
C. Inability of an individual to control urination at night during sleep (bedwetting)
D. The presence of bilirubin in the urine
E. Increased output of urine
F. The presence of pus in the urine
G. The presence of glucose in the urine
H. The physical, chemical, and microscopic analysis of urine
I. The presence of ketone bodies in the urine
J. Act of voiding urine
K. An accumulation of large amounts of ketone bodies in the tissues and body fluids
L. The weight of a substance compared with the weight of an equal volume of a substance known as the standard
M. The unit that describes the acidity or alkalinity of a solution
N. The functional unit of the kidney
O. The inability to empty the bladder; urine is being produced normally but is not being voided
P. The immediate need to urinate
Q. To empty the bladder
R. Failure of the kidneys to produce urine
S. Difficult or painful urination
T. The condition of having to urinate often
U. Blood present in the urine
V. Excessive (voluntary) urination during the night
W. The inability to retain urine

B. Word Parts

Directions: Indicate the meaning of each word part in the space provided. List as many medical terms as possible that incorporate the word part in the space provided.

Word Part	Meaning of Word Part	Medical Terms That Incorporate Word Part
1. an-		
2. ur/o		
3. -ia		
4. bilirubino/o		
5. dys-		
6. glyc/o		
7. hemato/o		

Word Part	Meaning of Word Part	Medical Terms That Incorporate Word Part
8. keton/o		
9. -osis		
10. noct/i		
11. olig/o		
12. poly		
13. py/o		
14. supra		
15. pub/o		
16. -ic		

EVALUATION OF LEARNING

Directions: Fill in each blank with the correct answer.

1. Most of the urine (95%) is composed of what substance?

____

____

2. List two conditions that may cause polyuria.

____

____

3. List two conditions that may cause oliguria.

____

____

4. What type of urine specimen is required for the detection of a urinary tract infection (UTI)?

____

5. Why is a first-voided morning specimen often preferred for urine testing?

____

____

6. A 24-hour urine specimen is often used to diagnose what condition?

____

7. Why should a patient not void directly into a 24-hour urine specimen container that contains a preservative?

____

8. List three changes that may take place in a urine specimen if it is allowed to stand at room temperature for more than 1 hour.

____

____

____

9. Why does concentrated urine tend to be dark yellow?

____

____

10. List two factors that may cause a urine specimen to become cloudy.

____

____

11. A urine specimen that has been allowed to stand at room temperature for a long period of time will have what type of odor?

____

12. What is the purpose of testing the specific gravity of urine?

____

13. What is the normal range for the specific gravity of urine?

____

14. What is the difference between qualitative and quantitative test results?

____

____

____

15. What may cause an increase in the pH of urine?

____

____

16. Why does urine become more alkaline if it is not preserved?

____

____

____

17. What may cause glycosuria?

____

____

18. What conditions may cause proteinuria?

___

___

19. What may cause ketosis?

___

___

20. What conditions may cause bilirubin to appear in the urine?

___

___

21. What may cause blood to appear in the urine?

___

___

22. Why should a nitrite test not be performed on a urine specimen that has been left standing at room temperature?

___

___

23. How should urine reagent strips be stored?

___

___

24. What is the purpose of performing a microscopic examination of the urine?

___

___

___

25. Why is a first-voided urine specimen recommended for a microscopic examination of the urine?

___

___

26. What effect does concentrated urine have on red blood cells in it?

___

___

27. What is a urinary cast?

___

___

28. What is the name of the vaginal infection caused by yeast?

29. List three reasons for performing a pregnancy test.

30. What is the name of the hormone that is present in the urine and blood only of a pregnant woman?

31. List five guidelines that should be followed when performing a pregnancy test.

CRITICAL THINKING ACTIVITIES

A. First-Voided Specimen

You have instructed Jim Pratt to collect a first-voided morning urine specimen, which is to be brought to the medical office for testing. Mr. Pratt asks the following questions. Respond to them in the spaces provided.

1. Why is a first-voided specimen desired?

2. Why must the specimen be preserved until it is brought to the medical office?

B. Clean-Catch Specimen

You have just instructed Ann Berger to obtain a clean-catch midstream specimen at the medical office. Mrs. Berger asks the following questions. Respond to them in the spaces provided.

1. What is the purpose of cleansing the urinary meatus?

2. Why must a front-to-back motion be used to clean the urinary meatus?

3. Why must a small amount of urine first be voided into the toilet?

4. Why should the inside of the specimen cup not be touched?

____

____

C. Urine Testing Kit Instructions

Obtain the package insert instructions that come with any type of commercially prepared diagnostic kit for the chemical testing of urine (e.g., Multistix 10 SG). Using the instructions, answer the following questions in the spaces provided. (*Note:* A package insert for Multistix 10 SG can be obtained on the Internet by performing a search for *Multistix 10 SG product insert*).

1. What is the brand name of the test?

____

2. This test assists in the diagnosis of what conditions?

____

____

____

3. What type of urine specimen is recommended for this test?

____

____

____

4. This test is used to detect the presence of what substances?

____

____

____

5. Explain the proper storage and handling of this test.

____

____

____

6. List any substances or techniques that may interfere with obtaining an accurate reading (e.g., not reading the test at the prescribed time).

____

____

____

D. Crossword Puzzle: Urinalysis

Directions: Complete the crossword puzzle using the clues provided.

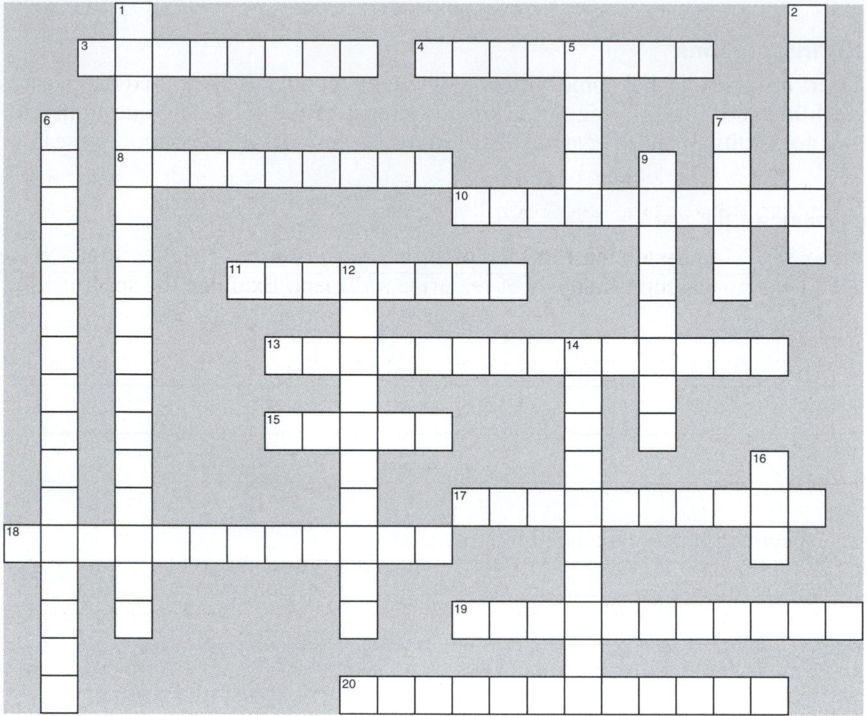

Across

3 Cause of oliguria
4 Cause of glycosuria
8 Yellow urine pigment
10 Treatment for UTI
11 Deteriorates urine strips
13 Security for urine drug testing
15 Neutral pH
17 Specimen for C & S
18 Normal cause of hematuria
19 Specimen for pregnancy test
20 24-hour specimen can diagnose cause of this

Down

1 Bed-wetting
2 Symptom of UTI
5 UTI bacteria
6 Exactly!
7 Most of urine
9 This drug causes polyuria
12 Cause of ketonuria
14 Physical, chemical, and microscopic
16 Makes pregnancy test positive

PRACTICE FOR COMPETENCY

Procedure 30-1: Clean-Catch Midstream Urine Specimen. Collection instructions: Instruct an individual in the procedure for collecting a clean-catch midstream specimen, and record the procedure in the chart provided.

Procedure 30-A: Color and Appearance of a Urine Specimen. Assess the color and appearance of a urine specimen, and record the results in the chart provided.

Procedure 30-2: Chemical Testing of Urine Using the Multistix 10 SG Reagent Strip.

a. Perform a Multistix 10 SG quality control testing procedure, and record results on the quality control log on the next page.

b. Perform a chemical assessment of a urine specimen using a Multistix 10 SG reagent strip. Record the results on the laboratory report form provided. Circle any abnormal results.

Procedure 30-3: Prepare a Urine Specimen for Microscopic Examination of Urine. Practice the procedure for preparing a urine specimen for a microscopic analysis of the urine sediment. Examine the specimen, and record the results in the chart provided.

Procedure 30-4: Urine Pregnancy Test. Perform a urine pregnancy test, and record results in the chart provided.

CHART	
Date	

Chart	
Date	

URINALYSIS QUALITY CONTROL LOG		
Name of Test: ________ Date: ________	Name of Control: ________ Lot #: ________ Exp. Date: ________	Technician: ________
TEST	EXPECTED RESULT (specified in product insert accompanying the control)	CONTROL RESULT
Glucose		
Bilirubin		
Ketone		
Specific gravity		
Blood		
pH		
Protein		
Urobilinogen		
Nitrite		
Leukocytes		

Multistix® *10 SG Reagent Strips for Urinalysis*

PATIENT

DATE TIME

LEUKOCYTES	NEGATIVE ☐		TRACE ☐	SMALL + ☐	MODERATE ++ ☐	LARGE +++ ☐	
NITRITE	NEGATIVE ☐		POSITIVE ☐	POSITIVE ☐	(Any degree of uniform pink color is found)		
UROBILINOGEN	NORMAL 0.2 ☐	NORMAL 1 ☐	mg/dL 2 ☐	4 ☐	8 ☐	(1mg = approx. 1 BU)	
PROTEIN	NEGATIVE ☐	TRACE ☐	mg/dL 30 * ☐	100 ++ ☐	300 +++ ☐	2000 OR MORE ☐	
pH	5.0 ☐	6.0 ☐	6.5 ☐	7.0 ☐	7.5 ☐	8.0 ☐	8.5 ☐
BLOOD	NEGATIVE ☐	NON-HEMOLYZED TRACE ☐	NON-HEMOLYZED MODERATE ☐	HEMOLYZED TRACE ☐	SMALL + ☐	MODERATE ++ ☐	LARGE +++ ☐
SPECIFIC GRAVITY	1.000 ☐	1.006 ☐	1.010 ☐	1.015 ☐	1.020 ☐	1.025 ☐	1.030 ☐
KETONE	NEGATIVE ☐	mg/dL	TRACE 5 ☐	SMALL 15 ☐	MODERATE 40 ☐	LARGE 80 ☐	LARGE 160 ☐
BILIRUBIN	NEGATIVE ☐		SMALL + ☐	MODERATE ++ ☐	LARGE +++ ☐		
GLUCOSE	NEGATIVE ☐	g/L (%) mg/dL	1/10 tr.) 100 ☐	1/6 250 ☐	1/2 500 ☐	1 1000 ☐	2 or more 2000 or more ☐

(Modified and printed by permission of Siemens Healthcare Diagnostics, Deerfield, Ill, 60015.)

Multistix® *10 SG Reagent Strips for Urinalysis*

PATIENT

DATE TIME

LEUKOCYTES	NEGATIVE ☐		TRACE ☐	SMALL + ☐	MODERATE ++ ☐	LARGE +++ ☐	
NITRITE	NEGATIVE ☐		POSITIVE ☐	POSITIVE ☐	(Any degree of uniform pink color is found)		
UROBILINOGEN	NORMAL 0.2 ☐	NORMAL 1 ☐	mg/dL 2 ☐	4 ☐	8 ☐	(1mg = approx. 1 BU)	
PROTEIN	NEGATIVE ☐	TRACE ☐	mg/dL 30 * ☐	100 ++ ☐	300 +++ ☐	2000 OR MORE ☐	
pH	5.0 ☐	6.0 ☐	6.5 ☐	7.0 ☐	7.5 ☐	8.0 ☐	8.5 ☐
BLOOD	NEGATIVE ☐	NON-HEMOLYZED TRACE ☐	NON-HEMOLYZED MODERATE ☐	HEMOLYZED TRACE ☐	SMALL + ☐	MODERATE ++ ☐	LARGE +++ ☐
SPECIFIC GRAVITY	1.000 ☐	1.006 ☐	1.010 ☐	1.015 ☐	1.020 ☐	1.025 ☐	1.030 ☐
KETONE	NEGATIVE ☐	mg/dL	TRACE 5 ☐	SMALL 15 ☐	MODERATE 40 ☐	LARGE 80 ☐	LARGE 160 ☐
BILIRUBIN	NEGATIVE ☐		SMALL + ☐	MODERATE ++ ☐	LARGE +++ ☐		
GLUCOSE	NEGATIVE ☐	g/L (%) mg/dL	1/10 tr.) 100 ☐	1/6 250 ☐	1/2 500 ☐	1 1000 ☐	2 or more 2000 or more ☐

(Modified and printed by permission of Siemens Healthcare Diagnostics, Deerfield, Ill, 60015.)

EVALUATION OF COMPETENCY

Procedure 30-1: Clean-Catch Midstream Specimen Collection Instructions

Name: ______________________________ Date: ______________

Evaluated by: ______________________________ Score: ______________

Performance Objective

Outcome:	Instruct a patient in the procedure for collecting a clean-catch midstream urine specimen.
Conditions:	Given the following: sterile specimen container, personal antiseptic towelettes, and tissues.
Standards:	Time: 10 minutes. Student completed procedure in ________ minutes.
	Accuracy: Satisfactory score on the Performance Evaluation Checklist.

Performance Evaluation Checklist

Trial 1	Trial 2	Point Value	Performance Standards
		●	Sanitized hands.
		●	Greeted the patient and introduced yourself.
		●	Identified the patient and explained the procedure.
		●	Assembled equipment.
		●	Labeled specimen container.
			Instructed the female patient by telling her to
		●	Wash hands and open antiseptic towelettes.
		●	Remove lid from specimen container without touching inside of container or lid.
		●	Pull down undergarments and sit on the toilet.
		●	Expose the urinary meatus by spreading the labia apart with one hand.
		●	Cleanse each side of the urinary meatus with a front-to-back motion using a separate towelette on each side of the meatus.
		▷	Explained why a front-to-back motion should be used.
		●	After use, discard each towelette into toilet.
		●	Cleanse directly across the meatus using a third towelette and discard it.
		●	Void a small amount of urine into the toilet, while continuing to hold the labia apart.
		▷	Explained the purpose of voiding into the toilet.
		●	Without stopping the urine flow, collect the next amount of urine by voiding into the sterile container.
		●	Fill container approximately half full with urine without touching the inside of the container.

Trial 1	Trial 2	Point Value	Performance Standards
		▷	Stated why the inside of the container should not be touched.
		●	Void the last amount of urine into the toilet.
		●	Replace specimen container lid.
		●	Wipe area dry with a tissue, flush the toilet, and wash hands.
			Instructed the male patient by telling him to
		●	Wash hands and open antiseptic towelettes, and remove lid from specimen container.
		●	Pull down undergarments and stand in front of toilet.
		●	Retract the foreskin of the penis if uncircumcised.
		●	Cleanse area around the meatus and the urethral opening by wiping each side of the meatus with a separate antiseptic towelette.
		●	Cleanse directly across the meatus using a third antiseptic towelette.
		●	Discard each towelette into the toilet after use.
		●	Void a small amount of urine into the toilet.
		●	Collect the next amount of urine by voiding into the sterile container without touching the inside of the container.
		●	Fill container approximately half full with urine.
		●	Void the last amount of urine into the toilet.
		●	Replace lid on specimen container.
		●	Wipe area dry with a tissue, flush the toilet, and wash hands.
			Performed the following:
		●	Provided patient with instructions on what to do with specimen.
		●	Charted the procedure correctly.
		●	Tested specimen or prepared it for transport to an outside laboratory.
		Ⓐ	Explained to a patient the rationale for performance of a procedure.
		*	Completed the procedure within 10 minutes.
			TOTALS

CHART	
Date	

Evaluation of Student Performance

EVALUATION CRITERIA			COMMENTS
Symbol	**Category**	**Point Value**	
✶	Critical Step	16 points	
●	Essential Step	6 points	
Ⓐ	Affective Competency	6 points	
▷	Theory Question	2 points	
Score calculation: 100 points – ___ points missed ___ Score Satisfactory score: 85 or above			

2008 CAAHEP Competencies Achieved

Psychomotor (Skills)

☑ IV. 2. Report relevant information to others succinctly and accurately.

Affective (Behavior)

☑ III. 1. Display sensitivity to patient rights and feelings in collecting specimens.
☑ III. 2. Explain the rationale for performance of a procedure to the patient.

2015 CAAHEP Competencies Achieved

Psychomotor (Skills)

☑ V. 11. Report relevant information concisely and accurately.

Affective (Behavior)

☑ V. 4. Explain to a patient the rationale for performance of a procedure.

ABHES Competencies Achieved

☑ 8. f. Display professionalism through written and verbal communications.
☑ 10. e. (1). Instruct patient in the collection of clean-catch mid-stream urine specimen.

Notes

EVALUATION OF COMPETENCY

Procedure 30-A: Assessing Color and Appearance of a Urine Specimen

Name: ______________________________ Date: ____________________

Evaluated by: ______________________________ Score: ____________________

Performance Objective

Outcome:	Assess the color and appearance of a urine specimen.
Conditions:	Given a transparent container and a urine specimen.
Standards:	Time: 5 minutes. Student completed procedure in __________ minutes.
	Accuracy: Satisfactory score on the Performance Evaluation Checklist.

Performance Evaluation Checklist

Trial 1	Trial 2	Point Value	Performance Standards
			Color
		●	Sanitized hands and applied gloves.
		●	Transferred urine specimen to a transparent container.
		●	Assessed the color of the urine specimen.
		✶	The assessment was identical to the evaluator's assessment.
		●	Charted the results correctly.
			Appearance
		●	Assessed the appearance of the urine specimen in the transparent container.
		✶	The assessment was identical to the evaluator's assessment.
		●	Charted the results correctly.
		●	Properly disposed of urine specimen.
		●	Sanitized hands and removed gloves.
		Ⓐ	Incorporated critical thinking skills when performing patient assessment.
		Ⓐ	Reassured a patient of the accuracy of the test results.
		✶	Completed the procedure within 5 minutes.
			TOTALS

Chart	
Date	

Evaluation of Student Performance

EVALUATION CRITERIA			COMMENTS
Symbol	**Category**	**Point Value**	
∗	Critical Step	16 points	
●	Essential Step	6 points	
Ⓐ	Affective Competency	6 points	
▷	Theory Question	2 points	
Score calculation: 100 points − ___ points missed ___ Score Satisfactory score: 85 or above			

2008 CAAHEP Competencies Achieved

Psychomotor (Skills)
☑ I. 14. Perform urinalysis.

Affective (Behavior)
☑ II. 2. Distinguish between normal and abnormal test results.

2015 CAAHEP Competencies Achieved

Psychomotor (Skills)
☑ I. 11. c. Obtain specimen and perform CLIA waived urinalysis.
☑ II. 2. Differentiate between normal and abnormal test results.

Affective (Behavior)
☑ I. 1. Incorporate critical thinking skills when performing patient assessment.
☑ II. 1. Reassure a patient of the accuracy of the test results.

ABHES Competencies Achieved

☑ 10. b. (1). Perform selected CLIA-waived tests that assist with diagnosis and treatment; urinalysis.

EVALUATION OF COMPETENCY

Procedure 30-2: Chemical Testing of Urine with the Multistix 10 SG Reagent Strip

Name: ______________________________ Date: ______________

Evaluated by: ______________________________ Score: ______________

Performance Objective

Outcome:	Perform a chemical assessment of a urine specimen.
Conditions:	Given the following: disposable gloves, Multistix 10 SG reagent strips, urine container, laboratory report form, and a waste container.
Standards:	Time: 5 minutes. Student completed procedure in ________ minutes.
	Accuracy: Satisfactory score on the performance evaluation checklist.

Performance Evaluation Checklist

Trial 1	Trial 2	Point Value	Performance Standards
		•	If necessary, performed a quality control testing procedure.
		▷	Stated when a quality control procedure should be performed.
		•	Obtained a freshly voided urine specimen from patient.
		▷	Explained why the container used to collect the specimen should be clean.
		•	Sanitized hands.
		•	Assembled equipment.
		•	Checked expiration date of the reagent strips.
		▷	Stated why expiration date should be checked.
		•	Applied gloves.
		•	Removed a reagent strip from container and recapped immediately.
		▷	Explained why container should be recapped immediately.
		•	Did not touch the test areas with fingers.
		▷	Explained why the test areas should not be touched with fingers.
		•	Mixed the urine specimen thoroughly.
		•	Removed the lid and completely immersed the reagent strip in urine specimen.
		•	Removed the strip immediately and ran the edge against the rim of urine container. Started the timer.
		▷	Explained why excess urine should be removed from the strip.
		•	Held the reagent strip in a horizontal position and placed it as close as possible to the corresponding color blocks on color chart.
		▷	Explained why the strip should be held in a horizontal position.

Trial 1	Trial 2	Point Value	Performance Standards
		●	Read the results at the exact reading times specified on the color chart.
		▷	Explained why the results must be read at specified times.
		✶	The results were identical to the evaluator's results.
		●	Disposed of the strip in a regular waste container.
		●	Removed gloves and sanitized hands.
		●	Charted the results correctly.
		Ⓐ	Incorporated critical thinking skills when performing patient assessment.
		Ⓐ	Reassured a patient of the accuracy of the test results.
		✶	Completed the procedure within 5 minutes.
			TOTALS

CHART	
Date	

Evaluation of Student Performance

EVALUATION CRITERIA			COMMENTS
Symbol	**Category**	**Point Value**	
✶	Critical Step	16 points	
●	Essential Step	6 points	
Ⓐ	Affective Competency	6 points	
▷	Theory Question	2 points	
Score calculation: 100 points – ___ points missed ___ Score Satisfactory score: 85 or above			

2008 CAAHEP Competencies Achieved
Psychomotor (Skills) ☑ I. 11. Perform quality control measures. ☑ I. 14. Perform urinalysis. ***Affective (Behavior)*** ☑ II. 2. Distinguish between normal and abnormal test results.

2015 CAAHEP Competencies Achieved
Psychomotor (Skills)
☑ I. 10. Perform a quality control measure.
☑ I. 11. c. Obtain specimen and perform CLIA waived urinalysis.
☑ II. 2. Differentiate between normal and abnormal test results.
Affective (Behavior)
☑ I. 1. Incorporate critical thinking skills when performing patient assessment.
☑ II. 1. Reassure a patient of the accuracy of the test results.

ABHES Competencies Achieved
☑ 10. a. Practice quality control.
☑ 10. b. Perform selected CLIA-waived tests that assist with diagnosis and treatment: (1) urinalysis (6) kit testing (c) dip sticks.

Multistix® *10 SG* Reagent Strips for Urinalysis

PATIENT

DATE TIME

LEUKOCYTES	NEGATIVE ☐		TRACE ☐	SMALL + ☐	MODERATE ++ ☐	LARGE +++ ☐	
NITRITE	NEGATIVE ☐		POSITIVE ☐	POSITIVE ☐	(Any degree of uniform pink color is found)		
UROBILINOGEN	NORMAL 0.2 ☐	NORMAL 1 ☐	mg/dL 2 ☐	4 ☐	8 ☐	(1mg = approx. 1 BU)	
PROTEIN	NEGATIVE ☐	TRACE ☐	mg/dL 30 + ☐	100 ++ ☐	300 +++ ☐	2000 OR MORE ☐	
pH	5.0 ☐	6.0 ☐	6.5 ☐	7.0 ☐	7.5 ☐	8.0 ☐	8.5 ☐
BLOOD	NEGATIVE ☐	NON-HEMOLYZED TRACE ☐	NON-HEMOLYZED MODERATE ☐	HEMOLYZED TRACE ☐	SMALL + ☐	MODERATE ++ ☐	LARGE +++ ☐
SPECIFIC GRAVITY	1.000 ☐	1.006 ☐	1.010 ☐	1.015 ☐	1.020 ☐	1.025 ☐	1.030 ☐
KETONE	NEGATIVE ☐	mg/dL	TRACE 5 ☐	SMALL 15 ☐	MODERATE 40 ☐	LARGE 80 ☐	LARGE 160 ☐
BILIRUBIN	NEGATIVE ☐		SMALL + ☐	MODERATE ++ ☐	LARGE +++ ☐		
GLUCOSE	NEGATIVE ☐	g/L (%) mg/dL	+ 1/10 tr.) 100 ☐	1/6 250 ☐	1/2 500 ☐	1 1000 ☐	2 or more 2000 or more ☐

(Modified and printed by permission of Siemens Healthcare Diagnostics, Deerfield, Ill, 60015.)

Multistix® 10 SG Reageant Strips for Urinalysis

PATIENT

DATE TIME

LEUKOCYTES	NEGATIVE ☐		TRACE ☐	SMALL + ☐	MODERATE ++ ☐	LARGE +++ ☐	
NITRITE	NEGATIVE ☐		POSITIVE ☐	POSITIVE ☐	(Any degree of uniform pink color is found)		
UROBILINOGEN	NORMAL 0.2 ☐	NORMAL 1 ☐	mg/dL 2 ☐	4 ☐	8 ☐	(1mg = approx. 1 BU)	
PROTEIN	NEGATIVE ☐	TRACE ☐	mg/dL 30 * ☐	100 ++ ☐	300 +++ ☐	2000 OR MORE ☐	
pH	5.0 ☐	6.0 ☐	6.5 ☐	7.0 ☐	7.5 ☐	8.0 ☐	8.5 ☐
BLOOD	NEGATIVE ☐	NON-HEMOLYZED TRACE ☐	NON-HEMOLYZED MODERATE ☐	HEMOLYZED TRACE ☐	SMALL + ☐	MODERATE ++ ☐	LARGE +++ ☐
SPECIFIC GRAVITY	1.000 ☐	1.006 ☐	1.010 ☐	1.015 ☐	1.020 ☐	1.025 ☐	1.030 ☐
KETONE	NEGATIVE ☐	mg/dL	TRACE 5 ☐	SMALL 15 ☐	MODERATE 40 ☐	LARGE 80 ☐	LARGE 160 ☐
BILIRUBIN	NEGATIVE ☐		SMALL + ☐	MODERATE ++ ☐	LARGE +++ ☐		
GLUCOSE	NEGATIVE ☐	g/L (%) mg/dL	1/10 tr.) 100 ☐	1/6 250 ☐	1/2 500 ☐	1 1000 ☐	2 or more 2000 or more ☐

(Modified and printed by permission of Siemens Healthcare Diagnostics, Deerfield, Ill, 60015.)

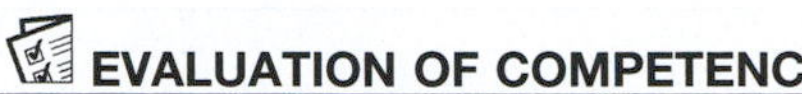

EVALUATION OF COMPETENCY

Procedure 30-3: Prepare a Urine Specimen for Microscopic Examination of Urine: Kova Method

Name: ________________________________ Date: ________________

Evaluated by: ____________________________ Score: ________________

Performance Objective

Outcome:	Prepare a urine specimen for microscopic analysis by the physician.
Conditions:	Given the following: disposable gloves; first-voided morning urine specimen; Kova urine centrifuge tube, cap, pipet, slide, and stain; test tube rack; urine centrifuge; mechanical stage microscope; and waste container.
Standards:	Time: 15 minutes. Student completed procedure in __________ minutes.
	Accuracy: Satisfactory score on the Performance Evaluation Checklist.

Performance Evaluation Checklist

Trial 1	Trial 2	Point Value	Performance Standards
		●	Sanitized hands.
		●	Assembled equipment.
		●	Applied gloves.
		●	Mixed urine specimen with pipet.
		▷	Stated the purpose of mixing the specimen.
		●	Poured urine specimen into urine centrifuge tube to the 12-mL mark.
		●	Capped the tube.
		●	Centrifuged specimen for 5 minutes.
		▷	Stated the purpose of centrifuging the specimen.
		●	Removed the tube from the centrifuge without disturbing the sediment.
		●	Removed the cap.
		●	Inserted Kova pipet into the urine tube and seated it firmly.
		●	Poured off the supernatant fluid.
		●	Removed pipet from the tube.
		●	Added one drop of Kova stain to the tube.
		▷	Stated the purpose of the stain.
		●	Placed pipet back in tube and mixed specimen thoroughly.
		●	Placed urine tube in test tube rack.

Trial 1	Trial 2	Point Value	Performance Standards
		●	Transferred a sample of the specimen to the Kova slide.
		●	Did not overfill or underfill the well of the Kova slide.
		●	Placed pipet in the urine tube.
		●	Allowed specimen to sit for 1 minute.
		▷	Explained the purpose of allowing the specimen to sit 1 minute.
		●	Properly focused the specimen under low power.
		●	Placed the slide on the stage of the microscope.
		●	Properly focused the specimen for the physician.
		●	Removed the slide from the stage when the physician is finished examining the specimen.
		●	Disposed of the slide and pipet in a regular waste container.
		●	Rinsed the remaining urine down the sink.
		●	Capped the empty urine tube and disposed of it in a regular waste container.
		●	Removed gloves and sanitized hands.
		Ⓐ	Explained to a patient the rationale for performance of a procedure.
		*	Completed the procedure within 15 minutes.
			TOTALS

Chart	
Date	

Evaluation of Student Performance

EVALUATION CRITERIA			COMMENTS
Symbol	Category	Point Value	
∗	Critical Step	16 points	
●	Essential Step	6 points	
Ⓐ	Affective Competency	6 points	
▷	Theory Question	2 points	
Score calculation: 100 points − ___ points missed ___ Score Satisfactory score: 85 or above			

2008 CAAHEP Competencies Achieved
Psychomotor (Skills) ☑ I. 11. Perform quality control measures. ☑ I. 14. Perform urinalysis. ***Affective (Behavior)*** ☑ III. 2. Explain the rationale for performance of a procedure to the patient.

2015 CAAHEP Competencies Achieved
Psychomotor (Skills) ☑ I. 9. Assist provider with patient exam. ***Affective (Behavior)*** ☑ V. 4. Explain to a patient the rationale for performance of a procedure.

ABHES Competencies Achieved
☑ 9. c. Assist provider with general/physical examination.

Notes

EVALUATION OF COMPETENCY

Procedure 30-4: Performing a Urine Pregnancy Test

Name: ______________________ Date: ______________

Evaluated by: ______________________ Score: ______________

Performance Objective

Outcome:	Perform a urine pregnancy test.
Conditions:	Given the following: disposable gloves, urine pregnancy testing kit, first-voided morning urine specimen, waste container.
Standards:	Time: 5 minutes. Student completed procedure in ________ minutes.
	Accuracy: Satisfactory score on the Performance Evaluation Checklist.

Performance Evaluation Checklist

Trial 1	Trial 2	Point Value	Performance Standards
		•	Sanitized hands.
		•	Assembled equipment.
		•	Checked the expiration date on the pregnancy test.
		▷	Explained why the expiration date should be checked.
		•	If necessary, ran controls on the pregnancy test.
		▷	Stated when controls should be run.
		•	Applied gloves.
		•	Mixed the urine specimen.
		•	Removed the test cassette from its pouch.
		•	Placed the test cassette on a clean, dry, level surface.
		•	Added 3 drops of urine to the well on the test cassette.
		•	Disposed of the pipet in a regular waste container.
		•	Waited 3 minutes and read the results.
		•	Interpreted the test results.
		*	The results were identical to the evaluator's results.
		▷	Described the appearance of a positive and a negative test result.
		▷	Explained what should be done if a blue control line does not appear.
		•	Disposed of the test cassette in a regular waste container.
		•	Removed gloves and sanitized hands.
		•	Charted the results correctly.
		Ⓐ	Incorporated critical thinking skills when performing patient assessment.

Trial 1	Trial 2	Point Value	Performance Standards
		Ⓐ	Reassured a patient of the accuracy of the test results.
		✶	Completed the procedure within 5 minutes.
			TOTALS

CHART	
Date	

Evaluation of Student Performance

EVALUATION CRITERIA			COMMENTS
Symbol	**Category**	**Point Value**	
✶	Critical Step	16 points	
●	Essential Step	6 points	
Ⓐ	Affective Competency	6 points	
▷	Theory Question	2 points	
Score calculation: 100 points − ___ points missed ___ Score Satisfactory score: 85 or above			

2008 CAAHEP Competencies Achieved
Psychomotor (Skills) ☑ I. 11. Perform quality control measures. ☑ I. 16. Screen test results. ***Affective (Behavior)*** ☑ II. 2. Distinguish between normal and abnormal test results.

2015 CAAHEP Competencies Achieved
Psychomotor (Skills) ☑ I. 10. Perform a quality control measure. ☑ I. 11. c. Obtain specimen and perform CLIA waived urinalysis. ☑ II. 2. Differentiate between normal and abnormal test results. ***Affective (Behavior)*** ☑ I. 1. Incorporate critical thinking skills when performing patient assessment. ☑ II. 1. Reassure a patient of the accuracy of the test results.

ABHES Competencies Achieved
☑ 10. a. Practice quality control. ☑ 10. b. Perform selected CLIA-waived tests that assist with diagnosis and treatment: (6) kit testing (a) pregnancy.

31 Phlebotomy

CHAPTER ASSIGNMENTS

✓ After Completing	Date Due	Study Guide Pages	STUDY GUIDE ASSIGNMENTS (CTA = Critical Thinking Activity)	Possible Points	Points You Earned
		877	Pretest	10	
		 878 878	Term Key Term Assessment A. Definitions B. Word Parts (Add 1 point for each key term)	 16 13	
		879-883	Evaluation of Learning questions	41	
		883	CTA A: Antecubital Veins	5	
			Evolve Site: Got Blood? (Record points earned)		
		884-885	CTA B: Venipuncture-Vacuum Tube Method	15	
		885-886	CTA C: Venipuncture Situations	7	
		886	CTA D: Skin Puncture	8	
		887	CTA E: Crossword Puzzle	29	
			Evolve Site: Apply Your Knowledge questions	10	
			Evolve Site: Video Evaluation	42	
		877	Posttest	10	
			ADDITIONAL ASSIGNMENTS		
			TOTAL POINTS		

Notes

✓ When Assigned By Your Instructor	Study Guide Pages	Practices Required	LABORATORY ASSIGNMENTS (Procedure Number and Name)	Score*
	889-890	5	**Practice for Competency** 31-1: Venipuncture—Vacuum Tube Method Textbook reference: pp. 830-835	
	891-894		**Evaluation of Competency** 31-1: Venipuncture—Vacuum Tube Method	*
	889-890	5	**Practice for Competency** 31-2: Venipuncture—Butterfly Method Textbook reference: pp. 837-842	
	895-898		**Evaluation of Competency** 31-2: Venipuncture—Butterfly Method	*
	889-890	3	**Practice for Competency** 31-3: Skin Puncture—Disposable Semiautomatic Lancet Device Textbook reference: pp. 848-850	
	899-901		**Evaluation of Competency** 31-3: Skin Puncture—Disposable Semiautomatic Lancet Device	*
	889-890	3	**Practice for Competency** 31-A: Skin Puncture—Reusable Semiautomatic Lancet Device Textbook reference: p. 848	
	903-905		**Evaluation of Competency** 31-A: Skin Puncture—Reusable Semiautomatic Lancet Device	*
			ADDITIONAL ASSIGNMENTS	

Notes

Name ______________________________ Date ______________

PRETEST

True or False

_______ 1. An individual who collects blood specimens is known as a vampire.

_______ 2. The purpose of applying a tourniquet when performing venipuncture is to make the patient's veins stand out.

_______ 3. The tourniquet should be left on the patient's arm for at least 2 minutes before performing a venipuncture.

_______ 4. Serum is obtained from whole blood that has been centrifuged.

_______ 5. A 25-gauge needle is recommended for performing venipuncture.

_______ 6. The size of the evacuated tube used to obtain a venous blood specimen depends on the size of the patient's veins.

_______ 7. A correct order of draw for the vacuum tube method of venipuncture is red, lavender, gray, and green.

_______ 8. Veins are most likely to collapse in patients with large veins and thick walls.

_______ 9. Hemolysis of a blood specimen results in inaccurate test results.

_______ 10. When obtaining a capillary specimen, the first drop of blood should be used for the test.

POSTTEST

True or False

_______ 1. Venous reflux can be prevented by filling the evacuated tube to the exhaustion of the vacuum.

_______ 2. If the tourniquet is applied too tightly, inaccurate test results may occur.

_______ 3. The median cubital vein is the best vein to use for venipuncture.

_______ 4. On standing, a blood specimen to which an anticoagulant has been added separates into plasma, buffy coat, and blood cells.

_______ 5. Whole blood is obtained by using a tube containing an anticoagulant.

_______ 6. An evacuated glass tube with a lavender stopper contains EDTA.

_______ 7. A red-stoppered tube is used to collect a blood specimen for most blood chemistries.

_______ 8. Not filling a tube to the exhaustion of the vacuum can result in hemolysis of the blood specimen.

_______ 9. If the needle is removed from the arm before removing the tourniquet, the evacuated tube will not fill completely.

_______ 10. If a fibrin clot forms in the serum layer of a blood specimen, it will lead to inaccurate test results.

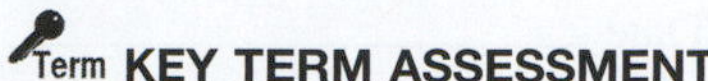

KEY TERM ASSESSMENT

A. Definitions

Directions: Match each key term with its definition.

_______ 1. Antecubital space
_______ 2. Anticoagulant
_______ 3. Buffy coat
_______ 4. Evacuated tube
_______ 5. Hematoma
_______ 6. Hemoconcentration
_______ 7. Hemolysis
_______ 8. Osteochondritis
_______ 9. Osteomyelitis
_______ 10. Phlebotomist
_______ 11. Phlebotomy
_______ 12. Plasma
_______ 13. Serum
_______ 14. Venipuncture
_______ 15. Venous reflux
_______ 16. Venous stasis

A. The liquid part of blood, consisting of a clear, straw-colored fluid that makes up approximately 55% of the blood volume
B. A substance that inhibits blood clotting
C. Health professional trained in the collection of blood specimens
D. The breakdown of blood cells
E. A closed glass or plastic tube that contains a premeasured vacuum
F. The temporary cessation or slowing of the venous blood flow
G. A thin, light-colored layer of white blood cells and platelets that lies between a top layer of plasma and a bottom layer of red blood cells when an anticoagulant has been added to a blood specimen
H. The surface of the arm in front of the elbow
I. Inflammation of bone and cartilage
J. An increase in the concentration of the nonfilterable blood components
K. Plasma from which the clotting factor fibrinogen has been removed
L. Incision of a vein for the removal of blood
M. Inflammation of the bone or bone marrow as a result of bacterial infection
N. A swelling or mass of coagulated blood caused by a break in a blood vessel
O. Puncturing of a vein
P. The backflow of blood (from an evacuated tube) into the patient's vein

B. Word Parts

Directions: Indicate the meaning of each word part in the space provided. List as many medical terms as possible that incorporate the word part in the space provided.

Word Part	Meaning of Word Part	Medical Terms That Incorporate Word Part
1. ante-		
2. anti-		
3. hemat/o		
4. -oma		
5. hem/o		
6. lysis		
7. oste/o		
8. myel/o		
9. -itis		
10. phleb/o		
11. -otomy		
12. ven/o		
13. -ous		

EVALUATION OF LEARNING

Directions: Fill in each blank with the correct answer.

1. List the three major areas of blood collection included in phlebotomy.

___

___

___

2. What is the purpose of performing a venipuncture?

___

___

3. List methods that can be used to perform a venipuncture.

___

___

___

4. What are the advantages of using the vacuum tube method of venipuncture?

___

___

5. When would the butterfly method of venipuncture be preferred over the vacuum tube method?

___

___

___

6. What reference source should be consulted for collection and handling requirements in the following situations?
   a. The specimen is being transported to an outside laboratory for testing:

   ___

   b. The specimen is being tested in the medical office:

   ___

7. Why should a patient be identified using two forms of identification?

___

___

8. What is a unique identifier?

___

9. Explain how to prevent venous reflux.

___

___

10. What is the purpose of the tourniquet?

11. Why are the antecubital veins preferred for performing a venipuncture?

12. After locating a suitable vein for venipuncture, what three qualities should be determined with respect to the vein?

13. List four techniques that can be used to make veins more prominent.

14. Why should the veins of the hand be used only as a last resort when performing a venipuncture?

15. How is a serum specimen obtained?

16. How is a whole blood specimen obtained?

17. List the three layers into which blood separates when it is mixed with an anticoagulant.

18. List the layers into which blood separates when an anticoagulant is not added to it.

19. List six OSHA safety precautions that must be followed when performing a venipuncture and separating serum or plasma from whole blood.

____

____

____

____

____

20. What are the ranges for the gauge and length of the needle used for the vacuum tube method of venipuncture?

____

____

21. What is the purpose of the flange on the plastic holder of the vacuum tube system?

____

____

22. What type of additive is present in each of the following evacuated tubes?

Red _______________

Red/gray speckled _______________

Lav _______________

Light blue _______________

Green _______________

Gray _______________

Royal blue _______________

23. What color stopper must be used to collect the blood specimen for each of the tests listed?

Complete blood count _______________

Prothrombin time _______________

Glucose tolerance test _______________

Most blood chemistry tests _______________

Blood gas determinations _______________

Lead testing _______________

24. Why is it important to use the correct order of draw when performing a venipuncture?

____

____

25. Why is it important to mix a tube containing an anticoagulant immediately after drawing it?

____

____

26. What are the ranges for the gauge and length of needle used for the butterfly method of venipuncture?

27. How can a vein be prevented from rolling when performing a venipuncture on the cephalic or basic veins?

28. What is typically observed when performing a venipuncture on a vein that collapses?

29. What are three ways in which a hematoma may occur?

30. List four ways to prevent a blood specimen from becoming hemolyzed.

31. List examples of substances dissolved in the serum of blood.

32. What is the purpose of performing laboratory tests on serum?

33. List the proper size tube that must be used to obtain the following serum specimens:

2 mL of serum

6 mL of serum

4 mL of serum

34. What is a fibrin clot, and why should it be avoided in a serum specimen?

35. How does a serum separator tube function in the collection of a serum specimen?

____

____

____

36. What is the preferred site for a skin puncture for the following individuals?

a. Adult ____

b. Infant ____

37. Why is it important not to penetrate the skin too deeply when performing a skin puncture?

____

____

38. How does the medical assistant determine the blade length to use to perform a skin puncture?

____

____

39. What are two examples of microcollection devices?

____

____

40. Why should a finger puncture not be performed on the index finger?

____

____

41. Why should the first drop of blood be wiped away when performing a finger puncture?

____

____

CRITICAL THINKING ACTIVITIES

A. Antecubital Veins

Practice palpating the antecubital veins on at least five classmates. Use a tourniquet applied to each person's arm, and ask the individual to clench his or her fist. Record the individual's name and which vein would be considered the best to use on each person when performing venipuncture.

	NAME	SUITABLE VEIN
1.		
2.		
3.		
4.		
5.		

B. Venipuncture—Vacuum Tube Method

Using the principles outlined in the vacuum tube venipuncture procedure, state what can happen under the following circumstances:

1. An evacuated tube is used that is past its expiration date.

2. The vacuum tube is not labeled.

3. The tourniquet is not applied tightly enough.

4. The tourniquet is left on for more than 1 minute.

5. The area that has just been cleansed with an antiseptic is not allowed to dry before the venipuncture is made.

6. The evacuated tube is inserted past the indentation in the plastic holder before the vein is entered.

7. An angle of less than 15 degrees is used when performing venipuncture.

8. An angle of more than 15 degrees is used when performing venipuncture.

9. The needle is moved after inserting it.

10. Venous reflux occurs when using an EDTA evacuated tube.

11. The vacuum tube is removed before it has filled to the exhaustion of the vacuum.

12. The needle is removed from the arm before the tourniquet has been removed.

13. A gauze pad is not placed slightly above the puncture site before removing the needle.

14. The patient bends the arm at the elbow after the needle is removed.

15. The patient lifts a heavy object after the procedure.

C. Venipuncture Situations

You are responsible for performing the venipunctures in your medical office. In the space provided, explain what you would do in each of the following situations:

1. The patient asks you if the venipuncture will hurt.

2. On palpating the patient's vein, you find that it feels stiff and hard.

3. You have attempted one venipuncture in a patient with small veins using the vacuum tube method of venipuncture; however, the vein collapsed, and you were unable to obtain blood.

4. The patient moves during the procedure, causing the needle to come out of his or her arm.

5. You have inserted the needle in the vein but notice a sudden swelling around the puncture site.

6. You inadvertently puncture the brachial artery after inserting the needle.

____

____

7. The patient begins to sweat and tells you that he or she feels warm and light-headed.

____

____

D. Skin Puncture

The medical assistant is performing a skin puncture on an adult patient to obtain a capillary blood specimen for a hemoglobin test. For each of the following situations, write C if the technique is correct and I if the technique is incorrect. If the technique is correct, explain the rationale for performing it that way; if incorrect, explain what might happen if the technique were performed in the incorrect manner.

_______ 1. Before making the puncture, the medical assistant asks the patient to rinse his or her hand in warm water.

____

____

_______ 2. The puncture is made with the patient in a standing position.

____

____

_______ 3. The site is allowed to dry thoroughly after it is cleansed with an antiseptic wipe.

____

____

_______ 4. The specimen is collected from the lateral part of the tip of the ring finger.

____

____

_______ 5. The puncture is made perpendicular to the lines of the fingerprint.

____

____

_______ 6. The depth of the puncture is 4 mm.

____

____

_______ 7. The first drop of blood is wiped away.

____

____

_______ 8. The puncture site is squeezed to obtain the blood specimen.

____

____

E. Crossword Puzzle: Phlebotomy

Directions: Complete the crossword puzzle using the clues provided.

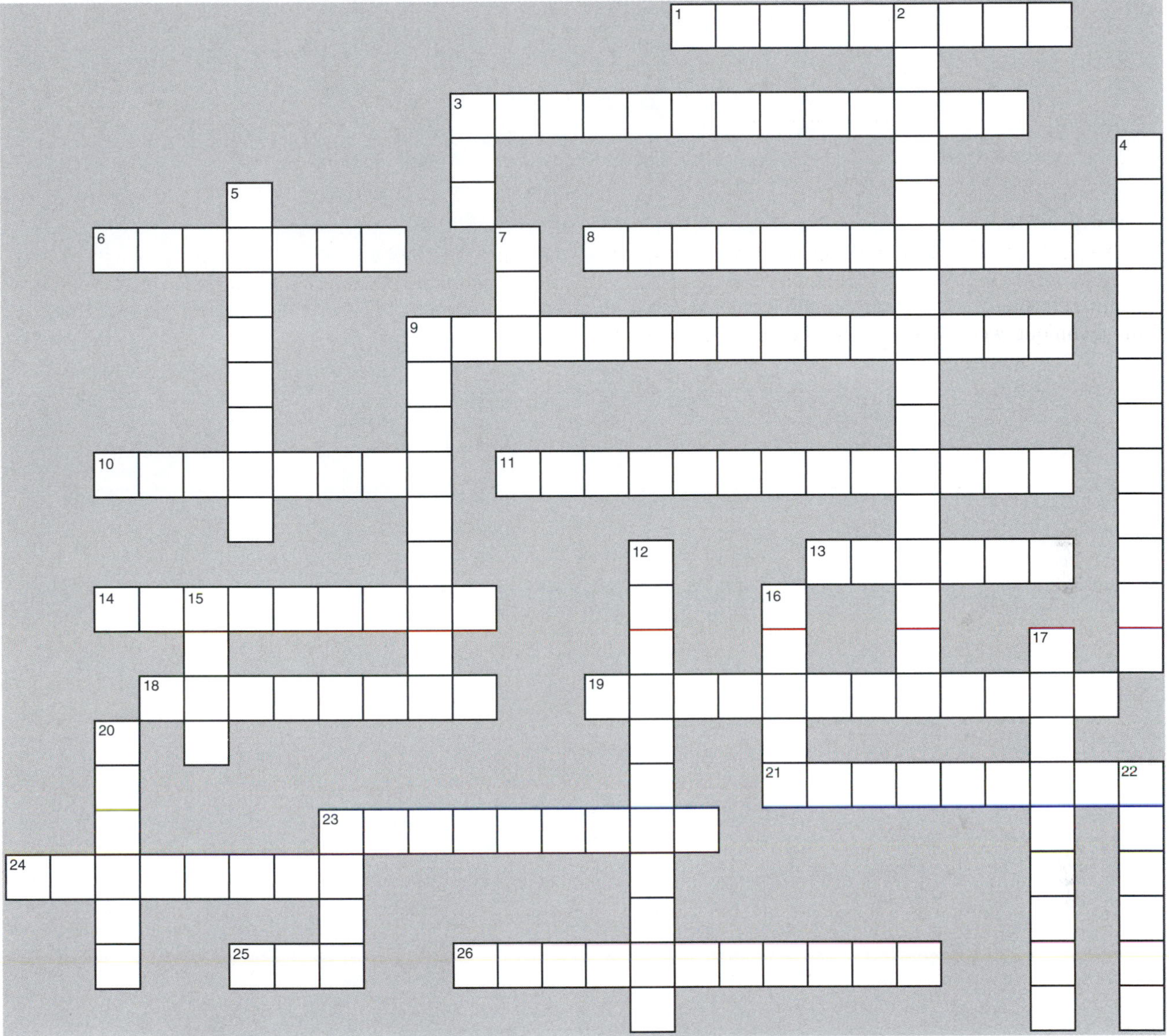

Across

1 What BP does during fainting
3 Makes RBCs clot quicker
6 Rolling vein
8 Best VP vein
9 Inflammation of bone and cartilage
10 Outdated tube problem
11 Inhibits blood clotting
13 Faint position
14 PT tube
18 EDTA tube
19 Backflow of blood
21 For small veins
23 Broken RBCs
24 Bad bruise
25 No additive tube
26 Based on size of pt's finger

Down

2 In front of the elbow
3 Select lavender tube for this test
4 Collects blood
5 First drop of capillary blood?
7 Contains a "separating" gel
9 Time limit for tourniquet
12 Do not use for skin puncture
15 Fluoride/oxalate tube
16 Don't use to palpate vein
17 WBCs and platelets
20 Fainting warning signal
22 Color of serum
23 Last choice veins

Notes

PRACTICE FOR COMPETENCY

Procedure 31-1: Venipuncture Vacuum Tube Method. Practice the procedure for collecting a venous blood specimen using the vacuum tube method. Record the procedure in the chart provided.

Procedure 31-2: Venipuncture Butterfly Method. Practice the procedure for collecting a venous blood specimen using the butterfly method. Record the procedure in the chart provided.

Procedure 31-3: Disposable Lancet. Obtain a capillary blood specimen using a disposable semiautomatic lancet device.

Procedure 31-A: Reusable Lancet. Obtain a capillary blood specimen using a reusable semiautomatic lancet.

Chart	
Date	

Chart	
Date	

EVALUATION OF COMPETENCY

Procedure 31-1: Venipuncture—Vacuum Tube Method

Name: ______________________ Date: ______________

Evaluated by: ______________________ Score: ______________

Performance Objective

Outcome:	Perform a venipuncture using the vacuum tube method.
Conditions:	Given the following: disposable gloves, tourniquet, antiseptic wipe, double-pointed needle, plastic holder, evacuated tubes with labels, gauze pad, adhesive bandage, biohazard sharps container, biohazard specimen bag, and a laboratory request form.
Standards:	Time: 10 minutes. Student completed procedure in ________ minutes. Accuracy: Satisfactory score on the Performance Evaluation Checklist.

Performance Evaluation Checklist

Trial 1	Trial 2	Point Value	Performance Standards
		●	Reviewed requirements for collecting and handling the blood specimen.
		●	Sanitized hands.
		●	Greeted the patient and introduced yourself.
		●	Identified the patient.
		●	Asked patient if he or she prepared properly.
			Prepared the equipment
		●	Assembled equipment.
		●	Selected the proper evacuated tubes.
		●	Checked the expiration date of the tubes.
		▷	Stated the purpose of checking the expiration date.
		●	Labeled the evacuated tubes.
		●	Completed a laboratory request form, if necessary.
		●	Screwed the plastic holder onto the Luer adapter and tightened securely.
		●	Opened the gauze packet.
		●	Positioned the evacuated tubes in the correct order of draw.
		●	Tapped evacuated tubes with a powdered additive below the stopper.
		▷	Stated the purpose for tapping the tube.
		●	Placed the first tube loosely in the plastic holder.

Trial 1	Trial 2	Point Value	Performance Standards
			Prepared the patient
		●	Explained the procedure to the patient and reassured patient.
		●	Performed a preliminary assessment of both arms.
		●	Correctly applied the tourniquet.
		●	Asked patient to clench fist.
		▷	Stated the purpose of the tourniquet and clenched fist.
		●	Assessed the veins of both arms.
		●	Determined the best vein to use.
		●	Positioned the patient's arm correctly.
		●	Thoroughly palpated the selected vein.
		●	Did not leave the tourniquet on for more than 1 minute.
		▷	Explained why the tourniquet should not be left on for more than 1 minute.
		●	Removed tourniquet and cleansed the puncture site.
		●	Allowed puncture site to air dry.
		▷	Explained why the site should be allowed to air dry.
		●	Did not touch the site after cleansing.
		●	Placed supplies within comfortable reach of the nondominant hand.
		●	Reapplied tourniquet and applied gloves.
			Performed the venipuncture
		●	Correctly positioned safety shield and removed cap from the needle.
		●	Properly held the venipuncture setup (bevel up) with the dominant hand.
		●	Positioned the tube with the label facing downward.
		▷	Explained why the label should face downward.
		●	Grasped the patient's arm and anchored the vein correctly.
		●	Positioned the venipuncture setup at a 15-degree angle to the arm, with the needle pointing in the same direction as the vein to be entered.
		●	Positioned the needle approximately $^{1}/_{8}$ inch below the place where the vein is to be entered.
		●	Told the patient that a small stick will be felt.
		●	With one continuous motion, entered the skin and then the vein.
		●	Stabilized the vacuum tube setup.
		▷	Stated why the vacuum tube setup should be stabilized.
		●	Pushed the tube forward slowly to the end of the holder using the flange.

Trial 1	Trial 2	Point Value	Performance Standards
		●	Allowed evacuated tube to fill to the exhaustion of the vacuum.
		▷	Explained why the tube should be allowed to fill to the exhaustion of the vacuum.
		●	Removed the tube from the plastic holder using the flange.
		●	Immediately and gently inverted tube 5 times if it contained a clot activator and 8 to 10 times if it contained an anticoagulant.
		●	Inserted the next tube into the holder using the flange.
		●	Continued until the last tube was filled.
		*	Removed the tourniquet and asked the patient to unclench fist.
		●	Removed the last tube from the holder.
		▷	Stated why the last tube should be removed.
		●	Placed gauze pad slightly above puncture site and withdrew the needle slowly and at the same angle as that for penetration.
		●	Immediately moved gauze over puncture site and applied pressure.
		●	Pushed safety shield forward with thumb until audible click is heard.
		●	Properly disposed of holder and needle in a biohazard sharps container.
		●	Instructed patient to apply pressure with the gauze pad for 1 to 2 minutes.
		▷	Stated why pressure should be applied.
		●	Applied adhesive bandage to puncture site.
		●	Placed tube in an upright position in a test tube rack.
		●	Removed gloves and sanitized hands.
		●	Charted the procedure correctly.
		●	Tested specimen or prepared specimen for transport according to medical office policy.
		Ⓐ	Applied critical thinking when performing patient assessment.
		Ⓐ	Showed awareness of a patient's concerns related to the procedure being performed.
		Ⓐ	Recognized the implications for failure to comply with Center for Disease Control (CDC) regulations in healthcare settings.
		*	Completed the procedure within 10 minutes.
			TOTALS

CHART	
Date	

Evaluation of Student Performance

EVALUATION CRITERIA			COMMENTS
Symbol	Category	Point Value	
∗	Critical Step	16 points	
●	Essential Step	6 points	
Ⓐ	Affective Competency	6 points	
▷	Theory Question	2 points	
Score calculation: 100 points − ____points missed ____Score Satisfactory score: 85 or above			

2008 CAAHEP Competencies Achieved
Psychomotor (Skills) ☑ I. 2. Perform venipuncture. ***Affective (Behavior)*** ☑ I. 1. Apply critical thinking skills in performing patient assessment and care. ☑ IV. I. Demonstrate empathy in communicating with patients, family, and staff.

2015 CAAHEP Competencies Achieved
Psychomotor (Skills) ☑ I. 2. b. Perform venipuncture. ☑ III. 10. Demonstrate proper disposal of biohazardous material a. sharps b. regulated waste. ***Affective (Behavior)*** ☑ I. 1. Apply critical thinking when performing patient assessment. ☑ I. 3. Show awareness of a patient's concerns related to the procedure being performed. ☑ III. 1. Recognize the implications for failure to comply with Center for Disease Control (CDC) regulations in healthcare settings.

ABHES Competencies Achieved
☑ 9. a. Practice standard precautions and perform disinfection/sterilization techniques. ☑ 10. c. Dispose of biohazardous materials. ☑ 10. d. (1). Collect, label and process specimens: Perform venipuncture.

EVALUATION OF COMPETENCY

Procedure 31-2: Venipuncture—Butterfly Method

Name: _______________________________ Date: _______________

Evaluated by: _______________________________ Score: _______________

Performance Objective

Outcome:	Perform a venipuncture using the butterfly method.
Conditions:	Given the following: disposable gloves, tourniquet, antiseptic wipe, winged infusion set, plastic holder, evacuated tubes with labels, gauze pad, adhesive bandage, biohazard sharps container, biohazard specimen bag, and a laboratory request form.
Standards:	Time: 10 minutes. Student completed procedure in __________ minutes.
	Accuracy: Satisfactory score on the Performance Evaluation Checklist.

Performance Evaluation Checklist

Trial 1	Trial 2	Point Value	Performance Standards
		•	Reviewed requirements for collecting and handling the blood specimen.
		•	Sanitized hands.
		•	Greeted the patient and introduced yourself.
		•	Identified patient.
		▷	Stated why the patient must be correctly identified.
		•	Asked patient if he or she prepared properly.
		▷	Explained why it is important for the patient to prepare properly.
			Prepared the equipment
		•	Assembled equipment.
		•	Selected the proper evacuated tubes.
		•	Checked the expiration date of the tubes.
		•	Labeled the evacuated tubes.
		•	Completed a laboratory request form, if necessary.
		•	Removed the winged infusion set from its package.
		•	Extended the tubing to its full length and stretched it.
		▷	Explained why the tubing should be extended and stretched.
		•	Screwed the plastic holder onto the Luer adapter and tightened it securely.
		•	Opened the gauze packet.
		•	Positioned the evacuated tubes in the correct order of draw.

Trial 1	Trial 2	Point Value	Performance Standards
		●	Tapped evacuated tubes with a powdered additive below the stopper.
		▷	Stated why tubes with powdered additives must be tapped.
		●	Placed the first tube loosely in the plastic holder with the label facing downward.
		▷	Explained why the label should be facing downward.
			Prepared the patient
		●	Explained the procedure to the patient and reassured patient.
		●	Performed a preliminary assessment of both arms.
		●	Correctly applied the tourniquet and asked patient to clench fist.
		●	Assessed the veins of both arms.
		●	Determined the best vein to use.
		●	Positioned the patient's arm correctly.
		▷	Stated why arm must be positioned correctly.
		●	Thoroughly palpated the selected vein.
		▷	Stated the purpose of palpating the vein.
		●	Did not leave the tourniquet on for more than 1 minute.
		●	Removed tourniquet and cleansed puncture site.
		●	Allowed puncture site to air dry.
		●	Did not touch the site after cleansing.
		●	Placed supplies within comfortable reach.
		●	Reapplied tourniquet and applied gloves.
			Performed the venipuncture
		●	Grasped the winged infusion set correctly.
		●	Removed the protective shield.
		●	Positioned the needle with the bevel up.
		▷	Explained why the bevel should be up.
		●	Grasped patient's arm and anchored the vein correctly.
		●	Positioned the needle at a 15-degree angle to arm, with needle pointing in the same direction as the vein to be entered.
		●	Positioned the needle approximately $^1/_8$ inch below the place where the vein is to be entered.
		●	Told the patient that a small stick will be felt.
		●	With one continuous motion, entered the skin and then the vein.
		▷	Explained why a continuous motion should be used.
		●	Decreased the angle of the needle to 5 degrees.

Trial 1	Trial 2	Point Value	Performance Standards
		●	Seated the needle.
		▷	Stated the purpose of seating the needle.
		●	Opened the butterfly wings and rested them flat against the skin.
		●	Kept the tube and holder in a downward position.
		●	Slowly pushed the tube forward to the end of the plastic holder.
		●	Allowed evacuated tube to fill to the exhaustion of the vacuum.
		▷	Explained why the tube should be filled to the exhaustion of the vacuum.
		●	Removed the tube from the plastic holder.
		●	Immediately and gently inverted evacuated tube 5 times if it contained a clot activator and 8 to 10 times if it contained an anticoagulant.
		▷	Explained why a tube with an anticoagulant must be inverted immediately.
		●	Inserted the next tube into the holder.
		●	Continued until the last tube was filled.
		*	Removed the tourniquet and asked the patient to unclench fist.
		▷	Stated why the tourniquet must be removed before the needle.
		●	Removed the last tube from the holder.
		●	Placed gauze pad slightly above puncture site. Grasped the setup just below the wings and withdrew the needle slowly and at the same angle as that for penetration.
		●	Immediately moved gauze over puncture site and applied pressure.
		●	Instructed the patient to apply pressure with the gauze.
		●	Activated the safety shield on the needle.
		●	Properly disposed of the winged infusion set and plastic holder in a biohazard sharps container.
		●	Continued to apply pressure for 1 to 2 minutes.
		●	Applied adhesive bandage.
		●	Placed the tubes in an upright position in a test tube rack.
		●	Removed gloves and sanitized hands.
		●	Charted the procedure correctly.
		●	Tested specimen or prepared specimen for transport according to medical office policy.
		Ⓐ	Applied critical thinking when performing patient assessment.
		Ⓐ	Showed awareness of a patient's concerns related to the procedure being performed.
		Ⓐ	Recognized the implications for failure to comply with Center for Disease Control (CDC) regulations in healthcare settings.
		*	Completed the procedure within 10 minutes.
			TOTALS

CHART	
Date	

Evaluation of Student Performance

EVALUATION CRITERIA			COMMENTS
Symbol	Category	Point Value	
✶	Critical Step	16 points	
●	Essential Step	6 points	
Ⓐ	Affective Competency	6 points	
▷	Theory Question	2 points	
Score calculation: 100 points – ____ points missed ____ Score Satisfactory score: 85 or above			

2008 CAAHEP Competencies Achieved
Psychomotor (Skills) ☑ I. 2. Perform venipuncture. ***Affective (Behavior)*** ☑ I. 1. Apply critical thinking skills in performing patient assessment and care. ☑ IV. I. Demonstrate empathy in communicating with patients, family, and staff.

2015 CAAHEP Competencies Achieved
Psychomotor (Skills) ☑ I. 2. b. Perform venipuncture. ☑ III. 10. Demonstrate proper disposal of biohazardous material a. sharps b. regulated waste. ***Affective (Behavior)*** ☑ I. 1. Apply critical thinking when performing patient assessment. ☑ I. 3. Show awareness of a patient's concerns related to the procedure being performed. ☑ III. 1. Recognize the implications for failure to comply with Center for Disease Control (CDC) regulations in healthcare settings.

ABHES Competencies Achieved
☑ 9. a. Practice standard precautions and perform disinfection/sterilization techniques. ☑ 10. c. Dispose of biohazardous materials. ☑ 10. d. (1). Collect, label and process specimens: Perform venipuncture.

EVALUATION OF COMPETENCY

Procedure 31-3: Skin Puncture—Disposable Semiautomatic Lancet Device

Name: ______________________________ Date: ______________

Evaluated by: ______________________________ Score: ______________

Performance Objective

Outcome:	Obtain a capillary blood specimen.
Conditions:	Given the following: disposable gloves, antiseptic wipe, CoaguChek lancet, gauze pad, and a biohazard sharps container.
Standards:	Time: 5 minutes. Student completed procedure in __________ minutes.
	Accuracy: Satisfactory score on the Performance Evaluation Checklist.

Performance Evaluation Checklist

Trial 1	Trial 2	Point Value	Performance Standards
		●	Sanitized hands.
		●	Greeted the patient and introduced yourself.
		●	Identified the patient.
		●	Asked patient if he or she prepared properly.
		●	Assembled equipment.
		●	Opened sterile gauze packet.
		●	Explained the procedure to the patient and reassured patient.
		●	Seated patient in chair.
		●	Extended the palmar surface of patient's hand facing up.
		●	Selected a puncture site.
		●	Warmed site if needed.
		▷	Explained why the site should be warmed.
		●	Cleansed puncture site and allowed it to air dry.
		▷	Explained why the site should be allowed to air dry.
		●	Did not touch the site after cleansing.
		●	Applied gloves.
		●	Firmly grasped patient's finger.
		●	Positioned the lancet firmly on the fingertip slightly to the side of center.
		●	Depressed the activation button without moving the lancet or finger.

Trial 1	Trial 2	Point Value	Performance Standards
		▷	Stated why the lancet and finger should not be moved.
		●	Disposed of lancet in biohazard sharps container.
		●	Waited a few seconds to allow blood flow to begin.
		●	Wiped away the first drop of blood with a gauze pad.
		▷	Stated why the first drop of blood should be wiped away.
		●	Allowed a second large, well-rounded drop of blood to form.
		●	Did not squeeze finger to obtain blood.
		●	Collected the blood specimen on a test strip or in the appropriate microcollection device.
		●	Instructed patient to hold a gauze pad over puncture site with pressure.
		●	Remained with patient until bleeding stopped.
		●	Applied an adhesive bandage if needed.
		●	Tested the blood specimen following the manufacturer's instructions.
		●	Removed gloves.
		●	Sanitized hands.
		Ⓐ	Applied critical thinking when performing patient assessment.
		Ⓐ	Showed awareness of a patient's concerns related to the procedure being performed.
		Ⓐ	Recognized the implications for failure to comply with Center for Disease Control (CDC) regulations in healthcare settings.
		*	Completed the procedure within 5 minutes.
			TOTALS

Evaluation of Student Performance

EVALUATION CRITERIA			COMMENTS
Symbol	**Category**	**Point Value**	
*	Critical Step	16 points	
●	Essential Step	6 points	
Ⓐ	Affective Competency	6 points	
▷	Theory Question	2 points	
Score calculation: 100 points – ____ points missed ____ Score Satisfactory score: 85 or above			

2008 CAAHEP Competencies Achieved
Psychomotor (Skills) ☑ I. 3. Perform capillary puncture. ***Affective (Behavior)*** ☑ IV. I. Demonstrate empathy in communicating with patients, family, and staff.

2015 CAAHEP Competencies Achieved
Psychomotor (Skills) ☑ I. 2. c. Perform capillary puncture. ☑ III. 10. Demonstrate proper disposal of biohazardous material a. sharps b. regulated waste. ***Affective (Behavior)*** ☑ I. 1. Apply critical thinking when performing patient assessment. ☑ I. 3. Show awareness of a patient's concerns related to the procedure being performed. ☑ III. 1. Recognize the implications for failure to comply with Center for Disease Control (CDC) regulations in healthcare settings.

ABHES Competencies Achieved
☑ 9. a. Practice standard precautions and perform disinfection/sterilization techniques. ☑ 10. c. Dispose of biohazardous materials. ☑ 10. d. (2). Collect, label, and process specimens: Perform capillary puncutre.

Notes

EVALUATION OF COMPETENCY

Procedure 31-A: Skin Puncture—Reusable Semiautomatic Lancet Device

Name: ______________________ Date: ______________

Evaluated by: ______________________ Score: ______________

Performance Objective

Outcome:	Obtain a capillary blood specimen.
Conditions:	Given the following: disposable gloves, antiseptic wipe, Glucolet II lancet device, sterile lancet/endcap, gauze pad, and a biohazard sharps container.
Standards:	Time: 10 minutes. Student completed procedure in ________ minutes.
	Accuracy: Satisfactory score on the Performance Evaluation Checklist.

Performance Evaluation Checklist

Trial 1	Trial 2	Point Value	Performance Standards
		•	Sanitized hands.
		•	Greeted the patient and introduced yourself.
		•	Identified patient.
		•	Asked patient if he or she prepared properly.
		•	Assembled equipment.
		•	Pushed the transparent barrel toward the release button until it clicked into place.
		•	Inserted lancet/endcap onto the lancet device.
		•	Opened sterile gauze packet.
		•	Explained the procedure to the patient and reassured patient.
		•	Seated patient in chair.
		•	Extended the palmar surface of patient's hand facing up.
		•	Selected a puncture site.
		•	Warmed site if needed.
		▷	Explained how patient's finger can be warmed.
		•	Cleansed puncture site and allowed it to air dry.
		•	Applied gloves.
		•	Twisted off plastic post from the endcap.
		•	Firmly grasped patient's finger.
		•	Placed the endcap firmly on the fingertip slightly to the side of center.

Trial 1	Trial 2	Point Value	Performance Standards
		●	Depressed the activation button without moving the Glucolet or finger.
		●	Wiped away the first drop of blood with a gauze pad.
		●	Allowed a second large, well-rounded drop of blood to form.
		▷	Explained why the finger should not be squeezed.
		●	Collected the blood specimen on a test strip or in the appropriate microcollection device.
		●	Instructed patient to hold a gauze pad over puncture site with pressure.
		●	Remained with patient until bleeding stopped.
		●	Applied an adhesive bandage if needed.
		●	Removed the endcap from the lancet device.
		●	Discarded the endcap in a biohazard waste container.
		●	Tested the blood specimen following the manufacturer's instructions.
		●	Removed gloves.
		●	Sanitized hands.
		●	Sanitized and disinfected the Glucolet.
		●	Stored Glucolet in its resting position.
		Ⓐ	Applied critical thinking when performing patient assessment.
		Ⓐ	Showed awareness of a patient's concerns related to the procedure being performed.
		Ⓐ	Recognized the implications for failure to comply with Center for Disease Control (CDC) regulations in healthcare settings.
		*	Completed the procedure within 5 minutes.
			TOTALS

Evaluation of Student Performance

EVALUATION CRITERIA			COMMENTS
Symbol	**Category**	**Point Value**	
*	Critical Step	16 points	
●	Essential Step	6 points	
Ⓐ	Affective Competency	6 points	
▷	Theory Question	2 points	
Score calculation: 100 points – ____ points missed ____ Score Satisfactory score: 85 or above			

2008 CAAHEP Competencies Achieved
Psychomotor (Skills)
☑ I. 3. Perform capillary puncture.
Affective (Behavior)
☑ IV. I. Demonstrate empathy in communicating with patients, family, and staff.

2015 CAAHEP Competencies Achieved
Psychomotor (Skills)
☑ I. 2. c. Perform capillary puncture.
☑ III. 10. Demonstrate proper disposal of biohazardous material a. sharps b. regulated waste.
Affective (Behavior)
☑ I. 1. Apply critical thinking when performing patient assessment.
☑ I. 3. Show awareness of a patient's concerns related to the procedure being performed.
☑ III. 1. Recognize the implications for failure to comply with Center for Disease Control (CDC) regulations in healthcare settings.

ABHES Competencies Achieved
☑ 9. a. Practice standard precautions and perform disinfection/sterilization techniques.
☑ 10. c. Dispose of biohazardous materials.
☑ 10. d. (2). Collect, label, and process specimens: Perform capillary puncutre.

Notes

32 Hematology

CHAPTER ASSIGNMENTS

✓ After Completing	Date Due	Study Guide Pages	STUDY GUIDE ASSIGNMENTS (CTA = Critical Thinking Activity)	Possible Points	Points You Earned
		911	Pretest	10	
		 912 912	Term Key Term Assessment A. Definitions B. Word Parts (Add 1 point for each key term)	 7 10	
		912-915	Evaluation of Learning questions	26	
		915-918	CTA A: Diseases	40	
		919	CTA B: Hematocrit	5	
		919	CTA C: Iron Content of Food	10	
		920	CTA D: Iron Deficiency Anemia	20	
		920	CTA E: Dear Gabby	10	
		921	CTA F: Crossword Puzzle	27	
			Evolve Site: Apply Your Knowledge questions	10	
			Evolve Site: Video Evaluation	38	
		911	Posttest	10	
			ADDITIONAL ASSIGNMENTS		
			TOTAL POINTS		

Notes

✓ When Assigned By Your Instructor	Study Guide Pages	Practices Required	LABORATORY ASSIGNMENTS (Procedure Number and Name)	Score*
	923-925	3	**Practice for Competency** 32-A: Hemoglobin Determination Textbook reference: pp. 855-857	
	927-929		**Evaluation of Competency** 32-A: Hemoglobin Determination	*
	923-925	3	**Practice for Competency** 32-1: Hematocrit Determination Textbook reference: pp. 858-860	
	931-933		**Evaluation of Competency** 32-1: Hematocrit Determination	*
	923-925	10	**Practice for Competency** 32-2: Preparation of a Blood Smear for a Differential Cell Count Textbook reference: pp. 863-865	
	935-937		**Evaluation of Competency** 32-2: Preparation of a Blood Smear for a Differential Cell Count	*
			ADDITIONAL ASSIGNMENTS	

Notes

Name ______________________________ Date ______________

PRETEST

True or False

_______ 1. The study of blood is known as serology.

_______ 2. The function of hemoglobin is to assist in blood clotting.

_______ 3. The normal hemoglobin range for a female is 12 to 16 g/dL.

_______ 4. A low hemoglobin reading occurs with polycythemia.

_______ 5. The normal hematocrit range for a female is 40% to 54%.

_______ 6. Leukocytosis is an abnormal increase in the number of leukocytes.

_______ 7. Strenuous exercise can result in an increase in the white blood cell count.

_______ 8. Leukemia can cause a decrease in the red blood cell count.

_______ 9. The normal range for neutrophils is 50% to 70%.

_______ 10. The PT test measures how long it takes for an individual's blood to form a clot.

POSTTEST

True or False

_______ 1. Red and white blood counts are included in a CBC.

_______ 2. The normal range for hemoglobin for an adult male is 14 to 18 g/dL.

_______ 3. An increase in the hemoglobin level occurs with CHF.

_______ 4. The term hematocrit means "to separate blood."

_______ 5. The buffy coat consists of red blood cells.

_______ 6. Hematocrit test results should be read at the top of the red blood cell column.

_______ 7. The normal adult range for a white blood cell count is 4500 to 11,000.

_______ 8. Leukopenia occurs when a patient has appendicitis.

_______ 9. The normal range for a red blood cell count for a woman is 4 to 5.5 million.

_______ 10. The function of warfarin is to inhibit the growth of bacteria in the body.

KEY TERM ASSESSMENT

A. Definitions

Directions: Match each key term with its definition.

_______ 1. Anemia
_______ 2. Anticoagulant
_______ 3. Hematology
_______ 4. Hemoglobin
_______ 5. Leukocytosis
_______ 6. Leukopenia
_______ 7. Polycythemia

A. An abnormal decrease in the number of white blood cells (less than 4500 per cubic millimeter of blood)
B. A disorder in which there is an increase in the red blood cell mass
C. A condition in which there is a decrease in the number of erythrocytes or in the amount of hemoglobin in the blood
D. The study of blood and blood-forming tissues
E. An abnormal increase in the number of white blood cells (greater than 11,000 per cubic millimeter of blood)
F. The protein- and iron-containing pigment of erythrocytes that transports oxygen in the body
G. A substance that inhibits blood clotting

B. Word Parts

Directions: Indicate the meaning of each word part in the space provided. List as many medical terms as possible that incorporate the word part in the space provided.

Word Part	Meaning of Word Part	Medical Terms That Incorporate Word Part
1. cyt/o		
2. -ia		
3. -osis		
4. anti-		
5. coagulant		
6. hemato/o		
7. -ology		
8. leuk/o		
9. -penia		
10. poly-		

EVALUATION OF LEARNING

Directions: Fill in each blank with the correct answer.

1. List the tests generally included in a complete blood cell count (CBC).

____

____

2. What is the normal hemoglobin range?

   a. Adult female: _______________________________

   b. Adult male: _______________________________

3. List five conditions that cause a decrease in the hemoglobin level.

____

____

____

4. What is the purpose of the hematocrit?

____

____

5. What is the normal hematocrit range?

   a. Adult female: _______________________________

   b. Adult male: _______________________________

6. What is the normal range for the white blood count for an adult?

____

7. List examples of conditions that may result in leukocytosis.

____

____

8. What is the normal range for the red blood count for an adult?

   a. Adult female: _______________________________

   b. Adult male: _______________________________

9. List the five types of white blood cells and the normal adult range for each.

____

____

____

10. What are the red blood cell indices?

____

____

11. What information is provided by the RBC indices?

____

____

12. What are the advantages of the following methods for performing a differential cell count?

   a. Automatic method: _______________________________

   b. Manual: _______________________________

13. Why must the white blood cells be stained when performing a manual differential cell count?

____

____

14. List the abbreviation for each of the following tests:
    a. Hematocrit ______________________
    b. Hemoglobin ______________________
    c. Differential cell count ______________________
    d. White blood cell count ______________________
    e. Red blood cell count ______________________

15. What does the PT test measure?

____

16. What is the PT adult reference range?

____

17. What is the purpose of performing an INR on a PT test?

____

____

18. What is the range for a PT/INR result of a healthy individual with a normal clotting ability?

____

19. What is the function of warfarin?

____

20. What are the most common conditions for which warfarin is prescribed?

____

____

21. What is the usual desired PT/INR range for a patient who is on warfarin therapy for a heart attack or stroke?

____

22. What is the goal of warfarin therapy?

____

____

23. How often should a patient on warfarin therapy have a PT/INR test performed?

____

24. What color-stoppered tube should be used to collect a specimen for a PT/INR test?

____

25. Why is it important to fill the blood tube for a PT/INR test to the exhaustion of the vacuum?

____

____

26. What are the advantages of PT/INR home testing?

____

____

CRITICAL THINKING ACTIVITIES

A. Diseases

1. You and your classmates work at a large clinic. It is National Disease Awareness Week. The physicians at your clinic ask you to develop informative, creative, and colorful brochures for patients about various diseases. Choose a condition from the list, and design a brochure using the blank Frequently Asked Questions (FAQ) brochure provided on the following page. Each student in the class should select a different disease. On a separate sheet of paper, write three true or false questions relating to the information in your brochure.
2. Present your brochure to the class. After all the brochures have been presented, each student should ask three questions to the entire class to see how well the class understands the diseases that were presented. (Note: Students can take notes during the presentations and refer to them when answering the questions.)

Conditions

1. Addison's disease
2. Amyotrophic lateral sclerosis
3. Aplastic anemia
4. Bell's palsy
5. Cirrhosis
6. Crohn's disease
7. Cushing's syndrome
8. Cystic fibrosis
9. Degenerative disc disease
10. Epilepsy
11. Hemolytic anemia
12. Hemophilia
13. Hernia
14. Hodgkin's disease
15. Hyperthyroidism
16. Hypothyroidism
17. Leukemia
18. Lupus erythematosus
19. Multiple sclerosis
20. Muscular dystrophy
21. Parkinson's disease
22. Peptic ulcer
23. Pernicious anemia
24. Polycythemia
25. Sickle-cell anemia
26. Ulcerative colitis

Notes

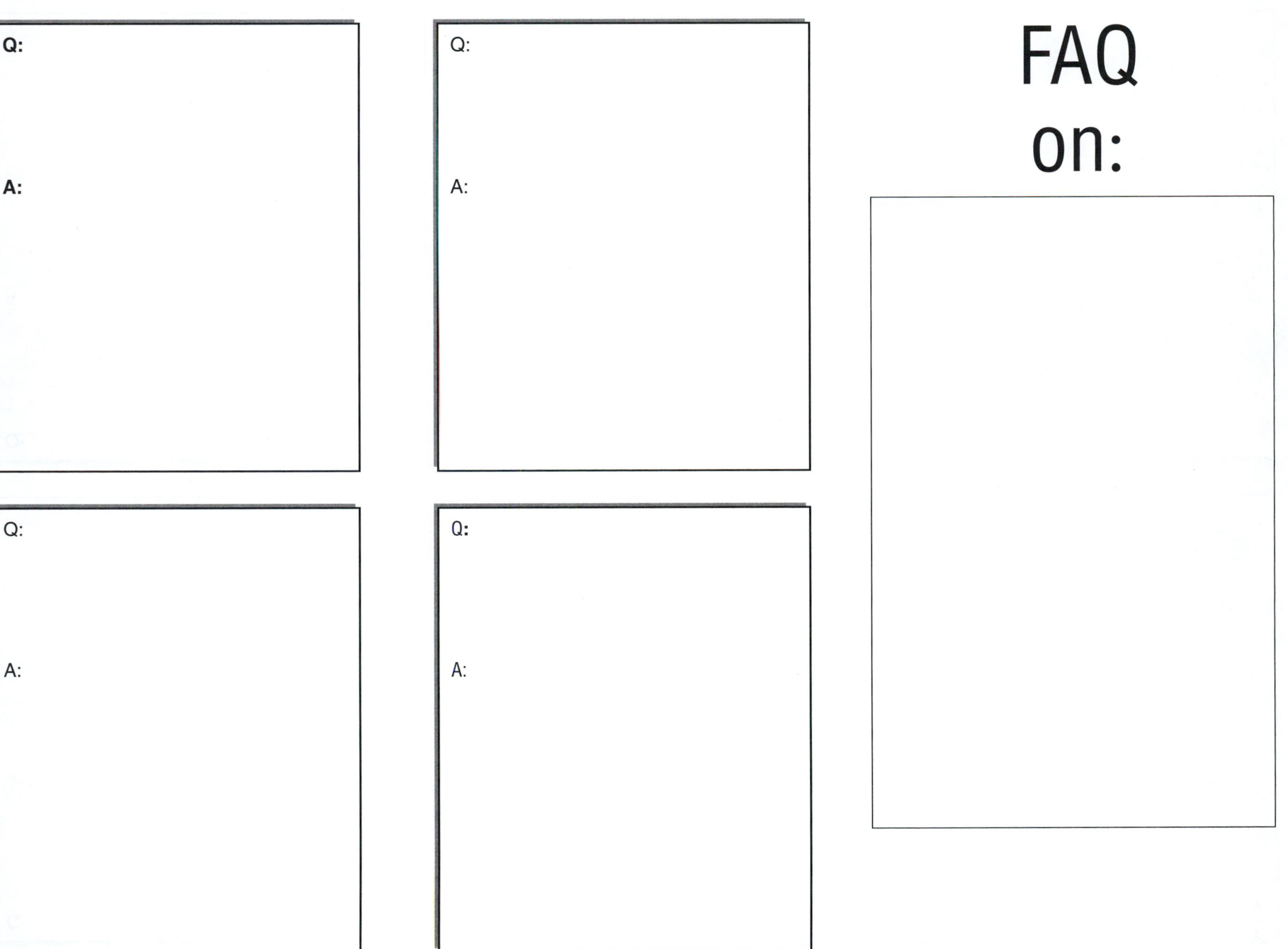
FAQ
on:
Q:
A:
Q:
A:
Q:
A:
Q:
A:

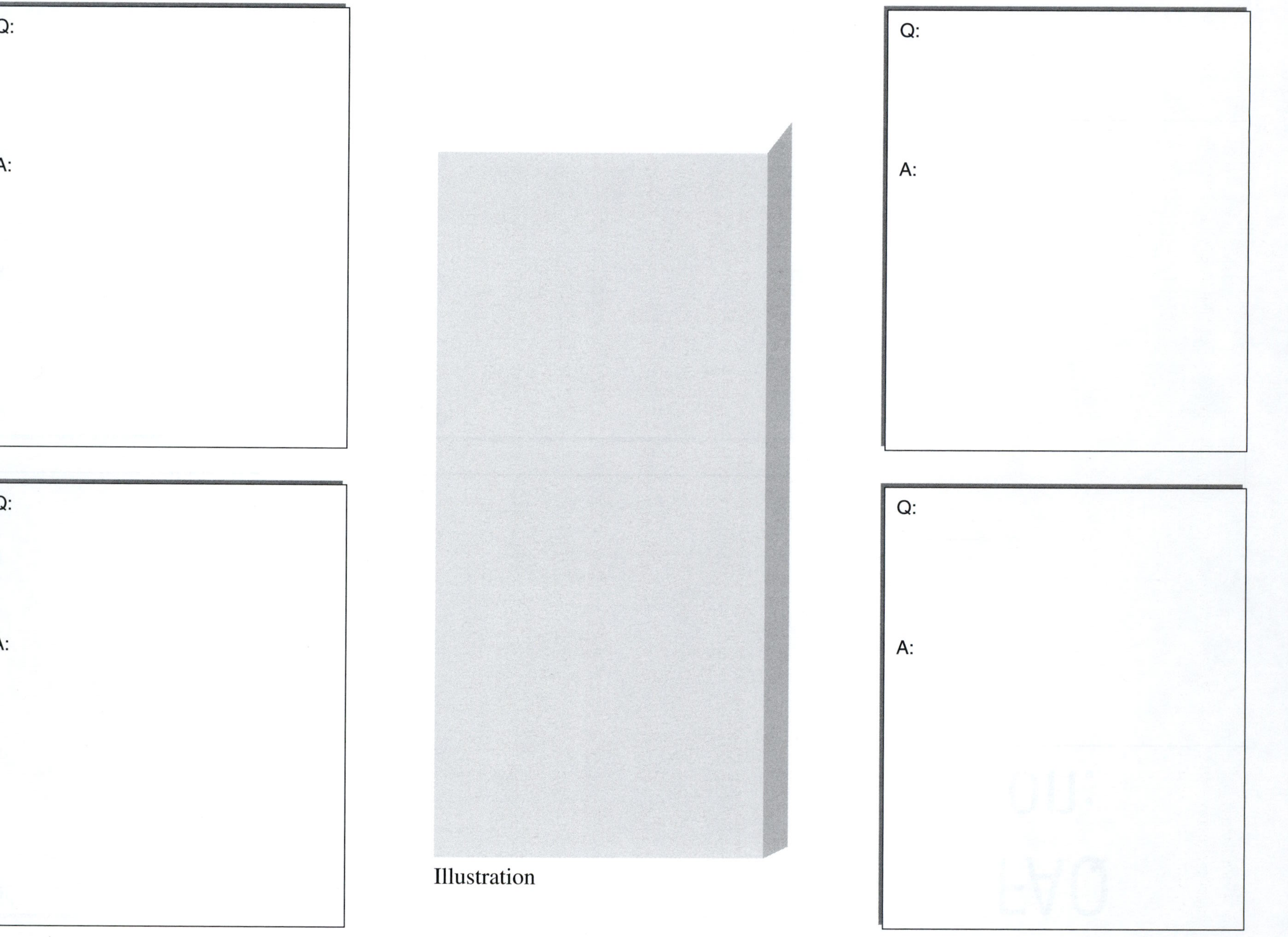
Q:
A:
Q:
A:
Illustration
Q:
A:
Q:
A:

B. Hematocrit

Label the layers of this microhematocrit capillary tube that has been centrifuged. Place an arrow at the point where you would take the hematocrit reading.

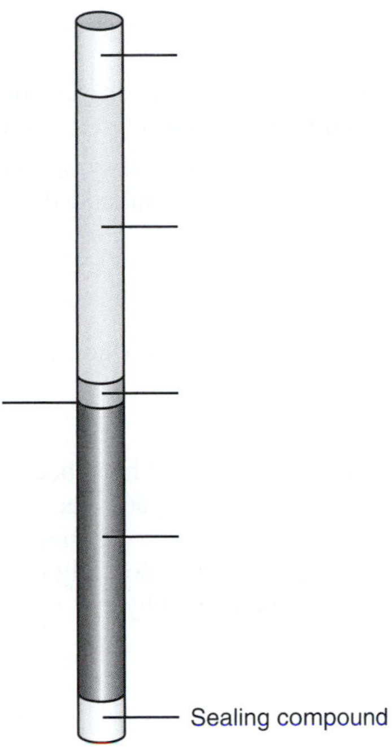

C. Iron Content of Food

Consuming food that is high in iron helps to prevent iron deficiency anemia. To become familiar with foods that are high in iron content and foods that contain little or no iron, plan the following two meals. One meal should be as high as possible in iron content and the other meal should not contain any iron at all.

Meal 1

____

____

____

____

____

Meal 2

____

____

____

____

____

D. Iron Deficiency Anemia

Create a profile of an individual who has iron deficiency anemia following these guidelines:

1. Using a blank piece of paper, colored pencils, crayons, or markers, draw a figure of an individual exhibiting iron deficiency anemia. Be as creative as possible.
2. Do not use any text on your drawing other than to label items you have drawn in your picture. (A picture is worth a thousand words!)
3. Try to include all of the symptoms of iron deficiency anemia in your drawing. The Iron Deficiency Anemia Patient Teaching Box on p. 790 in your textbook can be used as a reference source.
4. In the classroom, find a partner and trade drawings. Identify the symptoms of iron deficiency anemia in your partner's drawing. With your partner, discuss what treatment is recommended and also what this person could do to prevent iron deficiency anemia.

E. Dear Gabby

Gabby is attending her class reunion and wants you to fill in for her. In the space provided, respond to the following letter.

Dear Gabby,

I am a housewife with two adorable children, ages 2 and 4. I have been feeling rundown and tired lately, so I bought some vitamin pills at the drug store. They came individually packaged in foil and plastic. They are hard to open, so I cut each package and transferred the iron pills to a little plastic baggie. When I told my mother about what I thought was a great idea, she got very upset. She told me that I could possibly be putting my children at danger. She said that iron is poisonous to children and that I should not do that. Gabby, my mom has always been overprotective. Is this just another one of her episodes?

Signed,

Curious in Kansas

____

____

____

____

____

____

____

____

____

____

F. Crossword Puzzle: Hematology

Directions: Complete the crossword puzzle using the clues provided.

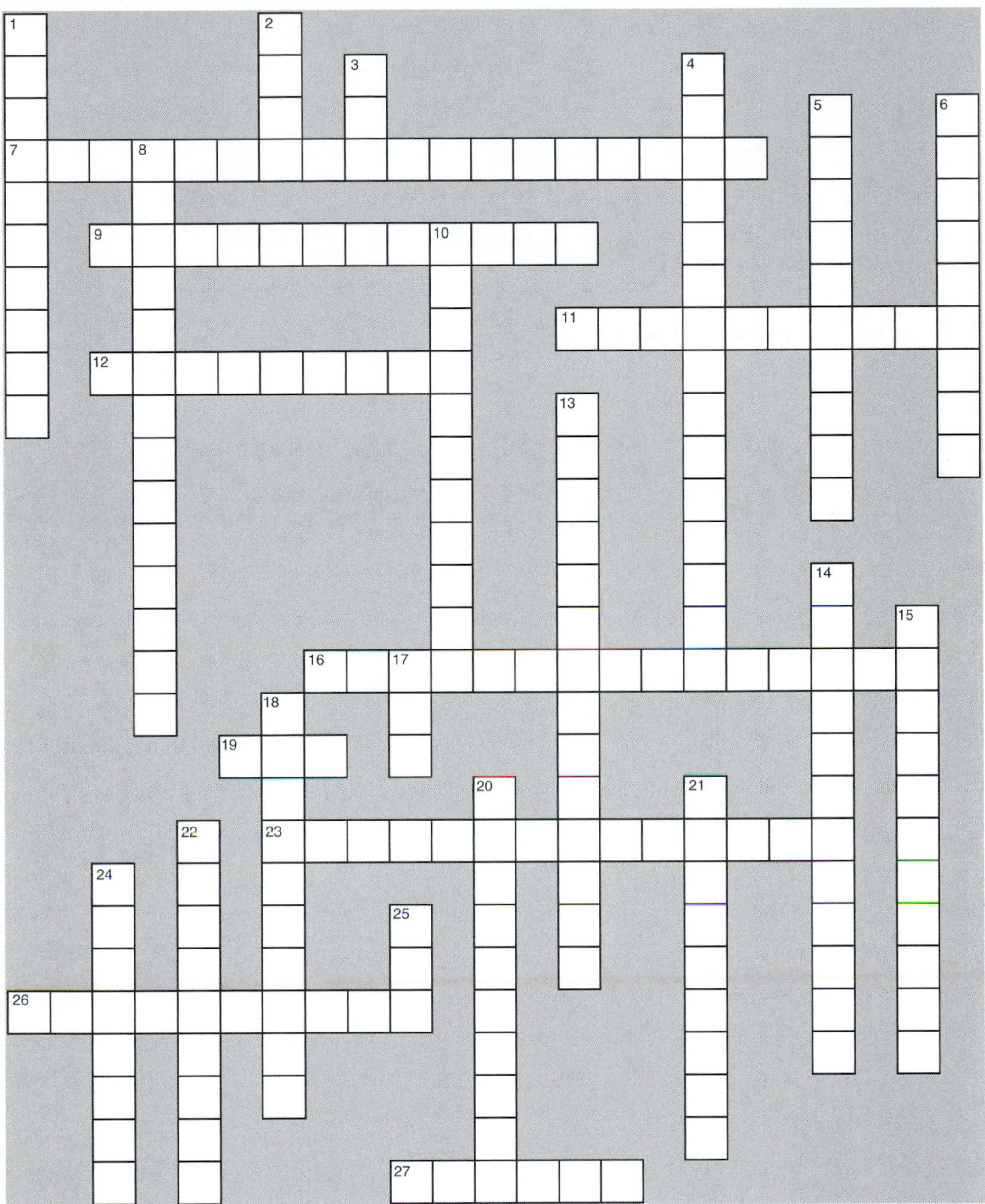

Across

7 Cause of blood pooling in heart
9 Condition of too many RBCs
11 Carries oxygen
12 Platelets and WBCs
16 Causes inaccurate PT/INR results
19 Common hematology test
23 Common cause of anemia
26 To separate blood
27 Liquid part of the blood

Down

1 Study of blood
2 Differential WBC count abbreviation
3 Hemoglobin abbreviation
4 Blood clotting test
5 Most numerous WBC
6 Symptom of anemia
8 Causes black stool
10 Red blood cell
13 May affect PT/INR test results
14 Above 11,000 WBCs
15 Indication for warfarin
17 aka thrombophlebitis
18 Calculations on CBC tests
20 Below 4500 WBCs
21 White blood cell
22 Color tube for PT/INR
24 Warfarin brand name
25 Hematocrit abbreviation

Notes

PRACTICE FOR COMPETENCY

Procedure 32-A: Hemoglobin Determination.

a. Run controls on a CLIA-waived hemoglobin analyzer, and record results on the quality control log on p. 925.

b. Perform a hemoglobin determination on a patient using a CLIA-waived hemoglobin analyzer, and record results in the chart provided. Circle any values that fall outside the normal range.

Procedure 32-1: Hematocrit Determination. Perform a hematocrit determination in duplicate, and record results in the chart provided. Circle any values that fall outside the normal range.

Procedure 32-2: Preparation of a Blood Smear for a Differential Cell Count. Prepare a blood smear for a differential white blood cell count.

CHART	
Date	

Chart	
Date	

QUALITY CONTROL HEMOGLOBIN LOG SHEET

Name of Meter ______________________ Control Lot Number: ______________

Low-Level Range: ______________________ Control Exp. Date: ______________

High-Level Range: ______________________

Date	Test Cards: Lot # and Expiration	Low-Level Value	Accept	Reject	High-Level Value	Accept	Reject	Technician

Notes

EVALUATION OF COMPETENCY

Procedure 32-A: Hemoglobin Determination

Name: ______________________ Date: ______________

Evaluated by: ______________________ Score: ______________

Performance Objective

Outcome:	Perform a hemoglobin determination.
Conditions:	Using a hemoglobin meter and operating manual and given the following: disposable gloves, antiseptic wipe, lancet, gauze pad, test cards, cod key, control solutions, quality control log, and a biohazard sharps container.
Standards:	Time: 10 minutes. Student completed procedure in ________ minutes.
	Accuracy: Satisfactory score on the Performance Evaluation Checklist.

Performance Evaluation Checklist

Trial 1	Trial 2	Point Value	Performance Standards
		●	Sanitized hands.
		●	Assembled equipment.
		●	Checked expiration date of test cards.
		●	Calibrated the hemoglobin meter.
		▷	Stated the purpose of calibrating the meter.
		●	Checked expiration date of control solution.
		●	Applied gloves and ran a low and high control.
		▷	Stated the purpose of running controls.
		●	Removed gloves and sanitized hands.
		●	Recorded control results in the quality control log.
		●	Greeted the patient and introduced yourself.
		●	Identified the patient and explained the procedure.
		●	Turned on the hemoglobin meter and checked the code number.
		●	Inserted a test card into the meter.
		●	Opened gauze packet.
		●	Cleansed puncture site and allowed it to air-dry.
		▷	Stated what happens to the blood drop if the site is not dry.
		●	Applied gloves and performed a finger puncture.

Trial 1	Trial 2	Point Value	Performance Standards
		●	Wiped away the first drop of blood.
		●	Collected the blood specimen.
		●	Placed a gauze pad over puncture site and applied pressure.
		●	Applied blood specimen to test card.
		●	Waited while hemoglobin meter analyzed the blood specimen.
		●	Read results on the display screen.
		▷	Stated the normal hemoglobin range for a female (12 to 16 g/dL) and a male (14 to 18 g/dL).
		●	Removed test card from meter.
		●	Properly disposed of test card in a biohazard waste container.
		●	Checked puncture site and applied adhesive bandage, if needed.
		●	Removed gloves and sanitized hands.
		●	Charted the test results correctly.
		*	Hemoglobin recording was identical to the reading on the digital display screen.
		Ⓐ	Explained to a patient the rationale for performance of a procedure.
		Ⓐ	Reassured a patient of the accuracy of the test results.
		*	Completed the procedure within 10 minutes.
			TOTALS

CHART	
Date	

Evaluation of Student Performance

EVALUATION CRITERIA			COMMENTS
Symbol	**Category**	**Point Value**	
✶	Critical Step	16 points	
●	Essential Step	6 points	
Ⓐ	Affective Competency	6 points	
▷	Theory Question	2 points	
Score calculation: 100 points – ___ points missed ___ Score Satisfactory score: 85 or above			

2008 CAAHEP Competencies Achieved
Psychomotor (Skills) ☑ I. 11. Perform quality control measures. ☑ I. 12. Perform hematology testing. ***Affective (Behavior)*** ☑ II. 2. Distinguish between normal and abnormal test results.

2015 CAAHEP Competencies Achieved
Psychomotor (Skills) ☑ I. 10. Perform a quality control measure. ☑ I. 11. a. Obtain specimens and perform CLIA waived hematology test. ☑ II. 2. Differentiate between normal and abnormal test results. ***Affective (Behavior)*** ☑ II. 1. Reassure a patient of the accuracy of the test results. ☑ V. 4. Explain to a patient the rationale for performance of a procedure.

ABHES Competencies Achieved
☑ 10. a. Practice quality control. ☑ 10. b. (2). Perform selected CLIA-waived tests that assist with diagnosis and treatment: hematology testing.

Notes

EVALUATION OF COMPETENCY

Procedure 32-1: Hematocrit

Name: ______________________________ Date: ______________

Evaluated by: ______________________________ Score: ______________

Performance Objective

Outcome:	Perform a hematocrit determination.
Conditions:	Given the following: microhematocrit centrifuge, disposable gloves, lancet, antiseptic wipe, gauze pad, capillary tubes, sealing compound, and a biohazard sharps container.
Standards:	Time: 10 minutes. Student completed procedure in ________ minutes.
	Accuracy: Satisfactory score on the Performance Evaluation Checklist.

Performance Evaluation Checklist

Trial 1	Trial 2	Point Value	Performance Standards
		•	Sanitized hands.
		•	Greeted the patient and introduced yourself.
		•	Identified the patient and explained the procedure.
		•	Assembled equipment.
		•	Opened gauze packet.
		•	Cleansed site with an antiseptic wipe and allowed it to air-dry.
		•	Applied gloves.
		•	Performed a finger puncture and discarded the lancet in a biohazard sharps container.
		•	Wiped away the first drop of blood.
		•	Massaged finger until large blood drop formed.
		•	Held one end of capillary tube horizontally but slightly downward next to the free-flowing puncture.
		•	Kept the tip of the pipet in the blood but did not allow it to press against the skin of the patient's finger.
		▷	Explained why the capillary tube should be kept in the blood specimen.
		•	Filled capillary tube (calibrated tubes filled to the calibration line; uncalibrated tubes filled approximately three-fourths full).
		▷	Explained why a tube with air bubbles is unacceptable.
		•	Filled a second capillary tube.
		▷	Stated why 2 capillary tubes must be filled.

Trial 1	Trial 2	Point Value	Performance Standards
		●	Placed gauze pad over puncture site and applied pressure.
		●	Sealed the dry end of each capillary tube.
		●	Checked puncture site and applied adhesive bandage, if needed.
		●	Placed capillary tubes in the microhematocrit centrifuge with the sealed end facing toward the outside.
		▷	Explained why the sealed end must face toward the outside.
		●	Balanced one tube with the other tube placed opposite it.
		●	Placed the cover over the capillary tubes and locked it securely.
		●	Centrifuged blood specimen for 3 to 5 minutes.
		▷	Explained the reason for centrifuging the blood specimen.
		●	Allowed centrifuge to come to a complete stop.
		●	Removed the protective cover from the capillary tubes.
		●	Read the results using the appropriate reading device.
		●	Determined if the results agreed within 4 percentage points.
		▷	Explained what to do if the results are not within 4 percentage points.
		●	Averaged the values of the two tubes together to derive the test results.
		*	Results were within ±1% of the evaluator's results.
		▷	Stated the normal hematocrit range for a female (37% to 47%) and a male (40% to 54%).
		●	Properly disposed of capillary tubes in a biohazard sharps container.
		●	Removed gloves and sanitized hands.
		●	Charted the test results correctly.
		●	Returned equipment.
		Ⓐ	Explained to a patient the rationale for performance of a procedure.
		Ⓐ	Reassured a patient of the accuracy of the test results.
		*	Completed the procedure within 10 minutes.
			TOTALS

CHART

Date	

Evaluation of Student Performance

EVALUATION CRITERIA			COMMENTS
Symbol	**Category**	**Point Value**	
∗	Critical Step	16 points	
●	Essential Step	6 points	
Ⓐ	Affective Competency	6 points	
▷	Theory Question	2 points	
Score calculation: 100 points – ____ points missed ____ Score Satisfactory score: 85 or above			

2008 CAAHEP Competencies Achieved
Psychomotor (Skills) ☑ I. 11. Perform quality control measures. ☑ I. 12. Perform hematology testing. ***Affective (Behavior)*** ☑ II. 2. Distinguish between normal and abnormal test results.

2015 CAAHEP Competencies Achieved
Psychomotor (Skills) ☑ I. 10. Perform a quality control measure. ☑ I. 11. a. Obtain specimens and perform CLIA waived hematology test. ☑ II. 2. Differentiate between normal and abnormal test results. ***Affective (Behavior)*** ☑ II. 1. Reassure a patient of the accuracy of the test results. ☑ V. 4. Explain to a patient the rationale for performance of a procedure.

ABHES Competencies Achieved
☑ 10. a. Practice quality control. ☑ 10. b. (2) Perform selected CLIA-waived tests that assist with diagnosis and treatment: hematology testing.

Notes

EVALUATION OF COMPETENCY

Procedure 32-2: Preparation of a Blood Smear for a Differential Cell Count

Name: ______________________ Date: ______________

Evaluated by: ______________________ Score: ______________

Performance Objective

Outcome:	Prepare a blood smear for a differential white blood cell count.
Conditions:	Given the following: disposable gloves, supplies to perform a finger puncture or venipuncture, slides with a frosted edge, slide container, biohazard specimen bag, laboratory request form, and a biohazard sharps container.
Standards:	Time: 10 minutes. Student completed procedure in __________ minutes.
	Accuracy: Satisfactory score on the Performance Evaluation Checklist.

Performance Evaluation Checklist

Trial 1	Trial 2	Point Value	Performance Standards
		●	Sanitized hands.
		●	Greeted the patient and introduced yourself.
		●	Identified the patient and explained the procedure.
		●	Assembled equipment.
		●	Labeled slides.
		●	Opened the gauze packet.
		●	Cleansed puncture site.
		●	Applied gloves.
		●	Performed a venipuncture or finger puncture.
		●	Placed a drop of blood in the middle of each slide approximately ¼ inch from the frosted edge of the slide.
		●	Held a spreader slide at a 30-degree angle to first slide in front of the drop of blood.
		▷	Stated what occurs if the angle is more than 30 degrees or less than 30 degrees.
		●	Moved the spreader slide until it touched the drop of blood.
		●	Spread the blood thinly and evenly across slide using the spreader slide.
		●	Prepared the second blood smear.
		●	Disposed of the spreader slide in a biohazard sharps container.
		●	Laid the blood smears on a flat surface and allowed them to dry.

Trial 1	Trial 2	Point Value	Performance Standards
		▷	Explained why the blood smears should be dried immediately.
		●	The length of the smear was approximately $1\frac{1}{2}$ inches.
		●	The smear was smooth and even, with no ridges, holes, lines, streaks, or clumps.
		●	The smear was not too thick or too thin.
		●	There was a feathered edge at the thin end of the smear.
		●	There was a margin on all sides of the smear.
		●	Placed the slides in a protective slide container.
		●	Placed lavender-stoppered tube and slide container in a biohazard specimen bag.
		●	Removed gloves and sanitized hands.
		●	Completed a laboratory request form.
		●	Placed lab request in outside pocket of specimen bag.
		●	Charted the procedure correctly.
		●	Filed copy of lab request in patient's chart.
		●	Placed specimen bag in appropriate location for pickup by lab courier.
		●	Charted the procedure correctly.
		Ⓐ	Explained to a patient the rationale for performance of a procedure.
		✶	Completed the procedure within 10 minutes.
			TOTALS

CHART	
Date	

Evaluation of Student Performance

EVALUATION CRITERIA			COMMENTS
Symbol	**Category**	**Point Value**	
✶	Critical Step	16 points	
●	Essential Step	6 points	
Ⓐ	Affective Competency	6 points	
▷	Theory Question	2 points	
Score calculation: 100 points – ___ points missed ___ Score Satisfactory score: 85 or above			

2008 CAAHEP Competencies Achieved
Psychomotor (Skills) ☑ I. 11. Perform quality control measures. ***Affective (Behavior)*** ☑ I. 1. Apply critical thinking skills in performing patient assessment and care.

2015 CAAHEP Competencies Achieved
Psychomotor (Skills) ☑ I. 10. Perform a quality control measure. ***Affective (Behavior)*** ☑ V. 4. Explain to a patient the rationale for performance of a procedure.

ABHES Competencies Achieved
☑ 10. a. Practice quality control ☑ 10. d. Collect, label, and process specimens.

Notes

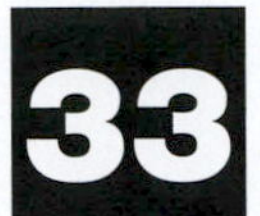

Blood Chemistry and Immunology

CHAPTER ASSIGNMENTS

✓ After Completing	Date Due	Study Guide Pages	STUDY GUIDE ASSIGNMENTS (CTA = Critical Thinking Activity)	Possible Points	Points You Earned
		943	Pretest	10	
		944	Key Term Assessment	10	
		944-949	Evaluation of Learning questions	47	
		949-952	CTA A: Type 2 Diabetes	40	
		953	CTA B: Oral Glucose Tolerance Test (2 points each)	10	
		953	CTA C: Coronary Artery Disease	20	
		953-954	CTA D: Cholesterol and Saturated Fat (5 points each)	15	
			Evolve Site: The Right Chemistry (Record points earned)		
		954	CTA E: Rh Incompatibility (5 points each)	20	
		955	CTA F: Crossword Puzzle	22	
			Evolve Site: Immunologic Tests (Record points earned)		
			Evolve Site: Apply Your Knowledge questions	10	
			Evolve Site: Video Evaluation	16	
		943	Posttest	10	
			ADDITIONAL ASSIGNMENTS		
			TOTAL POINTS		

Notes

✓ When Assigned By Your Instructor	Study Guide Pages	Practices Required	LABORATORY ASSIGNMENTS (Procedure Number and Name)	Score*
	957-960	3	**Practice for Competency** 33-A: Performing a Blood Chemistry Test Textbook reference: pp. 871-874	
	961-963		**Evaluation of Competency** 33-A: Performing a Blood Chemistry Test	*
	957-960	3	**Practice for Competency** 33-1: Blood Glucose Measurement Using the Accu-Chek Advantage Glucose Meter Textbook reference: pp. 883-886	
	965-967		**Evaluation of Competency** 33-1: Blood Glucose Measurement Using the Accu-Chek Advantage Glucose Meter	*
	957-960	3	**Practice for Competency** 33-B: Rapid Mononucleosis Testing (QuickVue + Mono Test) Textbook reference: pp. 891-893	
	969-971		**Evaluation of Competency** 33-B: Rapid Mononucleosis Testing (QuickVue + Mono Test)	*
			ADDITIONAL ASSIGNMENTS	

Notes

Name ____________________ Date ____________

PRETEST

True or False

_______ 1. The function of glucose in the body is to build and repair tissue.

_______ 2. Insulin is required for normal use of glucose in the body.

_______ 3. An abnormally low level of glucose in the body is known as hypoglycemia.

_______ 4. The hemoglobin A_{1C} test measures the average amount of blood glucose over a 3-month period.

_______ 5. Most of the cholesterol found in the blood comes from the intake of dietary cholesterol.

_______ 6. The primary use of the cholesterol test is to screen for the presence of coronary artery disease.

_______ 7. LDL picks up cholesterol from ingested fats and the liver and carries it to the cells.

_______ 8. An antibody is a substance that is capable of combining with an antigen.

_______ 9. Mononucleosis is transmitted through coughing and sneezing.

_______ 10. Symptoms of infectious mononucleosis include severe fatigue, fever, and sore throat.

POSTTEST

True or False

_______ 1. Serum is required for most blood chemistry tests.

_______ 2. The normal range for a fasting blood glucose level is 120 to 160 mg/dL.

_______ 3. The oral glucose tolerance test is used to assist in the diagnosis of diabetes mellitus.

_______ 4. Before meals, it is recommended that the blood glucose level for a diabetic patient be 60 to 80 mg/dL.

_______ 5. The recommended hemoglobin A_{1C} level for a patient with diabetes is 4% to 6%.

_______ 6. The buildup of plaque (due to high cholesterol) on the walls of arteries is known as thrombophlebitis.

_______ 7. An HDL cholesterol level greater than 50 mg/dL is a risk factor for coronary artery disease.

_______ 8. The triglyceride test requires that the patient not eat or drink for 12 hours before the test.

_______ 9. The RPR test is a screening test for syphilis.

_______ 10. The varicella virus causes infectious mononucleosis.

Term KEY TERM ASSESSMENT

Directions: Match each key term with its definition.

_______ 1. Agglutination
_______ 2. Analyte
_______ 3. Antibody
_______ 4. Antigen
_______ 5. Glycogen
_______ 6. HDL cholesterol
_______ 7. Hyperglycemia
_______ 8. Hypoglycemia
_______ 9. LDL cholesterol
_______ 10. Lipoprotein

A. An abnormally high level of glucose in the blood
B. A complex molecule consisting of protein and a lipid fraction such as cholesterol
C. The form in which carbohydrate is stored in the body
D. A lipoprotein consisting of protein and cholesterol that removes excess cholesterol from the cells
E. An abnormally low level of glucose in the blood
F. A lipoprotein, consisting of protein and cholesterol, that picks up cholesterol and delivers it to the cells
G. A substance that is capable of combining with an antigen resulting in an antigen-antibody reaction
H. Substance capable of stimulating the formation of antibodies
I. A substance that is being identified or measured in a laboratory test.
J. Clumping of blood cells

EVALUATION OF LEARNING

Directions: Fill in each blank with the correct answer.

1. What type of specimen is required for most blood chemistry tests?

____

2. What is the purpose of quality control?

____

____

3. What is the purpose of calibrating a blood chemistry analyzer?

____

____

4. At a minimum, when should a calibration check be performed on a blood chemistry analyzer?

____

5. What is the purpose of running a control on a blood chemistry analyzer?

____

____

6. List three reasons why a control may not produce expected results.

____

____

7. When running controls on a blood chemistry analyzer, what should be done if the controls do not perform as expected?

____

8. What is the function of glucose in the body?

____

____

9. Explain the function of insulin in the body.

____

____

10. List the abbreviation for each of the following tests:
    a. Fasting blood glucose _______________
    b. Two-hour postprandial blood glucose _______________
    c. Oral glucose tolerance test _______________

11. What type of patient preparation is required for a fasting blood glucose test?

____

____

12. List two reasons for performing a fasting blood glucose test.

____

13. What is prediabetes?

____

____

14. What are the values recommended by the American Diabetes Association for interpreting fasting blood glucose results?
    a. Normal _______________
    b. Prediabetes _______________
    c. Diabetes _______________

15. What type of patient preparation is required for a 2-hour postprandial blood glucose test?

____

____

16. Describe the procedure for performing a 2-hour postprandial blood glucose test.

____

____

17. What is the purpose of an oral glucose tolerance test?

____

____

18. What type of patient preparation is required for an oral glucose tolerance test?

19. Describe the procedure for an oral glucose tolerance test.

20. Define hypoglycemia and list three conditions that may cause it to occur.

21. Why is it important for an insulin-dependent diabetic to perform self-monitoring of blood glucose (SMBG)?

22. What is the ideal insulin testing schedule for SMBG?

23. What type of damage can occur to the body from prolonged high glucose levels in blood?

24. List three advantages of blood glucose monitoring at home.

25. What is the recommended blood glucose level for a diabetic during the following times of the day:
   a. Before meals
   b. One to 2 hours after meals
   c. At bedtime

26. What information is provided by a hemoglobin A_{1C} test?

27. What is the normal A_{1C} range for an individual without diabetes?

28. What is the recommended A_{1C} percentage for an individual with diabetes?

29. What are the storage requirements for blood glucose reagent test strips?

30. When should the calibration (coding) procedure be performed on a glucose meter?

31. What is cholesterol?

32. List the two main sources of cholesterol in the blood.

33. What is atherosclerosis, and why is it a health risk?

34. Why is LDL cholesterol referred to as bad cholesterol and HDL referred to as good cholesterol?

35. What does a total cholesterol test measure?

36. List the ranges for each of the following cholesterol categories:
    a. Desirable cholesterol level
    b. Borderline cholesterol level
    c. High cholesterol level

37. At what level is HDL cholesterol considered a risk factor for coronary heart disease?

38. What is the primary use of the cholesterol test?

39. What type of patient preparation is required for a triglyceride test?

40. List the ranges for each of the following triglyceride categories:

a. Normal

b. Borderline high

c. High

d. Very high

41. What conditions result in elevated blood triglycerides?

42. What is the purpose of performing a BUN?

43. What is the definition of immunology?

44. List three examples of antigens.

45. What is the purpose of performing each of the following serologic tests?

a. Rheumatoid factor

b. Antistreptolysin test

c. C-reactive protein

____

____

d. ABO and Rh blood typing

____

____

46. How is infectious mononucleosis transmitted?

____

____

47. What are the symptoms of infectious mononucleosis?

____

____

CRITICAL THINKING ACTIVITIES

A. Type 2 Diabetes

You are working for a physician specializing in internal medicine. The physician is concerned about the increased numbers of patients developing type 2 diabetes mellitus. He asks you to design a colorful, creative, and informative brochure on type 2 diabetes using the brochure format provided on the next page. This brochure will be published and placed in the waiting room to provide patients with education on type 2 diabetes. The diabetes Internet sites listed under On the Web at the end of Chapter 33 in your textbook can be used to complete this activity.

Notes

FAQ ON:

Q: A:

Q: A:

Q: A:

Q: A:

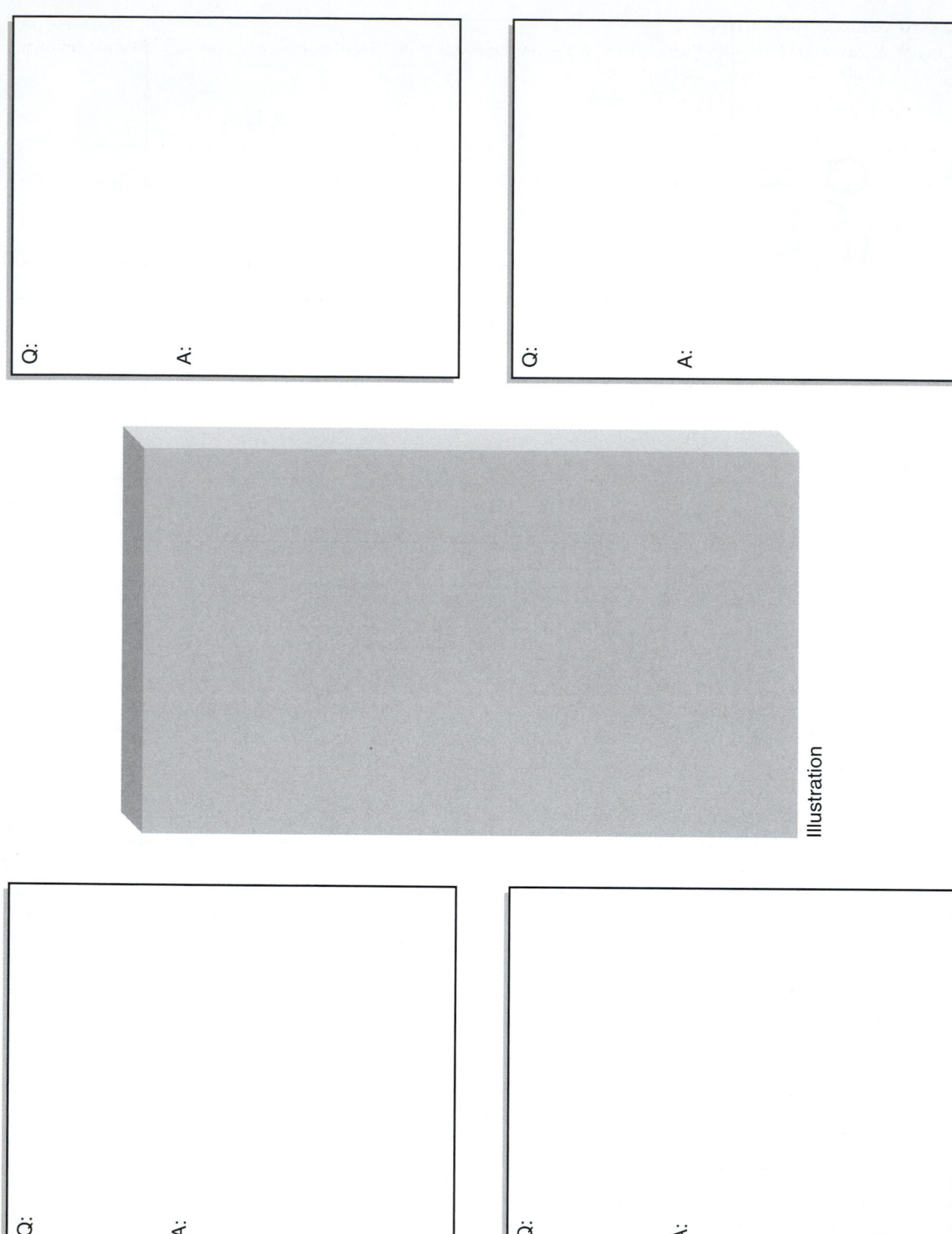

Q:
A:
Q:
A:
Illustration
Q:
A:
Q:
A:

B. Oral Glucose Tolerance Test

Marty Wolf has arrived at your office for an oral glucose tolerance test. What should you tell her regarding the following subjects? Explain the reason for each answer.

1. Consumption of food and fluid

____

____

2. Water consumption

____

____

3. Smoking

____

____

4. Leaving the test site

____

____

5. Activity

____

____

C. Coronary Artery Disease

Create a profile of an individual who is at risk for coronary artery disease (CAD) following these guidelines:

1. Using a blank piece of paper, colored pencils, crayons, or markers, draw a figure of an individual exhibiting risk factors for CAD. Be as creative as possible.
2. Do not use any text on your drawing other than to label items you have drawn in your picture. (A picture is worth a thousand words!)
3. Try to include at least eight risk factors for CAD in your drawing. The Highlight on Coronary Heart Disease with a Focus on Coronary Artery Disease box on p. 816 in your textbook can be used as a reference source.
4. In the classroom, find a partner and trade drawings. Identify the risk factors for CAD in your partner's drawing. With your partner, discuss what this person could do to lower his or her chances of developing CAD.

D. Cholesterol and Saturated Fat

Using a reference source, complete the following activities:

1. Create a dinner meal that is as high as possible in saturated fat and cholesterol.

____

____

____

____

____

2. Create a dinner meal that is as low as possible in saturated fat and cholesterol.

3. Choose a fast-food restaurant, and plan a meal that is as low as possible in saturated fat and cholesterol.

E. Rh Incompatibility

Erythroblastosis fetalis is a blood disorder of the newborn. It usually is caused by incompatibility between the infant's blood and the mother's blood. Using a reference source, answer the following questions regarding this condition in the space provided.

1. Explain how Rh incompatibility between the mother and her infant can cause this condition to occur.

2. Describe the symptoms associated with erythroblastosis fetalis.

3. Explain the treatment used for this condition.

4. How can this condition be prevented?

F. Crossword Puzzle: Blood Chemistry and Immunology

Directions: Complete the crossword puzzle using the clues provided.

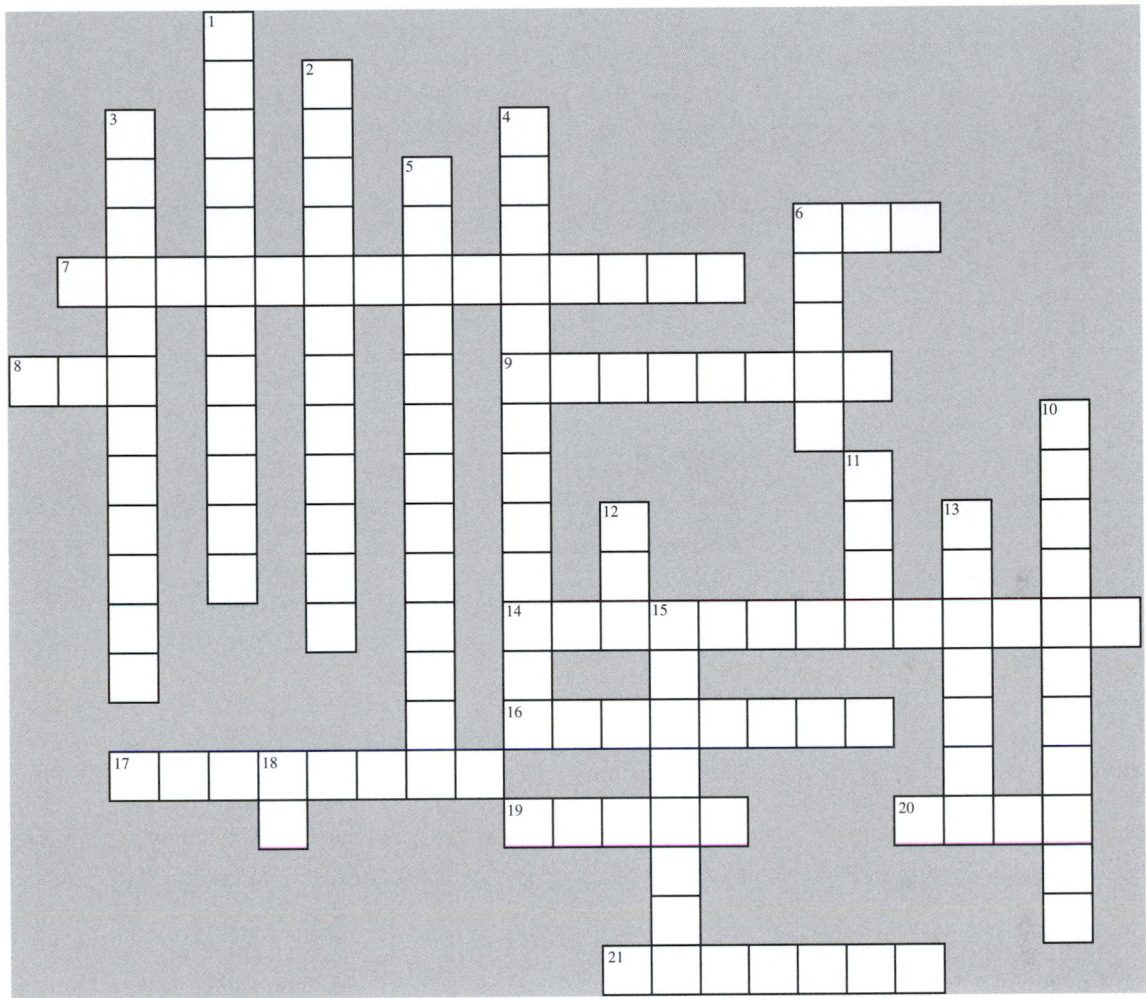

Across

6 Bad cholesterol
7 Cholesterol: 200-239
8 Good cholesterol
9 Stored glucose
14 Kissing disease
16 Combines with an antigen
17 Increases HDL cholesterol
19 Keep diabetic A1c below this
20 Series of glucose tests
21 Provides energy for body

Down

1 #1 killer in the U.S.
2 Raises cholesterol level
3 Low BG
4 High BG
5 Desirable: <150 mg/dL
6 Makes cholesterol
10 FBG: 100-125 mg/dL
11 Syphilis test
12 Detects renal disease
13 Risk factor for CAD
15 Unsaturated fat (ex)
18 Rheumatoid arthritis test

Notes

PRACTICE FOR COMPETENCY

Procedure 33-A: Blood Chemistry Test. Perform a blood chemistry test, and record results in the chart provided. Examples of blood chemistry tests: cholesterol, triglycerides, and BUN.

Procedure 33-1: Blood Glucose Measurement.

a. Run controls on a CLIA-waived glucose meter, and record results on the quality control log on p. 959.

b. Perform a fasting blood glucose test, and record results in the chart provided.

Procedure 33-B: Rapid Mononucleosis Test.

a. Run controls on a CLIA-waived mono, and record results on the quality control log on p. 960.

b. Perform a rapid mononucleosis test, and record results in the chart provided.

Chart	
Date	

Chart

Date	

QUALITY CONTROL LOG
BLOOD GLUCOSE

NAME OF METER	CONTROLS
Test Strips: Lot Number: ____________ Exp Date: ____________ Code Number: ____________	**Low-Level Control:** Lot Number: ____________ Exp Date: ____________ Expected Range: ____________ **High-Level Control:** Lot Number: ____________ Exp Date: ____________ Expected Range: ____________

Date	Low-Level Control	Accept	Reject	High-Level Control	Accept	Reject	Technician

QUALITY CONTROL LOG
MONONUCLEOSIS TEST

Date	Name of Test	Control Lot #	Control Expiration Date	External Positive Control	External Negative Control	Technician

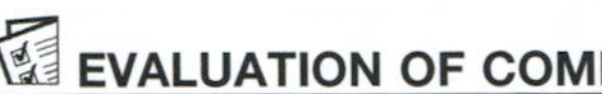

EVALUATION OF COMPETENCY

Procedure 33-A: Performing a Blood Chemistry Test

Name: ______________________ Date: ______________

Evaluated by: ______________________ Score: ______________

Performance Objective

Outcome:	Perform a fasting blood glucose test.
Conditions:	Given the following: disposable gloves, an antiseptic wipe, a lancet, gauze pad, -quality control log, and a biohazard sharps container. Using an automated blood chemistry -analyzer and operating manual.
Standards:	Time: 10 minutes. Student completed procedure in __________ minutes.
	Accuracy: Satisfactory score on the Performance Evaluation Checklist.

Performance Evaluation Checklist

Trial 1	Trial 2	Point Value	Performance Standards
		•	Sanitized hands.
		•	Assembled equipment.
		•	Calibrated the blood chemistry analyzer.
		•	Applied gloves and ran controls.
		•	Recorded results in the quality control log.
		•	Sanitized hands.
		•	Greeted the patient and introduced yourself.
		•	Identified patient and explained the procedure.
		•	Applied gloves.
		•	Performed a finger puncture.
		•	Collected the specimen according to manufacturer's instructions.
		•	Placed a gauze pad over the puncture site and applied pressure.
		•	Inserted the specimen into blood chemistry analyzer according to manufacturer's instructions.
		•	Operated the blood chemistry analyzer according to manufacturer's instructions.
		•	Read the results on digital display screen.
		•	Properly disposed of used materials.
		•	Checked puncture site and applied adhesive bandage if needed.
		•	Removed gloves.

Trial 1	Trial 2	Point Value	Performance Standards
		●	Sanitized hands.
		●	Charted the test results correctly.
		✶	The recording was identical to the reading on the digital display screen.
		Ⓐ	Explained to a patient the rationale for performance of a procedure.
		Ⓐ	Reassured a patient of the accuracy of the test results.
		✶	Completed the procedure within 10 minutes.
			TOTALS

CHART	
Date	

Evaluation of Student Performance

EVALUATION CRITERIA			COMMENTS
Symbol	**Category**	**Point Value**	
✶	Critical Step	16 points	
●	Essential Step	6 points	
Ⓐ	Affective Competency	6 points	
▷	Theory Question	2 points	
Score calculation: 100 points – ___ points missed ___ Score Satisfactory score: 85 or above			

2008 CAAHEP Competencies Achieved
Psychomotor (Skills) ☑ I. 11. Perform quality control measures. ☑ I. 13. Perform chemistry testing. ☑ II. 2. Maintain laboratory test results using flow sheets. ***Affective (Behavior)*** ☑ II. 2. Distinguish between normal and abnormal test results.

2015 CAAHEP Competencies Achieved
Psychomotor (Skills) ☑ I. 10. Perform a quality control measure. ☑ I. 11. b. Obtain specimens and perform CLIA waived chemistry test. ☑ II. 2. Differentiate between normal and abnormal test results. ☑ II. 3. Maintain lab test results using flow sheets. ***Affective (Behavior)*** ☑ II. 1. Reassure a patient of the accuracy of the test results. ☑ V. 4. Explain to a patient the rationale for performance of a procedure.

ABHES Competencies Achieved
☑ 10. a. Practice quality control. ☑ 10. b. (3) Perform selected CLIA-waived tests that assist with diagnosis and treatment: chemistry testing.

Notes

EVALUATION OF COMPETENCY

Procedure 33-1: Blood Glucose Measurement Using the Accu-Chek Advantage Glucose Meter

Name: ______________________ Date: ______________

Evaluated by: ______________________ Score: ______________

Performance Objective

Outcome:	Perform a fasting blood glucose test.
Conditions:	Given the following: disposable gloves, Accu-Chek Advantage glucose meter, reagent test strips, check strip, code key, control solutions, lancet, antiseptic wipe, gauze pad, quality control log, and a biohazard sharps container.
Standards:	Time: 10 minutes. Student completed procedure in __________ minutes.
	Accuracy: Satisfactory score on the Performance Evaluation Checklist.

Performance Evaluation Checklist

Trial 1	Trial 2	Point Value	Performance Standards
		•	Sanitized hands.
		•	Assembled equipment.
		•	Checked the expiration date on container of test strips.
		•	Calibrated the meter using the code key.
		▷	Stated the purpose of calibrating the meter.
		•	Ran a low and high control.
		▷	Stated the purpose for running controls.
		•	Recorded results in the quality control log.
		•	Sanitized hands.
		•	Greeted the patient and introduced yourself.
		•	Identified the patient and explained the procedure.
		•	Asked the patient if he or she prepared properly.
		▷	Stated the preparation required for a fasting blood glucose test.
		•	Removed a test strip from the container.
		•	Immediately replaced the lid of the container.
		▷	Explained why the lid should be replaced immediately.
		•	Gently inserted the test strip into the test strip guide.
		•	Checked that the code number matches the code number on the test strip container.

Trial 1	Trial 2	Point Value	Performance Standards
		●	Opened gauze packet.
		●	Cleansed the puncture site with an antiseptic wipe and allowed it to dry.
		●	Applied gloves.
		●	Performed a finger puncture.
		●	Disposed of the lancet in the biohazard sharps container.
		●	Wiped away the first drop of blood with a gauze pad.
		▷	Explained why the first drop of blood should be wiped away.
		●	Placed the patient's hand in a dependent position and gently massaged finger until a large drop of blood formed.
		●	Applied the drop of blood to the yellow target area of the test strip.
		●	Completely filled the yellow target area with blood.
		▷	Explained what to do if the yellow area is not completely covered with blood.
		●	Placed a gauze pad over puncture site and applied pressure.
		●	Observed the digital display of the test results.
		▷	Stated the normal range for a fasting blood glucose level (70 to 99 mg/dL).
		●	Removed the test strip from the meter and discarded it in a biohazard waste container.
		●	Turned off the meter.
		●	Checked puncture site and applied adhesive bandage, if needed.
		●	Removed gloves and sanitized hands.
		●	Charted the test results correctly.
		*	The recording was identical to the reading on the digital display screen.
		●	Properly stored the glucose meter.
		Ⓐ	Explained to a patient the rationale for performance of a procedure.
		Ⓐ	Reassured a patient of the accuracy of the test results.
		*	Completed the procedure within 10 minutes.
			TOTALS

Evaluation of Student Performance

EVALUATION CRITERIA			COMMENTS
Symbol	**Category**	**Point Value**	
∗	Critical Step	16 points	
●	Essential Step	6 points	
Ⓐ	Affective Competency	6 points	
▷	Theory Question	2 points	
Score calculation: 100 points – ____ points missed ____ Score Satisfactory score: 85 or above			

2008 CAAHEP Competencies Achieved
Psychomotor (Skills) ☑ I. 11. Perform quality control measures. ☑ I. 13. Perform chemistry testing. ☑ II. 2. Maintain laboratory test results using flow sheets. ***Affective (Behavior)*** ☑ II. 2. Distinguish between normal and abnormal test results.

2015 CAAHEP Competencies Achieved
Psychomotor (Skills) ☑ I. 10. Perform a quality control measure. ☑ I. 11. b. Obtain specimens and perform CLIA waived chemistry test. ☑ II. 2. Differentiate between normal and abnormal test results. ☑ II. 3. Maintain lab test results using flow sheets. ***Affective (Behavior)*** ☑ II. 1. Reassure a patient of the accuracy of the test results. ☑ V. 4. Explain to a patient the rationale for performance of a procedure.

ABHES Competencies Achieved
☑ 10. a. Practice quality control. ☑ 10. b. (3) Perform selected CLIA-waived tests that assist with diagnosis and treatment: chemistry testing.

Notes

EVALUATION OF COMPETENCY

Procedure 33-B: Rapid Mononucleosis Testing (QuickVue + Mono Test)

Name: ______________________ Date: ______________

Evaluated by: ______________________ Score: ______________

Performance Objective

Outcome:	Perform a rapid mononucleosis test.
Conditions:	Given the following: disposable gloves, the supplies needed to perform a finger puncture, a mononucleosis testing kit, and a biohazard container.
Standards:	Time: 10 minutes. Student completed procedure in ________ minutes.
	Accuracy: Satisfactory score on the Performance Evaluation Checklist.

Performance Evaluation Checklist

Trial 1	Trial 2	Point Value	Performance Standards
		•	Sanitized hands.
		•	Assembled equipment.
		•	Checked the expiration date on the testing kit.
		•	Applied gloves and ran a positive and a negative control, if necessary.
		•	Removed gloves and recorded results in the quality control log.
		•	Greeted the patient and introduced yourself.
		•	Identified the patient and explained the procedure.
		•	Cleansed the puncture site and allowed it to air dry.
		•	Applied gloves.
		•	Performed a finger puncture.
		•	Disposed of the lancet in a biohazard sharps container.
		•	Wiped away the first drop of blood.
		•	Collected the blood specimen with a capillary tube.
		•	Placed a gauze pad over puncture site and applied pressure.
		•	Dispensed the blood specimen into the add well on the test cassette.
		•	Added 5 drops of developing solution to the add well.
		•	Waited 5 minutes and read the results.
		▷	Described the appearance of a positive and negative test result.
		•	Disposed of the test cassette in a biohazard waste container.

Trial 1	Trial 2	Point Value	Performance Standards
		●	Checked puncture site and applied adhesive bandage, if needed.
		●	Removed gloves.
		●	Sanitized hands.
		●	Charted the results correctly.
		●	The results were identical to the evaluator's results.
		Ⓐ	Explained to a patient the rationale for performance of a procedure.
		Ⓐ	Reassured a patient of the accuracy of the test results.
		✶	Completed the procedure within 10 minutes.
			TOTALS

CHART	
Date	

Evaluation of Student Performance

EVALUATION CRITERIA			COMMENTS
Symbol	**Category**	**Point Value**	
✶	Critical Step	16 points	
●	Essential Step	6 points	
Ⓐ	Affective Competency	6 points	
▷	Theory Question	2 points	
Score calculation: 100 points − ___ points missed ___ Score Satisfactory score: 85 or above			

2008 CAAHEP Competencies Achieved
Psychomotor (Skills) ☑ I. 11. Perform quality control measures. ☑ I. 13. Perform immunology testing. ***Affective (Behavior)*** ☑ II. 2. Distinguish between normal and abnormal test results.

2015 CAAHEP Competencies Achieved
Psychomotor (Skills) ☑ I. 10. Perform a quality control measure. ☑ I. 11. d. Obtain specimens and perform CLIA waived immunology test. ☑ II. 2. Differentiate between normal and abnormal test results. ***Affective (Behavior)*** ☑ II. 1. Reassure a patient of the accuracy of the test results. ☑ V. 4. Explain to a patient the rationale for performance of a procedure.

ABHES Competencies Achieved
☑ 10. a. Practice quality control. ☑ 10. b. (4) Perform selected CLIA-waived tests that assist with diagnosis and treatment: immunology testing.

Notes

34 Medical Microbiology

CHAPTER ASSIGNMENTS

✓ After Completing	Date Due	Study Guide Pages	STUDY GUIDE ASSIGNMENTS (CTA = Critical Thinking Activity)	Possible Points	Points You Earned
		977	Pretest	10	
		978	Term Key Term Assessment	15	
		978-981	Evaluation of Learning questions	27	
		982	CTA A: Stages of an Infectious Disease	20	
			Evolve Site: Microscope Identification (Record points earned)		
		983	CTA B: Disease and Infection Control	10	
		983	CTA C: Sensitivity Testing	12	
		984	CTA D: Crossword Puzzle	21	
			Evolve Site: Apply Your Knowledge questions	10	
			Evolve Site: Video Evaluation	15	
		977	Posttest	10	
			ADDITIONAL ASSIGNMENTS		
			TOTAL POINTS		

Notes

✓ When Assigned By Your Instructor	Study Guide Pages	Practices Required	LABORATORY ASSIGNMENTS (Procedure Number and Name)	Score*
	985-986	3	**Practice for Competency** 34-1: Using the Microscope Textbook reference: pp. 903-905	
	987-989		**Evaluation of Competency** 34-1: Using the Microscope	*
	985-986	3	**Practice for Competency** 34-2: Collecting a Throat Specimen Textbook reference: p. 908	
	991-994		**Evaluation of Competency** 34-2: Collecting a Throat Specimen	*
	985-986	3	**Practice for Competency** 34-A: Rapid Strep Testing Textbook reference: p. 909	
	995-997		**Evaluation of Competency** 34-A: Rapid Strep Testing	*
			ADDITIONAL ASSIGNMENTS	

Notes

Name ______________________________ Date ______________

PRETEST

True or False

_______ 1. Microbiology is the scientific study of microorganisms and their activities.

_______ 2. A disease that can be spread from one person to another is known as an infectious disease.

_______ 3. Droplet infection is the transfer of pathogens from a fine spray emitted from a person already infected with the disease.

_______ 4. Streptococci are round bacteria that grow in pairs.

_______ 5. Chickenpox is caused by a virus.

_______ 6. The course adjustment on a microscope is used to obtain precise focusing of an object.

_______ 7. The purpose of transport media is to provide nutrients for the multiplication of the specimen.

_______ 8. A throat specimen should be collected from the tonsillar area and posterior pharynx.

_______ 9. A wet mount is used to examine microorganisms in the living state.

_______ 10. A smear is material spread on a slide for microscopic examination.

POSTTEST

True or False

_______ 1. Microorganisms that reside in the body but do not cause disease are known as transient flora.

_______ 2. The invasion of the body by a pathogenic microorganism is known as infection.

_______ 3. The interval of time between the invasion by a pathogen and the first symptoms of disease is known as the prodromal period.

_______ 4. Staphylococcal infections usually result in pus formation.

_______ 5. Escherichia coli normally reside in the urinary tract.

_______ 6. The high-power objective has a magnification of 40×.

_______ 7. Examination of urine sediment requires the use of the oil immersion objective.

_______ 8. A sequela to streptococcal sore throat is rheumatic fever.

_______ 9. The purpose of sensitivity testing is to identify the type of microorganism present.

_______ 10. When viewed under a microscope, gram-positive bacteria appear pink or red.

Term KEY TERM ASSESSMENT

Directions: Match each key term with its definition.

_______ 1. Bacilli
_______ 2. Cocci
_______ 3. Contagious
_______ 4. Culture
_______ 5. Culture medium
_______ 6. Incubate
_______ 7. Incubation period
_______ 8. Infectious disease
_______ 9. Inoculate
_______ 10. Microbiology
_______ 11. Normal flora
_______ 12. Sequelae
_______ 13. Smear
_______ 14. Specimen
_______ 15. Spirilla

A. A disease caused by a pathogen that produces harmful effects on its host
B. Capable of being transmitted directly or indirectly from one person to another
C. To introduce microorganisms into a culture medium for growth and multiplication
D. Bacteria that have a round shape
E. The scientific study of microorganisms and their activities
F. Material spread on a slide for microscopic examination
G. Morbid (secondary) condition occurring as a result of a less serious primary infection
H. A mixture of nutrients in which microorganisms are grown in the laboratory
I. The interval of time between invasion by a pathogenic microorganism and the appearance of the first symptoms of the disease
J. Bacteria that have a spiral or curved shape
K. Harmless, nonpathogenic microorganisms that normally reside in many parts of the body but do not cause disease
L. Bacteria that have a rod shape
M. The propagation of a mass of microorganisms in a laboratory culture medium
N. In microbiology, the act of placing a culture in a chamber that provides optimal growth requirements for the multiplication of the organisms, such as the proper temperature, humidity, and darkness
O. A small sample or part taken from the body to show the nature of the whole

EVALUATION OF LEARNING

Directions: Fill in each blank with the correct answer.

1. What occurs when pathogens invade the body, and what is the response of the body to the invasion?

____

____

2. What is droplet infection?

____

____

3. What is the prodromal period of an infectious disease?

____

____

4. List three infectious diseases caused by Staphylococcus aureus.

____

____

5. List three infectious diseases caused by different types of streptococci.

____

____

6. List three infectious diseases caused by different types of bacilli.

____

____

7. In what part of the body do E. coli bacteria normally reside?

____

8. List four infectious diseases caused by different viruses.

____

____

9. Explain the purpose of each of the following parts of a microscope:

Stage

____

____

Substage condenser

____

____

Iris diaphragm

____

____

Coarse adjustment

____

____

Fine adjustment

____

____

Ocular lens

____

____

10. Describe the function of each of the following objective lenses:

Low power

____

____

High power

Oil immersion

11. What is the purpose of using oil with the oil-immersion objective?

12. List five guidelines that should be followed for proper care of the microscope.

13. List five common areas of the body from which a microbiologic specimen may be obtained.

14. List two ways to prevent contamination of a specimen with extraneous microorganisms.

15. List two precautions a medical assistant should take to prevent infecting herself or himself with a microbiologic specimen.

16. Why should a specimen be processed as soon as possible after it is collected?

17. What is the purpose of a transport medium?

18. How should a collection and transport system be stored?

19. Describe the procedure for collecting a wound specimen.

____

____

20. A throat specimen is used to perform tests that assist in the diagnosis of what conditions?

____

____

21. Why is it important to diagnose and treat streptococcal pharyngitis as early as possible?

____

____

22. What type of reaction is used to identify streptococci with the direct antigen identification test?

____

23. What is the advantage of using the direct antigen identification test to diagnose streptococci compared with a culture test?

____

____

24. What is the purpose of performing a sensitivity test on a bacterial culture?

____

25. List two reasons for examining a microorganism in the living state.

____

____

26. What is the purpose of staining a smear?

____

____

27. What color do the following bacteria exhibit in a Gram-stained smear?

Gram-positive bacteria: ______________________________

Gram-negative bacteria: ______________________________

CRITICAL THINKING ACTIVITIES

A. Stages of an Infectious Disease

Your physician wants you to design a poster to hang in the office that outlines the stages of an infectious disease. Complete this project using the following diagram in your study guide.

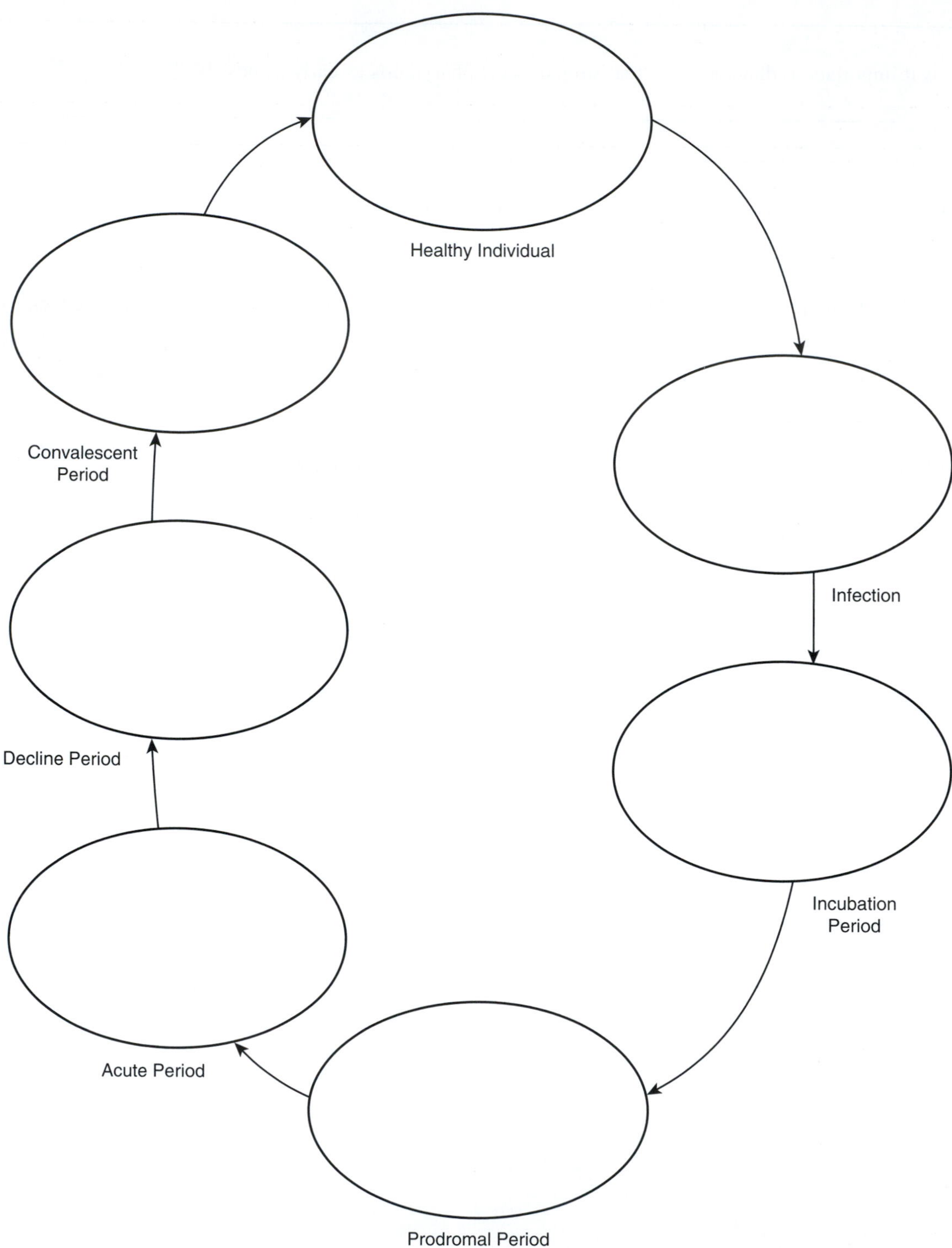

B. Disease and Infection Control

Obtain a current journal article on disease and infection control. The Internet sites listed under On the Web at the end of Chapter 34 in your textbook can be used to locate an article. List the important parts of your article below.

___

___

___

___

___

___

___

___

___

___

C. Sensitivity Testing

Refer to Figure 34-7 of the textbook. Place a check mark next to each antibiotic that is effective against the pathogen growing on the culture medium in the Petri plate.

_______ 1. azithromycin

_______ 2. cephalothin

_______ 3. ciprofloxacin

_______ 4. cefprozil

_______ 5. clarithromycin

_______ 6. doxycycline

_______ 7. erythromycin

_______ 8. nitrofurantoin

_______ 9. norfloxacin

_______ 10. penicillin

_______ 11. sulfisoxazole

_______ 12. tetracycline

D. Crossword Puzzle: Medical Microbiology

Directions: Complete the crossword puzzle using the clues provided.

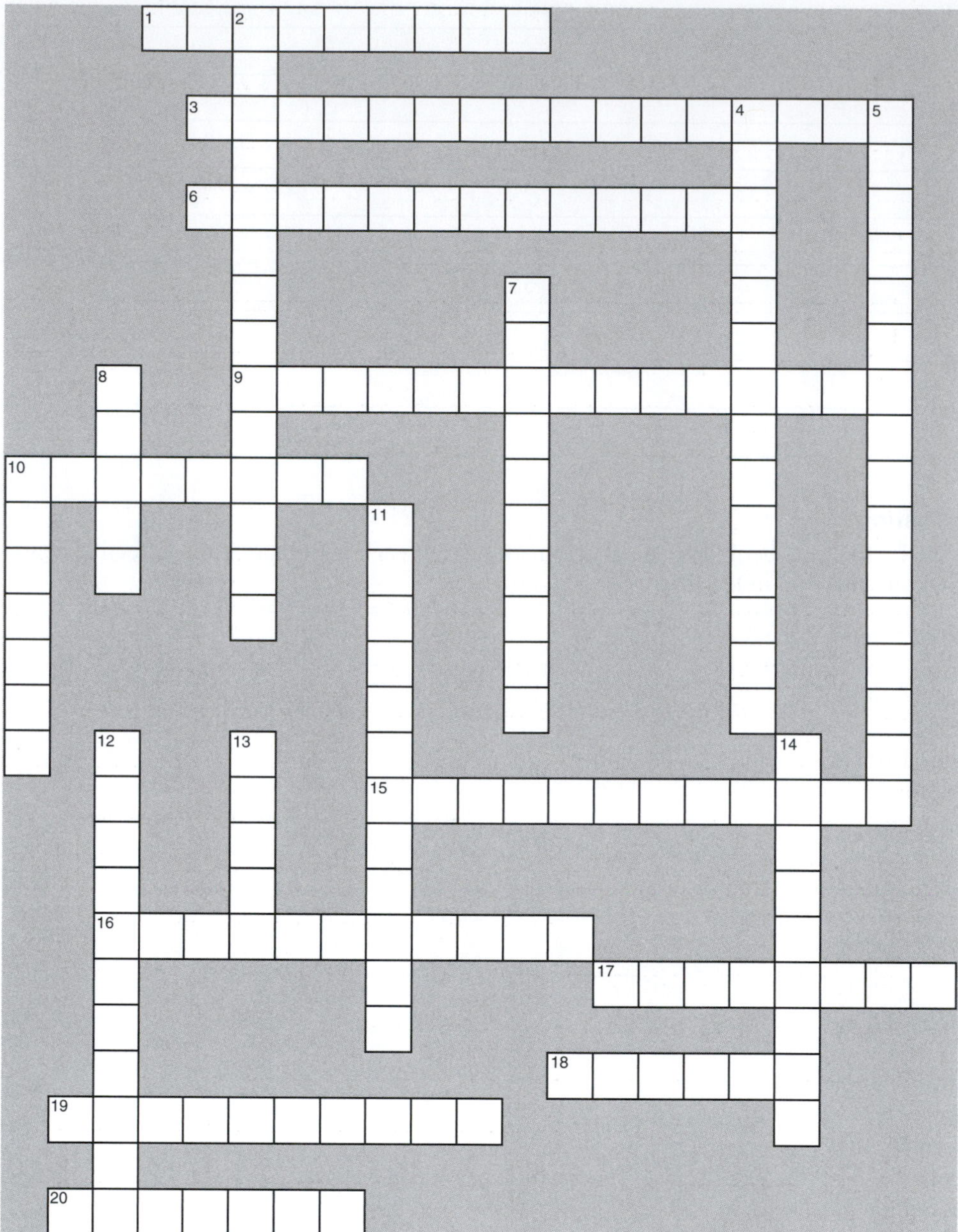

Across

1 Invasion by pathogens
3 Between invasion and first symptoms
6 Absent when present
9 Which antibiotic?
10 Sample of the body
15 Second line natural defense mechanism
16 Treatment for strep throat
17 Disease-producing MO
18 Color of gram-positive bacteria
19 Can catch it!
20 Rod-shaped bacteria

Down

2 For precise focusing
4 Sequela to strep throat
5 Way to transmit pathogens
7 It's everywhere!
8 Material spread on a slide
10 Secondary condition
11 Study of microorganisms
12 Harmless MOs residing in body
13 Round bacteria
14 Magnifies 40x

PRACTICE FOR COMPETENCY

Procedure 34-1: Using the Microscope. Practice using a microscope.

Procedure 34-2: Collecting a Throat Specimen. Obtain a throat specimen using a sterile cotton swab or a collection and transport system. Record the procedure in the chart provided.

Procedure 34-A: Rapid Strep Testing. Perform a strep test using a rapid strep testing kit, and record results in the chart provided.

CHART	
Date	

Chart

Date	

EVALUATION OF COMPETENCY

Procedure 34-1: Using the Microscope

Name: ______________________________ Date: ______________

Evaluated by: ______________________________ Score: ______________

Performance Objective

Outcome:	Use a microscope.
Conditions:	Given a microscope, lens paper, specimen slide, tissue or gauze, immersion oil, xylene, and a soft cloth.
Standards:	Time: 15 minutes. Student completed procedure in ________ minutes.
	Accuracy: Satisfactory score on the Performance Evaluation Checklist.

Performance Evaluation Checklist

Trial 1	Trial 2	Point Value	Performance Standards
		●	Cleaned the ocular and objective lenses with lens paper.
		●	Turned on the light source.
		●	Rotated the nosepiece to the low-power objective.
		●	Used the coarse adjustment to provide sufficient working space for placing the slide on the stage.
		●	Placed the slide on the stage, specimen side up, and secured it.
		●	Positioned the low-power objective until it almost touched the slide using the coarse adjustment.
		●	Observed this step.
		▷	Explained why this step should be observed.
		●	Looked through the ocular lens.
		●	Brought the specimen into coarse focus using the coarse adjustment knob.
		●	Observed the specimen until it came into coarse focus.
		●	Used the fine-adjustment knob to bring the specimen into sharp, clear focus.
		●	Adjusted the light as needed using the iris diaphragm.
		●	Rotated the nosepiece to the high-power objective.
		●	Used the fine-adjustment knob to bring the specimen into a precise focus.
		●	Did not use the coarse-adjustment knob to focus the high-power objective.
		▷	Explained why the coarse-adjustment knob should not be used for focusing at this point.

Trial 1	Trial 2	Point Value	Performance Standards
		●	Examined the specimen as required by the test or procedure being performed.
		●	Turned off the light after use.
		●	Removed the slide from the stage.
		●	Cleaned the stage with a tissue or gauze.
		●	Properly cared for and stored the microscope.
			Using the oil-immersion objective:
		●	Rotated the nosepiece to the oil-immersion objective.
		●	Placed the objective to one side.
		●	Placed a drop of immersion oil on the slide directly over the center opening in the stage.
		●	Moved the oil-immersion objective into place.
		●	Made sure the objective did not touch the stage or slide.
		●	Used the coarse adjustment to position the oil-immersion objective.
		●	Brought the objective down until the lens touched the oil but did not come in contact with the slide.
		●	Looked through the eyepiece.
		●	Focused slowly using the coarse objective until the object was visible.
		●	Used the fine adjustment to bring the object into sharp focus.
		●	Adjusted the light as needed using the iris diaphragm.
		●	Examined the specimen as required by the test or procedure being performed.
		●	Turned off the light after use.
		●	Removed the slide from the stage.
		●	Cleaned the oil-immersion objective with lens paper.
		▷	Explained why the lens must be cleaned immediately.
		●	Cleaned the oil from the slide by immersing it in xylene and wiping it with a soft cloth.
		*	Completed the procedure within 15 minutes.
			TOTALS

Evaluation of Student Performance

EVALUATION CRITERIA			COMMENTS
Symbol	**Category**	**Point Value**	
✶	Critical Step	16 points	
●	Essential Step	6 points	
Ⓐ	Affective Competency	6 points	
▷	Theory Question	2 points	
Score calculation: 100 points – ____ points missed ____ Score Satisfactory score: 85 or above			

2008 CAAHEP Competencies Achieved
Psychomotor (Skills) ☑ I. 10. Assist physician with patient care.

2015 CAAHEP Competencies Achieved
Psychomotor (Skills) ☑ I. 9. Assist provider with patient exam.

ABHES Competencies Achieved
☑ 9. c. Assist provider with general/physical examination.

Notes

EVALUATION OF COMPETENCY

Procedure 34-2: Collecting a Throat Specimen

Name: ______________________________ Date: ______________

Evaluated by: ______________________________ Score: ______________

Performance Objective

Outcome:	Collect a throat specimen.
Conditions:	Given the following: disposable gloves, tongue depressor, sterile swab, collection and transport system, laboratory request form, and a biohazard specimen bag.
Standards:	Time: 5 minutes. Student completed procedure in __________ minutes.
	Accuracy: Satisfactory score on the Performance Evaluation Checklist.

Performance Evaluation Checklist

Trial 1	Trial 2	Point Value	Performance Standards
			Throat specimen—sterile swab for strep testing in medical office
		•	Sanitized hands.
		•	Assembled equipment.
		•	Greeted the patient and introduced yourself.
		•	Identified the patient and explained the procedure.
		•	Positioned patient and adjusted light.
		•	Applied gloves.
		•	Removed the sterile swab from its peel-apart package, being careful not to contaminate it.
		•	Depressed patient's tongue with tongue depressor.
		•	Placed swab at the back of patient's throat and firmly rubbed it over lesions or white or inflamed areas of the tonsillar area and posterior pharynx.
		▷	Explained why swab should be rubbed over suspicious looking areas.
		•	Constantly rotated swab as the specimen was being obtained.
		▷	Described why a rotating motion should be used.
		•	Did not allow swab to touch any area other than throat.
		▷	Explained why swab should not be allowed to touch any areas other than throat.
		•	Kept patient's tongue depressed and withdrew swab and removed tongue depressor.
		•	Disposed of the tongue depressor.

Trial 1	Trial 2	Point Value	Performance Standards
		●	Performed the rapid strep test according to the directions accompanying the rapid strep testing kit.
		●	Removed gloves and sanitized hands.
		●	Charted the test results correctly.
		*	Completed the procedure within 5 minutes.
			Throat specimen—collection and transport system
		●	Sanitized hands.
		●	Greeted the patient and introduced yourself.
		●	Identified the patient and explained the procedure.
		●	Positioned patient and adjusted light.
		●	Applied gloves.
		●	Checked the expiration date on the peel-apart package.
		●	Peeled open the package and removed the cap from the collection tube.
		●	Removed the cap/swab unit from the peel-apart package.
		●	Depressed the patient's tongue with tongue depressor.
		●	Placed swab at the back of patient's throat and firmly rubbed it over lesions or white or inflamed areas of the tonsillar area and posterior pharynx.
		●	Constantly rotated swab as the specimen was being obtained.
		●	Did not allow swab to touch any area other than the collection site.
		●	Kept patient's tongue depressed and withdrew swab and removed tongue depressor.
		●	Disposed of the tongue depressor.
		●	Inserted swab into the collection tube.
		●	Pushed cap or swab in as far as it will go.
		●	Made sure the cap was tightly in place.
		●	Removed gloves and sanitized hands.
		●	Labeled tube.
		●	Completed a laboratory request form.
		●	Placed tube in a biohazard specimen transport bag.
		●	Placed laboratory request in outside pocket of bag.
		●	Charted the procedure.
		●	Transported specimen to the laboratory within 24 hours.
		▷	Explained why the specimen must be transported within 24 hours.

Trial 1	Trial 2	Point Value	Performance Standards
		Ⓐ	Explained to a patient the rationale for performance of a procedure.
		Ⓐ	Showed awareness of a patient's concerns related to the procedure being performed.
		✶	Completed the procedure within 5 minutes.
			TOTALS

CHART	
Date	

Evaluation of Student Performance

EVALUATION CRITERIA			COMMENTS
Symbol	**Category**	**Point Value**	
✶	Critical Step	16 points	
●	Essential Step	6 points	
Ⓐ	Affective Competency	6 points	
▷	Theory Question	2 points	
Score calculation: 100 points – ____ points missed ____ Score Satisfactory score: 85 or above			

2008 CAAHEP Competencies Achieved
Psychomotor (Skills) ☑ III. 7. Obtain specimens for microbiological testing. ***Affective (Behavior)*** ☑ III. 1. Display sensitivity to patient rights and feelings in collecting specimens. ☑ III. 2. Explain the rationale for performance of a procedure to the patient. ☑ III. 3. Show awareness of patients' concerns regarding their perceptions related to the procedures being performed.

2015 CAAHEP Competencies Achieved
Psychomotor (Skills) ☑ I. 11. e. Obtain specimens and perform CLIA waived microbiology test. ***Affective (Behavior)*** ☑ I. 3. Show awareness of a patient's concerns related to the procedure being performed. ☑ V. 4. Explain to a patient the rationale for performance of a procedure.

ABHES Competencies Achieved
☑ 10. d. (4) Collect, label, and process specimens: Obtain throat specimens for microbiologic testing.

EVALUATION OF COMPETENCY

Procedure 34-A: Rapid Strep Testing

Name: ______________________ Date: ______________

Evaluated by: ______________________ Score: ______________

Performance Objective

Outcome:	Perform a rapid strep test.
Conditions:	Given the following: disposable gloves, tongue blade, a QuickVue rapid strep testing kit, controls, manufacturer's instructions, quality control log, and a biohazard sharps container.
Standards:	Time: 10 minutes. Student completed procedure in ________ minutes.
	Accuracy: Satisfactory score on the Performance Evaluation Checklist.

Performance Evaluation Checklist

Trial 1	Trial 2	Point Value	Performance Standards
		●	Sanitized hands.
		●	Assembled equipment.
		●	Checked the expiration date on the testing kit.
		●	Applied gloves and ran a positive and negative control, if needed.
		▷	Stated when controls should be run.
		●	Disposed of test cassettes and swabs in a biohazard waste container.
		●	Removed gloves and sanitized hands.
		●	Recorded results in the quality control log.
		●	Greeted the patient and introduced yourself.
		●	Identified the patient and explained the procedure.
		●	Positioned patient and adjusted light.
		●	Sanitized hands and applied gloves.
		●	Removed test cassette from its foil pouch, and placed it on a clean, dry, level surface.
		●	Removed the sterile swab from its peel-apart package.
		●	Depressed patient's tongue with tongue depressor.
		●	Placed swab at the back of patient's throat and firmly rubbed it over lesions or white or inflamed areas of the tonsillar area and posterior pharynx.
		●	Constantly rotated swab as the specimen was being obtained.
		▷	Stated why the swab should be rotated.

Trial 1	Trial 2	Point Value	Performance Standards
		●	Did not allow swab to touch any area other than throat.
		●	Kept patient's tongue depressed and withdrew swab.
		●	Removed tongue depressor and discarded it.
		●	Inserted the swab completely into the swab chamber.
		●	Squeezed the extraction bottle once to break the glass ampule.
		●	Vigorously shook the extraction bottle five times.
		●	Filled the swab chamber to the rim.
		●	Started the timer.
		●	Waited 5 minutes and read the results.
		▷	Described the appearance of a positive and negative result.
		▷	Described the appearance of an invalid result.
		▷	Explained what to do if an invalid result occurs.
		*	The results were identical to the evaluator's results.
		●	Disposed of the test cassette and swab in a biohazard waste container.
		●	Removed gloves and sanitized hands.
		●	Recorded results in patient's chart.
		Ⓐ	Explained to a patient the rationale for performance of a procedure.
		Ⓐ	Showed awareness of a patient's concerns related to the procedure being performed.
		Ⓐ	Reassured a patient of the accuracy of the test results.
		*	Completed the procedure within 10 minutes.
			TOTALS

CHART	
Date	

Evaluation of Student Performance

EVALUATION CRITERIA			COMMENTS
Symbol	**Category**	**Point Value**	
∗	Critical Step	16 points	
●	Essential Step	6 points	
Ⓐ	Affective Competency	6 points	
▷	Theory Question	2 points	
Score calculation:	100 points – ____ points missed ____ Score		
Satisfactory score: 85 or above			

2008 CAAHEP Competencies Achieved
Psychomotor (Skills) ☑ I. 11. Perform quality control measures. ☑ III. 7. Obtain specimens for microbiological testing. ☑ III. 8. Perform CLIA-waived microbiology testing. ***Affective (Behavior)*** ☑ II. 2. Distinguish between normal and abnormal test results. ☑ III. 1. Display sensitivity to patient rights and feelings in collecting-specimens. ☑ III. 3. Show awareness of patients' concerns regarding their perceptions related to the procedures being-performed.

2015 CAAHEP Competencies Achieved
Psychomotor (Skills) ☑ I. 10. Perform a quality control measure. ☑ I. 11. e. Obtain specimens and perform CLIA waived microbiology test. ☑ II. 2. Differentiate between normal and abnormal test results. ***Affective (Behavior)*** ☑ I. 3. Show awareness of a patient's concerns related to the procedure being performed. ☑ II. 1. Reassure a patient of the accuracy of the test results. ☑ V. 4. Explain to a patient the rationale for performance of a procedure.

ABHES Competencies Achieved
☑ 10. a. Practice quality control. ☑ 10. b. Perform selected CLIA-waived tests that assist with diagnosis and treatment: (2) microbiology testing (6) kit testing (b) quick strep.

Notes

35 Nutrition

✓ After Completing	Date Due	Study Guide Pages	STUDY GUIDE ASSIGNMENTS (CTA = Critical Thinking Activity)	Possible Points	Points You Earned
		1001	Pretest	10	
		 1002 1003	Key Term Assessment A. Definitions B. Word Parts (Add 1 point for each key term)	 27 20	
		1003-1014	Evaluation of Learning questions	90	
		1015	CTA A: Nutrition Density	8	
		1015	CTA B: Sodium	10	
		1016-1019	CTA C: MyPlate	17	
		1019	CTA D: Nutrition Facts Panel Analysis	14	
		1020	CTA E: Nutrition and Disease	13	
		1020	CTA F: Ingredients List	15	
		1021	CTA G: Crossword Puzzle	20	
			Apply Your Knowledge Questions	10	
		1001	Posttest	10	
			ADDITIONAL ASSIGNMENTS		
			TOTAL POINTS		

✓ When Assigned By Your Instructor	Study Guide Pages	Practices Required	LABORATORY ASSIGNMENTS (Procedure Number and Name)	Score*
		3	**Practice for Competency** 35-A: Instruct a Patient According to Patient's Special Dietary Needs Textbook reference: pp. 915-943	
	1023-1026		**Evaluation of Competency** 35-A: Instruct a Patient According to Patient's Special Dietary Needs	*

Name ______________________________ Date ______________

PRETEST

True or False

_______ 1. A food with a high nutrient density is high in calories and low in nutrients.

_______ 2. Carbohydrates provide 4 kilocalories of energy per gram.

_______ 3. Ingested glucose that is not needed for energy is stored for later use in the form of glycogen.

_______ 4. Fat transports water soluble vitamins in the body.

_______ 5. Saturated fat is liquid at room temperature and comes primarily from plant sources.

_______ 6. The fat soluble vitamins include A, D, E, and K.

_______ 7. Food labeling is required for most packaged foods.

_______ 8. One pound of body fat is equal to 2,000 calories.

_______ 9. An individual with lactose intolerance is allergic to milk.

_______ 10. Common food allergens include milk, eggs, wheat, and peanuts.

POSTTEST

True or False

_______ 1. An enriched food has vitamins and minerals added to it to replace those lost during the processing of that food.

_______ 2. Micronutrients include vitamins and minerals.

_______ 3. Lactose is a monosaccharide.

_______ 4. Soluble fiber helps to lower the blood cholesterol level.

_______ 5. The function of protein is to build, maintain, and repair body tissue.

_______ 6. Minor minerals are found in the body in levels of 5 grams or higher.

_______ 7. Approximately 60 to 65% of an adult's total body weight is made up of water.

_______ 8. The treatment of obesity involves a combination of nutrition therapy, a physical exercise program, and a behavior modification plan.

_______ 9. The TLC eating plan provides recommendations for a heart healthy diet.

_______ 10. Celiac disease may result in damage to the intestinal villi.

Term KEY TERM ASSESSMENT

A. Definitions

Directions: Match each key term with its definition.

_______ 1. Antioxidant
_______ 2. Atherosclerosis
_______ 3. Bariatrics
_______ 4. Cholesterol
_______ 5. Complete protein
_______ 6. Disaccharide
_______ 7. Empty calorie food
_______ 8. Essential amino acid
_______ 9. Gluten
_______ 10. Glycogen
_______ 11. Incomplete protein
_______ 12. Kilocalorie
_______ 13. Lactose
_______ 14. Macronutrient
_______ 15. Micronutrient
_______ 16. Mineral
_______ 17. Monosaccharide
_______ 18. Nonessential amino acid
_______ 19. Nutrient
_______ 20. Nutrition
_______ 21. Nutrition therapy
_______ 22. Obesity
_______ 23. Percent daily value
_______ 24. Saturated fat
_______ 25. Triglycerides
_______ 26. Unsaturated fat
_______ 27. Vitamin

A. A food that provides calories but little or no nutrients. Also known as a low nutrient density food.
B. The amount of heat needed to raise the temperature of 1 kilogram of water 1 degree Celsius. (Often referred to as a calorie).
C. A chemical substance found in food that is needed by the body for survival and well-being.
D. The percentage of a nutrient provided by a single serving of a food item compared to how much is required for the entire day.
E. Buildup of fibrous plaques of fatty deposits and cholesterol on the inner walls of an artery that causes narrowing, obstruction, and hardening of the artery.
F. An organic compound that is required in small amounts by the body for normal growth and development.
G. A white waxy, fatlike substance that is essential for normal functioning of the body.
H. A type of protein found in certain grains such as wheat, rye, and barley.
I. A type of protein found in certain grains such as wheat, rye, and barley.
J. The chemical form in which most fat exists in food, as well as in the body.
K. An antioxidant is a molecule that inhibits the oxidation of other molecules.
L. A medical condition in which there is an excessive accumulation of body fat to the extent where it may have an adverse effect on the health and well-being of an individual.
M. A simple carbohydrate consisting of two sugar units.
N. A nutrient required in relatively large amounts by the body. Includes carbohydrates, fat, and protein.
O. A naturally occurring inorganic substance this is essential to the proper functioning of the body.
P. The branch of medicine that deals with the treatment and control of obesity and diseases associated with obesity.
Q. An amino acid that is required by the body, but cannot be manufactured by the body and must be obtained from food.
R. A protein that contains all of the essential amino acids needed by the body.
S. Nutrition is the study of nutrients in food including how the body uses them and their relationship to health.
T. A simple carbohydrate consisting of one sugar unit.
U. The form in which carbohydrate is stored in the body.
V. An amino acid that is required by the body that can be synthesized by the body in sufficient quantities to meet its needs.
W. A protein that lacks one or more of the essential amino acids needed by the body.
X. A type of fat that is liquid at room temperature and comes primarily from plant sources.
Y. A disaccharide which consists of two sugar units and is found in milk and milk products.
Z. A type of fat that is solid at room temperature and comes primarily from animal sources.
AA. A nutrient required in very small amounts by the body. Includes vitamins and minerals.

B. Word Parts

Directions: Indicate the meaning of each word part in the space provided. List as many medical terms as possible that incorporate the word part in the space provided.

Word Part	Meaning of Word Part	Medical Terms That Incorporate Word Part
1. anti-		
2. ox/i		
3. ather/o		
4. -sclerosis		
5. bar/o		
6. -iatrics		
7. di-		
8. saccharide		
9. glyc/o		
10. -gen		
11. kilo-		
12. lact/o		
13. -ose		
14. macr/o		
15. micr/o		
16. mono-		
17. non-		
18. satur-		
19. tri-		
20. vit/a		

EVALUATION OF LEARNING

Directions: Fill in each blank with the correct answer.

1. What benefits can be derived from good nutrition?

____

____

2. List examples of tasks performed by the medical assistant that required a knowledge of basic nutrition principles.

____

____

3. Define the term diet.

____

4. What are the responsibilities of a dietitian?

5. What is the difference between an enriched food and a fortified food?

   a. Enriched food:

   b. Fortified food:

6. What is malnutrition?

7. What is nutrient density?

8. How many kilocalories per gram are provided by each of the following macronutrients?

   a. Carbohydrate:

   b. Fat:

   c. Protein:

9. List specific examples of body functions that require an energy source.

10. What are two functions of insulin in the body?

11. What is the difference between a simple carbohydrate and a complex carbohydrate?

    a. Simple carbohydrate:

    b. Complex carbohydrate:

12. What sugar units are included in the following simple carbohydrate categories?

    a. Monosaccharides:

    b. Disaccharides:

13. What are some examples of empty calorie foods?

14. What are some examples of foods that are classified as complex carbohydrates?

____

____

15. Why can't fiber be used as an energy source by the body?

____

____

16. What are the advantages of soluble fiber in the diet? What are some examples of food sources containing soluble fiber?

____

____

____

17. What are the advantages of insoluble fiber in the diet? What are some examples of food sources containing insoluble fiber?

____

____

____

18. What functions are performed by fat in the body?

____

____

19. What are some examples of foods that are high in saturated fat?

____

____

20. List examples of food sources that include the following type of fat?

a. Monounsaturated fat: _______________

b. Polyunsaturated fat: _______________

21. What is the purpose of adding trans fat to a food item? What are some examples of foods that may contain high levels of trans fat?

____

____

____

22. What is the disadvantage of trans fat?

____

____

23. What is the function of cholesterol in the body? What are some examples of foods that contain cholesterol?

____

____

24. What may occur in an individual with a high blood cholesterol level?

____

____

25. What is the daily cholesterol recommendation for each of the following individuals?

a. Average individual: ______________________

b. Individual with heart disease: ______________________

26. What conditions may result in elevated triglyceride levels?

____

____

27. What are the functions of protein in the body? What are some rich food sources of protein?

____

____

____

28. What does protein break down into through the process of digestion?

____

29. What is the difference between an essential amino acid and a nonessential amino acid?

a. Essential amino acid: ______________________

b. Nonessential amino acid: ______________________

30. What is the difference between a complete protein and an incomplete protein? List food sources of each.

a. Complete protein: ______________________

Food Sources: ______________________

b. Incomplete protein: ______________________

Food Sources: ______________________

31. What is the difference between a water soluble vitamin and a fat soluble vitamin?

a. Water soluble vitamin: ______________________

b. Fat soluble vitamin: ______________________

32. What may result from an excessive consumption of the fat soluble vitamins?

____

____

33. What is the overall function of the B vitamins?

____

____

34. What are rich food sources of many of the B vitamins?

____

____

35. What is the function of vitamin C?

____

____

36. Identify diseases and conditions that may result from a deficiency of the following vitamins?

a. B_1 (Thiamine): ______________________

b. B_2 (Riboflavin): ______________________

c. B_3 (Niacin): ______________________

d. B_5 (Pantothenic): ______________________

e. B_6 (Pyridoxine): ______________________

f. B_7 (Biotin): ______________________

g. B_{12} (Folic acid): ______________________

h. C (Ascorbic acid): ______________________

37. Identify the function, food sources, and deficiency diseases and conditions of each of the following fat soluble vitamins.

a. Vitamin A

Function: ______________________

Food Sources: ______________________

Deficiency Diseases/Conditions: ______________________

____

b. Vitamin D

Function: ______________________

Food Sources: ______________________

Deficiency Diseases/Conditions: ______________________

____

c. Vitamin E

Function: ______________________

Food Sources: ______________________

Deficiency Diseases/Conditions: ______________________

____

d. Vitamin K

Function: ___

Food Sources: ___

Deficiency Diseases/Conditions: ___

___

38. What effect do free radicals have on body cells? What may occur as a result of this?

___

___

39. What is the difference between a major mineral and a minor mineral?

a. Major mineral: ___

b. Minor mineral: ___

40. Identify the function, food sources, and deficiency diseases and conditions of each of the following major minerals.

a. Calcium

Function: ___

Food Sources: ___

Deficiency Diseases/Conditions: ___

___

b. Magnesium

Function: ___

Food Sources: ___

Deficiency Diseases/Conditions: ___

___

Deficiency Diseases/Conditions: ___

___

c. Phosphorus

Function: ___

Food Sources: ___

Deficiency Diseases/Conditions: ___

___

d. Potassium

Function: ___

Food Sources: ___

Deficiency Diseases/Conditions: ___

___

e. Chloride

Function: ____________________

Food Sources: ____________________

Deficiency Diseases/Conditions: ____________________

____

f. Sodium

Function: ____________________

Food Sources: ____________________

Deficiency Diseases/Conditions: ____________________

____

41. Identify the function, food sources, and deficiency diseases and conditions of each of the following minor minerals.

a. Iron

Function: ____________________

Food Sources: ____________________

Deficiency Diseases/Conditions: ____________________

____

b. Copper

Function: ____________________

Food Sources: ____________________

Deficiency Diseases/Conditions: ____________________

____

c. Zinc

Function: ____________________

Food Sources: ____________________

Deficiency Diseases/Conditions: ____________________

____

d. Manganese

Function: ____________________

Food Sources: ____________________

Deficiency Diseases/Conditions: ____________________

____

e. Fluoride

Function: ____________________

Food Sources: ____________________

Deficiency Diseases/Conditions: ____________________

____

f. Selenium

Function: ____________________

Food Sources: ____________________

Deficiency Diseases/Conditions: ____________________

____

g. Iodine

Function: ____________________

Food Sources: ____________________

Deficiency Diseases/Conditions: ____________________

____

h. Chromium

Function: ____________________

Food Sources: ____________________

Deficiency Diseases/Conditions: ____________________

____

42. What are the functions of water in the body?

____

____

____

43. What percentage of an adult's total body weight is made up of water?

____

44. How is water lost from the body?

____

____

45. What is the major objective of the MyPlate and the 2010 Dietary Guidelines for Americans?

____

____

____

46. What are the recommended MyPlate proportions for the following food groups?

a. Fruits and vegetables: ____________________

b. Protein: ____________________

c. Grains: ____________________

d. Dairy: ____________________

47. What type of food requires a food label and what type does not require a food label?

a. Food requiring a food label: ___

b. Food not requiring a food label: ___

48. What are the seven basic sections of the Nutrition Facts panel?

___

___

___

___

49. What are the interpretation guidelines for the percent daily value of the following?

a. Low nutrient level: ___

b. Good nutrient level: ___

c. High or rich nutrient level: ___

50. What nutrients should be limited in the diet?

___

51. What nutrients should be obtained in adequate amounts in the diet?

___

52. In what order are the ingredients listed on a food label (in the ingredient list)?

___

53. What benefits are provided by the ingredient list?

___

___

___

54. List some terms that are used to describe added sugar in the ingredient list?

___

___

55. What terms are used to describe trans fat in the ingredient list?

___

___

56. What type of foods typically have a short ingredient list? What type of foods typically have a lengthy ingredient list?

a. Short ingredient list: ___

b. Lengthy ingredient list: ___

57. What is weight management?

58. What is the primary cause of obesity?

59. What diseases are associated with overweight and obesity?

60. What three components should be included in the treatment of obesity?

61. What is a calorie deficit and how does it contribute to weight loss?

62. How many calories make up one pound of body fat?

63. What are the disadvantages of a fad diet?

64. What are the characteristics of a fad diet?

65. How does physical exercise contribute to weight loss?

66. How does a behavior modification plan assist in weight loss?

67. How many minutes per week should a healthy adult spend in moderate-intensity physical exercise?

68. What may result from atherosclerosis of the coronary arteries?

69. According to the TLC eating plan, what is the daily recommended intake for each of the following?

a. Total fat: ______________________________

b. Saturated fat: ______________________________

c. Dietary fiber: ______________________________

d. Cholesterol: ______________________________

e. Sodium: ______________________________

70. What are some examples of foods that are high in cholesterol?

____

71. What can occur if hypertension is not brought under control?

____

____

72. How does a low sodium diet help to lower blood pressure?

____

____

73. What causes type 1 diabetes?

____

____

74. What are the six food groups included in the diabetic exchange list system?

____

____

75. What is the biggest risk factor for the development of type 2 diabetes?

____

76. What is insulin resistance?

____

____

77. What is lactose intolerance?

____

78. What is the cause of lactose intolerance?

____

79. What are the symptoms of lactose intolerance?

____

____

80. What is the treatment for lactose intolerance?

81. What is gluten intolerance?

82. What is celiac disease?

83. What are the symptoms of gluten intolerance?

84. What are some examples of foods that:

   a. Contain gluten:

   b. Are gluten-free:

85. What are the most common food allergens?

86. What are the symptoms of a food allergy?

87. What is an elimination diet?

88. What is a rotation diet?

89. How does denaturation assist in treating food allergies?

90. How do supplemental digestive enzymes assist in treating food allergies?

CRITICAL THINKING ACTIVITIES

A. Nutrient Density

1. List 3 examples of snacks you consume that have a high nutrient density.

   a. ______________________________

   b. ______________________________

   c. ______________________________

2. List 3 examples of snacks you consume that have a low nutrient density (empty calorie foods).

   a. ______________________________

   b. ______________________________

   c. ______________________________

3. List advantages and disadvantages of high nutrient density snacks.

   ____

   ____

   ____

4. List advantages and disadvantages of empty calorie foods.

   ____

   ____

   ____

B. Sodium

Review the Nutrition Facts Panel on five packaged foods. In the space provided, list the name of the food item and the amount of sodium included in one serving. Place a checkmark next to each food item that is high in sodium.

Name of Food **Amount of Dietary Fiber**

a. ______________________________

b. ______________________________

c. ______________________________

d. ______________________________

e. ______________________________

C. My Plate

Create a breakfast, lunch, and dinner meal for yourself according to the MyPlate guidelines. Indicate your food group choices in the spaces provided in the appropriate (breakfast, lunch, or dinner) MyPlate illustration.

1. Breakfast

2. Lunch

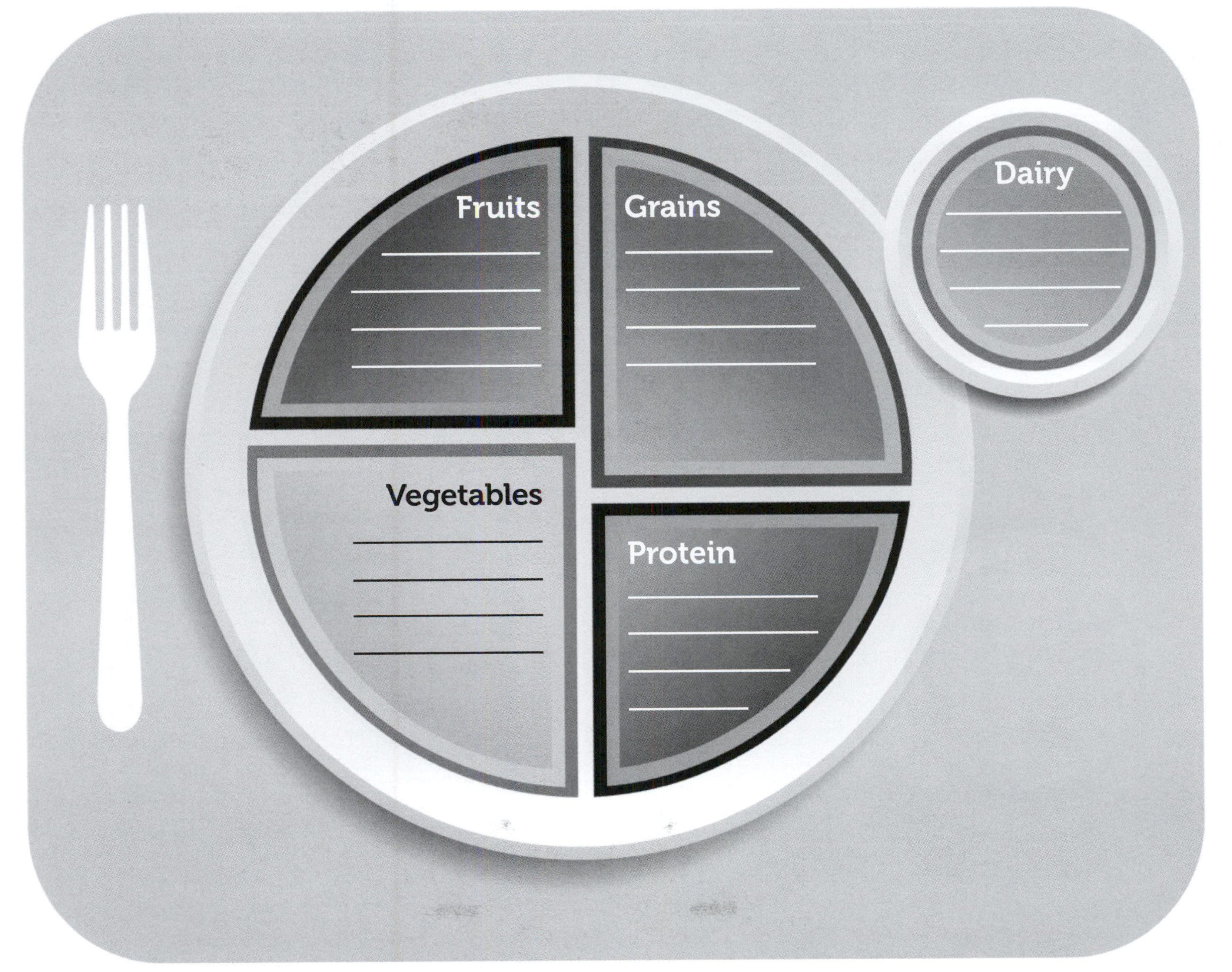

(Modified from U.S. Department of Agriculture: ChooseMyPlate, 2011, www.choosemyplate.gov.)

3. Dinner

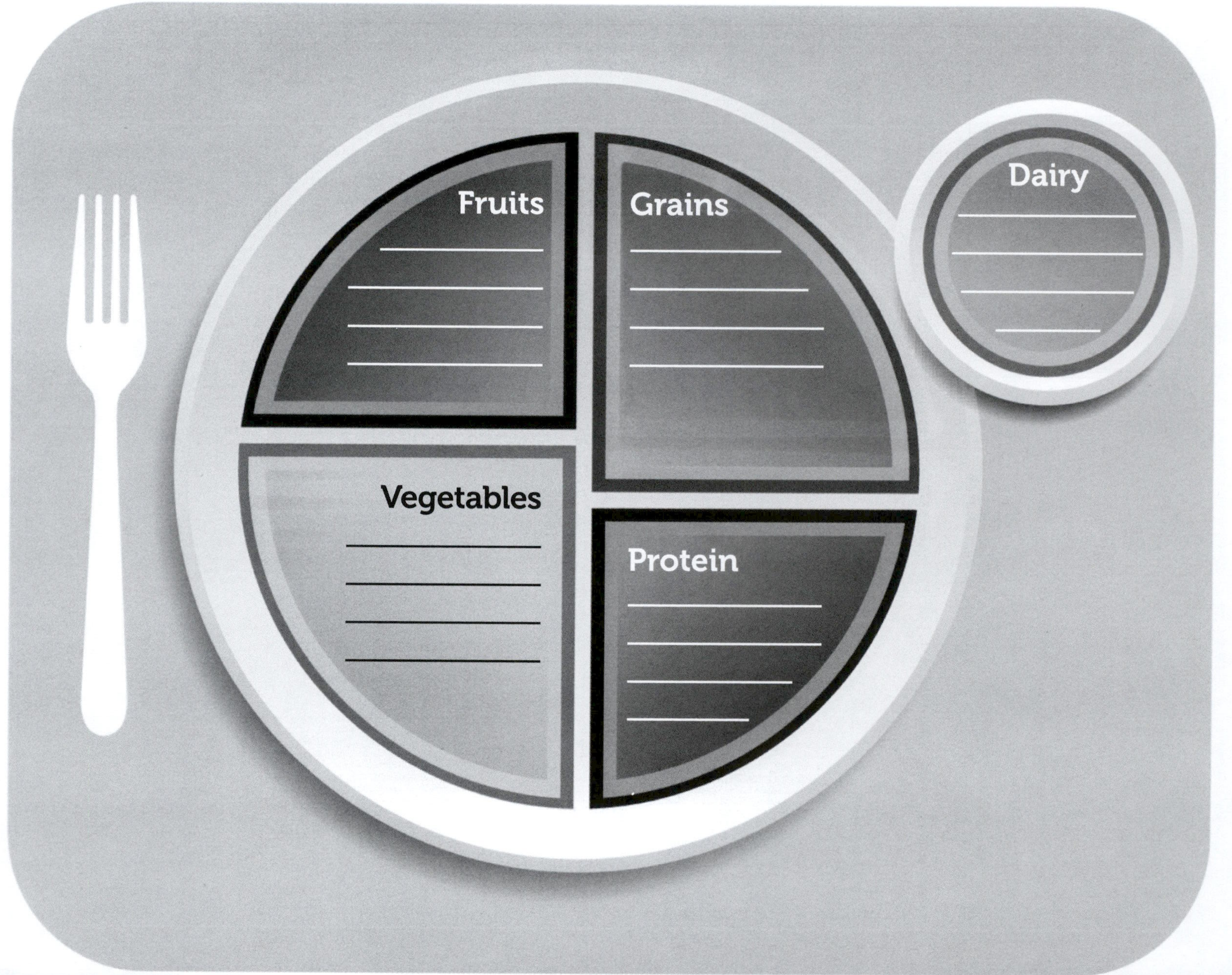

4. Compare each of the breakfast, lunch, and dinner MyPlate meals with the meals you typically consume. In the space provided below, discuss the similarities and differences between the meals.

____

____

____

D. Nutrition Facts Panel Analysis

Refer to the Nutrition Facts Panel in your textbook (Figure 35-10) and answer the following questions:

1. How many calories are in one serving of this food item? ______________________
2. How many calories in this food item come from fat? ______________________
3. How many servings are included in the package? ______________________
4. What makes up one serving of this food item? ______________________
5. How many total calories are in the package? ______________________
6. How many total grams of fat are in one serving of this food item? ______________________
7. What is the %DV of saturated fat in this food item? ______________________
8. What is the %DV of sodium in this food item? ______________________
9. Would this food item be considered a rich source of fiber? ______________________
10. Would this food item be considered a rich source of Vitamin A? ______________________
11. Would this food item be considered a rich source of Vitamin C? ______________________
12. Would this food item be considered a rich source of calcium? ______________________
13. Should an individual on a low sodium diet avoid this food item? ______________________
14. Do you consider this food item a healthy food choice? Explain the rationale for your answer.

____

____

____

E. Nutrition and Disease

The chart below lists the nutrients included on a nutrition facts panel. For each nutrient, indicate a disease or condition that may require a modification in consumption of that nutrient. Indicate if the nutrient should be increased or decreased by placing a checkmark in the appropriate box.

Nutrient	Disease or Condition	Increase	Decrease
1. Total fat			
2. Saturated fat			
3. Trans fat			
4. Cholesterol			
5. Sodium			
6. Total Carbohydrate			
7. Dietary Fiber			
8. Sugars			
9. Proteins			
10. Vitamin A			
11. Vitamin C			
12. Calcium			
13. Iron			

F. Ingredients List

1. Obtain an ingredient list from an unprocessed healthy food (usually has a short ingredient list) and list the ingredients of the food item below:

____

____

____

2. Obtain an ingredient list from a highly processed food (usually has a long ingredient list) and list the ingredients of the food item below:

____

____

____

____

3. Compare the ingredients in these two lists (unprocessed food and processed food) and discuss your findings below:

____

____

____

G. Crossword Puzzle: Nutrition

Directions: Complete the crossword puzzle using the clues provided.

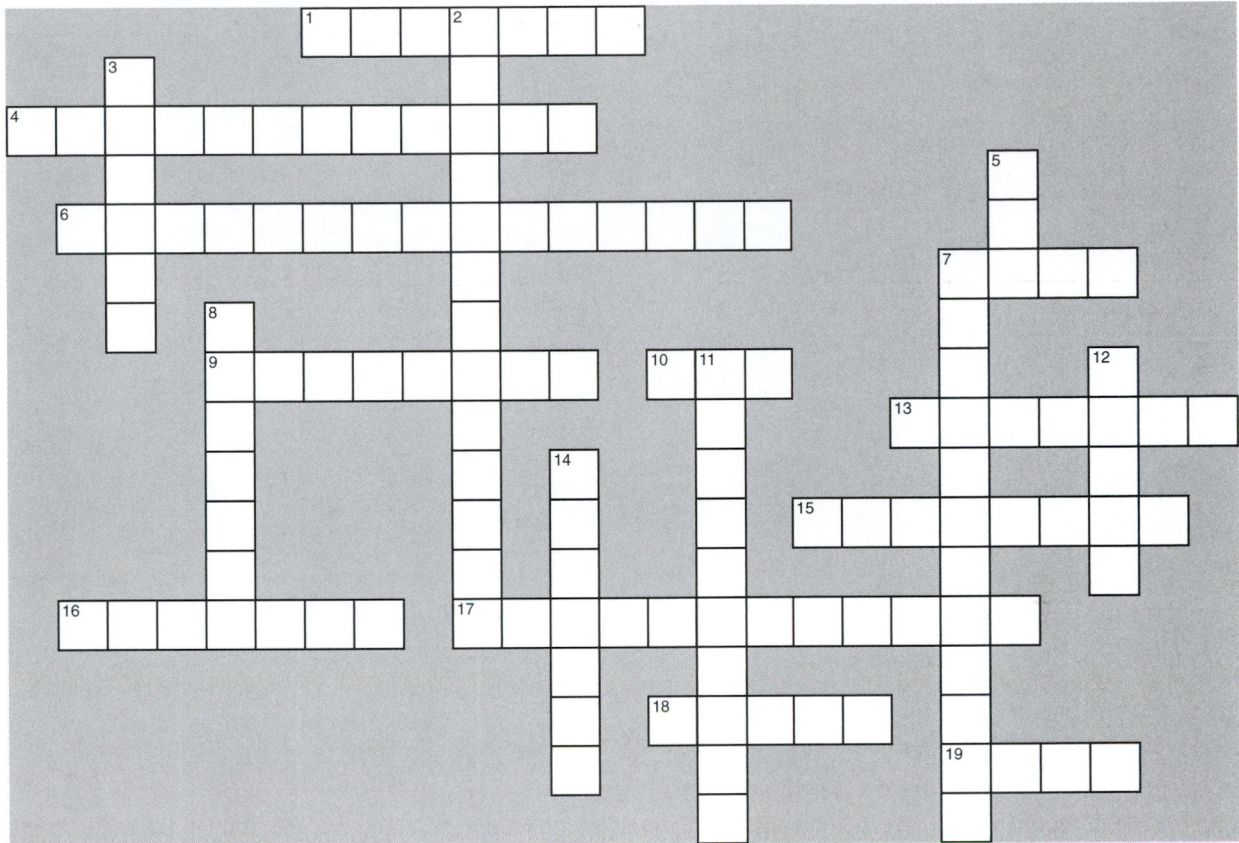

Across

1 Builds, maintains, and repairs tissue
4 Poor nutrition
6 Condition of artery plaque
7 Daily food and drink
9 Chemical substance in food needed by body
10 Provides 9 kcal/gram
13 Breaks down lactose
15 Storage product for glucose
16 Common food allergen
17 Solid fat
18 Celiac disease damages this
19 Eating plan to prevent and control hypertension

Down

2 Chemical form of fat
3 Wheat protein
5 Correlates with total body fat
7 Two sugar units
8 Enables glucose to enter a cell
11 Makes up protein
12 Makes up 60% to 65% of an adult
14 Milk sugar

Notes

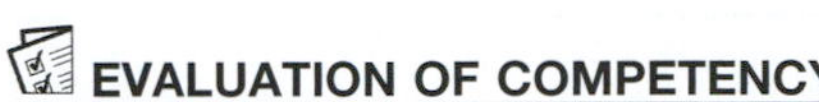

EVALUATION OF COMPETENCY

Procedure 35-A: Instruct a Patient According to Patient's Special Dietary Needs

Name: ______________________________ Date: ____________________

Evaluated by: ______________________________ Score: ____________________

Performance Objective

Outcome:	Instruct a patient according a patient's specialized dietary needs.
Conditions:	Given the following: Scenario, a Nutrition Facts Panel (Figure 35-10 in textbook), and Ingredients List (Figure 35-11 in textbook). **Scenario:** Based upon a thorough health history, physical examination, and laboratory test results, Dr. Cedy has determined that a patient is malnourished because of unhealthy food choices. The patient consumes approximately 2,000 kcal per day and has a BMI of 24 which within normal body weight. Dr. Cedy wants you to instruct the patient in reading a food label to assist the patient in making healthier food choices.
Standards:	Time: 10 minutes. Student completed procedure in __________ minutes. Accuracy: Satisfactory score on the performance evaluation checklist.

Performance Evaluation Checklist

Trial 1	Trial 2	Point Value	Performance Standards
		•	Greeted the patient and introduced yourself.
		•	Identified the patient.
		•	Informed the patient that you will be providing instructions on reading a food label to assist the patient in making healthier food choices.
		•	Explained that the food label is required for most packaged food.
			Using Figure 35-10 in your textbook, instructed the patient on each section of the nutrition facts panel
		•	1. **Serving Size:** Explained the serving size and servings per package section including the following:
		•	a. The serving size represents the size of a single serving.
		•	b. The total number of servings in the package are included in this section.
		•	c. A packaged food frequently contains more than one serving.
		•	d. The serving size is presented in familiar units such as cups or pieces.
		•	e. The amount of calories and nutrients listed on the remainder of the label are based on one serving.
		•	f. This section allows a comparison of similar foods with the same serving size to determine which is a healthier choice.
		•	2. **Amount of Calories:** Explained the amount of calories section including the following:
		•	a. The amount of calories represents the total number of calories in one serving.

Trial 1	Trial 2	Point Value	Performance Standards
		•	b. The number of calories is listed on the left side and the number of calories from fat is listed on the right side.
		•	c. It is important to pay attention to the number of calories consumed. If two servings are consumed, this doubles the amount of calories and nutrients consumed.
		•	3. **Percent Daily Value:** Explained the percent daily value section including the following:
		•	a. Indicates the percentage of a nutrient provided by a single serving of a food item compared with how much is required for the entire day.
		•	b. Provides information on whether a nutrient in one serving contributes a little or a lot of that nutrient to the total daily diet which helps to make informed food choices.
		•	c. The %DV is based on a 2,000 kcal/day diet.
		•	d. Each nutrient is based on 100% of the recommended daily amount for that nutrient.
		•	e. Interpretation guidelines for %DV include the following: • Low nutrient level: 5% DV or less • Good nutrient level: 10% to 19% DV • High or rich nutrient level: 20% DV or more
		•	4. **Nutrients Which Should be Limited:** Explained which nutrients are important to health but should be limited in the diet. Included the following:
		•	a. Nutrients to limit include total fat (including saturated fat and trans fat), cholesterol, and sodium.
		•	These nutrients should be limited because they contribute to health problems such as heart disease, some cancers, and hypertension.
		•	b. Foods should be selected with a low %DV of these nutrients (5% DV or less).
		•	5. **Nutrients Which Should be Obtained in Adequate Amounts:** Explained which nutrients should be obtained in adequate amounts. Included the following:
		•	a. Nutrients to obtain in adequate amounts include dietary fiber, vitamin A, vitamin C. calcium, and iron.
		•	Consuming adequate amounts of these nutrients improves health and helps reduce the risk of certain diseases and conditions.
		•	b. The patient should strive to achieve a 100% DV of these nutrients each day.
		•	c. Foods should be selected with a high %DV of these nutrients (20% DV or more).
		•	6. **Footnote With Daily Values:** Explained the footnote section including the following:
		•	a. The daily values listed for total fat, saturated fat, cholesterol, and sodium are considered the maximum upper limits that should be consumed each day.
		•	b. The daily value for dietary fiber is considered the minimum level to try to reach each day.

Trial 1	Trial 2	Point Value	Performance Standards
		●	c. Relayed the DV amount for each nutrient for a 2,000 kcal/day diet to the patient.
		●	7. **Additional Nutrients:** Explained the additional nutrients section including the following:
		●	a. Total carbohydrates consist of both simple and complex carbohydrates.
		●	b. Sugars include the simple carbohydrates.
		●	c. Dietary fiber is a complex carbohydrate.
		●	d. The remaining carbohydrate comes from starches.
		●	e. A %DV for protein is not required on a food label since most Americans consume more protein than they need.
			Using Figure 35-11 in your textbook, instructed the patient on the ingredient list
		●	Explained that the ingredients are listed in descending order of weight from highest to lowest.
		●	Stated that the first ingredient makes up the largest proportion of the food by weight than any other ingredient
		●	Explained that the ingredient list can assist in making healthy food choices.
		●	Explained that added sugar and trans fat appear in the ingredient list under a number of different names.
		●	Provided the patient with examples of names used to describe sugar and trans fat.
		●	Explained that the ingredient list allows the consumer to scan for ingredients that may cause food allergies.
		●	Explained that unprocessed foods typically have a short and simple ingredient list.
		●	Explained that processed foods typically have a lengthy list of ingredients that include chemical terms.
		●	Answered any questions the patient had regarding food labels.
		Ⓐ	Showed awareness of patient's concerns regarding a dietary change.
		Ⓐ	Demonstrated: a. empathy b. active listening c. nonverbal communication
		●	Charted the procedure correctly.
		✶	Completed the procedure within 10 minutes.
			TOTALS

CHART	

Evaluation of Student Performance

EVALUATION CRITERIA			COMMENTS
Symbol	**Category**	**Point Value**	
∗	Critical Step	16 points	
●	Essential Step	6 points	
Ⓐ	Affective Competency	6 points	
▷	Theory Question	2 points	
Score calculation: 100 Points – ____ Points missed ____ Score Satisfactory score: 85 or above			

2008 CAAHEP Competencies Achieved
Psychomotor (Skills) ☑ IV. 5. Instruct patients according to their needs to promote health -maintenance and disease prevention. ☑ IV. 9. Document patient education. ***Affective (Behavior)*** ☑ I. 2. Use language/verbal skills that enable patients' understanding. ☑ IV. 3. Use appropriate body language and other nonverbal skills in communicating with patients, family, and staff.

2015 CAAHEP Competencies Achieved
Psychomotor (Skills) ☑ IV. 1. Instruct a patient according to patient's special dietary needs. ***Affective (Behavior)*** ☑ IV. 1. Show awareness of patient's concerns regarding a dietary change. ☑ V. 1. Demonstrate: a. empathy b. active listening c. nonverbal communication

ABHES Competencies Achieved
☑ 2. d. Apply a system of diet and nutrition 1) Explain the importance of diet and nutrition 2) Educate patients regarding proper diet and nutrition guidelines 3) Identify categories of patients that require special diets or diet modifications

36 Emergency Preparedness and Protective Practices

CHAPTER ASSIGNMENTS

✓ After Completing	Date Due	Study Guide Pages	STUDY GUIDE ASSIGNMENTS (CTA = Critical Thinking Activity)	Possible Points	Points You Earned
		1031	Pretest	10	
		1032	Term Key Term Assessment	14	
		1032-1038	Evaluation of Learning questions	60	
		1038	CTA A: Disasters	20	
		1038-1039	CTA B: Personal Safety Plan	30	
		1039	CTA C: Disaster Planning in the Medical Office	30	
		1040	CTA D: Fire Hazards	20	
		1040	CTA E: Methods of Fire Protection and Prevention	20	
		1040	CTA F: Use of Fire Extinguisher	20	
		1040-1042	CTA G: Table-Top Fire Drill	60	
		1043	CTA H: Table-top Mock Emergency Events	60	
		1043	CTA I: Community Resources	8	
		1044	CTA J: Crossword Puzzle	20	
			e Evolve Site: Apply Your Knowledge questions	10	
		1031	Posttest	10	
			ADDITIONAL ASSIGNMENTS		
			TOTAL POINTS		

Notes

✓ When Assigned By Your Instructor	Study Guide Pages	Practices Required	LABORATORY ASSIGNMENTS (Procedure Number and Name)	Score*
	1045	5	**Practice for Competency** 36-1: Demonstrating Proper Use of a Fire Extinguisher Textbook reference: pp. 957-958	
	1047-1048		**Evaluation of Competency** 36-1: Demonstrating Proper Use of a Fire Extinguisher	*
	1045	4	**Practice for Competency** 36-2: Participating in a Mock Exposure Event Textbook reference: pp. 959-962	
	1049-1052		**Evaluation of Competency** 36-2: Participating in a Mock Exposure Event	*
			ADDITIONAL ASSIGNMENTS	

Notes

Name ____ Date ____________________

PRETEST

True or False

_______ 1. A flood is an example of a man-made disaster.

_______ 2. A positive reaction to a disaster involves the triggering of resources to meet the challenge.

_______ 3. During the alarm phase of the general adaptation syndrome (GAS), the body prepares for fight or flight.

_______ 4. During the recovery phase of the GAS, epinephrine is released into the bloodstream.

_______ 5. Hyperventilation may occur during severe anxiety.

_______ 6. Emergency exit routes must be at least 60 inches wide.

_______ 7. An oxygen tank is an example of an ignition source.

_______ 8. A fire door prevents the spread of fire from one area of a building to another.

_______ 9. The number, size, location, and type of fire extinguishers in a medical office are determined by the owner of the building.

_______ 10. The sequence of events that should be included in responding to a fire include: rescue, activate, confine, and extinguish/evacuate.

POSTTEST

True or False

_______ 1. A man-made disaster is caused by the natural processes of the earth.

_______ 2. Stress is the body's response to threat or change.

_______ 3. Epinephrine causes a decrease in the blood pressure.

_______ 4. Anxiety is a feeling of worry or uneasiness.

_______ 5. The responsibility of an emergency evacuation coordinator is to take charge of and manage evacuation procedures.

_______ 6. A secondary exit route is the quickest and easiest way to exit a building in an emergency.

_______ 7. The elements that must exist in order for a fire to occur include a fuel source, ignition source, and carbon dioxide.

_______ 8. A flammable material catches on fire easily.

_______ 9. A portable fire extinguisher can be used to fight a large fire that is out of control.

_______ 10. The batteries in a smoke detector should be changed every 6 months.

KEY TERM ASSESSMENT

Directions: Match each key term with its definition.

_______ 1. Anxiety
_______ 2. Disaster
_______ 3. Emergency action plan
_______ 4. Emergency preparedness
_______ 5. Evacuation
_______ 6. Evacuation procedures
_______ 7. Exit route
_______ 8. Fire extinguisher
_______ 9. Fire prevention plan
_______ 10. Fire protection
_______ 11. HAZMAT
_______ 12. Man-made disaster
_______ 13. Natural disaster
_______ 14. Stress

A. The process of making plans to prevent, respond, and recover from an emergency situation
B. A feeling of worry or uneasiness, often triggered by an event that is perceived as having an uncertain outcome
C. The implementation of safety measures to reduce the unwanted effects of fire
D. A sudden event that causes damage or loss of life
E. A catastrophic event that is caused by nature or the natural process of the earth
F. A written document that describes that actions that employees should take to ensure their safety if a fire or other emergency situation occurs
G. A continuous and unobstructed path of travel from any point within a workplace to a place of safety
H. A planned systemic retreat of people to safety in an emergency situation
I. An event that causes serious damage through intentional or negligent human actions or the failure of a man-made system
J. The body's response to threat or change
K. A written document that identifies flammable and combustible materials stored in the workplace and ways to control workplace fire hazards
L. A portable device that discharges an agent designed to extinguish a fire
M. An acronym that refers to materials that pose a danger to health or the environment and must be handled with protective equipment.
N. Clear step-by-step procedures for the rapid, efficient, and safe removal of individuals from a building during an emergency.

EVALUATION OF LEARNING

1. Why is it important for medical offices to plan ahead for a disaster or serious emergency?

____

____

2. What causes a natural disaster?

____

____

3. What are some examples of natural disasters?

____

____

4. What is a man-made disaster?

____

5. What are some examples of man-made disasters?

____

____

6. What does a positive reaction to a disaster involve?

7. When do individuals usually react negatively to a disaster?

8. What characteristics of a disaster tend to cause the most serious psychological effects?

9. What occurs during the alarm phase of the GAS?

10. What changes occur in the body when epinephrine stimulates the sympathetic nervous system?

11. What occurs during the resistance phase of the GAS?

12. How long does the resistance phase last?

13. What are some examples of stress-related symptoms that may occur during the resistance phase?

14. What occurs during the recovery phase of the GAS?

15. What occurs during the exhaustion phase of GAS?

16. What is anxiety?

17. Why is it important to learn and practice emergency procedures?

18. How might severe anxiety be a problem in an emergency situation?

____

____

19. What are the symptoms of severe anxiety?

____

____

20. How should the medical assistant respond to a patient exhibiting severe anxiety?

____

____

21. What should the medical assistant do if an emergency occurs at his or her workplace?

____

____

22. What is the purpose of an emergency action plan?

____

____

23. What methods are typically used in the medical office to report emergency situations and/or alert employees to the presence of an emergency situation?

____

____

____

24. According to OSHA, when is it acceptable to use direct voice communication to alert employees of an emergency situation?

____

____

25. What is the responsibility of an emergency evacuation coordinator?

____

____

26. According to OSHA, what three components must be included in an emergency evacuation plan?

____

____

____

27. What type of evacuation is typically required for the following?

a. Large fire: _______________

b. Small waste basket fire: _______________

c. Tornado: _______________

28. List five guidelines (as stipulated by OSHA) that must be followed with respect to exit routes?

29. What is the difference between a primary and secondary exit route?

a. Primary exit route:

b. Secondary exit route:

30. What information should be included on an evacuation floor plan?

31. Why is it important to account for all building occupants following an emergency evacuation?

32. What is an evacuation warden?

33. List examples of how a fire may start in the medical office.

34. What three elements must exist in order for a fire to occur?

35. Explain the difference between a flammable and a combustible material and list examples of each.

a. Flammable material:

Examples:

b. Combustible material:

Examples:

36. List five examples of fuel sources that may be found in the medical office.

37. List examples of common ignition sources.

38. What effect will oxygen released from an oxygen tank have on a fire?

39. What is the purpose of a fire prevention plan?

40. List methods of fire prevention in the medical office for each of the following categories:

a. Flammable and combustible materials:

b. Electrical equipment and appliances:

c. Inspection and maintenance:

41. What is the purpose of fire protection?

42. Explain how sprinklers are activated.

43. What is the purpose of a fire door?

44. What occurs when a fire alarm is activated?

45. What type of testing and maintenance should be performed on battery-operated smoke detectors?

46. What are some examples of fire extinguishing agents?

47. What are the two primary functions of a fire extinguisher?

48. List the fuel sources included in the following fire classifications:

Class A: ___

Class B: ___

Class C: ___

Class D: ____________________

Class K: ____________________

49. Where are fire extinguishers usually located?

____

50. Why is it important to properly maintain a fire extinguisher?

____

51. What is the purpose of the tag attached to a fire extinguisher?

____

52. Identify the steps that should be taken in operating a fire extinguisher following the PASS format.

P: ____________________

A: ____________________

S: ____________________

S: ____________________

53. Describe the steps that should be taken in responding to a fire following the RACE format.

R: ____________________

A: ____________________

C: ____________________

E: ____________________

54. What information should be included in the training of employees on the emergency action plan as required by OSHA?

____

____

____

____

55. When must the emergency action plan be reviewed with each employee?

____

____

____

56. What is the purpose of an emergency practice drill?

____

____

57. Why is it important to conduct fire drills?

____

____

58. Who determines whether or not fire drills must be held at a facility?

59. What is the difference between a fire drill and a disaster drill?

60. What role does the medical assistant serve in developing and implementing an emergency action plan?

CRITICAL THINKING ACTIVITIES

A. Disasters

1. Indicate a major natural disaster and a man-made disaster that has occurred in your community and/or state.
2. Provide a brief description and damage caused by each of these disasters. (*Note:* An Internet search using the terms: "Disasters in (name of your state)" will assist you in completing this activity.)
3. Natural disaster:

4. Man-made disaster:

B. Personal Safety Plan

1. Choose a natural disaster (e.g., tornado, hurricane, flood, blizzard) or man-made disaster (e.g., fire, power outage, burglary) that might occur in your locale.
2. Develop and outline a personal safety plan for responding to the disaster in your home environment. Include information on what you would do before, during, and after the disaster occurred. The following website can assist you in locating information to complete this activity: www.redcross.org, www.fema.gov
   a. Name of disaster: ____________________
   b. Personal Safety Plan Response:

      Before: ____________________

During: ____

____

____

After: ____

____

____

C. Disaster Planning in the Medical Office

1. Choose a natural disaster or man-made disaster that might occur in your locale.
2. Outline step-by-step emergency procedures for responding to the disaster in a medical office setting using the form presented below.

The following websites can assist you in locating information to complete this activity:

www.redcross.org

www.fema.gov

www.osha.gov/Publications/osha3088.pdf

www.osha.gov/SLTC/emergencypreparedness

DISASTER PLANNING IN THE MEDICAL OFFICE
Name of Disaster: ______________________   **Step-by-Step Emergency Procedure Response:**
1.
2.
3.
4.
5.
6.
7.
8.
9.
10.
11.
12.

D. Fire Hazards

Perform a survey of your home to determine if there are any fire hazards. If so, list these hazards and what steps should be taken to correct them. Table 36-1 in your textbook and the following websites will assist you in completing this activity: www.fire-extinguisher101.com/hazards.html, www.usfa.fema.gov/citizens/home_fire_prev/cooking.shtm, hartfordauto.thehartford.com/Safe-Driving/Home-Safety/Fire-Safety.

Fire Hazard: **Steps Needed to Correct:**

____

____

____

____

E. Methods of Fire Protection and Prevention

Survey the interior of a health care facility (or other type of commercial building) in your community and indicate the fire protection and prevention methods in place at this facility. List these below:

____

____

____

____

F. Use of Fire Extinguisher

Perform an Internet search for a video of the operation of a fire extinguisher. Write a short paragraph below describing the video.

____

____

____

____

G. Table-Top Fire Drill

Participate in a table-top fire drill by completing the following:

1. Each student should create a small "paper-doll" figure out of paper, cardboard, felt, and other materials (e.g., a tongue blade or popsicle stick). The figure should be free-standing (be able to stand by itself).
2. Form a group of students and assemble around a table or other flat surface.
3. Place the Evacuation Floor Plan (provided on page 1042 of this study guide) in the center of the table.
4. Locate and review the purpose of the following using the evacuation floor plan:
   a. Primary exit route
   b. Secondary exit route
   c. Fire alarm pull stations
   d. Portable fire extinguishers
   e. Emergency exit doors
   f. Wheelchair accessible exits
   g. Assembly areas
   h. Shelter-in-place areas

5. Choose a student (paper-doll) to play the role of the emergency evacuation coordinator. which includes the following responsibilities:
   a. Calling emergency responders
   b. Identifying safe evacuation routes
   c. Ensuring evacuation wardens are performing their duties
   d. Coordinating with emergency responders
5. Select students (paper-dolls) to play the role of patients with various types of conditions.
6. Select students (paper-dolls) to play the role of evacuation wardens. Assign various duties to these students as outlined in Table 36-2 of your textbook.
7. Place the various paper-doll figures in various rooms on the Evacuation Floor Plan.
8. Designate a fire that has erupted in one of the rooms on the floor plan.
7. Locate Procedure 36-2: Participating in a Mock Exposure Event in your textbook and go to the following subheading: CONDUCT THE FIRE DRILL.
8. Conduct a table-top fire drill following the step-by-step procedures listed under Conduct the Fire Drill. Explain the principle for performing each step in the drill after performing it.
9. Evaluate the fire drill by completing the Fire Drill Evaluation Form below.

FIRE DRILL EVALUATION FORM

Date: ______________________ **Completed By:** ______________________

S	U	Evaluation Criteria:
		The fire drill was completed in an orderly, efficient, and timely manner.
		Building occupants and emergency responders were immediately alerted to the emergency situation.
		Evacuation wardens effectively completed their duties.
		Patients and visitors were escorted to the nearest exits and assembly area.
		Each building occupant was accounted for following the evacuation.
		Emergency responders were provided with appropriate information.

STRENGTHS:

CONCERNS:	MEANS OF IMPROVEMENT:

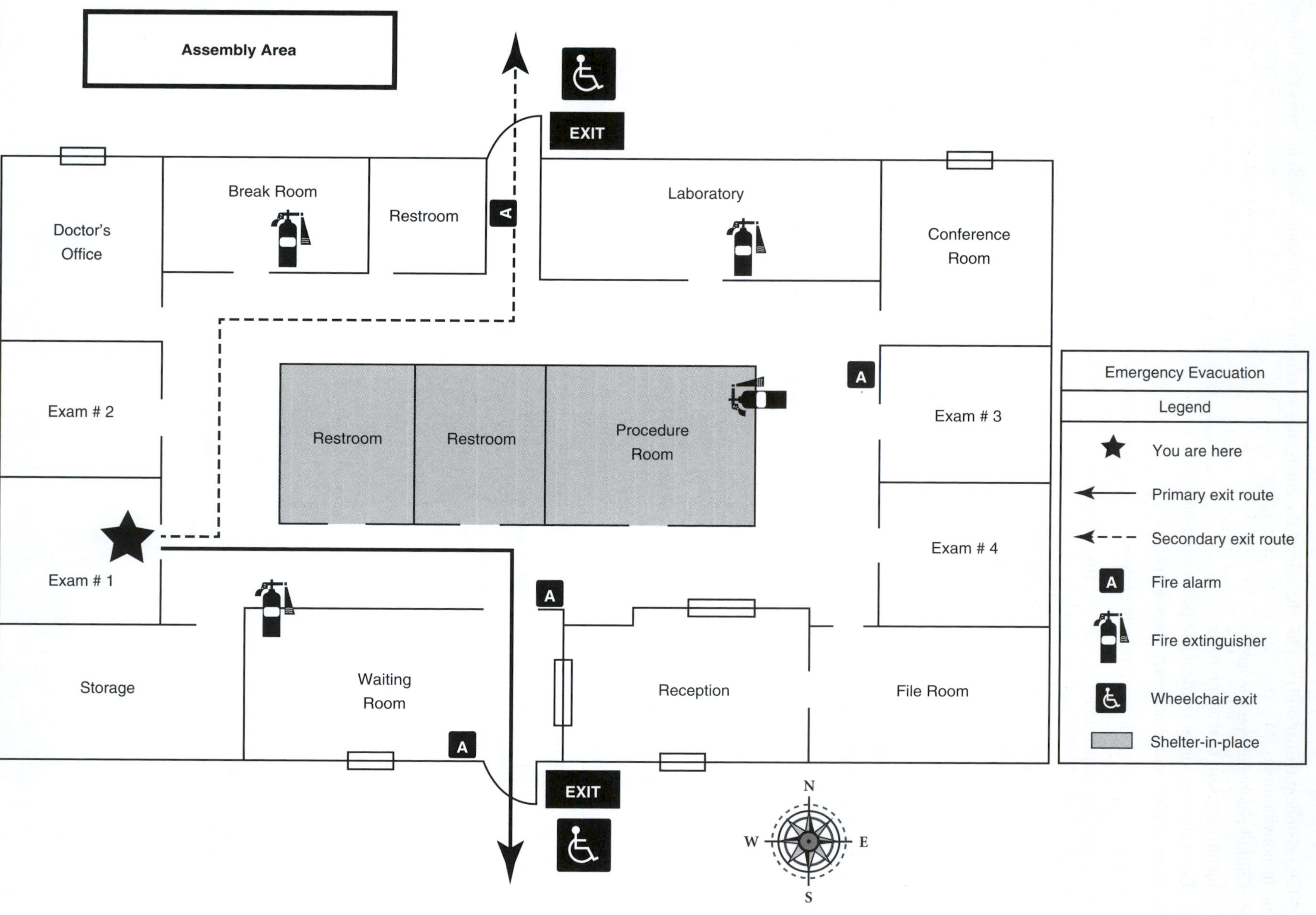

Evacuation Floor Plan.

H. Table-Top Mock Exposure Events

Repeat the activity described above in Critical Thinking Activity G: Table-Top Fire Drill using a step-by-step emergency procedure plan developed by a group member as outlined in CTA C. The group member who created the emergency plan should take the role of the evacuation coordinator. If time permits, participate in as many mock exposure events as possible using emergency plans developed by other members of your group. Evaluate the timeliness and effectiveness of each emergency event and record the key points below:

____

____

____

____

____

I. Community Resources

Look up and indicate below the name and telephone number of the following:

1. Emergency Management Services (will usually be 911): ____________________
2. Poison Control Center: ____________________
3. Local hospital(s): ____________________
4. Local health department: ____________________
5. State health department: ____________________
6. State HAZMAT response team: ____________________
7. Local area emergency management (LEMA) office: ____________________
8. Local chapter of the American Red Cross: ____________________
9. Citizen Corps Council or Citizen Emergency Response Team (if any): ____________________

J. Crossword Puzzle: Emergency Preparedness and Protective Practices

Directions: Complete the crossword puzzle using the clues provided.

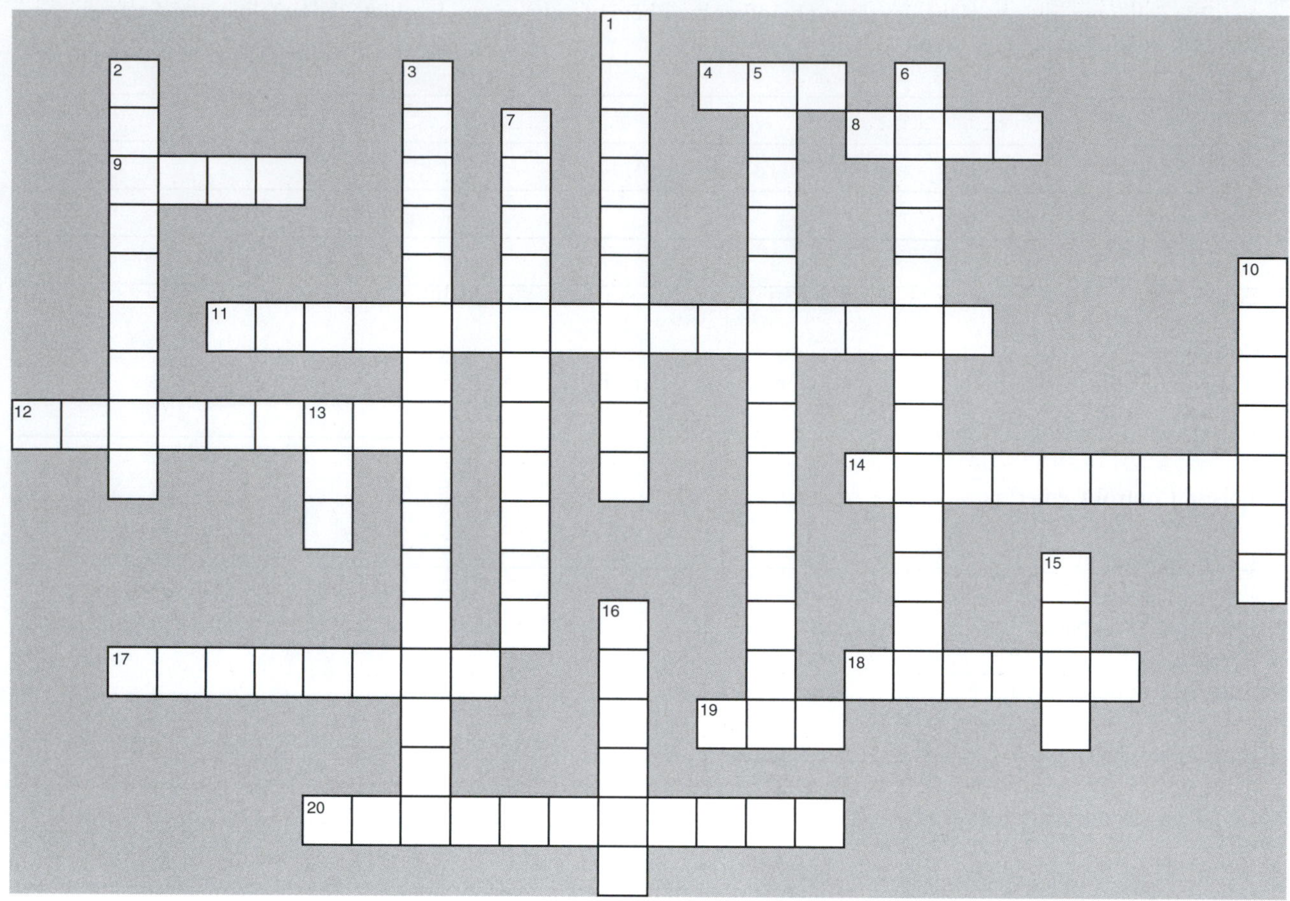

Across

4 Actions to take in an emergency
8 Man-made disaster
9 How to respond to a fire
11 Severe anxiety symptom
12 Natural disaster
14 Catches on fire easily
17 Increases blood glucose
18 Caused by threat or change
19 Reaction to stress
20 Helps to control anxiety

Down

1 Planned emergency retreat
2 Fire alerter
3 Quickest way to exit
5 Releases epinephrine
6 Alarm reaction response
7 Stimulates sympathetic NS
10 Worry or uneasiness
13 Multipurpose fire extinguisher
15 Fire extinguisher procedure
16 Fire element

PRACTICE FOR COMPETENCY

Procedure 36-1: Demonstrating Proper Use of a Fire Extinguisher: Demonstrate the proper use of a fire extinguisher in a role-playing situation using a discharged fire extinguisher.

Using the information printed on the label of the fire extinguisher (or owner's manual), complete the information requested below:

1. What is the brand name of the extinguisher?

____

2. What type of extinguishing agent is contained in the extinguisher (e.g., dry chemical, foam, carbon dioxide)?

____

3. What types of fire classification(s) is this extinguisher capable of extinguishing?

____

4. What type of precautions should be observed with this extinguisher?

____

____

5. What are the storage requirements for the fire extinguisher?

____

____

6. What should be done with the fire extinguisher after it has been discharged?

____

____

7. What type of care and maintenance is required for this extinguisher?

____

____

____

Procedure 36-2: Participating in a Mock Exposure Event:

a. Prepare for participating in a mock exposure (fire drill) event by first completing Critical Thinking Activity G: Table-Top Fire Drill.

b. Participate in a mock exposure (fire drill) event at a facility designated by your instructor.

Notes

EVALUATION OF COMPETENCY

Procedure 36-1: Demonstrating Proper Use of a Fire Extinguisher

Name: ______________________________ Date: ______________

Evaluated by: ______________________________ Score: ______________

Performance Objective

Outcome:	Demonstrate use of a fire extinguisher in a role-playing situation.
Conditions:	Given the following: Portable multipurpose (ABC) fire extinguisher that has been discharged and a poster, flashing light or other indicator to indicate the location of the fire.
Standards:	Time: 5 minutes. Student completed procedure in ________ minutes. Accuracy: Satisfactory score on the Performance Evaluation Checklist.

Performance Evaluation Checklist

Trial 1	Trial 2	Point Value	Performance Standards
		●	Identified a safe evacuation route before approaching the fire.
		▷	Stated the reason for identifying a safe evacuation route.
		●	Removed the fire extinguisher from its mounting device.
		●	Held the fire extinguisher upright with the nozzle pointing away from you.
		●	Stood 6 to 8 feet from the fire, keeping the back to the exit.
		▷	Explained the reason for standing at 6 to 8 feet from the fire and keeping the back to the exit.
		●	Performed a quick assessment of the fire to determine if an attempt should be made to extinguish it with a fire extinguisher.
		▷	Stated when an attempt to extinguish a fire with a fire extinguisher should not be made.
		●	Pulled the safety pin straight out from the handle of the fire extinguisher.
		▷	Stated the purpose of the tamper-proof seal and the safety pin.
		●	Aimed the nozzle at the base of the fire (not the flames).
		▷	Stated why the nozzle should be directed at the base of the fire.
		●	Squeezed the handle slowly and continuously to release the extinguishing agent.
		▷	Stated what occurs if the pressure is released from the handle.
		●	Swept the extinguisher evenly from side to side at the base of the fire.
		▷	Stated why a sweeping motion should be used.
		●	Moved closer to the fire gradually as it began to smoulder.
		●	Continued to discharge the extinguishing agent until the fire was completely out.

Trial 1	Trial 2	Point Value	Performance Standards
		▷	Stated what should be done if the fire grows larger.
		●	Backed away from the extinguished fire and continued to watch the area.
		▷	Stated the reason for continuing to watch the area.
		Ⓐ	Demonstrated self-awareness in responding to an emergency situation.
		*	Completed the procedure within 5 minutes.
			TOTALS

Evaluation of Student Performance

EVALUATION CRITERIA			COMMENTS
Symbol	**Category**	**Point Value**	
*	Critical Step	16 points	
●	Essential Step	6 points	
Ⓐ	Affective Competency	6 points	
▷	Theory Question	2 points	
Score calculation: 100 points − ____ points missed ____ Score Satisfactory score: 85 or above			

2008 CAAHEP Competencies Achieved

Psychomotor (Skills)

☑ XI. 1. Comply with safety signs, symbols, and labels.
☑ XI. 5. b. Demonstrate proper use of the following equipment: Fire extinguishers.

Affective (Behavior)

☑ IX. 2. Demonstrate self awareness in responding to emergency situations and care.

2015 CAAHEP Competencies Achieved

Psychomotor (Skills)

☑ XII. 1. Comply with: a. safety signs b. symbols c. labels.
☑ XII. 2. b. Demonstrate proper use of fire extinguishers.

Affective (Behavior)

☑ XII. 2. Demonstrate self-awareness in responding to an emergency situation.

ABHES Competencies Achieved

☑ 9. g. Recognize and respond to medical office emergencies.

EVALUATION OF COMPETENCY

Procedure 36-2: Participating in a Mock Exposure Event

Name: ______________________________ Date: ______________________

Evaluated by: ______________________________ Score: ______________________

Performance Objective

Outcome:	Participate in a mock exposure event.
Conditions:	Given the following: scenario, a poster, flashing light or other indicator to indicate the location of the fire, evacuation floor plan, employee roster, patient log-in sheet, pen, and paper.
Standards:	Time: 20 minutes. Student completed procedure in __________ minutes. Accuracy: Satisfactory score on the Performance Evaluation Checklist.

Performance Evaluation Checklist

Trial 1	Trial 2	Point Value	Performance Standards
			PRE-DRILL ACTIVITIES:
		●	Made a list of the names and phone numbers that may be needed in the event of a fire.
		●	Located and reviewed the purpose of the following using the evacuation floor plan: a. Primary exit route b. Secondary exit route c. Fire alarm pull stations d. Portable fire extinguishers e. Emergency exit doors f. Wheelchair accessible exits g. Shelter-in-place areas h. Assembly areas
		●	Located and reviewed the purpose of the following: a. Sprinklers b. Smoke detectors c. Fire doors d. Exit signs
		●	Evaluated primary and secondary exit routes for the following: a. Clearly marked and well-lit b. Unobstructed and free of clutter c. Exit doors are free of decorations or signs that obscure visibility of the exit d. Exit doors are unlocked from the inside e. Exit doors open outwards f. Fire extinguishers are in place and clearly identified g. Evacuation floor plans are posted in multiple locations
		●	Assigned an emergency evacuation coordinator to perform the following: a. Calling emergency responders b. Identifying safe evacuation routes c. Ensuring evacuation wardens are performing their duties d. Coordinating with emergency responders

Trial 1	Trial 2	Point Value	Performance Standards
		●	Compiled an employee roster.
		●	Assigned evacuation wardens
		●	Assigned individuals to play the role of patients.
		●	Compiled a patient log-in sheet.
			CONDUCTED THE FIRE DRILL:
		●	Rescued anyone in immediate danger of the fire.
		●	Performed the following if an individual's clothes are on fire: a. Instructed person to stop, drop, and roll b. Covered the person with a blanket or clothing to extinguish the flames.
		●	Activated the fire alarm.
		●	Immediately notified emergency responders.
		▷	Stated the information that should be relayed to the medical dispatcher.
		●	Closed doors and windows in the immediate area of the fire.
		▷	Stated the purpose of closing doors and windows.
		●	Extinguished the fire with a fire extinguisher if it is small and confined.
		▷	Explained what to do if the fire is too large to extinguish.
		●	Performed evacuation duties and evacuated the area immediately.
		▷	Stated why it is important to evacuate immediately.
		●	Shut down all electrical equipment and appliances in the immediate area.
		●	Before exiting a door, felt the door with the back of the hand. Performed the following if an exit door is warm: a. Did not open the door. b. Called 911 to report your location. c. Placed clothing or towels along the bottom of the door. d. Stayed calm and waited to be rescued. e. Did not break the window.
		●	Exited by the primary exit route.
		▷	Explained what to do if the primary route is blocked.
		●	Exited by stairways only.
		▷	Explained why an elevator should not be used during a fire.
		●	Closed doors after a room is evacuated and placed an "X" on the door.
		●	Escorted patients to the designated assembly area.
		●	Accounted for all building occupants.
		▷	Stated the reason for accounting for all building occupants.
		●	Kept building occupants together in the assembly area and did not allow them to block access to the building.

Trial 1	Trial 2	Point Value	Performance Standards
		●	Did not allow building occupants to re-enter the building and to not leave until dismissed.
		●	Provided emergency responders with necessary information.
			POST-DRILL ACTIVITIES
		●	Evaluated the effectiveness of the fire drill.
		●	Identified the strengths, concerns and means of improvement of the fire drill.
		●	Documented the results of the fire drill.
		▷	Stated the purpose of evaluating and documenting the results of the fire drill.
		Ⓐ	Recognized the physical and emotional effects on persons involved in an emergency situation.
		Ⓐ	Demonstrated self-awareness in responding to an emergency situation.
		*	Completed the procedure within 20 minutes.
			TOTALS

FIRE DRILL EVALUATION FORM

Date: ______________________ **Completed By:** ______________________

S	U	Evaluation Criteria:
		The evacuation was completed in an orderly, efficient, and timely manner.
		Building occupants and emergency responders were immediately alerted to the situation.
		Evacuation wardens effectively completed their duties.
		Patients and visitors were escorted to the nearest exits and assembly area.
		Each building occupant was accounted for following the evacuation.
		Emergency responders were provided with appropriate information.

STRENGTHS:

CONCERNS:	MEANS OF IMPROVEMENT:

Evaluation of Student Performance

EVALUATION CRITERIA			COMMENTS
Symbol	**Category**	**Point Value**	
*	Critical Step	16 points	
●	Essential Step	6 points	
Ⓐ	Affective Competency	6 points	
▷	Theory Question	2 points	
Score calculation: 100 points − ___ points missed ___ Score Satisfactory score: 85 or above			

2008 CAAHEP Competencies Achieved

Psychomotor (Skills)

☑ XI. 1. Comply with safety signs, symbols, and labels.
☑ XI. 2. Evaluate the work environment to identify safe vs. unsafe working conditions.
☑ XIII. 3. Develop a personal (patient and employee) safety plan.
☑ XI. 4. Develop an environmental safety plan.
☑ XI. 5. b. Demonstrate proper use of the following equipment: Fire extinguisher.
☑ XI. 6. Participate in a mock environmental exposure event with documentation of steps taken.
☑ XI. 7. Explain an evacuation plan for a physician's office.
☑ XI. 8. Demonstrate methods of fire prevention in the healthcare setting.
☑ XI. 12. Maintain a current list of community resources for emergency preparedness.

Affective (Behavior)

☑ I. 1. Apply critical thinking skills in performing patient assessment and care.
☑ 1.2. Use language/verbal skills that enable patients' understanding.
☑ XI. 1. Recognize the effects of stress on all persons involved in emergency situations.
☑ XI. 2. Demonstrate self awareness in responding to emergency situations.

2015 CAAHEP Competencies Achieved

Psychomotor (Skills)

☑ V. 9. Develop a current list of community resources related to patients' healthcare needs.
☑ V. 11. Report relevant information concisely and accurately.
☑ XII. 1. Comply with: a. safety signs b. symbols c. labels.
☑ XII. 2. b. Demonstrate proper use of fire extinguishers.
☑ XII. 4. Participate in a mock exposure event with documentation of specific steps.
☑ XII. 5. Evaluate the work environment to identify unsafe working conditions.

Affective (Behavior)

☑ XII. 1. Recognize the physical and emotional effects on persons involved in an emergency situation.
☑ XII. 2. Demonstrate self-awareness in responding to an emergency situation.

ABHES Competencies Achieved

☑ 4. e. Perform risk management procedures.
☑ 9. g. Recognize and respond to medical office emergencies.
☑ 9. i. Identify community resources and complementary and Alternative Medicine practice (CAM).
☑ 9. j. Make adaptations with patients with special needs.

37 Emergency Medical Procedures and First Aid

CHAPTER ASSIGNMENTS

✓ After Completing	Date Due	Study Guide Pages	STUDY GUIDE ASSIGNMENTS (CTA = Critical Thinking Activity)	Possible Points	Points You Earned
		1055	Pretest	10	
		1056	Term Key Term Assessment	16	
		1056-1061	Evaluation of Learning questions	27	
		1061	CTA A: First-Aid Kit	10	
		1061	CTA B: EMD Information	5	
		1062	CTA C: Emergency Care (2 points each)	6	
		1062-1063	CTA D: Emergency Situations (3 points each)	33	
		1055	Posttest	10	
			ADDITIONAL ASSIGNMENTS		
			TOTAL POINTS		

Notes

Name ______________________________ Date ______________

PRETEST

True or False

_______ 1. A specially equipped cart for holding and transporting medications, equipment, and supplies needed in an emergency is known as a crash cart.

_______ 2. Symptoms of an asthmatic attack include dyspnea and wheezing.

_______ 3. Symptoms of a heart attack include sudden weakness on one side of the body.

_______ 4. Another name for a stroke is a coronary occlusion.

_______ 5. Arterial bleeding is characterized by a slow and steady flow of blood that is dark red.

_______ 6. A laceration is an example of a closed wound.

_______ 7. Symptoms of a fracture include pain, swelling, deformity, and loss of function.

_______ 8. A sprain is a tearing of ligaments at a joint.

_______ 9. Heat stroke is a life-threatening emergency.

_______ 10. Insulin enables glucose to enter the body's cells and be converted to energy.

POSTTEST

True or False

_______ 1. When providing emergency care, you should obtain information about what happened from bystanders.

_______ 2. Emphysema is a progressive lung disorder in which there is a loss of elasticity of the alveoli of the lungs.

_______ 3. Symptoms that may occur with hyperventilation include rapid and deep respirations and tachycardia.

_______ 4. The first priority for hypovolemic shock is to control bleeding.

_______ 5. Status asthmaticus is the type of shock caused by a reaction of the body to a substance to which an individual is highly allergic.

_______ 6. Another name for a nosebleed is epistaxis.

_______ 7. The type of fracture in which the broken ends of the bone are forcefully jammed together is a green-stick fracture.

_______ 8. The type of seizure in which the abnormal electrical activity is localized into very specific areas of the brain is a tonic-clonic seizure.

_______ 9. Chipmunks have a high incidence of rabies.

_______ 10. Emergency care for insulin shock is to give the patient sugar immediately.

KEY TERM ASSESSMENT

Directions: Match each key term with its definition.

_______ 1. Burn
_______ 2. Crash cart
_______ 3. Crepitus
_______ 4. Dislocation
_______ 5. Emergency medical services
_______ 6. First aid
_______ 7. Fracture
_______ 8. Hypothermia
_______ 9. Poison
_______ 10. Pressure point
_______ 11. Seizure
_______ 12. Shock
_______ 13. Splint
_______ 14. Sprain
_______ 15. Strain
_______ 16. Wound

A. A network of community resources, equipment, and personnel that provides care to victims of injury or sudden illness
B. Any substance that causes illness, injury, or death if it enters the body
C. An injury to the tissues caused by exposure to thermal, chemical, electrical, or radioactive agents
D. Any device that immobilizes a body part
E. A grating sensation caused by fractured bone fragments rubbing against each other
F. A sudden episode of involuntary muscular contractions and relaxation, often accompanied by changes in sensation, behavior, and level of consciousness
G. A stretching or tearing of muscles or tendons caused by trauma
H. The immediate care that is administered to an individual who is injured or suddenly becomes ill before complete medical care can be obtained
I. A break in the continuity of an external or internal surface caused by physical means
J. A specially equipped cart for holding and transporting medications, equipment, and supplies needed for performing lifesaving procedures in an emergency
K. Any break in a bone
L. The failure of the cardiovascular system to deliver enough blood to all the vital organs of the body
M. An injury in which one end of a bone making up a joint is separated or displaced from its normal anatomic position
N. A life-threatening condition in which the temperature of the entire body falls to a dangerously low level
O. A site on the body where an artery lies close to the surface of the skin and can be compressed against an underlying bone to control bleeding
P. Trauma to a joint that causes tearing of ligaments

EVALUATION OF LEARNING

Directions: Fill in each blank with the correct answer.

1. What is the purpose of first aid?

____
____
____
____

2. What is the purpose of the office crash cart?

____
____
____
____

3. What is the difference between an EMT-basic and an EMT-paramedic?

4. What are the responsibilities of an emergency medical dispatcher?

5. List five OSHA Standards that should be followed when administering first aid.

6. What is the reason for performing each of the following during an emergency situation?

   a. Remaining calm and speaking in a normal tone of voice

   b. Making sure it is safe before approaching the patient

   c. Following OSHA Standards when providing emergency care

   d. Activating the emergency medical services

   e. Not moving the patient unnecessarily

   f. Checking the patient for a medical alert tag

7. What are the symptoms of asthma?

8. What is emphysema?

9. What are the symptoms of hyperventilation?

10. What are the symptoms of a heart attack?

11. What are the symptoms of a stroke?

12. What is the cause of the following types of shock?

   a. Hypovolemic

   b. Cardiogenic

   c. Neurogenic

   d. Anaphylactic

   e. Psychogenic

13. What are the characteristics of each of the following types of external bleeding?

   a. Capillary

   b. Venous

c. Arterial

14. What is the difference between an open wound and a closed wound?

15. What are the signs and symptoms of a fracture?

16. What are the characteristics of each of the following types of fractures?

a. Impacted

b. Greenstick

c. Transverse

d. Oblique

e. Comminuted

f. Spiral

17. What are the characteristics of each of the following types of burns?

a. Superficial

b. Partial thickness

c. Full thickness

18. What is the difference between a partial seizure and a generalized seizure?

19. List two examples of each of the following types of poisoning:

a. Ingested

b. Inhaled

c. Absorbed

d. Injected

20. What spiders (found in the United States) have bites that can result in serious or life-threatening reactions?

21. What species of snakes (found in the United States) are poisonous?

22. What animals tend to have a high incidence of rabies?

23. What factors place an individual at higher risk for developing heat- and cold-related injuries?

24. What areas of the body are most susceptible to frostbite?

25. What is the difference between type 1 diabetes and type 2 diabetes?

26. What is insulin shock, and what causes it to occur?

27. What is a diabetic coma, and what causes it to occur?

CRITICAL THINKING ACTIVITIES

A. First-Aid Kit

You are assembling a first-aid kit. What supplies should be included in your kit? Identify one use for each of the supplies you list.

B. EMD Information

Jeff Stickler suddenly develops weakness in his left arm and leg, has difficulty speaking, and has a severe headache and dizziness. You immediately call the Emergency Medical Services (EMS). What information should you be prepared to relay to the emergency medical dispatcher (EMD)?

C. Emergency Care

In which of the following emergency situations would you be legally permitted to administer first aid? Explain your answers.

1. A patient is unconscious and bleeding profusely.

2. You identify yourself and state your level of training and what you plan to do. You ask the patient if it is alright to administer emergency care. The patient responds by saying, "Yes, please help me."

3. You ask the patient if you can administer emergency care, but the patient refuses your help.

D. Emergency Situations

Explain what you would do in each of the following situations.

1. Holly Murphy falls while roller skating. She comes down hard on her left arm, which begins to swell and discolor. Holly guards her arm and complains of intense pain.

2. John Phillips is mowing the grass and mows over a yellow jacket nest. He is stung twice and soon starts complaining of intense itching and exhibits erythema and hives on his arms, torso, and face.

3. Steve Williams complains of severe indigestion and squeezing pain in the chest. He is short of breath and perspiring profusely.

4. Clara Miller is playing basketball and is accidentally hit in the face with the ball. Her nose begins bleeding profusely.

5. Debbie Carter, age 4 years, finds some children's chewable vitamins that have been left open on a table. She eats about 10 of them.

6. Rita Preston accidentally cuts her finger with a knife while preparing dinner. Her finger begins bleeding profusely.

7. Jose Perez is jogging on a cinder track. He falls and scrapes his left knee on the cinders.

8. Charlotte Lambert is getting ready to perform a piano recital for her entire church congregation. Suddenly she starts breathing very rapidly and deeply and complains that she feels light-headed and dizzy.

9. Bruce Jones is a diabetic. He is in a hurry and forgets to eat breakfast. He begins exhibiting behavior similar to that of someone who is intoxicated.

10. Debra Murray is delivering newspapers and is bitten by a strange dog. The bite causes several puncture marks and slight bleeding.

____

____

____

____

11. Tanya Howe is playing tennis on a hot and humid day and begins to feel weak and nauseous. Her skin feels cold and clammy, and she is sweating profusely and complains of dizziness.

____

____

____

____

38 The Medical Record

CHAPTER ASSIGNMENTS

✓ After Completing	Date Due	Study Guide Pages	STUDY GUIDE ASSIGNMENTS (CTA = Critical Thinking Activity)	Possible Points	Points You Earned
		1069	Pretest	10	
		1070	Key Term Assessment	23	
		1070-1076	Evaluation of Learning questions	50	
		1076	CTA A: General Procedure Consent Form	4	
		1077	CTA B: Medical Records Release Form	4	
		1077	CTA C: Chief Complaint	6	
		1078	CTA D: Crossword Puzzle	23	
		1097-1103	Taking Patient Symptoms: Supplemental Education for Chapter 38 (5 points for each problem)	30	
			Evolve Site: Apply Your Knowledge questions	10	
			Evolve Site: Video Evaluation	6	
		1069	Posttest	10	
			ADDITIONAL ASSIGNMENTS		
			TOTAL POINTS		

Notes

✓ When Assigned By Your Instructor	Study Guide Pages	Practices Required	LABORATORY ASSIGNMENTS (Procedure Number and Name)	Score*
	1079	1	**Practice for Competency** 38-1: Completion of a Procedure Consent Form Textbook reference: p. 1001	
	1087-1088		**Evaluation of Competency** 38-1: Completion of a Procedure Consent Form	*
	1081	1	**Practice for Competency** 38-2: Release of Medical Information Textbook reference: pp. 1001-1002	
	1089-1091		**Evaluation of Competency** 38-2: Release of Medical Information	*
	1083-1086	2	**Practice for Competency** 38-3: Obtaining Patient History and Formulating Chief Complaint Textbook reference: pp. 1017-1018	
	1093-1096		**Evaluation of Competency** 38-3: Obtaining Patient History and Formulating Chief Complaint	*
			ADDITIONAL ASSIGNMENTS	

Notes

Name ______________________________ Date ______________

PRETEST

True or False

_______ 1. The medical record serves as a legal document.

_______ 2. The purpose of progress notes is to update the medical record with new information.

_______ 3. The patient registration record consists of a list of the problems associated with the patient's illness.

_______ 4. All OTC medications taken by the patient should be documented on the medication record form.

_______ 5. A consultation report is a narrative report of a clinical opinion about a patient's condition by a practitioner other than the primary physician.

_______ 6. A report of the analysis of body specimens is known as a diagnostic report.

_______ 7. Medical impressions are conclusions drawn from an interpretation of data.

_______ 8. A source-oriented medical record is arranged by patient problems.

_______ 9. Diabetes mellitus is an example of a familial disease.

_______ 10. Pain is an example of an objective symptom.

POSTTEST

True or False

_______ 1. The purpose of HIPAA is to provide patients with more control over the use and disclosure of their health information.

_______ 2. The health history provides subjective data about a patient to assist the physician in arriving at a diagnosis.

_______ 3. Physical therapy helps a patient with a disability learn new skills to perform the activities of daily living.

_______ 4. A copy of the patient's emergency room report is sent to the patient's family physician.

_______ 5. When a medical assistant (MA) witnesses a patient's signature on a form, it means that the MA is verifying that the patient understands the information on the form.

_______ 6. SOAP is the acronym for the format used to organize POR progress notes.

_______ 7. The chief complaint is the symptom causing the patient the most trouble.

_______ 8. The social history includes information on the patient's lifestyle, such as health habits and living environment.

_______ 9. Vital signs are often documented on a flow sheet in the electronic health record (EHR).

_______ 10. When a procedure has been performed, it should be documented within 24 hours.

KEY TERM ASSESSMENT

Directions: Match each key term with its definition.

_______ 1. Attending physician
_______ 2. Chief Complaint
_______ 3. Consultation report
_______ 4. Diagnosis
_______ 5. Diagnostic procedure
_______ 6. Digital image
_______ 7. Discharge summary report
_______ 8. Documenting
_______ 9. Electronic medical record
_______ 10. Familial
_______ 11. Flow sheet
_______ 12. Health history
_______ 13. Home health care
_______ 14. Inpatient
_______ 15. Medical record
_______ 16. Medical record format
_______ 17. Objective symptom
_______ 18. Physical examination
_______ 19. Problem
_______ 20. Reverse chronological order
_______ 21. SOAP
_______ 22. Subjective symptom
_______ 23. Symptom

A. A collection of subjective data about a patient
B. A narrative report of an opinion about a patient's condition by a practitioner other than the attending physician
C. Any condition that requires further observation, diagnosis, management, or patient education
D. A picture that is stored electronically to allow viewing on a computer
E. The process of making written or electronic entries about a patient in the medical record
F. The way a medical record is organized
G. Any change in the body or its functioning that indicates the presence of disease
H. Progress notes including the following categories: subjective, objective, assessment, plan
I. A health record that is stored on a computer
J. A brief summary of the significant events of a patient's hospitalization
K. A written record of the important information regarding a patient
L. A paper document or electronic screen that allows similar data to be recorded and viewed chronologically
M. Arranging documents with the most recent document on top or in the front.
N. The scientific method of determining and identifying a patient's condition
O. A report of the objective findings from the physician's assessment of each body system
P. Occurring in or affecting members of a family more frequently than would be expected by chance
Q. The physician responsible for the care of a hospitalized patient
R. A procedure performed to assist in the diagnosis, management, or treatment of a patient's condition
S. A patient who has been admitted to the hospital for at least one overnight stay
T. A statement of the most important symptom or symptoms for which a patient is seeking care
U. A symptom felt by the patient but not observed by an examiner
V. A symptom that can be observed by an examiner
W. The provision of medical and nonmedical care in a patient's home or place of residence

EVALUATION OF LEARNING

Directions: Fill in each blank with the correct answer.

1. List three functions of the medical record.

____

2. What is the meaning of the acronym HIPAA?

____

3. What is the purpose of the HIPAA privacy rule?

____

4. Who must comply with HIPAA?

____

5. What is a Notice of Privacy Practices (NPP)?

____

____

6. List examples of when HIPAA does not require written consent for the use or disclosure of a patient's health information in the following categories:

   a. Treatment: ______________________________

   b. Payment: ______________________________

   c. Health care operations: ______________________________

7. What are the two most common types of medical records?

____

8. Briefly describe how the Health Information Technology for Economic and Clinical Health (HITECH) Act has accelerated the adoption of electronic health records.

____

____

9. Describe each of the following medical record formats:

   Source-oriented record ______________________________

   ____

   Problem-oriented record ______________________________

   ____

   Electronic health record ______________________________

   ____

10. What is reverse chronological order?

____

____

11. List and describe the four parts of a POR.

____

____

____

____

12. What is the function of the problem list? ______________________________

13. What two general categories of information are included on a patient registration record?

14. What does the term "meaningful use" refer to?

15. When is a procedure consent form required?

16. What is the purpose of a procedure consent form?

17. What information must the patient receive before signing a procedure consent form?

18. What does witnessing a signature mean? What does it not mean?

19. When must a patient complete a medical records release form?

20. What information must be included on a medical records release form?

21. Why are correspondence and messages filed or documented in a patient's medical record?

22. List three uses of the health history.

23. What is the purpose of the physical examination?

24. What is an advantage of the EMR related to allergies?

25. List three categories of medication that may be included in a medication record.

26. What is the purpose of progress notes?

27. What is the purpose of a laboratory report?

28. List five examples of diagnostic procedure reports.

29. How can the EMR facilitate continuity of care?

30. What information is included in a consultation report?

31. List five examples of home health services.

32. What is the purpose of a therapeutic service report?

33. What is the difference between physical therapy and occupational therapy?

34. What is the purpose of an operative report?

35. What is the purpose of the discharge summary report?

36. Why is a copy of the emergency room report sent to the patient's family physician?

37. What are the seven parts of the health history?

38. What is a chief complaint?

39. What guidelines should be followed in recording the chief complaint?

40. What is the current illness, and how is this information obtained?

41. List five examples of information included in the past medical history.

42. List three examples of familial diseases.

43. Explain the importance of the social history.

44. What is the purpose of the review of systems (ROS)?

45. List the general guidelines for documenting in a patient's medical record.

46. List the specific guidelines for documenting in the paper-based medical record.

47. What type of information is documented on flow sheets in the medical record?

48. List three examples of subjective symptoms.

49. List three examples of objective symptoms.

50. Why should the following be updated and/or documented in the patient's medical record?

a. Allergies and current medications

b. Procedures performed on the patient

c. Specimens collected from the patient

d. Laboratory tests ordered for the patient

e. Instructions given to the patient regarding medical care

CRITICAL THINKING ACTIVITIES

A. General Procedure Consent

Refer to the general procedure consent (see Figure 38-4) in your textbook, and answer the following questions.

1. When is a general procedure consent form used to obtain informed consent?

2. What information must be filled in in boxes 1 and 2 before this form is given to a patient?

3. What should the medical assistant do if a patient asks what complications might occur after the proposed procedure?

4. If the medical assistant signs the form as a witness, what does that mean?

B. Medical Records Release Form

Refer to the medical records release form (see Figure 38-5) in your textbook, and answer the following questions.

1. What medical information is protected by law and cannot be released unless specifically authorized by the patient?

____

____

2. List three reasons why a patient may authorize the release of his or her medical information.

____

____

____

3. After this form is completed and signed, how long is it valid before it expires?

____

4. What must the patient do if he or she wants to revoke the authorization?

____

____

C. Chief Complaint

Indicate whether each of the following statements is an incorrect (I) or correct (C) example of recording a chief complaint (CC). If the example is incorrect, explain which recording guideline is not being followed.

_______ 1. CC: Low back pain ____

_______ 2. CC: Sore throat and fever for the past 2 days ____

_______ 3. CC: Dyspnea, paleness, and fatigue, similar to that associated with anemia, which have lasted for 2 weeks

____

_______ 4. CC: Poor health for the past several months ____

_______ 5. CC: Weakness and fatigue related to poor eating habits and lack of exercise

____

_______ 6. CC: Heart palpitations occurring after drinking coffee in the morning before work

____

____

D. Crossword Puzzle: The Medical Record

Directions: Complete the crossword puzzle using the clues provided.

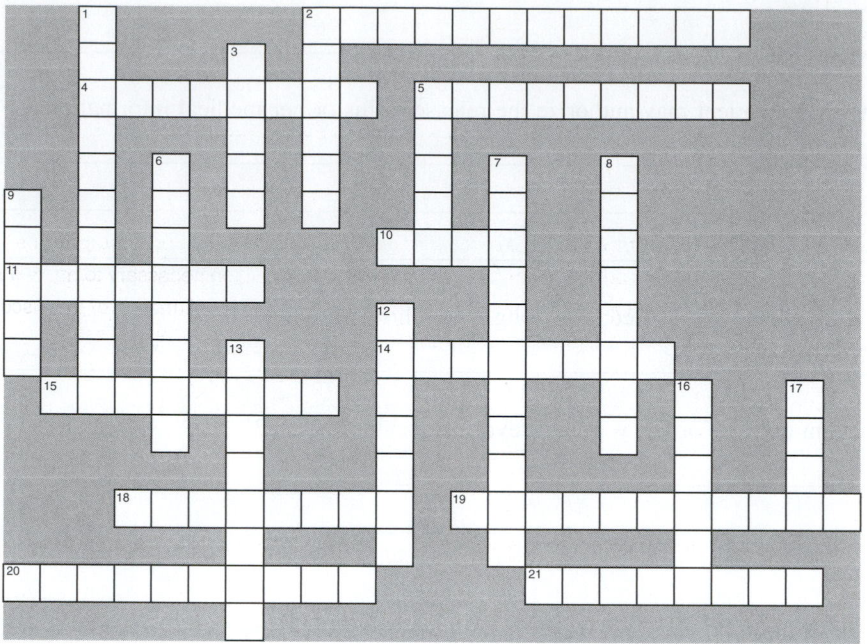

Across

2 Stool is hard and dry
4 Blue skin due to lack of O_2
5 Nosebleed
10 Skin eruption
11 Dizziness
14 No appetite
15 Yellow skin
18 Severe itching
19 Involuntary contractions of muscles
20 Gas
21 Head pain

Down

1 Fast pulse rate
2 Shivering
3 May be productive or nonproductive
5 Fluid retention
6 Ejection of stomach contents
7 Decreased H_2O levels in the body
8 Red face
9 Elevated temp
12 Bad all over
13 Loose, watery stools
16 Sensation of stomach discomfort
17 Feeling of distress or suffering

PRACTICE FOR COMPETENCY

Procedure 38-1: Completion of a Procedure Consent Form. Complete the consent to treatment form using a classmate as the patient.

WALDEN-MARTIN

FAMILY MEDICAL CLINIC

1234 ANYSTREET ANYTOWN, ANYSTATE 1234

PHONE 123-123-1234 FAX 123-123-5678

General Procedure Consent

Patient Name: ______________________ **Date:** ______________________

The Doctor has discussed with you your condition and the recommended surgical or medical procedures to be performed. This discussion was intended to ensure that you had the opportunity to receive the information necessary to make a reasoned and informed decision whether or not to consent to the procedure. This document is written confirmation of the discussion and contain some of the more significant medical information discussed.

1. Based on this discussion, I understand the following condition may exist in my case:

2. I understand the procedure proposed for treating or diagnosing my condition is:

3. I have been informed of the purpose and reasonable expected benefits of the proposed procedure, the possibility of success or failure, major problems of recuperation, the reasonably anticipated consequences if the procedure is not performed, and the available alternatives.

4. I understand that all surgical and therapeutic procedures involve some risks including pain, scarring, bleeding and infection.

5. I am aware that in the practice of medicine, other unexpected risks or complications not discussed may or may not further acknowledge that no guarantees or promises have been made to me concerning the results of any procedures. Although the benefits are judged to outweigh the risks, should any complications occur, any one of them could be permanent. I heareby voluntarily give my authority and consent to the doctor to perform the proposed procedure described above.

6. I have been given the opportunity to ask questions about my condition, alternative forms of treatment, risk treatment, the procedure to be used, and the risks and hazards involved. I believe I have sufficient information to give this informed consent.

I understand I have read and fully understand the contents of this form, that the disclosure referred to above were made to me and that ass blanks and statement requiring insertion or completion were filled in before I signed my name below.

Patient Signature: ______________________ **Date:** ______________________

If a patient is a minor or unable to give consent,
Signature of person authorized to consent for patient:

Relationship to Patient: ______________________

Witness: ______________________ **Date:** ______________________

Notes

Procedure 38-2: Release of Medical Information. Complete the medical records release form using a classmate as the patient.

WALDEN-MARTIN

FAMILY MEDICAL CLINIC
1234 ANYSTREET ANYTOWN, ANYSTATE 1234
PHONE 123-123-1234 FAX 123-123-5678

Medical Records Release

Patient Name: ______________________ **Date of Birth:** ______________________

SSN: ______________________ **Phone:** ______________________

Address: ______________________

I, ______________________ authorize ______________________

Walden-Martin Family Medical Clinic to disclose/release the following information (check all applicable):

- ☐ All records
- ☐ Abstract/summary
- ☐ Laboratory/pathology records
- ☐ Pharmacy/prescription records
- ☐ X-ray/radiology records
- ☐ Other
- ☐ Billing records

***Note:** If these records contain any information from previous providers or information about HIV/AIDS status, cancer diagnosis, drug alcohol abuse, or sexually transmitted disease, you are hereby authorizing disclosure of this information. A copy of this signed authorization must be given to the individual.*

These records are for services provided on the following date(s):

Please send the records listed above to (use additional sheets if necessary):

Name: ______________________ **Phone:** ______________________

Address: ______________________ **Fax:** ______________________

The information may be used/disclosed for each of the following purposes:

- ☐ At patient's request
- ☐ For employment purposes
- ☐ For patient's health care
- ☐ Other
- ☐ For payment/insurance

This authorization shall expire no later than:__________or upon the following event __________, and may not be valid for greater than one year from the date of signature for medical records.

I understand that after the custodial of records discloses my health information, it may no longer be protected by federal privacy laws. I understand that this authorization is voluntary and I may refuse to sign this authorization which will not affect my ability to obtain treatment; receive payment; or eligibility for benefits unless allowed by law. By signing below I represent and warrant that I have authority to sign this document and authorize the use or disclosure of protected health information and that there are no claims or orders that would prohibit, limit, or otherwise restrict my ability to authorize the use or disclosure of this protected health information.

______________________ ______________________

Patient signature
(or patient's personal representative)

Date:

______________________ ______________________

Printed name of patient representative

Representative's authority to sign for patient
(i.e. parent, guardian, power of attorney, executor)

Notes

Procedure 38-3: Obtaining Patient History and Formulating Chief Complaint. Complete the health history form (pp. 1084-1085) using yourself as the patient.

Enter a Medical History in SimChart® for the Medical Office

Enter a medical history using the Simulation Playground of SimChart® for the Medical Office.

Select a patient of the same sex and approximate age as yourself. Click on **Comprehensive Visit** and select **New Patient**. Select **Health History** on from the **Record** tab. Click the **Add New** button under **Past Medical History, Past Hospitalizations**, and **Past Surgeries** to add and save each piece of information from your health history form. Save the page and move to the **Social and Family History** tab. Click the **Add New** button under **Family History: Who lives in the home, Paternal**, and **Maternal** to add information about family members using your health history form and save the information for each. Then complete all other information requested under health history and save the page. If you have a completed prenatal health history form you can practice entering the information by selecting the **Pregnancy History** tab. (See Study Guide Chapter 23: The Gynecologic Examination and Patient Care for a pregnancy history form or the textbook if you have questions about the information or terms related to the pregnancy history.)

A

PATIENT HEALTH HISTORY

IDENTIFICATION DATA Please print the following information.

Name ______ Today's date ______

Address ______ ___ Male ___ Female

______ ___ Married ___ Separated ___ Divorced ___ Widowed ___ Single

Telephone ______ ______ Date of Birth ______

B

PAST HISTORY

Have you ever had the following: (Circle "no" or "yes", leave blank if uncertain)

Measles ___ no yes	Heart Disease ___ no yes	Diabetes ___ no yes	Hemorrhoids ___ no yes
Mumps ___ no yes	Arthritis ___ no yes	Cancer ___ no yes	Asthma ___ no yes
Chickenpox ___ no yes	Sexually Transmitted Disease ___ no yes	Polio ___ no yes	Allergies ___ no yes
Whooping Cough ___ no yes	Anemia ___ no yes	Glaucoma ___ no yes	Eczema ___ no yes
Scarlet Fever ___ no yes	Bladder Infections ___ no yes	Hernia ___ no yes	AIDS or HIV+ ___ no yes
Diphtheria ___ no yes	Epilepsy ___ no yes	Blood or Plasma Transfusions ___ no yes	Infectious Mono ___ no yes
Pneumonia ___ no yes	Migraine Headaches ___ no yes	Back Trouble ___ no yes	Bronchitis ___ no yes
Rheumatic Fever ___ no yes	Tuberculosis ___ no yes	High Blood Pressure ___ no yes	Mitral Valve Prolapse no yes
Stroke ___ no yes	Ulcer ___ no yes	Thyroid Disease ___ no yes	Any other disease ___ no yes Please list: ______
Hepatitis. ___ no yes	Kidney Disease ___ no yes	Bleeding Tendency ___ no yes	

MAJOR HOSPITALIZATIONS: If you have ever been hospitalized for any major medical illness or operation, write in your most recent hospitalizations below.

Hospitalizations	Year	Operation or illness	Name of hospital	City and state
1st Hospitalization				
2nd Hospitalization				
3rd Hospitalization				
4th Hospitalization				

TESTS AND IMMUNIZATIONS: Mark an X next to those that you have had.

Tests:

- ☐ TB Test
- ☐ Rectal/Hemoccult
- ☐ Sigmoidoscopy
- ☐ Colonoscopy
- ☐ Electrocardiogram
- ☐ Chest X-ray
- ☐ Mammogram
- ☐ Pap Test

Immunizations:

- ☐ Influenza
- ☐ Hepatitis B
- ☐ Tetanus
- ☐ MMR
- ☐ Polio

CURRENT MEDICATIONS: List the following that you are currently taking: Prescription medications, over-the-counter (OTC) medications, vitamin supplements, and herbal supplements. ☐ None

Medication ______ Frequency ______

ALLERGIES: List all allergies (foods, drugs, environment). ☐ None

ACCIDENTS/ INJURIES: Describe all serious accidents, severe injuries, head injury, or fractrures. Include the date each occurred. ☐ None

Accident/Injury: ______ Date: ______

C

FAMILY HISTORY

For each member of your family, follow the purple or blue line across the page and check boxes for:
1. Their present state of health
2. Any illnesses they have had

	Good Health	Poor Health	Deceased	If deceased, write in age and cause of death.	Allergies or Asthma	Diabetes	Heart Disease	Stroke	Cancer	High Blood Pressure	Glaucoma	Arthritis	Ulcer	Kidney Disease	Mental Health Problems	Alcohol/Drug Abuse	Obesity	High Cholesterol	Thyroid Disease
Father:																			
Mother:																			
Brothers/Sisters:																			

D

SOCIAL HISTORY

EDUCATION ______ High school ______ College ______ Post graduate

Occupation ______________________ Years ______

Previous occupations ______________________ Years ______

______________________ Years ______

Have you ever been exposed to any of the following in your environment?

☐ Excess dust (coal, lime, rock) ☐ Cleaning fluids/solvents ☐ Radiation ☐ Other toxic materials

☐ Sand ☐ Hair spray ☐ Insecticides

☐ Chemicals ☐ Smoke or auto exhaust fumes ☐ Paints

Please answer the follwing questions by placing an X in the box in front of the word Yes or No, except where you are asked for specific information. This information is obviously highly confidential and will be released to other health professionals or insurance carriers ONLY with your consent.

DIET:

Do you eat a good breakfast? ☐ Yes ☐ No

Do you snack between meals (soft drinks, chips, candy bars)? ☐ Yes ☐ No

Do you eat fresh fruits and vegetables each day? ☐ Yes ☐ No

Do you eat whole grain breads and cereals? ☐ Yes ☐ No

Is your diet high in fat content? ☐ Yes ☐ No

Is your diet high in cholesterol content? ☐ Yes ☐ No

Is your diet high in salt content? ☐ Yes ☐ No

Are you allergic to any foods? ☐ Yes ☐ No

How many glasses of water do you drink each day? ______

How would you describe your overall eating habits? ☐ Excellent ☐ Good ☐ Fair ☐ Poor

PERSONAL HISTORY:

Do you find it hard to make decisions? ☐ Yes ☐ No

Do you find it hard to concentrate or remember? ☐ Yes ☐ No

Do you feel depressed? ☐ Yes ☐ No

Do you have difficulty relaxing? ☐ Yes ☐ No

Do you have a tendency to worry a lot? ☐ Yes ☐ No

Have you gained or lost much weight recently? ☐ Yes ☐ No

Do you lose your temper often? ☐ Yes ☐ No

Are you disturbed by any work or family problems? ☐ Yes ☐ No

Are you having sexual difficulties? ☐ Yes ☐ No

Have you ever considered committing suicide? ☐ Yes ☐ No

Have you ever desired or sought psychiatric help? ☐ Yes ☐ No

EXERCISE:

Do you exercise on a regular basis? ☐ Yes ☐ No

Does your job require strenuous, sustained physical work? ☐ Yes ☐ No

SLEEP PATTERNS:

Do you seem to feel exhausted or fatigued most of the time? ☐ Yes ☐ No

Do you have difficulty either falling asleep or staying asleep? ☐ Yes ☐ No

USE OF TOBACCO/ALCOHOL/CAFFEINE/DRUGS: Amt:

How much do you smoke per day? ☐ Cigarettes __ ☐ Cigars/pipes __

☐ Don't smoke

Do you take two or more alcoholic drinks per day? ☐ Yes ☐ No

Do you drink six or more cups of coffee or tea per day? ☐ Yes ☐ No

Are you a regular user of sleeping pills, marijuana, tranquilizers, pain killers, etc? ☐ Yes ☐ No

Have you ever used heroin, cocaine, LSD, PCP, etc? ☐ Yes ☐ No

List any country outside the USA you have visited in the past six months? ______________

When did you have your last physical examination? ______

Practice obtaining patient symptoms by completing Taking Patient Symptoms: Supplemental Education for Chapter 38 (pp. 1097-1103 in this study guide).

Enter the Chief Complaint in SimChart® for the Medical Office

Enter the chief complaint in SimChart® for the Medical Office by choosing **Chief Complaint** from the **Record** tab for the same patient you used for to enter the patient history. (Note that only one Chief Complaint can be entered for an encounter). As part of this activity practice performing a review of systems by asking a classmate questions to determine if they have the symptoms at the bottom of the **Chief Complaint** screen. Enter the answers and save the screen. Explain any unfamiliar terms to your simulated patient.

EVALUATION OF COMPETENCY

Procedure 38-1: Completion of a Procedure Consent Form

Name: ______________________________ Date: ______________

Evaluated by: ______________________________ Score: ______________

Performance Objective

Outcome:	Complete a procedure consent form.
Conditions:	Given procedure consent form, a clipboard and a pen.
Standards:	Time: 10 minutes. Student completed procedure in ________ minutes.
	Accuracy: Satisfactory score on the Performance Evaluation Checklist.

Performance Evaluation Checklist

Trial 1	Trial 2	Point Value	Performance Standards
		●	Typed or printed required information on the procedure consent form.
		●	Confirmed that the physician discussed the procedure with the patient.
		▷	Explained why the procedure should be discussed with the patient before the form is signed.
		●	Greeted the patient, identified the patient by full name and date of birth, and introduced yourself.
		Ⓐ	Explained the rationale for asking the patient to read and sign the form in language that the patient could understand.
		●	Gave the consent form to the patient to read.
		●	Asked if the patient had any questions.
		●	Listened carefully and responded appropriately to patient concerns or questions.
		▷	Explained why the patient should be referred back to the physician if they had questions.
		▷	Explained the patient's rights in respect to the proposed procedure.
		●	Asked the patient to sign the form.
		●	Witnessed the patient's signature and dated the form.
		▷	Explained what witnessing a signature means.
		●	Provided the patient with a copy of the completed form.
		✶	Filed the original form in the patient's paper medical record or scanned the original form into the EHR.
		Ⓐ	Protected the integrity of the medical record.
		✶	Completed the procedure within 10 minutes.
			TOTALS

Evaluation of Student Performance

EVALUATION CRITERIA			COMMENTS
Symbol	**Category**	**Point Value**	
✶	Critical Step	16 points	
●	Essential Step	6 points	
Ⓐ	Affective Competency	6 points	
▷	Theory Question	2 points	
Score calculation: 100 points − ____ points missed ____ Score Satisfactory score: 85 or above			

2008 CAAHEP Competencies Achieved
Psychomotor (Skills) ☑ IV. 2. Report relevant information to others succinctly and accurately. ☑ IV. 4. Explain general office policies. ☑ IX. 1. Respond to issues of confidentiality. ☑ IX. 3. Apply HIPAA rules in regard to privacy/release of information. ☑ IX. 7. Document accurately in the patient record. ☑ IX. 8. Apply local, state, and federal health care legislation and regulation appropriate to the medical assisting practice setting. ***Affective (Behavior)*** ☑ IX. 1. Demonstrate sensitivity to patient rights. ☑ IX. 3. Recognize the importance of local, state, and federal legislation and regulations in the practice setting.

2015 CAAHEP Competencies Achieved
Psychomotor (Skills) ☑ V. 4. a. Coach patients regarding office policies. ☑ V.11. Report relevant information concisely and accurately. ☑ VI.6. Utilize an EMR. ☑ X. 2. Apply HIPAA rules in regard to a. privacy, b. release of information. ☑ X. 3. Document patient care accurately in the patient record. ***Affective (Behavior)*** ☑ V.4. Explain to a patient the rationale for performance of a procedure. ☑ X.2. Protect the integrity of the medical record.

ABHES Competencies Achieved
☑ 4.a. Follow documentation guidelines. ☑ 8.a. Gather and process documents. ☑ 8. f. Display professionalism through written and verbal communications.

EVALUATION OF COMPETENCY

Procedure 38-2: Release of Medical Information

Name: ______________________________ Date: ______________

Evaluated by: ______________________________ Score: ______________

Performance Objective

Outcome:	1. Assist a patient in the completion of a medical records release form. 2. Release information according to a completed medical records release form.
Conditions:	Given a medical records release form and the patient's medical record.
Standards:	Time: 15 minutes. Student completed procedure in ________ minutes. Accuracy: Satisfactory score on the Performance Evaluation Checklist.

Performance Evaluation Checklist

Trial 1	Trial 2	Point Value	Performance Standards
			Completion of a release of information form
		▷	Explained patient rights in respect to the information contained in the medical record.
		●	Greeted the patient and introduced yourself.
		●	Identified the patient by full name and date of birth.
		Ⓐ	Explained the procedure to follow if you do not recognize the patient.
		●	Coached the patient about the office policy for release of the medical record.
		●	Explained the rationale for asking the patient to read and sign the form in language that the patient could understand.
		●	Provided the patient with a medical records release form.
		●	Asked the patient to complete the form.
		●	Provided assistance if needed.
		●	Checked to make sure all information was completed.
		●	Asked the patient to sign the form.
		●	Witnessed the patient's signature and dated the form if required by office policy.
		●	Provided the patient with a copy of the completed form.
		●	Copied the medical information requested on the form or printed the information from the EHR.
		*	Released only the information requested.
		●	Included a copy of the completed form with the medical information.

Trial 1	Trial 2	Point Value	Performance Standards
		●	Documented what information was released along with the date of release.
		●	Signed the release form with your name and credentials verifying you were the individual releasing the information.
		✶	Filed the original document and the release form in the patient's medical record.
		Ⓐ	Protected the integrity of the medical record.
		●	Sent the medical information according to the medical office policy.
			Mailed or faxed requests
		●	Checked the expiration date on the release of medical information form.
		▷	Explained the procedure to follow if the form is expired.
		●	Verified the signature on the form.
		▷	Stated what to do if in doubt regarding the authenticity of the signature.
		●	Copied or printed the information requested on the form.
		✶	Released only the information requested.
		●	Documented what information was released along with the date of release.
		●	Signed the document with your name and credentials.
		●	Filed the original document and the release form in the patient's medical record.
		●	Sent the medical information according to the medical office policy.
		✶	Completed the procedure within 15 minutes.
			TOTALS

Evaluation of Student Performance

EVALUATION CRITERIA			COMMENTS
Symbol	**Category**	**Point Value**	
✶	Critical Step	16 points	
●	Essential Step	6 points	
Ⓐ	Affective Competency	6 points	
▷	Theory Question	2 points	
Score calculation: 100 points – ___ points missed ___ Score Satisfactory score: 85 or above			

2008 CAAHEP Competencies Achieved
Psychomotor (Skills) ☑ IV. 2. Report relevant information to others succinctly and accurately. ☑ IV. 4. Explain general office policies. ☑ IX. 1. Respond to issues of confidentiality. ☑ IX. 3. Apply HIPAA rules in regard to a. privacy, b. release of information. ☑ IX. 7. Document patient care accurately in the patient record. ***Affective (Behavior)*** ☑ IX.1. Demonstrate sensitivity to patient rights. ☑ IX. 3. Recognize the importance of local, state, and federal legislation in the practice setting.

2015 CAAHEP Competencies Achieved
Psychomotor (Skills) ☑ V. 4. a. Coach patients regarding office policies. ☑ V.11. Report relevant information concisely and accurately. ☑ VI.6. Utilize an EMR. ☑ X. 2. Apply HIPAA rules in regard to a. privacy, b. release of information. ☑ X. 3. Document patient care accurately in the patient record. ***Affective (Behavior)*** ☑ V.4. Explain to a patient the rationale for performance of a procedure. ☑ X.2. Protect the integrity of the medical record.

ABHES Competencies Achieved
☑ 4. a. Follow documentation guidelines. ☑ 4. b. Institute federal and state guidelines when releasing medical records or information. ☑ 4. f. Comply with federal, state, and local health laws and regulations as they relate to health care settings. ☑ 8. a. Gather and process documents. ☑ 8. f. Display professionalism through written and verbal communications.

Notes

EVALUATION OF COMPETENCY

Procedure 38-3: Obtaining Patient History and Formulating Chief Complaint

Name: ______________________________ Date: ______________

Evaluated by: ______________________________ Score: ______________

Performance Objective

Outcome:	1. Obtain a patient history using reflection, restatement, and clarification techniques. 2. Formulate and document the patient's chief complaint and/or patient symptoms.
Conditions:	Given the following: medical record of the patient to be interviewed, a patient history form and a black ink pen or computer with access to the EHR.
Standards:	Time: 20 minutes. Student completed procedure in __________ minutes. Accuracy: Satisfactory score on the Performance Evaluation Checklist.

Performance Evaluation Checklist

Trial 1	Trial 2	Point Value	Performance Standards
		●	Assembled equipment.
		●	Made sure the correct patient record was obtained or viewed on the computer.
		●	Escorted the patient to a quiet room.
		●	In a calm and friendly manner and introduced yourself.
		●	Identified the patient by full name and date of birth.
		●	Asked the patient to be seated.
		Ⓐ	Seated yourself facing the patient at a distance of 3 to 4 feet.
		▷	Explained how this seating arrangement facilitated communication and maintained self-boundaries.
			Used effective communication skills
		●	Used the patient's name of choice.
		Ⓐ	Demonstrated genuine interest and concern for the patient.
		Ⓐ	Maintained appropriate eye contact.
		●	Used terminology the patient could understand. When medical terminology was used, pronounced correctly and explained as needed.
		●	Listened carefully and attentively to the patient.
		●	Paid attention to the patient's nonverbal messages and used appropriate body language.
		●	Avoided judgmental comments.

Trial 1	Trial 2	Point Value	Performance Standards
		●	Avoided rushing the patient.
		Ⓐ	Used feedback techniques including reflection, restatement, and clarification as necessary.
			Reviewed and/or documented the patient history on the patient history form or in the EHR
		●	Recorded or reviewed the past history on the patient history form or in the EHR. Included pregnancy history for a female patient if documenting in SimChart® for the Medical Office.
		●	Reviewed and/or documented the family history
		●	Reviewed and/or documented the social history including information about the use of tobacco products and smoking status.
		●	Reviewed and/or recorded allergies on the patient history form or by entering each allergy using the **Add Allergy** button in SimChart® for the Medical Office and saving every screen as indicated.
		●	Reviewed and/or recorded all the patient's current medications including prescription medications, over-the-counter medications, and vitamins/supplements using the **Add Medication** button in SimChart® for the Medical Office and saving every screen as indicated.
			Obtained and documented the chief complaint
		●	Used an open-ended question to obtain the chief complaint.
		▷	Explained why an open-ended question should be used.
		●	Limited the CC to one or two symptoms.
		●	Referred to a specific rather than a vague symptom.
		●	Documented concisely and briefly.
		●	Used medical terminology correctly in documentation.
		●	Used the patient's own words as much as possible.
		●	Included the duration of the symptom.
		●	Obtained additional information regarding the chief complaint using what, when, and where questions.
		●	Clarified as needed using reflection, restatement or summarizing what the patient had said. Repeated in simpler language if the patient did not appear to understand.
		●	If documenting in the EHR, filled in each field of the **Chief Complaint** screen with concise, pertinent information.
		●	Thanked the patient and proceeded to the next step in the patient workup.
		●	Informed the patient approximately how long they would have to wait for the physician.

Trial 1	Trial 2	Point Value	Performance Standards
		●	Placed the paperwork (including a paper medical record) in the appropriate location for review by the physician.
		✶	Completed the procedure within 20 minutes.
			TOTALS

DOCUMENTATION OF CHIEF COMPLAINT FOR THE EHR	
Chief Complaint:	
History of Present Illness:	
Location:	Timing:
Quality:	Context:
Severity:	Modifying Factors:
Duration:	Associated Signs and Symptoms

Evaluation of Student Performance

EVALUATION CRITERIA			COMMENTS
Symbol	**Category**	**Point Value**	
✶	Critical Step	16 points	
●	Essential Step	6 points	
Ⓐ	Affective Competency	6 points	
▷	Theory Question	2 points	
Score calculation: 100 points – ___ points missed ___ Score Satisfactory score: 85 or above			

2008 CAAHEP Competencies Achieved

Psychomotor (Skills)

☑ IV. 1. Use reflection, restatement, and clarification techniques to obtain a patient history.
☑ IV. 3. Use medical terminology correctly and pronounced accurately to communicate information to providers and patients.
☑ IX. 7. Document accurately in the patient record.

Affective (Behavior)

☑ IV. 3. Use appropriate body language and other nonverbal skills in communicating with patients, family, and staff.
☑ IV. 9. Recognize and protect personal boundaries in communicating with others.

2015 CAAHEP Competencies Achieved

Psychomotor (Skills)

☑ V. 1. Use feedback techniques to obtain patient information including a. reflection, b. restatement, and c. clarification.
☑ V. 3. Use medical terminology correctly and pronounced accurately to communicate information to providers and patients.
☑ V.11 Report relevant information concisely and accurately.

Affective (Behavior)

☑ V.1. Demonstrate: a. empathy, b. active listening, c. nonverbal communication
☑ V.2. Demonstrate the principles of self-boundaries.

ABHES Competencies Achieved

☑ 3. d. Define and use medical abbreviations when appropriate and acceptable.
☑ 4. a. Follow documentation guidelines.
☑ 7.b. Utilize electronic medical records (EMR) and practice management systems.
☑ 8. a. Gather and process documents.
☑ 8. f. Display professionalism through written and verbal communication.
☑ 9. b. Obtain vital signs, obtain patient history, and formulate chief complaint.

TAKING PATIENT SYMPTOMS: SUPPLEMENTAL EDUCATION FOR CHAPTER 38

Taking a patient's symptoms is a frequent and important responsibility of the medical assistant, who must have a thorough knowledge of symptoms and related terminology. A symptom is defined as any change in the body or its functioning that indicates the presence of disease. The medical assistant can observe objective symptoms presented by the patient, such as coughing, rash, and swelling. The medical assistant must rely on information relayed by the patient to obtain data on subjective symptoms. Examples of subjective symptoms include pain, pruritus, and vertigo.

This section is designed as supplemental education for Chapter 38 (The Medical Record) in your textbook. Completion of the exercises in this section can assist you in recording a patient's symptoms effectively and thoroughly, which is essential to an accurate diagnosis by the physician.

Learning Objectives

After completing this section, you should be able to do the following:

1. Explain the purpose of analyzing a symptom.
2. State the seven basic types of information that must be obtained to analyze a symptom.
3. Analyze a symptom by using direct questions.

Analysis of a Symptom

Before a symptom can be analyzed, the chief complaint (CC) must first be identified. The chief complaint is the patient's reason for seeking care or the symptom causing the patient the most trouble. An open-ended question should be used to elicit the chief complaint from the patient, and it should be documented following the documentation guidelines presented in your textbook (pp. 1011-1021). The next step is to analyze the chief complaint in detail from the time of its onset. The purpose of this is to provide a complete description of the current status of the chief complaint.

Analyzing the chief complaint requires a combination of good listening and writing skills. The medical assistant must know what information should be recorded for each symptom and the questions to ask the patient to obtain this information. A list of symptoms, explanation of the information required for each symptom, and examples of questions to ask the patient are provided.

Type of Information Required

The following information is needed for each symptom to provide a full description of the current status of the chief complaint:

1. Location of the symptom. This refers to the specific area of the body where the symptom is located. Locating the symptom is the first step in determining the cause of the patient's disease. The patient may refer to the location in general terms, such as the head, arm, stomach, or back. The medical assistant must be more specific than this and determine the exact location using descriptions, such as "occurs in the lower back" or "occurs under the sternum." Several questions can assist in accomplishing this.
   - Where exactly does it hurt?
   - Can you show me where it hurts?
   - Do you feel it anywhere else?

2. Quality of the symptom. The quality of the symptom includes a complete and concise description of the symptom. The medical assistant should use informative terms to describe the character of each symptom. For example, if the patient complains of pain, the character of the pain must be included. Several terms can be used to describe pain.
   - Burning
   - Aching
   - Sharp
   - Dull
   - Throbbing
   - Cramp-like
   - Squeezing

   If the patient has vomited, the medical assistant should indicate the color, odor, and consistency of the vomitus. If the patient has a cough, the medical assistant should indicate if it is productive or nonproductive and whether blood is present. Refer to the table of terms on p. 1103 of this manual, which can assist in describing symptoms. Specific examples of questions that are helpful in determining the quality of the symptom are as follows:
   - Describe it (the symptom) to me as fully as possible.
   - What is it (the symptom) like?

3. Severity of the symptom. Severity refers to the quantitative aspect of the symptom. It includes the following:
   - Intensity of the symptom (e.g., mild, moderate, severe)
   - Number (e.g., of convulsions, of nosebleeds)
   - Volume (e.g., of vomitus, of blood, of mucus)
   - Size or extent (e.g., of the rash, edema, lumps, or masses)

   This information assists the physician in determining the extensiveness or seriousness of the illness. Questions to determine severity are often specific to that symptom. For example, if the patient has a productive cough, the medical assistant should determine how much phlegm is being coughed up (e.g., teaspoon, half of a cup). At first, this area may appear difficult, but as you practice taking symptoms, you will learn what questions to ask the patient, and it eventually it will become automatic. The examples at the end of this section and the student practice problems provide guidance in developing skill in this area. Some examples of general questions that can be used to determine the severity of a symptom are as follows:
   - How bad is it (the symptom)?
   - Does it (the symptom) limit your normal activities?

4. Chronology and timing of the symptom. Chronology and timing include a sequential account of the symptom up to the time the patient came to the medical office for treatment. This information is important in determining the duration of the symptom and change in it since it first occurred. Chronology and timing include the following four areas:
   a. Date of onset: The date of onset of the symptom should be indicated, if possible, as a calendar date and clock time. The patient may need some time to recall this information. Examples of questions that help obtain this information are as follows:
      - When did you experience this (the symptom) for the first time?
      - Exactly when did this begin?

   b. Duration: The duration of the symptom refers to how long the symptom lasts after it occurs; for example: 10 minutes, 2 hours, continuously. Examples of questions to obtain this information are as follows:
      - How long does it last after occurring?
      - For what length of time do you experience this symptom?

   c. Frequency: The frequency of the symptom refers to how often the symptom occurs, such as twice daily or a single attack every 2 weeks. Examples of questions to obtain this information are as follows:
      - How often does it occur?
      - How often has the symptom recurred?

   d. Change over time: This area refers to any change in the symptom since it first occurred. A change in a symptom reflects the nature of the underlying disease, which assists the physician in making a diagnosis. Examples of questions to obtain this information are as follows:
      - Has the symptom changed since it first occurred?
      - Is it (the symptom) getting better, worse, or staying the same?

5. Manner of onset. The manner of onset refers to what the patient was doing when the symptom first occurred and exactly what was experienced by the patient when the symptom began. These data help provide information on the pathologic process responsible for the symptom. For example, the patient might have been lifting a heavy object before experiencing low back pain. This information helps the physician in making an accurate diagnosis. Examples of questions that are helpful in determining the manner of onset are as follows:
   - What exactly did you experience when it (the symptom) first occurred?
   - What was the first thing you noticed?
   - Did it (the symptom) come on suddenly or gradually?
   - What were you doing when it (the symptom) began?
   - Where were you when this happened?
   - How were you feeling before it (the symptom) began?

6. Modifying factors. Symptoms are often influenced by activities or physiologic processes, such as physical exercise, change in weather, bodily functions (e.g., bowel movements, eating, coughing), pregnancy, emotional states, and fatigue. Some activities may aggravate the symptom while others may alleviate it. These influences may help to determine what is causing the problem. For example, pain that becomes worse after the patient eats but is relieved after taking an antacid assists the physician in focusing on gastrointestinal disorders. Questions to assist in determining modifying factors are as follows:
   - Does anything make it (the symptom) better?
   - Does anything make it worse?
   - What have you done to make it better?
   - What did you do to help it?
   - Are you taking any medication for it? Did it help?

7. Associated symptoms. There is usually more than one symptom associated with a disease process. Determining these additional symptoms gives the physician a complete picture of the illness. Examples of questions that help to identify the presence of additional symptoms are as follows:
   - Are you having any other symptoms?
   - What other problems have you noticed since you became ill?

Examples

The following examples illustrate how to analyze a symptom. The chief complaint is listed first, followed by questions to ask the patient from the seven basic categories of information.

Example: *Chief complaint: Headaches that began 2 months ago*

1. Using your finger, point to the location of the headache.
2. Describe the pain. Is it sharp, dull, throbbing?
3. Are you able to carry on normal activities when you have a headache?
4. Is it sometimes more severe than usual?
5. When exactly did your headaches begin?
6. How long does your headache last when it occurs?
7. How often do you get a headache?
8. Since your headaches began, have they gotten better or worse, or have they stayed the same?
9. What were you doing the first time you experienced a headache?
10. What was your health status before your headaches began?
11. Do you get a headache before, during, or after a particular activity, such as reading or watching TV?
12. Does anything make your headache better?
13. Are you taking any medication for your headache? Does it help?
14. Have you had any other problems since your headaches began, such as nausea, vomiting, dizziness, or problems with vision?

Example: *Chief complaint: The patient has been coughing for the past 3 days.*

1. Does it hurt when you cough? Where? Show me with one of your fingers.
2. What is the cough like?
3. Can you cough for me?
4. Do you bring up any phlegm when you cough? What color is it? Is blood present?
5. Describe the pain. Is it sharp, dull, squeezing?
6. Do you become exhausted when you cough?
7. How much phlegm do you bring up? A teaspoon? Half a cup?

8. How much blood is present in the phlegm?

9. When did your cough first begin?

10. Does it seem like an attack? How long does the attack last?

11. How often do you get a coughing attack?

12. Does your cough seem to be getting better or worse?

13. What was the first thing you noticed when you became ill?

14. How were you feeling before your symptoms began?

15. Is there anything that makes your cough better?

16. Is there anything that makes your cough worse?

17. Do you cough more at night or during the day?

18. Are you taking any medication for it? Does it help?

19. Are you having any other problems?

Practice Problems

In the space provided, indicate examples of direct questions to ask the patient to obtain the necessary information for the symptoms presented in the chief complaint.

Problem 1

Chief complaint: *Earache and fever for the past 2 days*

Questions:

___

___

___

___

___

___

___

___

___

___

Problem 2

Chief complaint: *Rash with itching that began 3 days ago*

Questions:

____

____

____

____

____

____

____

____

____

____

Problem 3

Chief complaint: *Pain during urination that began yesterday*

Questions:

____

____

____

____

____

____

____

____

____

____

Problem 4

Chief complaint: *Low back pain for the past 3 months*

Questions:

Problem 5

Chief complaint: *Sore throat and fever for the past 24 hours*

Questions:

Problem 6

Chief complaint: *Chest pain that occurred this morning*

Questions:

Terms for Describing Symptoms

Pain

Burning, aching, sharp, dull, throbbing, cramping, squeezing

Radiating, transient, constant

Localized, superficial, deep

Respirations

Rapid, irregular, shallow, deep, labored, gasping, noisy, wheezing

Apnea, dyspnea, orthopnea

Discomfort, pain, cyanosis, cough

Cough

Nonproductive, productive

Persistent, dry, hacking, barking, spasmodic

Phlegm: color, consistency, presence or absence of blood

Exhausting or painful

Cardiovascular System

Pain, palpitations

Sharp, radiating

Dyspnea, orthopnea

Cyanosis

Gastrointestinal System

Abdomen: flaccid, rigid, distended

Appetite: anorexia, intolerance to foods

Heartburn, pain after eating, belching, nausea, vomiting, flatulence, change in bowel habits, constipation, diarrhea, black stools

Urine or Stool

Abnormality: color, odor, consistency, frequency

Contents: sediment, mucus, blood

Elimination: urgency, nocturia, pain, burning

Skin

Rash: pruritus, red, swelling, distribution

Lesions: color, character, distribution

Pallor: flushing, jaundice, warm, dry, cold, clammy

Ecchymosis, petechiae, cyanosis, edema

Pruritus, sweating, change in color, bruises easily

Ears

Pain, loss of hearing, tinnitus, vertigo

Discharge, infection

Eyes

Itching, burning, blurry vision, seeing double, photophobia

Discharge, watering, infection

Notes

39 Patient Reception

CHAPTER ASSIGNMENTS

✓ After Completing	Date Due	Study Guide Pages	STUDY GUIDE ASSIGNMENTS (CTA = Critical Thinking Activity)	Possible Points	Points You Earned
		1109	Pretest	10	
		1110	Key Term Assessment	5	
		1110-1112	Evaluation of Learning questions	18	
		1112	CTA A: Privacy Practices	5	
		1112	CTA B: Verifying Insurance and Referrals	8	
		1113	CTA C: Patient Informational Material	20	
			Evolve Site: Apply Your Knowledge questions	10	
			Evolve Site: Video Evaluation	8	
		1109	Posttest	10	
			ADDITIONAL ASSIGNMENTS		
			TOTAL POINTS		

Notes

✓ When Assigned By Your Instructor	Study Guide Pages	Practices Required	LABORATORY ASSIGNMENTS (Procedure Number and Name)	Score*
	1115	3	**Practice for Competency** 39-1: Opening the Medical Office Textbook reference: pp. 1027-1028	
	1121-1122		**Evaluation of Competency** 39-1: Opening the Medical Office	*
	1115	3	**Practice for Competency** 39-2: Closing the Medical Office Textbook reference: p. 1028	
	1123-1124		**Evaluation of Competency** 39-2: Closing the Medical Office	*
	1116-1119	3	**Practice for Competency** 39-3: Obtaining New Patient Information Textbook reference: pp. 1035-1036	
	1125-1127		**Evaluation of Competency** 39-3: Obtaining New Patient Information	*
	1119	3	**Practice for Competency** 39-4: Explaining Office Policies and Procedures Textbook reference: pp. 1037-1038	
	1129-1130		**Evaluation of Competency** 39-4: Explaining Office Policies and Procedures	*
			ADDITIONAL ASSIGNMENTS	

Notes

Name ______________________________ Date ______________

PRETEST

True or False

_______ 1. The first thing the medical assistant (MA) does when opening the office is to unlock the file cabinets, medical record files, and medicine cabinets.

_______ 2. After opening the office, the MA should be sure that the telephones are switched to the day message or call the answering service.

_______ 3. An electronic task system consists of a folder for each month and a folder for each day.

_______ 4. Some types of insurance require authorization every time the patient visits the primary care physician.

_______ 5. A radio, CD player, television, or DVD player is usually turned on in the morning before patients arrive.

_______ 6. The autoclave is often run just before closing the medical office so that instruments can dry overnight.

_______ 7. Only one person at a time should be permitted to stand at the reception desk to check in.

_______ 8. A new patient must sign a form acknowledging receipt of HIPAA privacy practices.

_______ 9. Only the top side of the insurance card must be photocopied.

_______ 10. If a patient has managed care insurance, a referral form may be required to see a physician other than the primary care provider.

POSTTEST

True or False

_______ 1. As soon as the MA has opened the office, he or she usually runs the autoclave.

_______ 2. After opening the office, the MA should check the fax machine for faxes that may have arrived overnight.

_______ 3. A tickler file is used to remind the MA of tasks to be done on a specific day.

_______ 4. The medical assistant must place a telephone call in order to obtain authorization for an office visit if a patient has Medicaid or Medicare.

_______ 5. Holders for patient information brochures are often located in the waiting room.

_______ 6. The MA turns off all equipment as the last thing when closing the office.

_______ 7. A sliding glass window between the waiting room and reception desk helps maintain patient confidentiality.

_______ 8. A new patient must sign a form providing consent for treatment and release of information.

_______ 9. Insurance companies usually require authorization every time the patient sees the primary care physician.

_______ 10. If the patient has a copayment, it is usually collected before the patient sees the physician.

Term KEY TERM ASSESSMENT

Directions: Match each key term with its definition.

_______ 1. Assignment of benefits

_______ 2. Call-in times

_______ 3. Copayment

_______ 4. Medicaid

_______ 5. Tickler file

A. A fixed amount of money that the patient is responsible to pay at each visit

B. A chronological file containing reminders of things to be done

C. Authorization given by the patient to allow the insurance company to make payments directly to the health care provider

D. Blocks of time when a physician accepts telephone calls from patients

E. A federal and state insurance program for low-income patients

EVALUATION OF LEARNING

Directions: Fill in each blank with the correct answer.

1. List five activities that the MA must perform to open the office.

____

____

2. How does the MA prepare the telephone system for patient calls at the beginning of the day?

____

____

3. How should the MA prepare for the day's activities in the medical office?

____

____

4. If an office uses paper medical records, how are they prepared before patients arrive?

____

____

____

5. What should the MA do to be sure the waiting room is ready for patients?

____

____

6. How does the MA check equipment and prepare supplies at the beginning of the day?

____

____

____

7. List seven tasks that the MA should perform when closing the medical office.

____

____

____

8. How does the medical office identify which patients have arrived for appointments?

____

____

9. What is the function of a sliding glass window between the reception desk and the patient waiting area?

____

10. Identify at least three statements or forms that a new patient must sign before being examined by the physician.

____

____

11. What is required by the HIPAA legislation related to notifying patients about privacy practices?

____

____

12. How does the MA verify a patient's identity and insurance information?

____

____

____

____

13. When does a patient need a written or electronic referral form?

____

14. What information is included in a written or electronic referral form?

____

____

15. What information must be obtained from an established patient who is checking in?

____

____

16. What is a copayment, and when is a copayment usually collected?

____

17. What are at least eight pieces of information about a medical practice that might be found on a website or in an informational brochure?

____

____

____

____

____

18. What are three reasons that a physician might not be accepting new patients?

____

____

CRITICAL THINKING ACTIVITIES

A. Privacy Practices

Obtain a printed sample Notice of Privacy Practices from a medical office either from your own physician or from the Internet. Many organizations post their privacy statements on their websites. Using the copy of the privacy practices statement, highlight the sections where the following required content is included. Then write a brief statement stating whether your example contains all required information or not.

1. How the medical office may use and disclose protected health information about an individual.
2. The individual's rights with respect to the information and how the individual may exercise these rights, including how the individual may complain to the medical office.
3. The medical office's legal duties with respect to the information, including a statement that the medical office is required by law to maintain the privacy of protected health information.
4. How individuals can obtain further information about the medical office's privacy policies.
5. The effective date of the Notice of Privacy Practices.

B. Verifying Insurance and Referrals

Based on information in the chapter, choose the following methods necessary to verify that the patient's insurance will cover charges and that the patient has a completed referral form if necessary. Enter the letter(s) of the correct step(s) the MA must take when a patient checks in. Some situations require more than one answer.

a. Ask to see the patient's insurance card (or card of the insured party).

b. Ask to see and scan or make a photocopy of the patient's insurance card (or card of the insured party).

c. Check that the patient has current insurance using a card reader, fax, computer, or telephone.

d. Use a telephone or computer to verify insurance coverage and/or obtain preauthorization.

e. Check to see that there is a completed referral form.

f. Explain that the patient will be responsible for the bill because insurance will not cover the service(s).

1. An established patient has an appointment with his or her primary care physician. ________________
2. A new patient has an appointment with a primary care physician. ________________
3. A new patient with managed care insurance has an appointment with a cardiologist. ________________
4. An established patient with Medicaid has an appointment for a blood pressure check. ________________
5. An established patient tells the MA that she has changed insurance since the last visit. ________________
6. A new patient with managed care insurance visits a dermatologist for a minor surgical procedure. ________________
7. A mother brings an infant to the pediatrician for his or her first well-baby checkup. ________________
8. An established patient is being scheduled for a cosmetic laser procedure. ________________

C. Patient Informational Material

1. Create a patient information brochure or use a word processing program to create two or more web pages for a physician in private practice. Assume that the location of the office is at the same address as your medical assisting school. Include the following information:
   - Physician's name, credentials, and specialty
   - Brief statement of the physician's philosophy of patient care
   - Directions to the office, parking, and access to public transportation, if any
   - General statement that most insurance is accepted and that copayments are expected at the time of the visit
   - Policy regarding cancellation of appointments
   - Name of a local hospital that the physician is affiliated with
   - Description of how medication refills are handled

2. Compare your patient informational material with that of at least two of your classmates and discuss how this material could be used by the medical office.

Notes

PRACTICE FOR COMPETENCY

Procedure 39-1: Opening the Medical Office. Practice opening the office.

A. Make a list of tasks to open the office:

____

____

____

____

____

____

Procedure 39-2: Closing the Medical Office. Practice closing the office.

A. Make a list of tasks to close the office:

____

____

____

____

____

____

New Patient Information Form. Complete the new patient information form using yourself as the patient. Use the form to practice Procedure 39-3.

REGISTRATION
(PLEASE PRINT)

Home Phone: ____________ Today's Date: ____________

PATIENT INFORMATION

Name ____________ Last Name First Name Initial Soc. Sec.# ____________

Address ____________

City ____________ State ____________ Zip ____________

Single ___ Married ___ Widowed ___ Separated ___ Divorced ___ Sex M___ F___ Age ___ Birthdate ____________

Patient Employed by ____________ Occupation ____________

Business Address ____________ Business Phone ____________

By whom were you referred? ____________

In case of emergency who should be notified? ____________ Last Name Relationship to Patient Phone ____________

PRIMARY INSURANCE

Person Responsible for Account ____________ Last Name First Name Initial

Relation to Patient ____________ Birthdate ____________ Soc. Sec.# ____________

Address (if different from patient's) ____________ Phone ____________

City ____________ State ____________ Zip ____________

Person Responsible Employed by ____________ Occupation ____________

Business Address ____________ Business Phone ____________

Insurance Company ____________

Contract # ____________ Group # ____________ Subscriber # ____________

Name of other dependents covered under this plan ____________

ADDITIONAL INSURANCE

Is patient covered by additional insurance? ___ Yes ___ No

Subscriber Name ____________ Relationship to Patient ____________ Birthdate ____________

Address (if different from patient's) ____________ Phone ____________

City ____________ State ____________ Zip ____________

Subscriber Employed by ____________ Business Phone ____________

Insurance Company ____________

Contract # ____________ Group # ____________ Subscriber # ____________

Name of other dependents covered under this plan ____________

ASSIGNMENT AND RELEASE

I, the undersigned, certify that I (or my dependent) have insurance coverage with ____________ Name of Insurance Company(ies)

and assign directly to Dr. ____________ insurance benefits, if any, otherwise payable to me for services rendered. I understand that I am financially responsible for all charges whether or not paid by insurance. I hereby authorize the doctor to release all information necessary to secure the payment of benefits. I authorize the use of this signature on all insurance submissions.

____________ Responsible Party Signature ____________ Relationship ____________ Date

ORDER# 58-8426 • © 1996 BIBBERO SYSTEMS, INC. • PETALUMA, CALIFORNIA • TO REORDER CALL TOLL FREE: (800) 242-9330

(Courtesy Bibbero Systems, Inc., Petaluma, Calif. [800] 242-2396; Fax [800] 242-9330; www.bibbero.com.)

Acknowledgment of Receipt of Notice of HIPAA Privacy Practices Form. Complete the Acknowledgment of Receipt of Notice of HIPAA Privacy Practices Form using yourself as the patient. Use the form to practice Procedure 39-3.

Acknowledgment of Receipt of the Notice of Privacy Practices

Please Review Carefully

The Notice of Privacy Practices tells you how **[Practice Name]** uses and discloses information about you. Not all situations will be described. We are required to give you a notice of our privacy practices for the information we collect and keep about you. We reserve the right to revise this notice, and you can obtain a copy of any revision upon written request.

I, ____, have been given a copy of the **Notice of Privacy Practices.**

______________________________	__________	____________________
Patient or Legal Guardian's Signature	Date	Relationship to Patient

______________________________	______________________________
Print Patient's Name	Print Name of Legal Guardian (if any)

______________________________________	__________
Signature of Witness (If signed with an "X" or mark)	Date

Effective Date: April 14, 2003

WALDEN-MARTIN

FAMILY MEDICAL CLINIC
1234 ANYSTREET ANYTOWN, ANYSTATE 1234
PHONE 123-123-1234 FAX 123-123-5678

PATIENT INFORMATION FORM – ADDITIONAL INFORMATION

Patient Name: ______________________ Date: ______________

1. Do you have a written Advanced Directive/Living Will or Healthcare Power of Attorney in place? If yes, please plan to bring a copy with you to your next appointment for us to scan into your record.

☐ YES ☐ NO

If no, would you like information regarding your patient rights in making healthcare decisions?

☐ YES ☐ NO

2. May we send you email or text messages

☐ YES ☐ NO

Email address: ______________________

Cell phone # for text messages: ______________________

3. What is your Ethnicity?
   - ☐ Hispanic or Latino
   - ☐ Not Hispanic or Latino
   - ☐ Decline to Specify

4. What is your race?
   - ☐ American Indian or Alaska Native
   - ☐ Asian
   - ☐ Black or African American
   - ☐ Decline to Specify
   - ☐ Native Hawaiian/Other Pacific Islander
   - ☐ White

5. What is your preferred language for communication?

Patient Signature: ______________________ Date: ______________

Procedure 39-3: Obtaining New Patient Information. Practice obtaining new patient information from classmates using the forms they completed on the previous pages. Review a classmate's form to be sure it is complete. Explain what information is needed if there is missing information.

Enter a New Patient into SimChart® for the Medical Office

Practice entering the information from your own form into SimChart® for the Medical Office using the Simulation Playground. Create an imaginary name for the patient. Click the **Patient Demographics** icon and perform a patient search to be sure that a record does not already exist. Then click the **Add Patient** button. Enter the information in the required fields using the **Patient, Guarantor**, and **Insurance** tabs. Save the information on each tab before moving to the next tab. After completing all three tabs, click the Save Patient button.

Procedure 39-4: Explaining Office Policies and Procedures. Using the patient information brochure prepared for Critical Thinking Activity C, practice orienting classmates (as simulated new patients) to office policies and procedures. Discuss adaptations that might need to be made for patients from different cultural backgrounds, different developmental levels, and if barriers to communication exist.

Notes

EVALUATION OF COMPETENCY

Procedure 39-1: Opening the Medical Office

Name: ______________________ Date: ______________

Evaluated by: ______________________ Score: ______________

Performance Objective

Outcome:	Open the medical office.
Conditions:	In a medical office.
Standards:	Time: 15 minutes. Student completed procedure in ________ minutes.
	Accuracy: Satisfactory score on the Performance Evaluation Checklist.

Performance Evaluation Checklist

Trial 1	Trial 2	Point Value	Performance Standards
		•	Entered the office and disarmed any alarm system.
		•	Turned on the lights.
		•	Adjusted heat or air conditioning to a comfortable setting.
		•	Unlocked the door for patients and visitors to enter.
		•	Turned on computers, printers, copier, and/or other machines.
		•	Called answering service for messages or listened to messages from voice mail or office answering machine.
		•	Wrote down complete message information on message forms.
		•	Arranged messages in order of importance.
		•	Dealt with urgent messages or calls.
		•	Pulled paper medical records for routine messages about patients.
		•	Clipped each message about a patient to the correct medical record.
		•	Placed routine messages in appropriate location(s) for office staff to review.
		•	Reviewed the day's activities and noted any special tasks.
		•	Counted the money in the cash drawer and recorded the amount.
		•	Checked the office for safety hazards.
		•	Straightened up the waiting room and turned on radio, television, or DVD player.
		•	Refilled holder of patient information brochures as needed.
		•	Printed appointment lists as needed.
		•	Pulled medical records as needed for the day's appointments.

Trial 1	Trial 2	Point Value	Performance Standards
		●	Arranged paper medical records in order of appointments.
		●	Printed or stamped the date on progress notes of paper medical records as needed.
		●	Printed any necessary paperwork required by an electronic medical record system.
		●	Prepared charge slips and clipped to patient records, if office policy.
		●	Checked biohazard waste containers and changed or discarded properly.
		●	Ran or emptied the autoclave as needed.
		*	Completed the procedure within 15 minutes.
			TOTALS

Evaluation of Student Performance

EVALUATION CRITERIA			COMMENTS
Symbol	Category	Point Value	
*	Critical Step	16 points	
●	Essential Step	6 points	
Ⓐ	Affective Competency	6 points	
▷	Theory Question	2 points	
Score calculation: 100 points – ___ points missed ___ Score Satisfactory score: 85 or above			

2008 CAAHEP Competencies Achieved
Psychomotor (Skills) ☑ V. 9. Perform routine maintenance of office equipment with documentation. ☑ XI. 2. Evaluate the work environment to identify safe vs. unsafe working conditions. ***Affective (Behavior)*** ☑ V. 2. Implement time management principles to maintain effective office function.

2015 CAAHEP Competencies Achieved
Psychomotor (Skills) ☑ VI. 8. Perform routine maintenance of administrative or clinical equipment. ☑ XII. 5. Evaluate the work environment to identify safe vs. unsafe working conditions.

ABHES Competencies Achieved
☑ 8.e.1. Perform routine maintenance of administrative equipment.

EVALUATION OF COMPETENCY

Procedure 39-2: Closing the Medical Office

Name: ______________________ Date: ______________________

Evaluated by: ______________________ Score: ______________________

Performance Objective

Outcome:	Open the medical office.
Conditions:	In a medical office.
Standards:	Time: 15 minutes. Student completed procedure in ________ minutes.
	Accuracy: Satisfactory score on the Performance Evaluation Checklist.

Performance Evaluation Checklist

Trial 1	Trial 2	Point Value	Performance Standards
		•	Made sure examination rooms were clean and contained all necessary supplies.
		•	Ran the autoclave if needed.
		•	Printed a patient schedule for the next day.
		•	Pulled paper medical records for the next day.
		•	Printed charge slips and clipped to the medical records, if office policy.
		•	Made sure cabinets or rooms containing medical records were locked.
		•	Balanced the cash drawer and prepared the bank deposit. Made bank deposit at the end of the day.
		•	Locked the cash drawer or placed the cash fund in the office safe.
		•	Activated the night telephone system by switching telephone message or calling the answering service.
		•	Turned off office machines including computers, printers, and photocopier.
		•	Unplugged coffee pot, toaster, or other machines that might pose a fire hazard.
		•	Locked door used for patients and visitors.
		•	Turned heat or air conditioning to night setting.
		•	Turned off the lights.
		•	Armed the security system.
		•	Made sure that staff exit door was locked securely.
		*	Completed the procedure within 15 minutes.
			TOTALS

Evaluation of Student Performance

EVALUATION CRITERIA			COMMENTS
Symbol	**Category**	**Point Value**	
✶	Critical Step	16 points	
●	Essential Step	6 points	
Ⓐ	Affective Competency	6 points	
▷	Theory Question	2 points	
Score calculation: 100 points – ____ points missed ____ Score Satisfactory score: 85 or above			

2008 CAAHEP Competency Achieved
Affective (Behavior) ☑ V. 2. Implement time management principles to maintain effective office function.

2015 CAAHEP Competency Achieved
Psychomotor ☑ III.5. Perform sterilization procedures.

ABHES Competency Achieved
☑ 9.a. Practice standard precautions and perform disinfection/sterilization techniques.

EVALUATION OF COMPETENCY

Procedure 39-3: Obtaining New Patient Information

Name: ________________________ Date: ________________

Evaluated by: ________________________ Score: ________________

Performance Objective

Outcome:	Obtain new patient information, obtain consents, and validate insurance coverage.
Conditions:	Given the following: clipboard, pen, new patient information form, Notice of Privacy Practices form, receipt of Notice of Privacy Practices form, consent for release of protected health information (optional), photocopier, insurance card reader (optional), telephone, medical record, computer, and scanner.
Standards:	Time: 10 minutes. Student completed procedure in ________ minutes.
	Accuracy: Satisfactory score on the Performance Evaluation Checklist.

Performance Evaluation Checklist

Trial 1	Trial 2	Point Value	Performance Standards
		•	Placed a new patient information form on a clipboard with a pen.
		•	Asked a new patient to complete the form and return it.
		▷	Explained why patient privacy must be maintained and identified measures to maintain it.
		•	Verified that the form was complete and signed by the patient or authorized representative.
		•	Asked to see the insurance card of the patient or insured individual.
		•	Photocopied both sides of the insurance card or scanned the insurance card to the office computer system.
		•	Placed the photocopy of the insurance card in the patient's medical record if a paper medical record was used.
		•	Confirmed patient eligibility for insurance as needed using a card reader, computer or telephone.
		•	Verified that there was a completed referral form as needed.
		•	Verified patient's identification using a photo ID or two other forms of identification (if it is office policy)
		•	Displayed sensitivity when communicating with patient regarding third party requirements.
		•	Displayed sensitivity when discussing the patient's financial responsibility, if the visit would not be completely covered by insurance.
		•	Gave the patient a copy of the Notice of Privacy Practices or made it available for the patient to read.

Trial 1	Trial 2	Point Value	Performance Standards
		✶	Asked the patient to sign the form indicating receipt of the Notice of Privacy Practices.
		●	Signed the Notice of Privacy Practices form as a witness.
		●	Asked the patient to read and sign any consent for release of personal health information used by the office.
		●	Inserted new forms into the paper medical record or scanned forms to the office computer system.
		●	Placed the medical record (or other paperwork) and charge slip to indicate that the patient has been checked in.
		●	Asked the patient to have a seat and indicated the probable wait time.
		●	Transferred information from the new patient information form to the patient's computer account (or validated that information obtained by telephone was correct.)
		●	Scanned patient forms according to office policy (if the office uses an electronic medical record).
		✶	Maintained professionalism and used appropriate body language in communicating with patients, family and staff.
		✶	Maintained patient confidentiality through the entire procedure.
		✶	Completed the procedure within 10 minutes.
			TOTALS

Evaluation of Student Performance

EVALUATION CRITERIA			COMMENTS
Symbol	**Category**	**Point Value**	
✶	Critical Step	16 points	
●	Essential Step	6 points	
Ⓐ	Affective Competency	6 points	
▷	Theory Question	2 points	
Score calculation: 100 points – ___ points missed ___ Score Satisfactory score: 85 or above			

2008 CAAHEP Competencies Achieved
Psychomotor (Skills) ☑ VII. 1. Apply both managed care policies and procedures. ☑ VII. 2. Apply third party guidelines. ☑ VII. 6. Verify eligibility for managed care services. ☑ IX. 1. Respond to issues of confidentiality. ☑ IX. 3. Apply HIPAA rules in regard to the privacy/release of information. ***Affective (Behavior)*** ☑ IV. 3. Use appropriate body language and other nonverbal skills in communicating with patients, family and staff. ☑ IX. 3. Recognize the importance of local, state, and federal legislation and regulations in the practice setting.

2015 CAAHEP Competencies Achieved
Psychomotor (Skills) ☑ VI.7. Input patient data utilizing a practice management system. ☑ VII.3. Obtain accurate patient billing information. ☑ VII. 4. Inform a patient of financial obligations for services rendered. ☑ VIII.2. Verify eligibility for services including documentation. ☑ X.2.a. Apply HIPAA rules in regard to privacy. ***Affective (Behavior)*** ☑ VII.2. Display sensitivity when requesting payment for services rendered. ☑ VIII.3. Display sensitivity when communicating with patients regarding third party requirements.

ABHES Competency Achieved
☑ 4. c. Follow established policies when initiating or terminating medical treatment. ☑ 4. f. Comply with federal, state and local health laws and regulations. ☑ 8. c.2. Differentiate managed care: i.e. HOM, PPO, IPA including referrals and pre-certification. ☑ 8. f. Display professionalism through written and verbal communication.

Notes

EVALUATION OF COMPETENCY

Procedure 39-4: Explaining Office Policies and Procedures

Name: ______________________ Date: ______________________

Evaluated by: ______________________ Score: ______________________

Performance Objective

Outcome:	Orient a new patient to the medical office.
Conditions:	Given the following: patient information booklet, map, list of points to cover.
Standards:	Time: 10 minutes. Student completed procedure in ________ minutes.
	Accuracy: Satisfactory score on the Performance Evaluation Checklist.

Performance Evaluation Checklist

Trial 1	Trial 2	Point Value	Performance Standards
		•	Offered to give or send a patient information booklet if one is available.
		•	Took the patient's cultural background, developmental life stage, and potential barriers to communication into consideration when coaching the patient about office policies.
		•	Identified the name, credentials, and specialty of each physician who would accept new patients.
		•	Offered information as required about languages spoken in the office and any additional services that would be available.
		•	Identified the location of the office, gave directions, and discussed parking as needed.
		•	Told the patient if the office accepted his or her medical insurance plan.
		•	Discussed expectations for payment of the patient's bill.
		•	Described how far in advance to make and/or cancel appointments.
		•	Told the patient how to contact the office.
		•	Informed the patient if the physician had specific call-in times.
		•	Explained how prescription refills would be handled.
		•	Identified hospital affiliation(s) of the office physician(s).
		•	Asked if there were other questions and responded-appropriately.
		•	Applied active listening skills when communicating with the patient and/or family.
		*	Completed the procedure within 10 minutes.
			TOTALS

Evaluation of Student Performance

EVALUATION CRITERIA			COMMENTS
Symbol	**Category**	**Point Value**	
∗	Critical Step	16 points	
●	Essential Step	6 points	
Ⓐ	Affective Competency	6 points	
▷	Theory Question	2 points	
Score calculation: 100 points – ___ points missed ___Score Satisfactory score: 85 or above			

2008 CAAHEP Competencies Achieved
Psychomotor (Skills) ☑ IV. 4. Explain general office policies. ***Affective (Behavior)*** ☑ IV. 2. Apply active listening skills. ☑ IV. 7. Demonstrate recognition of the patient's level of understanding in communication. ☑ VII. 3. Communicate in language the patient can understand regarding-managed care and insurance plans.

2015 CAAHEP Competencies Achieved
Psychomotor (Skills) ☑ V.4.a. Coach patients regarding office policies ☑ V.5. Coach patients appropriately considering a. cultural diversity, b. developmental life state, c. communication barriers. ***Affective (Behavior)*** ☑ V.1.b. Demonstrate active listening

ABHES Competency Achieved
☑ 8. 2.f. Display professionalism through written and verbal communication.

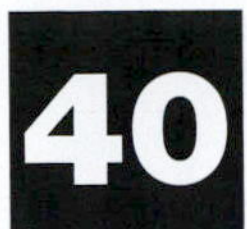

Medical Office Computerization

CHAPTER ASSIGNMENTS

✓ After Completing	Date Due	Study Guide Pages	STUDY GUIDE ASSIGNMENTS (CTA = Critical Thinking Activity)	Possible Points	Points You Earned
		1133	Pretest	10	
		1134	Term Key Term Assessment—Part I	24	
		1135	Term Key Term Assessment—Part II	21	
		1135-1142	Evaluation of Learning questions	66	
		1142	CTA A: Computer System	7	
		1142-1143	CTA B: Computer Monitor	5	
		1143	CTA C: Storage Size	7	
			Evolve Site: Apply Your Knowledge questions	10	
		1133	Posttest	10	
			ADDITIONAL ASSIGNMENTS		
			TOTAL POINTS		

Notes

Name ______________________________ Date ______________

PRETEST

True or False

_______ 1. Computers that are linked together are known as a network.

_______ 2. The transfer of data to the computer for processing is known as input.

_______ 3. Spreadsheet software consists of an electronic ledger designed to perform mathematical calculations quickly.

_______ 4. The information in RAM (random access memory) is permanently stored on the computer.

_______ 5. A monitor should be cleaned by wiping it gently with a soft, lint free cloth or a commercial wipe.

_______ 6. The Internet is a global system of interconnected computer networks.

_______ 7. Printed output from a computer is known as hard copy.

_______ 8. A USB flash drive stores information in the form of magnetized particles.

_______ 9. Antivirus software monitors all files for malicious software designed to penetrate a computer network without consent.

_______ 10. Paper documents are entered into a patient's EHR by scanning them into the computer.

POSTTEST

True or False

_______ 1. A program that consists of raw, unorganized facts about subject matter is entered into the computer for processing.

_______ 2. An operating system assists the computer in carrying out its tasks.

_______ 3. The mainboard directs the step-by-step operation of all the processing functions.

_______ 4. One gigabyte (GB) is equal to 1000 megabytes (MB).

_______ 5. The screen size of a typical desktop monitor is larger than the screen size of a laptop computer.

_______ 6. The monitor should be placed so that the top of the monitor is about 4 inches below eye level.

_______ 7. Grime can be removed from a computer keyboard using a can of compressed inert gas.

_______ 8. When a computer is turned off, all the information in RAM is lost.

_______ 9. The reports system allows the user to customize a medical management program to meet the specific requirements of a medical office.

_______ 10. A system that protects a computer network from unauthorized access by users on the Internet is known as a firewall.

Term KEY TERM ASSESSMENT—PART I

Directions: Match each computer term with its definition.

_______ 1. App
_______ 2. Backup
_______ 3. Broadband
_______ 4. Cloud computing
_______ 5. Computer
_______ 6. Computer system
_______ 7. Data
_______ 8. Data processing
_______ 9. Digital subscriber line (DSL)
_______ 10. Documentation
_______ 11. Email
_______ 12. Encryption
_______ 13. Firewall
_______ 14. Hard disk drive
_______ 15. Hard copy
_______ 16. Hardware
_______ 17. Input
_______ 18. Input device
_______ 19. Internet
_______ 20. Main computer memory
_______ 21. Microcomputer
_______ 22. Microprocessor
_______ 23. Network
_______ 24. Operating system

A. Raw, unorganized facts about subject matter presented to the computer for processing
B. The "brain" of the computer housed in the main unit that interprets and executes the instructions that operate the computer
C. A written set of instructions accompanying an application program, designed to assist the user in operating the program
D. Technology that allows digital signals to be transmitted over telephone lines at high speed
E. A method of transmitting electronic data that handles a wide range of frequencies
F. A device for entering data into the computer (e.g., keyboard, mouse, scanner)
G. A small general purpose computer that relies on a tiny microprocessor chip to perform its processing functions
H. A storage device consisting of one or more rigid, nonflexible platters coated with a magnetically sensitive material and encased in a permanently sealed, air-tight container
I. A model where the Internet is used to store and access data and programs, and servers are not physically located at the same site as the computer
J. A system that protects a computer network from unauthorized access by users on its own network or another network, such as the Internet
K. A type of system software that performs tasks required by the computer to operate itself
L. All of the hardware and software components making up the computer
M. An electronic machine that has the ability to process data according to a program in order to produce a desired result
N. Printed output from a computer
O. A specialized program, often small enough to run on a mobile device
P. The part of the central processing unit (CPU) that is responsible for temporarily storing information until it is needed for processing
Q. The physical devices making up a computer system (e.g., main computer unit, keyboard, monitor, printer)
R. The transfer of data to the computer for processing
S. A duplicate copy of a program or data kept in case the original is damaged, lost, or destroyed
T. The changing of raw facts or data into usable information following a three-part sequence: input, processing, output
U. A method of composing, sending, receiving and storing messages sent over the Internet
V. A process by which electronic information is changed into an unreadable format
W. A group of computers that share data and resources
X. A global system of interconnected computer networks

KEY TERM ASSESSMENT—PART II

Directions: Match each computer term with its definition.

_______ 1. Optical disc
_______ 2. Optical disc drive
_______ 3. Output
_______ 4. Output device
_______ 5. Patient portal
_______ 6. Printing speed
_______ 7. Processing
_______ 8. Program
_______ 9. RAM (random-access memory)
_______ 10. Router
_______ 11. Sequential access memory
_______ 12. Server
_______ 13. Software
_______ 14. Solid state drive
_______ 15. Special keys
_______ 16. Storage capacity
_______ 17. Storage device
_______ 18. URL
_______ 19. User
_______ 20. Web browser
_______ 21. World Wide Web

A. A large computer that stores data and manages tasks for other computers on a network
B. A general term for the programs or instructions that tell a computer what to do
C. A set of instructions organized in a logical step-by-step sequence, which tells the computer how to perform a specific function
D. A wired or wireless device used to form or connect networks
E. The main computer memory of a microcomputer, which is used to temporarily store items until needed by the computer for processing
F. The number of pages per minute (ppm) generated by a printer
G. A device that transfers processed data to the user (e.g., computer monitor and printer)
H. A storage device consisting of a flat, round, portable disk that stores data using laser technology
I. Uses integrated circuits (flash memory) to store data permanently
J. The individual using the computer
K. A series of interlinked websites or files accessed via the Internet
L. A software program used to access the World Wide Web
M. Keys that issue commands to the computer to perform specific functions
N. A device installed in a drive bay on the main computer unit that uses a laser to read an optical disc or write onto (burn) an optical disc
O. The transfer of processed data back to the user
P. The manipulation and reorganization of data according to the instructions in a program
Q. The maximum amount of information that a device can hold, measured in bytes
R. Computer memory in which all stored data must be searched from beginning to end to locate the desired information
S. A device that permanently stores information for later retrieval by the computer
T. The characters and/or words used to access a specific website or file on the World Wide Web
U. An online application that allows patients to interact with and communicate with their healthcare providers

EVALUATION OF LEARNING

Directions: Fill in each blank with the correct answer.

Computer Concepts

1. What are the principal uses of a computer to perform administrative procedures in the medical office?

____

____

2. What is a computer network?

3. What are the three phases included in the data processing sequence?

4. Why must data be converted into an electronic code before being processed by the computer?

5. What are four examples of input devices?

6. List two examples of output devices.

7. What is the difference between system software and application software?

8. What is the function of an operating system?

9. What tasks are performed by the word processing function included in a medical practice management program?

10. What is spreadsheet software?

11. How does a practice management program work like a spreadsheet application program?

12. What are telecommunication functions included in a practice management program?

13. What is database management?

14. What functions can be performed by database management software?

15. What is the relationship between practice management software and and electronic health record when both are used in a medical office?

____

____

16. What is voice recognition software used for?

____

17. List five methods that practice management programs and/or electronic health records use to enter data.

____

____

18. Describe they type of data saved using the following file formats.

.bmp ____

.gif ____

.doc or .docx ____

.rtf ____

.txt ____

.xls or .xlsx ____

19. What are examples of documentation?

____

20. What computer hardware is necessary to perform administrative procedures in the medical office?

____

____

21. What is the function of the microprocessor (central processing unit or CPU)?

____

____

22. What is the difference in processing speed between a CPU with a 3-GHz chip and one with a 1.5-GHz chip?

____

23. What is the function of main memory (RAM)?

____

____

24. What items are commonly held in RAM?

____

____

25. What is the difference between random access and sequential access?

26. What happens to data in RAM when a computer is turned off?

27. How are units of storage capacity of a computer named?

28. Explain how to prevent overheating of the computer.

29. What is the primary cause of improper functioning of the computer?

30. What can happen if a liquid spills into the main computer unit?

31. What is the function of the computer monitor?

32. What are the advantages and disadvantages of a liquid crystal display (LCD) flat panel monitor?

33. How should the monitor be positioned to prevent back and neck tension?

34. What can be done to prevent eye strain when working with a computer monitor?

35. What is the difference between a glare filter and a privacy filter?

36. What are the functions and examples of the following special keys?

    a. Modifier keys

b. Lock keys

____

____

c. Navigation keys

____

____

37. How should the computer keyboard be positioned to prevent muscle fatigue?

____

38. How should the following parts of a keyboard be cleaned?

a. Surface of the keyboard: ____

b. Interior of the keyboard: ____

39. What should be done if water spills into the keyboard?

____

____

____

40. What types of printers are most commonly used in the medical office?

____

41. What are the advantages and disadvantages of an inkjet printer?

____

____

42. What are the advantages and disadvantages of a laser printer?

____

____

43. How should the outside casing of a printer be cleaned?

____

44. List examples of storage devices used with a microcomputer.

____

45. What method or organization is used to store and retrieve information from a hard disk?

____

46. What is the storage capacity range for a hard disk?

____

47. What is the difference between a hard disk and a solid state drive?

48. How does an optical disc store data?

49. Which type of optical disc holds more information, a CD or a DVD?

50. What makes up a USB (universal serial bus) flash drive?

Medical Office Computerization

1. What are the advantages of medical office computerization?

2. What is an audit trail?

3. What are the disadvantages of computerization of the medical office?

4. How does a medical office minimize the effects of a computer system malfunction?

5. What measures should be taken to promote the efficient running of a computerized medical office?

6. How do modern systems connect computers or networks to the Internet?

7. What is secure messaging within the EHR, and why is it more secure than e-mail?

8. What are the advantages of providing Internet access to patients using a patient portal?

9. What is encryption, and what standard has been required as of January 1, 2012, to transmit patient health information electronically?

____

____

10. What is an advantage of transmitting prescriptions electronically?

____

____

11. What procedures typically are performed by a medical assistant using an EHR?

____

____

____

12. How do physicians use the EHR?

____

____

____

____

13. Describe the following measures that maintain the security of the EHR.

    a. Authentication:

    ____

    b. Levels of authorization:

    ____

    c. Automatic logoff:

    ____

    d. Audit controls:

    ____

    e. Antivirus software:

    ____

    f. Firewall:

    ____

14. What is the purpose of making a backup of all records stored on a computer's hard disk?

____

____

15. What type of backup system is most commonly used for the medical office?

____

____

16. What are three important aspects of maintaining a computer system?

CRITICAL THINKING ACTIVITIES

A. Computer System

Observe a computer system, and complete the following questions.

1. What is the brand name of the computer?

2. What hardware is included with this computer system?

3. What application software is installed on this computer system?

4. What operating system is being used with this computer?

5. What input devices are included with this computer system?

6. What output devices are included with this computer system?

7. How many optical drives does this computer have?

B. Computer Monitor

Observe a computer monitor, and complete the following questions.

1. Is this a CRT (cathode ray tube) monitor or an LCD flat panel monitor?

2. What is the screen size (in inches) of this monitor?

3. What controls are present on the monitor? If there is a menu, what menu options are present?

4. Position the monitor correctly to prevent back and neck tension. Explain what steps you took to do this.

____

____

5. Adjust the brightness or contrast to determine the setting that works best for your viewing comfort. Explain what you did to accomplish this.

____

____

____

C. Storage Size

Arrange the following terms related to storage of computer data in order from the smallest unit to the largest unit in the left hand column. Write the approximate equivalent units to the next smaller unit in the right hand column. **Example:** 1 gigabyte (GB) is approximately 1000 megabytes (MG)

megabyte (MB)   kilobyte (KB)

terabyte(TB)   petabyte (PB)

byte   bit

gigabyte (GB)

Unit of storage (smallest to largest)	Approximate equivalent
1.	
2.	
3.	
4.	
5.	
6.	
7.	

Notes

41 Telephone Techniques

CHAPTER ASSIGNMENTS

✓ After Completing	Date Due	Study Guide Pages	STUDY GUIDE ASSIGNMENTS (CTA = Critical Thinking Activity)	Possible Points	Points You Earned
		1149	Pretest	10	
		1149	Term Key Term Assessment	4	
		1150-1152	Evaluation of Learning questions	28	
		1153	CTA A: Screening Telephone Calls	8	
		1153-1154	CTA B: Follow-up Questions	5	
		1154	CTA C: Telephone Messages When the Office is Closed	10	
		1154	CTA D: Outgoing Calls	3	
			Evolve Site: Apply Your Knowledge questions	10	
			Evolve Site: Video Evaluation	10	
		1149	Posttest	10	
			ADDITIONAL ASSIGNMENTS		
			TOTAL POINTS		

Notes

✓ When Assigned By Your Instructor	Study Guide Pages	Practices Required	LABORATORY ASSIGNMENTS (Procedure Number and Name)	Score*
	1155	3	**Practice for Competency** 41-1: Performing Telephone Screening Textbook reference: pp. 1071-1072	
	1161-1162		**Evaluation of Competency** 41-1: Performing Telephone Screening	*
	1155	3	**Practice for Competency** 41-2: Taking a Telephone Message Textbook reference: pp. 1072-1073	
	1163-1164		**Evaluation of Competency** 41-2: Taking a Telephone Message	*
	1156-1160	3	**Practice for Competency** 41-3: Taking Requests for Medication or Prescription Refills Textbook reference: pp. 1073-1074	
	1165-1166		**Evaluation of Competency** 41-3: Taking Requests for Medication or Prescription Refills	*
	1160	3	**Practice for Competency** 41-4: Telephoning a Patient for Follow-up Textbook reference: p. 1076	
	1167-1168		**Evaluation of Competency** 41-4: Telephoning a Patient for Follow-up	*
			ADDITIONAL ASSIGNMENTS	

Notes

Name ________________________________ Date ________________

PRETEST

True or False

_______ 1. The medical assistant (MA) should obtain a caller's name before placing the caller on hold.

_______ 2. A caller will not be able to pick up nonverbal cues during a telephone call with the medical office.

_______ 3. Call forwarding sends telephone calls to a different extension or telephone number.

_______ 4. Most medical offices rely only on voice mail during the night and weekends.

_______ 5. When taking a message about a patient, the medical assistant should include the patient's date of birth.

_______ 6. Physicians should not be contacted when out of the office using cell phones or pagers.

_______ 7. A telephone electronic routing system avoids placing incoming calls on hold.

_______ 8. A physician will accept a call from another physician, even if it interrupts a patient examination.

_______ 9. The MA may not take a message from a laboratory that includes the results of diagnostic tests.

_______ 10. If a patient requests a prescription refill, the MA should ask for the pharmacy name and telephone number or the mail-order prescription service.

POSTTEST

True or False

_______ 1. If a call is on hold, the MA should check back with the caller at least every 30 seconds.

_______ 2. When answering the telephone, the MA should first identify the practice and himself or herself.

_______ 3. Call park places a call on hold so that it can be retrieved from a different telephone.

_______ 4. Voice mail mailboxes each have a separate extension.

_______ 5. Medical assistants should transfer all calls from patients requesting medication refills to a licensed professional.

_______ 6. Physicians may have access to e-mail using their smartphones.

_______ 7. A telephone electronic routing system saves the expense of designating one person to answer incoming telephone calls.

_______ 8. Most physicians take calls from patients while they are seeing other patients.

_______ 9. Medical assistants routinely give patients the results of normal diagnostic tests over the telephone.

_______ 10. The MA may take a message if a patient wants a referral or a diagnostic test.

Term KEY TERM ASSESSMENT

Directions: Match each key term with its definition.

_______ 1. Enunciation

_______ 2. Pager

_______ 3. Smartphone

_______ 4. Voice mail

A. A method for delivery, storage, and retrieval of telephone messages that is built into the telephone system

B. An electronic device that notifies the recipient to receive a message or return a telephone call

C. The act of speaking clearly and concisely

D. A cell phone with computer capabilities

EVALUATION OF LEARNING

Directions: Fill in each blank with the correct answer.

1. Give examples of three ways the MA can display courtesy when answering the telephone in the medical office.

____

____

2. How can the MA project a pleasing telephone personality when talking to callers in the medical office?

____

____

3. How should the MA answer the office telephone?

____

____

4. Identify three ways to maintain proper body mechanics and avoid muscle strain when spending several minutes on the telephone.

____

____

____

5. How does the MA handle a second call when speaking to a caller on a multiline telephone?

____

____

____

6. Identify and describe four features of most telephone systems.

____

____

____

7. How is voicemail used in the medical office?

____

____

____

8. How can patients get assistance for an urgent situation that occurs when the office is closed?

____

____

9. What are two devices that may be used to maintain contact with the physician when he or she is not in the medical office?

____

10. What is AIDET an acronym for, and what does each initial of the acronym stand for?

____

____

11. What is an acronym that provides guidance when a customer or caller has a complaint, and what does each initial of the acronym stand for?

____

____

12. What is an electronic routing system for incoming telephone calls?

____

____

13. When answering incoming calls, what three types of calls take priority over other telephone calls?

____

____

14. Identify four types of calls that are usually handled by the MA.

____

____

____

15. List nine pieces of information that should be included if the MA takes a telephone message.

____

____

____

____

____

16. What are two ways an MA might take a message using a computer?

____

____

17. How should the MA handle a telephone call requesting test results?

____

____

____

18. If a patient or pharmacy calls with a request to have a prescription refilled or renewed, what specific information should the MA record on a telephone message?

____

____

____

19. How should the MA handle a call if the caller has a medical question?

20. How should the MA handle a call from another physician?

21. How should the MA handle a telephone call about a serious emergency?

22. If a telephone call concerns a possible case of poisoning, where should the caller be referred?

23. What should the MA do if a caller's condition does not seem to be a serious emergency, but the MA is not sure how urgent the problem is?

24. How should the MA handle a call if the caller asks for the physician but will not identify himself or herself?

25. How should the MA handle a call if the caller has a complaint about service received in the medical office?

26. What guidelines should the MA follow when calling a patient?

27. What guidelines should the MA follow related to personal telephone calls?

28. How is the telephone used to remind patients about appointments?

CRITICAL THINKING ACTIVITIES

A. Screening Telephone Calls

For each of the following telephone calls, choose the best action for the MA from the following options. Assume that Dr. Warner is in the office seeing patients and a registered nurse is also in the office.

a. Transfer the call to Dr. Warner

b. Transfer the call to a licensed professional, such as one of the physicians or a nurse

c. Handle the call

d. Tell the caller that Dr. Warner is seeing patients, and offer to take a message

_______ 1. The caller identifies himself as Dr. Stephen Miller and asks to speak to Dr. Warner.

_______ 2. The caller asks for Dr. Warner and states that she wants the results of an MRI done last week.

_______ 3. The caller says that she has a question about her bill.

_______ 4. The caller asks for an appointment because the practice has been recommended to her.

_______ 5. The caller says that her daughter, a patient of Dr. Warner, fell off a swing and screams when anyone touches her left arm.

_______ 6. The caller identifies herself as a pharmacist and asks for Dr. Warner.

_______ 7. The caller says that she is calling to get results of a blood test done that morning.

_______ 8. The caller asks for an appointment because she has a sore throat and fever of 101°F.

B. Follow-Up Questions

If you were the MA taking a message in each of the following examples, identify two questions you would ask the patient to complete the message.

1. Maria Burget, is calling because she wants to know the results of blood tests that were done for her daughter Isabella (DOB 7/23/2010) the previous week. Isabella is a patient of Dr. Martin. Mrs. Burget tells you that she is at work, and the best time to call is after 2:00 PM.

____

____

2. Moira Siever (DOB 1/24/1964) is calling to get a refill of her antidepressant which was prescribed by Dr. Martin. She takes one paroxetine tablet every morning. She only has two tablets left. She gives you her home telephone number and says that it is her day off.

____

____

3. A nurse calls from the hospital and says that she would like to obtain an order for a stronger pain medication for Jana Green (DOB 5/1/1936), a hospitalized patient. She gives you the telephone number of the nurse's station. She will be available until the end of the shift at 4:00 PM.

____

____

4. Maria Gomez calls about her son Pedro who fell at school and twisted his ankle. Mrs. Gomez picked her son up from school, and she would like to discuss the injury with his doctor. She gives you her home telephone number and cell phone number and says she will be available at any time.

____

____

5. A caller identifies himself as Robert Warner. He says that Dr. Walden contacted him to obtain information about purchasing new examination tables. He gives you his office telephone number and cell phone number.

____

____

C. Telephone Message When the Office is Closed

Create a telephone message for the Walden-Martin Family Medical Clinic to be used when the office is closed. The message should include instructions for an emergency, instructions if the caller needs medical advice, and instructions to leave a nonurgent message. If the caller wants a prescription refill, he or she should be referred to a different specific number to leave a detailed message.

____

____

____

____

____

____

D. Outgoing Calls

Explain the procedure for each of the following:

1. Calling a patient for an appointment reminder

____

____

2. Calling a pharmacy with a prescription refill

____

____

3. Placing a telephone call from a physician in the office to another physician

____

____

PRACTICE FOR COMPETENCY

Procedure 41-1: Performing Telephone Screening. Practice the procedure with a classmate as if you are an MA at Walden-Martin Family Medical Clinic. When you are the caller, choose one of the scenarios below without preparing your classmate ahead of time.

1. Pretend to be another physician calling to speak to Dr. Walden.
2. Pretend to be a patient calling for results of a laboratory or diagnostic test for your husband or mother.
3. Pretend to be a patient who wants directions to the office or who has questions about public transportation to the office.
4. Pretend to be a relative of Dr. Martin who wants to speak to the physician.
5. Pretend to be a patient experiencing severe chest pain or bleeding.

Procedure 41-2: Taking a Telephone Message. Practice the procedure with a classmate as if you are an MA at Walden-Martin Family Medical Clinic. When you are the caller, choose one of the scenarios below without telling your classmate ahead of time. One person should answer the calls for Dr. Walden, and the other should answer the calls for Dr. Martin. When you are the caller, provide a simulated telephone number or other information if the MA requests it. When you are the MA, inform the caller that the doctor is with a patient, offer to take a message, and complete a telephone message form making sure to ask for all necessary information. Take the messages on the message forms below and/or directly into SimChart® for the Medical Office.

1. You are calling from the Admitting Department at Memorial Hospital to get admitting orders from Dr. Martin for Ella Rainwater, DOB 7/11/1959. The patient is in the admitting department.
2. You are calling from the Nuclear Medicine Department at Memorial Hospital. You want to speak to Dr. Walden about a test you just did on Kyle Reeves (DOB 1/1/1996). You are concerned about the test because the results seem to be very abnormal.
3. You are calling to find out the results of a thyroid scan that you had at Memorial Hospital yesterday. Your physician is Dr. Martin.
4. You are calling to find out the results of a complete blood count and chemistry screen that were done at the laboratory 2 days ago. Your physician is Dr. Walden.
5. You cut your left hand with a knife, and you are a patient of Dr. Martin. It is a deep cut, about ¾ inch long. It does not bleed if you put pressure on it, but it does start to bleed again if you take the gauze square off. You want to know if you should come to the office or go to the emergency room.
6. A neighbor's child told you she saw your 3-year-old daughter eat several berries from a plant in the yard. The child does not seem ill, but you want to ask her doctor, Dr. Walden, what to do. Should you bring her to the office or take her to the emergency room? Can the doctor call you back?

Taking a Telephone Message using SimChart® for the Medical Office
Practice taking telephone messages using the Simulation Playground of SimChart® for the Medical Office. Use Emma Willis to take messages for Dr. Walden, and use Celia Tapia to take messages for Dr. Martin. After you have selected the patient, click on Phone Consultation. Fill out the Create New Encounter screen and save the message.

Procedure 41-3: Taking Requests for Medication or Prescription Refills. Practice this procedure with a classmate. One medical assistant should accept calls for Dr. Walden, and one should accept calls for Dr. Martin. Use information from the following simulated prescription labels to call for prescription refills. If the medication is an antibiotic or analgesic, when you are playing the part of the medical assistant, ask for symptoms that require the refill. Pretend to call one prescription to the pharmacy as authorized by your physician. Document the prescription refill you call to the pharmacy in the simulated paper medical record on p. 1160.

Furosemide 20 mg tab Generic equivalent for: Lasix Take 1 tablet daily West Street Pharmacy Pharmacy telephone: (123) 123-2211	Indomethacin 25 mg cap Take 1-2 capsules with food up to three times daily for moderate to severe pain Best Pharmacy Pharmacy telephone: (123) 123-6155
Tetracycline 250 mg cap (for acne) Take 1 capsule twice daily Walgreens Mail Service Pharmacy	Atorvastatin 20 mg tab Generic equivalent for: Lipitor Take 1 tablet every day Wide River Pharmacy Pharmacy telephone: (123) 123-1981
Crestor 10 mg tab Take 1 tablet by mouth every day Best Pharmacy Pharmacy telephone: (123) 123-6155	Atenolol 50 mg tab Take 1 tablet by mouth daily West Street Pharmacy Pharmacy telephone: (123) 123-2211

WALDEN-MARTIN
FAMILY MEDICAL CLINIC
1234 ANYSTREET ANYTOWN, ANYSTATE 1234
PHONE 123-123-1234 FAX 123-123-5678

Date:		Time:	
Caller:		Provider:	
Regarding Patient:		Patient Date of Birth:	

☐ PLEASE CALL ☐ INFORMATION ONLY ☐ RETURNED YOUR CALL ☐ REQUEST

Message:			
Pharmacy:			
Provider Recommendation:			
Action Documentation:			
Completed By:		Date/Time:	

WALDEN-MARTIN
FAMILY MEDICAL CLINIC
1234 ANYSTREET ANYTOWN, ANYSTATE 1234
PHONE 123-123-1234 FAX 123-123-5678

Date:		Time:	
Caller:		Provider:	
Regarding Patient:		Patient Date of Birth:	

☐ PLEASE CALL ☐ INFORMATION ONLY ☐ RETURNED YOUR CALL ☐ REQUEST

Message:			
Pharmacy:			
Provider Recommendation:			
Action Documentation:			
Completed By:		Date/Time:	

WALDEN-MARTIN
FAMILY MEDICAL CLINIC
1234 ANYSTREET ANYTOWN, ANYSTATE 1234
PHONE 123-123-1234 FAX 123-123-5678

Date: Time:

Caller: Provider:

Regarding Patient: Patient Date of Birth:

☐ PLEASE CALL ☐ INFORMATION ONLY ☐ RETURNED YOUR CALL ☐ REQUEST

Message:

Pharmacy:

Provider Recommendation:

Action Documentation:

Completed By: Date/Time:

WALDEN-MARTIN
FAMILY MEDICAL CLINIC
1234 ANYSTREET ANYTOWN, ANYSTATE 1234
PHONE 123-123-1234 FAX 123-123-5678

Date: Time:

Caller: Provider:

Regarding Patient: Patient Date of Birth:

☐ PLEASE CALL ☐ INFORMATION ONLY ☐ RETURNED YOUR CALL ☐ REQUEST

Message:

Pharmacy:

Provider Recommendation:

Action Documentation:

Completed By: Date/Time:

WALDEN-MARTIN
FAMILY MEDICAL CLINIC
1234 ANYSTREET ANYTOWN, ANYSTATE 1234
PHONE 123-123-1234 FAX 123-123-5678

Date:		Time:	
Caller:		Provider:	
Regarding Patient:		Patient Date of Birth:	

☐ PLEASE CALL ☐ INFORMATION ONLY ☐ RETURNED YOUR CALL ☐ REQUEST

Message:

Pharmacy:

Provider Recommendation:

Action Documentation:

Completed By: Date/Time:

WALDEN-MARTIN
FAMILY MEDICAL CLINIC
1234 ANYSTREET ANYTOWN, ANYSTATE 1234
PHONE 123-123-1234 FAX 123-123-5678

Date:		Time:	
Caller:		Provider:	
Regarding Patient:		Patient Date of Birth:	

☐ PLEASE CALL ☐ INFORMATION ONLY ☐ RETURNED YOUR CALL ☐ REQUEST

Message:

Pharmacy:

Provider Recommendation:

Action Documentation:

Completed By: Date/Time:

Record medication refills called to a pharmacy in the paper medical record below.

CHART	
Date	

Procedure 41-4: Telephoning a Patient for Follow-Up. Practice the procedure with a classmate as if you are an MA at Walden-Martin Family Medical Clinic. When you are the caller, choose one of the scenarios below without telling your classmate ahead of time. One person should choose the scenarios for Dr. Walden, and the other should choose the scenarios for Dr. Martin.

1. Dr. Martin has asked you to call the patient above who had a thyroid scan to schedule an appointment to discuss the test results. Give the patient an appointment this week.
2. Dr. Walden has asked you to call the patient who had a complete blood count and chemistry screen above and instruct the patient to repeat the blood tests in a week. The patient should also make an appointment with Dr. Gomez next week.
3. Dr. Martin has asked you to call the patient who had a knife cut and instruct her to come to the office to be seen. Ask how long it will take her to get to the office, and give her that appointment time.
4. Dr. Walden has asked you to call the patient whose child was seen eating berries. Ask the mother to get a sample of the plant leaves and berries if possible and call Poison Control. Give her the telephone number of the local Poison Control center.
5. Dr. Martin has asked you to call a patient and tell her that her throat culture is positive for strep, and that he has prescribed an antibiotic. Instruct the patient to pick up the medication at her usual pharmacy.
6. Dr. Walden has asked you to call a patient and tell him that he is prescribing a new medication for his cholesterol based on his recent blood test. The patient should pick up the medication at the pharmacy and make an appointment to follow up after 3 months.

EVALUATION OF COMPETENCY

Procedure 41-1: Performing Telephone Screening

Name: ______________________ Date: ______________

Evaluated by: ______________________ Score: ______________

Performance Objective

Outcome:	Screen telephone calls.
Conditions:	Given the following: telephone, message form (paper or electronic), pen or pencil, computer appointment schedule or appointment book, and clock or watch.
Standards:	Time: 15 minutes. Student completed procedure in ______ minutes.
	Accuracy: Satisfactory score in the Performance Evaluation Checklist.

Performance Evaluation Checklist

Trial 1	Trial 2	Point Value	Performance Standards
		•	Answered the telephone within the first three rings.
		•	Identified the medical office, gave name, and said, "How can I help you?"
		•	Listened as the caller identified the reason for the call.
		•	Decided promptly if it was a call that should be transferred.
		•	Asked for the caller's name if not given by the caller.
		•	Took a message if appropriate (see Procedure 41-2: Taking a Telephone Message).
		•	If necessary to transfer the call, placed the caller on hold.
		•	Told the person to whom the call would be transferred the caller's name and extension (if necessary).
		•	Asked questions to assess any problem requiring immediate care.
		•	Transferred an urgent call to a physician or licensed professional if possible or followed office guidelines.
		•	Instructed a caller whose health was at risk to call 911.
		•	Monitored calls on hold and returned to a caller on hold within 30–45 seconds if a transferred call was not picked up.
		•	Asked a caller for permission before placing on hold to take a new call.
		•	Gave a second caller the option to be placed on hold or have the call returned before returning to a previous call.
		•	Repeated important information before ending a call.
		•	Ended the call politely.
		Ⓐ	Demonstrated active listening skills.

Trial 1	Trial 2	Point Value	Performance Standards
		Ⓐ	Demonstrated respect for individual diversity including gender, race, religion, age, economic status.
		✶	Completed the procedure within 15 minutes.
			TOTALS

Evaluation of Student Performance

EVALUATION CRITERIA			COMMENTS
Symbol	**Category**	**Point Value**	
✶	Critical Step	16 points	
●	Essential Step	6 points	
Ⓐ	Affective Competency	6 points	
▷	Theory Question	2 points	
Score calculation: 100 points − ___ points missed ___ Score Satisfactory score: 85 or above			

2008 CAAHEP Competencies Achieved
Psychomotor (Skills) ☑ IV. 7. Demonstrate telephone techniques. ***Affective (Behavior)*** ☑ IV. 2. Apply active listening skills. ☑ IV. 7. Demonstrate recognition of the patient's level of understanding in communication.

2015 CAAHEP Competencies Achieved
Psychomotor (Skills) ☑ V.6. Demonstrate professional telephone techniques. ***Affective (Behavior)*** ☑ V.1.b. Demonstrate active listening. ☑ V. 3. Demonstrate respect for individual diversity including a. gender, b. race, c. religion, d. age, e. economic status.

ABHES Competencies Achieved
☑ 8. f. Display professionalism through written and verbal communication.

EVALUATION OF COMPETENCY

Procedure 41-2: Taking a Telephone Message

Name: ______________________ Date: ______________

Evaluated by: ______________________ Score: ______________

Performance Objective

Outcome:	Take a telephone message.
Conditions:	Given the following: telephone, paper or electronic message form, computer (for electronic form), pen, and clock or watch.
Standards:	Time: 5 minutes. Student completed procedure in ________ minutes.
	Accuracy: Satisfactory score in the Performance Evaluation Checklist.

Performance Evaluation Checklist

Trial 1	Trial 2	Point Value	Performance Standards
		•	Determined that the person being called was not available.
		•	Offered to take a message.
		•	Gave the caller a reason why the person could not take the call.
		•	Filled in complete information legibly on the paper telephone message form or the electronic message form.
		•	Documented the name of the caller and business affiliation, if appropriate..
		•	Documented the patient name (if not the caller) and patient date of birth as needed.
		•	Documented the date and time of the call.
		•	Documented the telephone number of the caller, including area code.
		•	Documented the reason for the call and information the caller included in the message.
		•	Initialed the paper message form.
		•	Left any response section blank for the intended recipient to complete.
		•	Verified information.
		•	Gave caller a time when the call might be returned or told caller that the message would be given to the intended recipient.
		•	Ended the call politely.
		•	Clipped a message related to a patient to the patient's paper medical record or saved an electronic message from a patient to the EHR.
		•	Placed a paper message where the intended recipient would expect to find it or transmitted an electronic message to the person being called.

Trial 1	Trial 2	Point Value	Performance Standards
		●	Performed follow up according to office procedure.
		Ⓐ	Demonstrated active listening skills.
		Ⓐ	Demonstrated respect for individual diversity including gender, race, religion, age, economic status.
		✶	Completed the procedure within 5 minutes.
			TOTALS

Evaluation of Student Performance

EVALUATION CRITERIA			COMMENTS
Symbol	**Category**	**Point Value**	
✶	Critical Step	16 points	
●	Essential Step	6 points	
Ⓐ	Affective Competency	6 points	
▷	Theory Question	2 points	
Score calculation:	100 points – ___ points missed ___ Score		
Satisfactory score: 85 or above			

2008 CAAHEP Competencies Achieved
Psychomotor (Skills) ☑ IV. 2. Report relevant information to others succinctly and accurately. ☑ IV. 7. Demonstrate telephone techniques. ***Affective (Behavior)*** ☑ IV. 2. Apply active listening skills. ☑ IV. 7. Demonstrate recognition of the patient's level of understanding in communication.

2015 CAAHEP Competencies Achieved
Psychomotor (Skills) ☑ V.6. Demonstrate professional telephone techniques. ☑ V. 7. Document telephone messages accurately. ☑ V.11. Report relevant information concisely and accurately. ***Affective (Behavior)*** ☑ V.1.b. Demonstrate active listening. ☑ V. 3. Demonstrate respect for individual diversity including a. gender, b. race, c. religion, d. age, e. economic status.

ABHES Competencies Achieved
☑ 8. f. Display professionalism through written and verbal communication.

EVALUATION OF COMPETENCY

Procedure 41-3: Taking Requests for Medication or Prescription Refills

Name: ______________________________ Date: ______________

Evaluated by: ______________________________ Score: ______________

Performance Objective

Outcome:	Take a message requesting medication or a prescription refill.
Conditions:	Given the following: telephone, paper or electronic message form, computer (for electronic form), pen, and clock or watch.
Standards:	Time: 5 minutes. Student completed procedure in ________ minutes. Accuracy: Satisfactory score in the Performance Evaluation Checklist.

Performance Evaluation Checklist

Trial 1	Trial 2	Point Value	Performance Standards
		•	Identified the caller and telephone number.
		•	Identified if the caller was a patient or a pharmacy.
		•	Wrote complete and legible information on the paper message form (or entered accurately on computer message form including the patient's date of birth.
		•	Included the name of the medication, dose per tablet or capsule, and number of tablets or capsules and times taken daily.
		•	Included the patient's name and telephone number (if the patient was the caller).
		•	Included pharmacy name and telephone number or name of mail order service.
		•	If the caller was the pharmacy, gave a time when the physician would be likely to approve the refill.
		•	Ended the call politely.
		•	Clipped the message to the patient's medical record or attached patient medical record to computer message.
		•	Placed the message for review by the physician or forwarded the message electronically.
		•	If the physician was available to take the call, pulled the patient's paper medical record before transferring the call.
		•	After performing any follow-up requested by the physician, filed a paper message in the patient's paper-based medical record.
		Ⓐ	Demonstrated active listening skills.

Trial 1	Trial 2	Point Value	Performance Standards
		Ⓐ	Demonstrated respect for individual diversity including gender, race, religion, age, economic status.
		✶	Completed the procedure within 5 minutes.
			TOTALS

Evaluation of Student Performance

EVALUATION CRITERIA			COMMENTS
Symbol	**Category**	**Point Value**	
✶	Critical Step	16 points	
●	Essential Step	6 points	
Ⓐ	Affective Competency	6 points	
▷	Theory Question	2 points	
Score calculation: 100 points – ___ points missed ___Score Satisfactory score: 85 or above			

2008 CAAHEP Competencies Achieved
Psychomotor (Skills) ☑ IV. 2. Report relevant information to others succinctly and accurately. ☑ IV. 7. Demonstrate telephone techniques. ***Affective (Behavior)*** ☑ IV. 2. Apply active listening skills. ☑ IV. 7. Demonstrate recognition of the patient's level of understanding in communication.

2015 CAAHEP Competencies Achieved
Psychomotor (Skills) ☑ V.6. Demonstrate professional telephone techniques. ☑ V. 7. Document telephone messages accurately. ☑ V.11. Report relevant information concisely and accurately. ***Affective (Behavior)*** ☑ V.1.b. Demonstrate active listening. ☑ V. 3. Demonstrate respect for individual diversity including a. gender, b. race, c. religion, d. age, e. economic status.

ABHES Competencies Achieved
☑ 8. f. Display professionalism through written and verbal communication.

EVALUATION OF COMPETENCY

Procedure 41-4: Telephoning a Patient for Follow-Up

Name: ______________________ Date: ______________

Evaluated by: ______________________ Score: ______________

Performance Objective

Outcome:	Telephone a patient for follow-up.
Conditions:	Given the following: telephone, scratch paper, pen or pencil, telephone number, instructions from the physician, and patient medical record as needed.
Standards:	Time: 5 minutes. Student completed procedure in ________ minutes.
	Accuracy: Satisfactory score in the Performance Evaluation Checklist.

Performance Evaluation Checklist

Trial 1	Trial 2	Point Value	Performance Standards
		●	Organized information that might be necessary during the telephone call.
		●	Wrote down telephone number including area code and country code as needed.
		●	Placed the telephone call.
		●	Asked for the patient or correct individual.
		●	Identified the medical practice and self.
		●	If call was not answered, left message on voicemail or answering machine, including name of medical office, own name, and telephone number.
		●	When speaking to the patient, gave information as instructed by the physician.
		●	Gave the patient only the information authorized by the physician.
		●	Repeated instructions if any were given.
		●	Ended call professionally and said "good-bye."
		Ⓐ	Applied active listening skills.
		Ⓐ	Demonstrated respect for individual diversity including gender, race, religion, age, economic status.
		✶	Completed the procedure within 5 minutes.
			TOTALS

Evaluation of Student Performance

EVALUATION CRITERIA			COMMENTS
Symbol	**Category**	**Point Value**	
∗	Critical Step	16 points	
●	Essential Step	6 points	
Ⓐ	Affective Competency	6 points	
▷	Theory Question	2 points	
Score calculation: 100 points − ___ points missed ___ Score Satisfactory score: 85 or above			

2008 CAAHEP Competencies Achieved
Psychomotor (Skills) ☑ IV. 7. Demonstrate telephone techniques. ***Affective (Behavior)*** ☑ IV. 2. Apply active listening skills. ☑ IV. 7. Demonstrate recognition of the patient's level of understanding in communication.

2015 CAAHEP Competencies Achieved
Psychomotor (Skills) ☑ V.6. Demonstrate professional telephone techniques. ***Affective (Behavior)*** ☑ V.1.b. Demonstrate active listening. ☑ V. 3. Demonstrate respect for individual diversity including a. gender, b. race, c. religion, d. age, e. economic status.

ABHES Competencies Achieved
☑ 8. f. Display professionalism through written and verbal communication.

42 Scheduling Appointments

CHAPTER ASSIGNMENTS

✓ After Completing	Date Due	Study Guide Pages	STUDY GUIDE ASSIGNMENTS (CTA = Critical Thinking Activity)	Possible Points	Points You Earned
		1173	Pretest	10	
		1174	Term Key Term Assessment	16	
		1174-1177	Evaluation of Learning questions	18	
		1177	CTA A: Computer-Generated Appointment Schedule	5	
		1177	CTA B: Methods of Scheduling	5	
		1177	CTA C: Appointment Schedule	5	
		1178	CTA D: Setting Priorities for Appointments	4	
		1178	CTA E: Scheduling Diagnostic Tests and Procedures	5	
			Evolve Site: Guided Practice: Preparing and Maintaining the Appointment Book	10	
			Evolve Site: Guided Practice: Scheduling a New Patient	10	
			Evolve Site: Guided Practice: Scheduling an Outpatient Diagnostic Test	10	
			Evolve Site: Guided Practice: Scheduling an Inpatient Admission and an Inpatient Surgical Procedure	10	
			Evolve Site: Apply Your Knowledge questions	10	

✓ After Completing	Date Due	Study Guide Pages	STUDY GUIDE ASSIGNMENTS (CTA = Critical Thinking Activity)	Possible Points	Points You Earned
			Evolve Site: Video Evaluation	16	
		1173	Posttest	10	
			ADDITIONAL ASSIGNMENTS		
			TOTAL POINTS		

✓ When Assigned By Your Instructor	Study Guide Pages	Practices Required	LABORATORY ASSIGNMENTS (Procedure Number and Name)	Score*
	1179-1183	3	**Practice for Competency** 42-1: Setting Up the Appointment Schedule Textbook reference: pp. 1084-1085	
	1191-1192		**Evaluation of Competency** 42-1: Setting Up the Appointment Schedule	*
	1183	3	**Practice for Competency** 42-2: Making an Appointment Textbook reference: p. 1088	
	1193-1194		**Evaluation of Competency** 42-2: Making an Appointment	*
	1183-1185	1	**Practice for Competency** 42-3: Managing the Appointment Schedule Textbook reference: pp. 1090-1091	
	1195-1196		**Evaluation of Competency** 42-3: Managing the Appointment Schedule	*
	1185-1188	1	**Practice for Competency** 42-4: Scheduling Inpatient or Outpatient Diagnostic Tests or Procedures Textbook reference: pp. 1093-1094	
	1197-1198		**Evaluation of Competency** 42-4: Scheduling Inpatient or Outpatient Diagnostic Tests or Procedures	*
	1188-1189	1	**Practice for Competency** 42-5: Scheduling Inpatient or Outpatient Admissions Textbook reference: pp. 1094-1095	
	1199-1200		**Evaluation of Competency** 42-5: Scheduling Inpatient or Outpatient Admissions	*
			ADDITIONAL ASSIGNMENTS	

Notes

Name ______________________________ Date ______________

PRETEST

True or False

_______ 1. If a patient fails to keep an appointment without notification, it should be noted in the medical record.

_______ 2. A new patient who requests a physical examination should be scheduled the same day or the next day if possible.

_______ 3. Most medical offices use some type of time-specified appointment system.

_______ 4. In the stream method of appointment scheduling, each patient is given a different appointment time.

_______ 5. An example of clustering patient appointments is making appointments for new patients.

_______ 6. In the appointment schedule, times when physicians are available to see patients are blocked.

_______ 7. Demographic data for new patients are usually obtained when scheduling the first appointment.

_______ 8. Many medical offices call patients a few days before an appointment as a reminder.

_______ 9. The physician can usually admit a patient to the hospital without insurance preauthorization.

_______ 10. Patients usually call the hospital to schedule their own surgery.

POSTTEST

True or False

_______ 1. A written appointment book must be kept to provide a legal record of appointments.

_______ 2. A patient with a sore throat and fever should be given a same-day appointment.

_______ 3. In wave scheduling, several patients are given the same appointment time.

_______ 4. The method of scheduling appointments with the least waiting time for patients is open hours.

_______ 5. Categorization refers to the practice of scheduling patients with similar problems back to back.

_______ 6. Most medical offices set up the appointment schedule for only the next 2 or 3 months.

_______ 7. If a patient makes an appointment while in the office, he or she should be given a written appointment reminder card.

_______ 8. All patients must obtain a referral from the primary care provider before making an appointment with a specialist.

_______ 9. If a medical assistant (MA) schedules a diagnostic test for a patient, he or she should also provide any written instructions about preparation for the test.

_______ 10. An ECG and complete blood count are usually required before a patient can have inpatient or outpatient surgery.

KEY TERM ASSESSMENT

Directions: Match each key term with its definition.

_______ 1. Appointment matrix
_______ 2. Blocked
_______ 3. Clustering
_______ 4. Double booking
_______ 5. Established patient
_______ 6. Hospice
_______ 7. Modified wave scheduling
_______ 8. New patient
_______ 9. No-show
_______ 10. Patient self-scheduling
_______ 11. Preadmission testing (PAT)
_______ 12. Preauthorization
_______ 13. Referral
_______ 14. Stream scheduling (single booking)
_______ 15. Triage
_______ 16. Wave scheduling

A. Allowing patients access to computer scheduling to schedule their own appointments
B. Grouping patients with similar problems or conditions on certain days or at certain times of the day
C. The process of sorting patients according to their need for care
D. Times that are crossed out of the appointment schedule (not available for appointments)
E. A patient who has never been seen by the physician or for billing purposes has not been seen within the past 3 years
F. A scheduling method that uses both fixed appointments and more than one patient scheduled for the same appointment time
G. In managed care, written authorization by the primary care physician for a patient to receive additional services
H. Booking two people into a single time slot
I. Scheduling three or four patients every half hour, who are seen in the order in which they arrive
J. A patient who has been seen by one of the physicians in the practice within the past 3 years
K. A form or arrangement for information, such as appointments
L. An appointment scheduling method where each patient is given a specific appointment time
M. Diagnostic tests that are performed before the patient is admitted for surgery or a diagnostic procedure
N. A person who does not appear for his or her appointment
O. A program or facility that provides care to terminally ill patients
P. Permission from a patient's insurance company for a test, procedure, or surgery

EVALUATION OF LEARNING

Directions: Fill in each blank with the correct answer.

1. Identify seven guidelines to follow when making appointments.

____

____

____

____

____

2. Identify two methods of scheduling appointments.

____

____

3. What is the purpose of the daily appointment schedule? How is it handled to preserve patient confidentiality?

____

____

____

4. Identify and describe each of the following types of appointment scheduling.

   a. Time-specified (stream) scheduling (single booking)

   ____

   b. Wave scheduling

   ____

   c. Modified wave scheduling

   ____

   d. Double booking

   ____

   e. Open booking

   ____

   f. Patient self-scheduling

   ____

   g. Clustering (categorization)

   ____

5. What factors must be considered when setting up the appointment schedule?

____

____

____

6. How are new patients treated differently from established patients when making appointments?

____

____

7. Identify eight types of medical problems for which patients would usually be given a same-day appointment.

____

____

____

____

8. Identify four categories of medical problems that are usually referred to an emergency department.

____

____

____

9. How should the MA handle a patient who comes to the office without an appointment?

10. What should an MA do if an appointment needs to be changed?

11. What should the MA do if a patient who has an appointment does not keep the appointment or call to cancel the appointment?

12. Identify three common methods to help patients remember appointments.

13. What is a referral?

14. How does an MA schedule a diagnostic test at a facility such as the hospital x-ray department?

15. What should the MA document in the patient's medical record after scheduling a diagnostic test for the patient?

16. How should the MA arrange for a patient to be admitted to the hospital?

17. Where will preadmission testing be performed before surgery?

18. If a patient is having inpatient surgery, how should the MA schedule it?

____

____

CRITICAL THINKING ACTIVITIES

A. Computer-Generated Appointment Schedule

Refer to the computer-generated appointment schedule (Figure 42-2) in your textbook, and answer the following questions. Note that the stars denote times that are booked for the patient identified above the stars.

1. How many minutes is an appointment with Dr. Warner for a well-baby visit? ______________
2. How many minutes is an appointment with Dr. Warner for a recheck? ______________
3. What times are blocked in the schedule? ______________
4. Who is the first patient scheduled after lunch? ______________
5. If the schedule continued, what would be the next available time? ______________

B. Methods of Scheduling

Refer to the comparison of single booking, wave scheduling, and modified wave scheduling (Figure 42-3) in your textbook, and answer the following questions.

1. In which method are all patients in the same hour given the same appointment time? ______________
2. In which method is each patient given a different appointment time? ______________
3. Which method makes it most likely that there will always be a patient waiting even if some patients are delayed or cancel? ______________
4. Which method(s) make it easier to work patients in while other patients undress or have diagnostic tests?

   ____
5. Which method decreases waiting time for the patient? ______________

C. Appointment Schedule

Refer to the computerized appointment schedule (Figure 42-4) in your textbook, and answer the following questions.

1. What time do all staff have scheduled lunch on Tuesday 6/2? ______________

   ____
2. What is the advantage of using color to create the schedule with a computer system? ______________
3. For what date and time has the appointment for Emma Willis been scheduled? What is the duration of the appointment ______________
4. When is the staff meeting scheduled? ______________
5. When is the appointment to see a pharmacy representative scheduled? What is the duration of the appointment? ______________

   ____

D. Setting Priorities for Appointments

Consider the following four patients who call the office on a day where there are no open appointments. Which patient(s) should be worked into the schedule today, and which patient(s) can be given appointments tomorrow? Give a reason for your answer.

1. Erma Willis, a 66-year-old woman, reports that she has a fever of 100°F and she also had nausea and diarrhea -during the previous night.

   ____

   ____

2. Diego Lupez, a 34-year-old man, reports that he fell at work that morning, injuring his right arm and shoulder. He can move his right arm and shoulder, but the pain is severe and seems to be getting worse.

   ____

   ____

3. Anna Richardson, a patient of Dr. Martin, calls about her father, Lawrence Sheehan, a 72-year-old man who is visiting from out of town. Mr. Sheehan has had angina pectoris for several years, but for the past 2 days he has been having more frequent and more severe episodes of chest pain. He had one episode that morning that was relieved by rest and his usual medication.

   ____

   ____

4. Monique Jones, a 29-year-old woman, calls complaining of generally feeling tired and without energy for the past 3 weeks. She is concerned because she expected to start feeling better before this.

   ____

   ____

E. Scheduling Diagnostic Tests and Procedures

Using yourself as a patient, answer the following questions that you might be asked when calling to schedule a diagnostic test or procedure:

1. What is the patient's name?
2. What is the patient's date of birth?
3. What is the patient's address and telephone number?
4. What type of insurance does the patient have? Insurance ID number?
5. Who is the patient's employer?

PRACTICE FOR COMPETENCY

Procedure 42-1: Setting Up the Appointment Schedule. Using one of the blank appointment schedule forms, set up the appointment schedule for Walden-Martin Family Medical Clinic.

1. Monday, October 12, 20XX: Dr. Martin is scheduled for hospital rounds at 9:00-10:00 AM and will begin appointments at 10:00 AM. Dr. Walden and Jean Burke, NP will begin seeing patients at 9:00 AM. All staff will take a one-hour lunch break beginning at 1:00 PM. Dr. Martin has a regular Monday meeting from 4:00 PM to 5:00 PM at the hospital. He will not return to the office. The appointment times from 2:45 PM through 3:00 PM are blocked out for all staff as catch-up time. Block the time from 8 AM to 9 AM every day because office hours start at 9:00.
2. Tuesday, October 13, 20XX: All practitioners will begin appointments at 9:00 AM. All staff will take a one-hour lunch break at noon. Dr. Walden has a meeting with a sales representative from 3:00 to 3:30 PM. Jean Burke, NP, will leave the office at 2:00 PM to attend a meeting that will last the rest of the afternoon.
3. Wednesday, October 15, 20XX: Dr. Martin and Dr. Walden will begin appointments at 9:00 AM. They will take their lunch break at noon. They will begin afternoon appointments at 1:00 PM. Jean Burke, NP will begin seeing patients at 9:30 AM, and the time between 9:00 AM and 9:30 AM should be blocked. The appointment times from 2:45 PM to 3:00 PM should be blocked as catch-up time for all three practitioners. The office closes at 3:30 PM on Wednesdays.

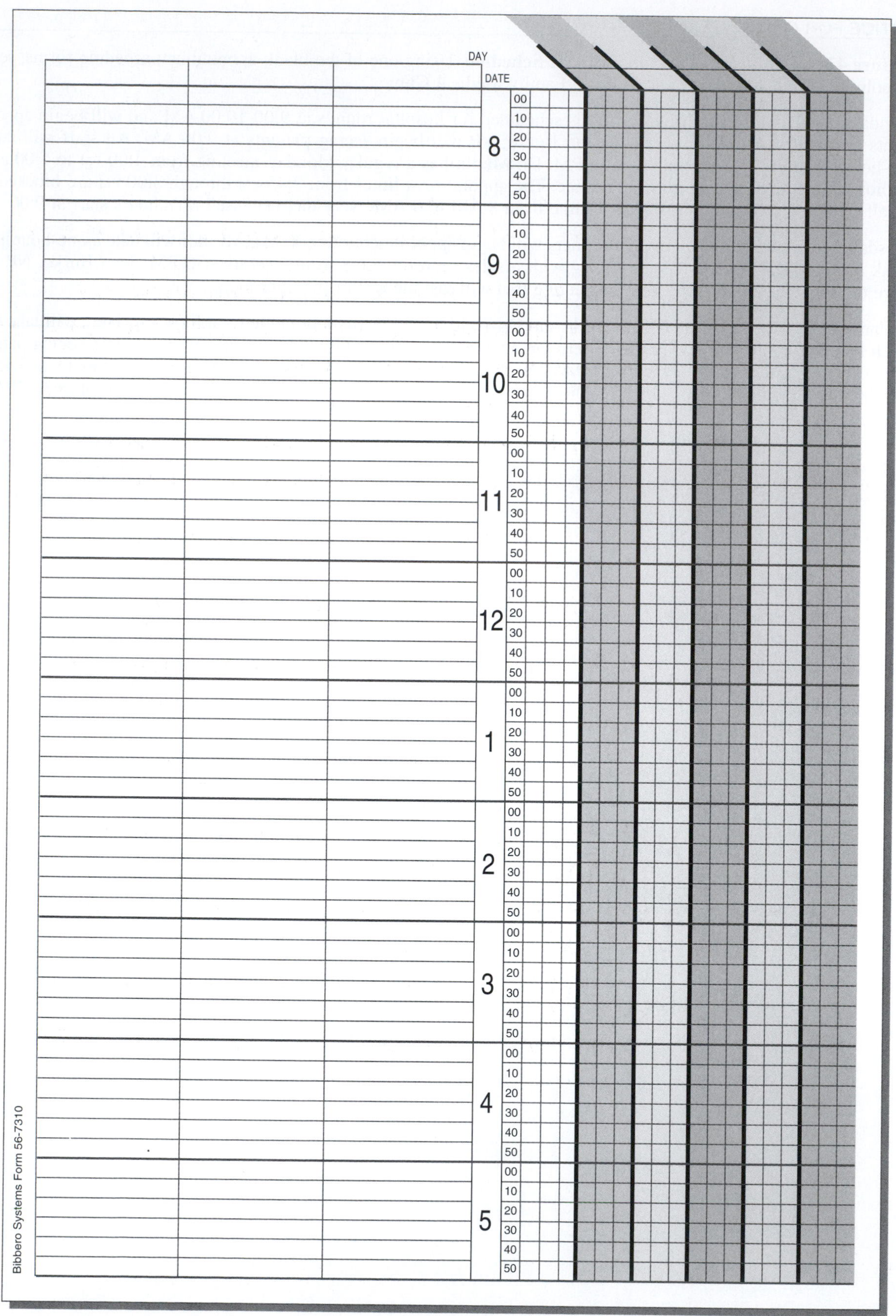
DAY

DATE

8 00 10 20 30 40 50

9 00 10 20 30 40 50

10 00 10 20 30 40 50

11 00 10 20 30 40 50

12 00 10 20 30 40 50

1 00 10 20 30 40 50

2 00 10 20 30 40 50

3 00 10 20 30 40 50

4 00 10 20 30 40 50

5 00 10 20 30 40 50

Bibbero Systems Form 56-7310

(Courtesy Bibbero Systems, Inc., Petaluma, Calif. [800] 242-2376; Fax [800] 242-9330; www.bibbero.com.)

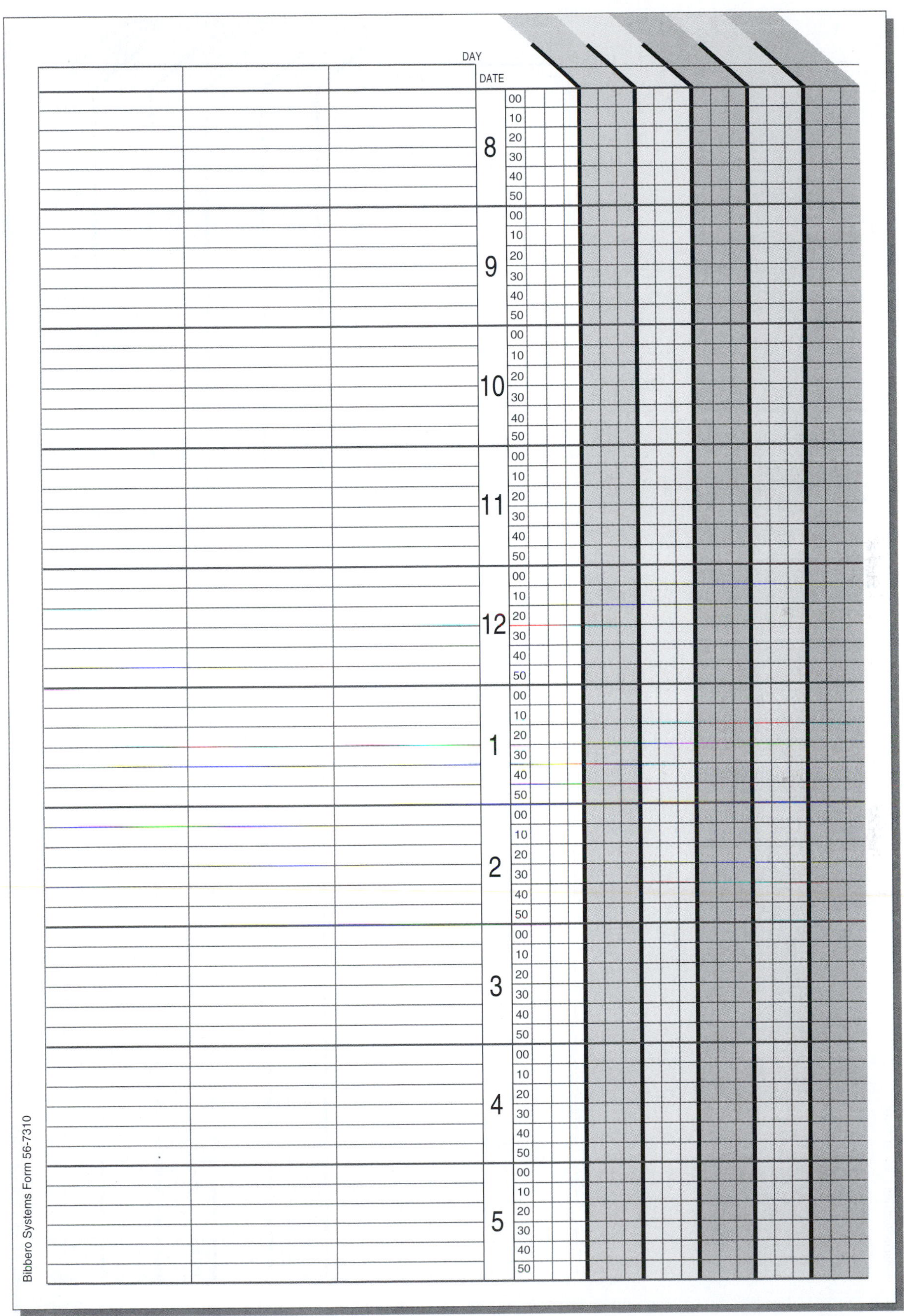

DAY
DATE

8 00 10 20 30 40 50
9 00 10 20 30 40 50
10 00 10 20 30 40 50
11 00 10 20 30 40 50
12 00 10 20 30 40 50
1 00 10 20 30 40 50
2 00 10 20 30 40 50
3 00 10 20 30 40 50
4 00 10 20 30 40 50
5 00 10 20 30 40 50

Bibbero Systems Form 56-7310

(Courtesy Bibbero Systems, Inc., Petaluma, Calif. [800] 242-2376; Fax [800] 242-9330; www.bibbero.com.)

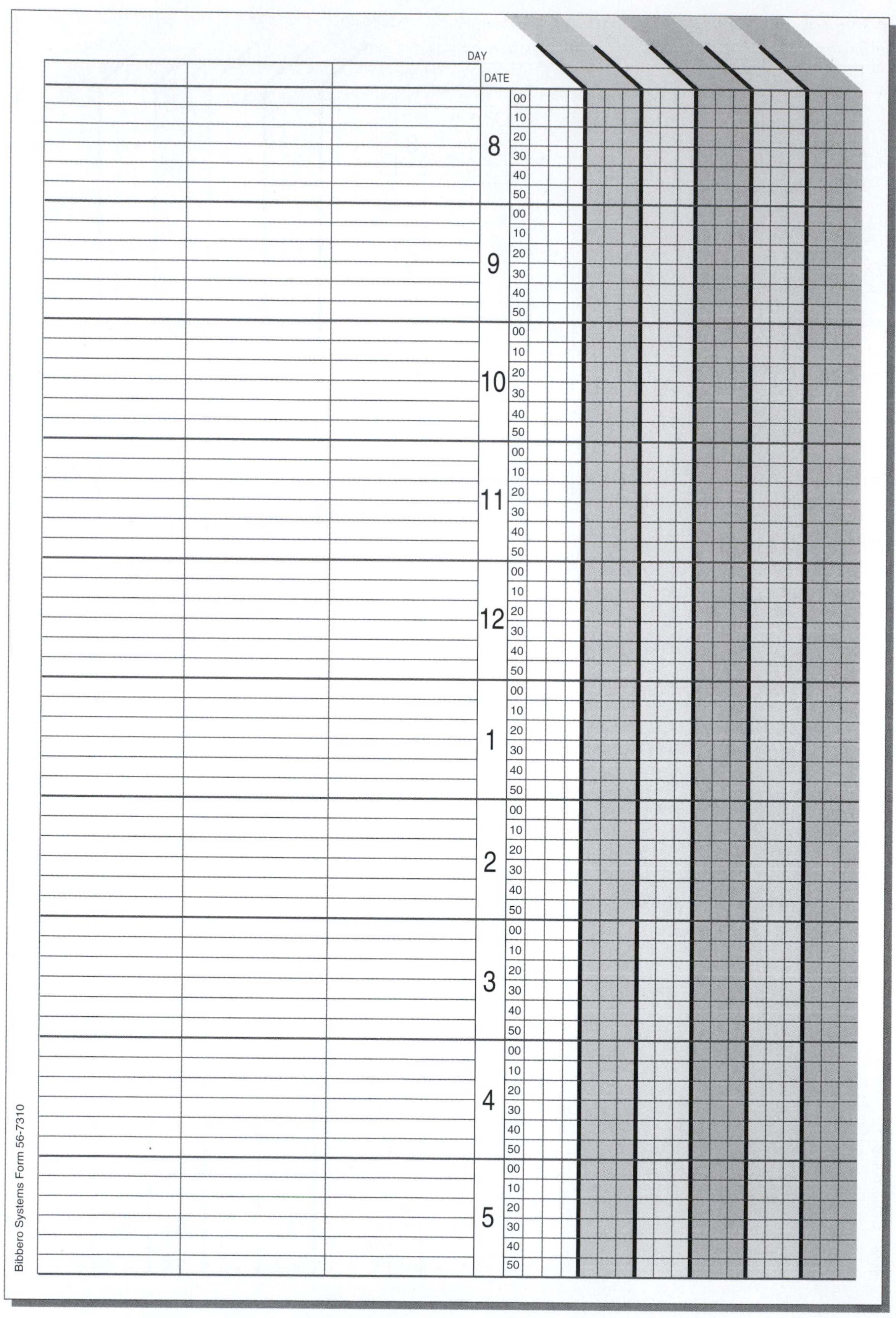

DAY

DATE

Hour	Minutes
8	00, 10, 20, 30, 40, 50
9	00, 10, 20, 30, 40, 50
10	00, 10, 20, 30, 40, 50
11	00, 10, 20, 30, 40, 50
12	00, 10, 20, 30, 40, 50
1	00, 10, 20, 30, 40, 50
2	00, 10, 20, 30, 40, 50
3	00, 10, 20, 30, 40, 50
4	00, 10, 20, 30, 40, 50
5	00, 10, 20, 30, 40, 50

Bibbero Systems Form 56-7310

(Courtesy Bibbero Systems, Inc., Petaluma, Calif. [800] 242-2376; Fax [800] 242-9330; www.bibbero.com.)

Set Up the Appointment Schedule Using SimChart® for the Medical Office

Use the information above to set up the appointment schedule for three days in the same week in October.

Click the **Add Appointment** button or anywhere within the calendar (in Calendar View) to open the **New Appointment** window.

Select the **Block** radio button, and then select the correct type of block from the **Block Type** dropdown menu. If you select "Other", enter a name for the type of block (e.g. Office Closed).

Select the correct practitioner from the **For** dropdown menu.

Select the date, start time and end time, and save your work.

If the same times are blocked on different days, click the **Recurrence** button and select the recurrence pattern (Daily, Weekly or Monthly) and the recurrence duration either by number of occurrences or by end date.

View the schedules for all providers by clicking on Provider View. (Note that you cannot add appointments in Provider View.)

Click the **Save** button.

Procedure 42-2: Making an Appointment. Schedule appointments for the following patients using the first appointment schedule (first day) you created for Procedure 42-1. Assume that established patients will be given 15-minute follow-up appointments and new patients will be given 30-minute new patient appointments (except for Jean Burke, NP, whose new patients are seen for 45 minutes). Use the abbreviation NEW for new patients and the abbreviation re √ for patients who are returning for follow-up. Include the patient's day telephone number. Make appointments back to back to avoid 15-minute gaps in the schedule. Make appointments in the order that patients call.

1. Celia Tapia, an established patient, calls for a follow-up appointment for diabetes with Dr. Martin. She is working and wants to come as late as possible. Her telephone number is 123-200-5006
2. Norma Washington makes a follow-up appointment following a fall last week. She is retired, and his telephone number is 123-754-4685. She wants to see Dr. Martin as early in the day as possible.
3. Diana Starr (DOB 7/2/1987) telephones for an appointment for an examination. She is a new patient who has recently moved to the area. Her home telephone has not yet been connected, but her work telephone number is 123-731-1998. She asks to see the nurse practitioner and requests a late afternoon appointment. Her insurance is Aetna (ID number 627W854, group number 7339), and her social security number is 111-20-2111. She works until 4:00 PM.
4. Douglas Wright (DOB 3/5/1948) telephones for an appointment because he has been having dizziness and feeling weak. He has never had an appointment with Dr. Walden before, but a friend told him that Dr. Walden is very experienced. He would prefer to come before lunch or as early in the day as possible. His telephone number is (123) 731-8282. His insurance is Medicare, and his ID number is 222-11-2111R. (His social security number is 222-11-2111). There is no group number for Medicare, so enter 0000 if entering into SimChart® for the Medical Office.
5. Casey Hernandez (DOB 10/08/2000) needs a follow-up appointment for headaches with Jean Burke, NP. She is in school and cannot arrive before 3:00. Her home telephone number is (123) 954-3578.

Make Appointments Using SimChart® for the Medical Office

Use the information above to make appointments on the first day you set up the appointment schedule in October.

Follow the directions given in the Medical Office Workflow handout that accompanies SimChart® for the Medical office.

If it is a new patient, click the Create New Patient button, fill in the required information given in the situation above, and save your work. Then continue to make the appointment.

Procedure 42-3: Managing the Appointment Schedule. Use the computer-generated appointment schedule on the following page to manage appointments for May 30, 20XX. Note that the appointment schedule is full because stars denote times that are booked for the patient identified above the stars. New patients with physical examinations are scheduled for 30 minutes, physical examinations for established patients are 20 minutes, and routine visits for established patients are also scheduled for 20 minutes. Assume that any patient will need 30 minutes to get to the office. Be sure to mark any cancellations who do not reschedule or any no-shows in red. If a patient cancels, you can give his or her appointment to another patient. Double book any patient with an urgent problem who must be seen today.

1. Robert Ricigliano calls at 8:00 AM to cancel his appointment at 9:00 AM. He doesn't want to reschedule at this time.
2. Douglas Wright telephones at 8:15 AM because he has been running a fever of 102°F since yesterday and has been off work. He would like to come as early as possible. His home telephone number is (490) 648-9010. He is a patient of Dr. Warner.
3. Lucille Morena calls at 9:00 AM to reschedule her appointment for next week. She is a new patient.

4. Peter Williams calls at 9:30 AM. He hurt his finger after slamming it in his car door this morning. He has gone to work, but it is hurting more now. It has swollen up, and he can't bend it. He would like to come in to see Dr. Warner. His work telephone number is (490) 932-6554.

5. Maria Santos calls at 10:00 AM to say that she has car trouble and won't be able to arrive by 11:00 AM. She asks if there is any way she could come after lunch.

Western Medical Center

Richard Warner, MD
Schedule for May 30, 20XX

Time	Name	Reason	Home Phone	Work Phone
9:00 AM	ROBERT RICIGLIANO	Physical exam	(490) 459-2811	(490) 459-6217
9:10 AM	*			
9:20 AM	*			
9:30 AM	JUNE ST. JAMES	BP & ECG	(490) 459-5807	(490) 459-9222
9:40 AM	*			
9:50 AM	DARLA SISSLE	Influenza vaccine	(490) 220-1156	
10:00 AM	Catch-up			
10:10 AM	*			
10:20 AM	LLOYD RIDLON	Recheck	(490) 459-4242	(490) 459-0419
10:30 AM	ESTELLE JORDAN	New patient	(490) 459-8249	(490) 459-1062
10:40 AM	*			
10:50 AM	*			
11:00 AM	MARIA SANTOS	Physical exam	(490) 459-0022	
11:10 AM	*			
11:20 AM	THOMAS MAXWELL	Recheck	(490) 459-4123	(490) 459-9201
11:30 AM	*			
11:40 AM	ROBIN SOTO	Well baby	(490) 459-1349	
11:50 AM	*			
12:00 PM	LUNCH			
12:10 PM	*			
12:20 PM	*			
12:30 PM	*			
12:40 PM	*			
12:50 PM	*			
1:00 PM	LUCILLE MORENA	Chem screen	(490) 459-6677	(490) 459-1566
1:10 PM	*			
1:20 PM	*			
1:30 PM	*			

Record the information about the cancelled appointment for Robert Ricigliano in the chart provided.

	CHART
Date	

Procedure 42-4: Scheduling Inpatient or Outpatient Diagnostic Tests or Procedures. Working with a classmate, call the ultrasound department of Memorial Hospital. One student should schedule the diagnostic test, and the other student should ask the questions and record information. Use the New Patient Information sheets for patient information.

Student 1: Schedule the first available time for a computed tomography (CT) scan of the head with contrast for Charles Latham. The patient has never had a procedure done at Memorial Hospital.

Diagnosis: Severe frontal headaches for 1 month. No known allergies.

Preparation for this test: No preparation

Questions to ask: Allergy to iodine or shellfish; ask female if she is pregnant

Student 2: Schedule the first available time for a barium swallow (x-ray) for Darlene Jordan. The patient has never had a procedure done at Memorial Hospital.

Diagnosis: Epigastric pain for two weeks. No known allergies.

Preparation for this test: NPO after midnight

Questions to ask: Ask female if she is pregnant

Record the information about the diagnostic test and instructions given to the patient below.

	CHART
Date	

Questions to ask when scheduling an x-ray or CT scan:

1. What is the test to be scheduled?
2. What date and time would the patient prefer?
3. What is the patient's name?
4. What is the patient's birth date?
5. What is the patient's address?
6. What city and zip?
7. What is the patient's telephone number?
8. What is the physician's name?
9. What insurance does the patient have?
10. Who is the insured?
11. What is the group (policy) number?
12. What is the ID (subscriber) number?
13. What is the diagnosis?
14. If female, could the patient be pregnant?
15. Does the patient have any allergies to medication or iodine?

New Patient Information

(Please Print) Physician: Richard Warner, MD
Home Phone: (490) 555-3319 Date: 9/14/20XX

PATIENT INFORMATION

Last Name LATHAM First CHARLES Initial R
Address 10971 CLARKWELL ROAD
City WESTERN State OH Zip 44770
Single ___ Married X Widowed ___ Separated ___ Divorced ___
Sex M X F ___ Age 49 Birth date 7/19/1961
Employer LATHAM PLUMBING
Occupation PLUMBER
In an emergency, who should be notified?
ANNA LATHAM (wife) Phone (490) 555-3319
Name Relationship

PRIMARY INSURANCE

Name of insured CHARLES LATHAM Responsible Party Yes X No ___
Relation to Patient SELF Birth date 7/19/1961
Address (if different from patient)
___ Phone ___
City ___ State ___ Zip ___

Insured employed by LATHAM PLUMBING
Occupation PLUMBER

Business Address 10971 CLARKWELL ROAD, WESTERN, OH 44770
Business Phone (490) 555-3320

Insurance Company STANDARD HEALTH INDEMNITY ID # 665514281
Policy (Group) # 594281

I the undersigned assign directly to Blackburn Primary Care Associates insurance benefits, if any, otherwise payable to me for services rendered. I understand that I am financially responsible for all charges whether or not paid by insurance. I hereby authorize the doctor to release all information necessary to secure the payment of benefits. I authorize the use of this signature on all insurance submissions.

Charles Latham self 10/25/20XX
Responsible party Signature Relationship Date

New Patient Information

(Please Print) Physician: *Richard Warner, MD*
Home Phone: *(490) 555-4810* Date: *9/14/20XX*

PATIENT INFORMATION

Last Name *JORDAN* First *DARLENE* Initial *L*
Address *617 HILLSIDE ROAD*
City *WESTERN* State *OH* Zip *44770*
Single ___ Married *X* Widowed ___ Separated ___ Divorced ___
Sex M ___ F *X* Age *30* Birth date *4/19/1980*
Employer *BEST SUPERMARKET*
Occupation *CASHIER*
In an emergency, who should be notified?
EDWARD JORDAN (husband) ___ Phone *(490) 555-4810*
Name Relationship

PRIMARY INSURANCE

Name of insured *EDWARD JORDAN* Responsible Party Yes *X* No ___
Relation to Patient *HUSBAND* Birth date *2/24/1978*
Address (if different from patient)
___ Phone ___
City ___ State ___ Zip ___

Insured employed by *MEYERS PHARMACY*
Occupation *PHARMACIST*

Business Address *428 MAIN STREET, WESTERN, OH 44770*
Business Phone *(490) 555-6192*

Insurance Company *STANDARD HEALTH HMO* ID # *28621954*
Policy (Group) # *86190*

I the undersigned assign directly to Blackburn Primary Care Associates insurance benefits, if any, otherwise payable to me for services rendered. I understand that I am financially responsible for all charges whether or not paid by insurance. I hereby authorize the doctor to release all information necessary to secure the payment of benefits. I authorize the use of this signature on all insurance submissions.

Darlene Jordan *self* *9/14/20XX*
Responsible party Signature Relationship Date

Procedure 42-5: Scheduling Inpatient or Outpatient Admissions. Working with a classmate, call Memorial Hospital to schedule an admission for a patient.

Student 1: Schedule an admission for Charles Latham. The patient will be admitted this afternoon, and admission orders will be faxed from the office. His wife will bring him to the hospital. Use the patient information form in Procedure 42-4.

Diagnosis: Pneumococcal pneumonia.

Insurance precertification number: M 200068AC

Student 2: Schedule an admission for Darlene Jordan. The patient will be arriving at the hospital by ambulance from home. Admission orders will be faxed from the office. Use the patient information form in Procedure 42-4.

Diagnosis: Hematemesis; R/O acute peptic ulcer with hemorrhage.

Insurance precertification number: 0011582

Record the information about the hospital admission below.

CHART	
Date	

Questions to ask when the MA is calling for hospital admission (answer telephone as Memorial Hospital Admitting Department):

1. What is the patient's name and address? ___
2. What is the patient's birth date? ___
3. What is the patient's admission diagnosis? ___
4. What type of insurance does the patient have? ___
5. What is/are the patient's insurance number(s)? ___
6. What is the physician's name? ___
7. How is the patient being transported? ___
8. When will the patient be admitted? ___
9. How will the physician's orders be provided? ___

Notes

EVALUATION OF COMPETENCY

Procedure 42-1: Setting Up the Appointment Schedule

Name: ______________________________ Date: ____________________

Evaluated by: ______________________________ Score: ____________________

Performance Objective

Outcome:	Set up an appointment schedule.
Conditions:	Given the following: appointment book or computer scheduling program, physician schedule, pen, and office calendar.
Standards:	Time: 15 minutes. Student completed procedure in ________ minutes.
	Accuracy: Satisfactory score on the Performance Evaluation Checklist.

Performance Evaluation Checklist

Trial 1	Trial 2	Point Value	Performance Standards
		•	Blocked times when the office would not be open.
		•	Blocked times when each individual physician would not be available to see patients, including lunch and hospital rounds.
		•	Blocked days or parts of days when individual physicians would be away from the office for vacation, conferences, or other scheduled events.
		•	For each physician, marked times scheduled for certain types of examinations or procedures.
		•	Blocked time for same-day appointments, catch-up time, and unexpected needs.
		∗	Completed an accurate appointment schedule.
		∗	Completed the procedure within 15 minutes.
			TOTALS

Evaluation of Student Performance

EVALUATION CRITERIA			COMMENTS
Symbol	**Category**	**Point Value**	
∗	Critical Step	16 points	
●	Essential Step	6 points	
Ⓐ	Affective Competency	6 points	
▷	Theory Question	2 points	
Score calculation: 100 points – ___ points missed ___ Score Satisfactory score: 85 or above			

2008 CAAHEP Competencies Achieved
Psychomotor (Skills) ☑ V. 1. Manage appointment schedule, using established priorities. ***Affective (Behavior)*** ☑ V. 2. Implement time management principles to maintain effective office function.

2015 CAAHEP Competency Achieved
Psychomotor (Skills) ☑ VI. 1. Manage appointment schedule, using established priorities.

ABHES Competencies Achieved
☑ 7.b. Utilize Electronic Medical Records (EMR) and Practice Management Systems ☑ 8 d. Apply scheduling principles

EVALUATION OF COMPETENCY

Procedure 42-2: Making an Appointment

Name: ______________________ Date: ______________

Evaluated by: ______________________ Score: ______________

Performance Objective

Outcome:	Make an appointment for a patient.
Conditions:	Given the following: appointment book or computer program, and pencil.
Standards:	Time: 10 minutes. Student completed procedure in ________ minutes.
	Accuracy: Satisfactory score on the Performance Evaluation Checklist.

Performance Evaluation Checklist

Trial 1	Trial 2	Point Value	Performance Standards
		•	Obtained physician name and scheduling preference from the patient.
		•	Found an open appointment of the correct length of time.
		•	Offered the patient a date and time for the appointment.
		•	Kept locating appointments until an acceptable date and time was found.
		•	Entered demographic data into computer for a new patient.
		•	Discussed cost of the visit with a new patient without insurance.
		•	Informed a new patient if a written referral form would be necessary.
		•	Recorded patient name, date of birth, reason for the visit, and daytime telephone number for an established patient or a new patient.
		•	Blocked out correct amount of time based on the reason for the visit. (Used pencil in a manual appointment book.)
		•	Repeated the information to the patient before ending the call.
		Ⓐ	Displayed sensitivity to patient preferences when making the appointment.
		•	Offered directions to the office if a new patient.
		*	Completed the procedure within 10 minutes.
			TOTALS

Evaluation of Student Performance

EVALUATION CRITERIA			COMMENTS
Symbol	Category	Point Value	
✶	Critical Step	16 points	
●	Essential Step	6 points	
Ⓐ	Affective Competency	6 points	
▷	Theory Question	2 points	
Score calculation: 100 points − ____ points missed ____Score Satisfactory score: 85 or above			

2008 CAAHEP Competencies Achieved
Psychomotor (Skills) ☑ V. 1. Manage appointment schedule, using established priorities. ***Affective (Behavior)*** ☑ V. 2. Implement time management principles to maintain effective office function.

2015 CAAHEP Competencies Achieved
Psychomotor (Skills) ☑ VI. 1. Manage appointment schedule, using established priorities. ***Affective (Behavior)*** ☑ VI. 1. Display sensitivity when managing appointments.

ABHES Competencies Achieved
☑ 7.b. Utilize Electronic Medical Records (EMR) and Practice Management Systems ☑ 8 d. Apply scheduling principles

EVALUATION OF COMPETENCY

Procedure 42-3: Managing the Appointment Schedule

Name: ______________________________ Date: ______________

Evaluated by: ______________________________ Score: ______________

Performance Objective

Outcome:	Review the appointment schedule, cancel an appointment, change an appointment, indicate a missed appointment and document cancellations and missed appointments.
Conditions:	Given the following: Appointment book or computer scheduling program, printed appointment schedule, and pen.
Standards:	Time: 10 minutes. Student completed procedure in ________ minutes. Accuracy: Satisfactory score on the Performance Evaluation Checklist.

Performance Evaluation Checklist

Trial 1	Trial 2	Point Value	Performance Standards
		•	Using the appointment schedule, made sure all medical records and necessary paperwork were prepared.
		•	Checked patients in on the official schedule as they arrived.
		•	Canceled an appointment on the day it was scheduled by drawing a line through the appointment in ink on the official paper schedule.
		•	Erased the canceled appointment in appointment book.
		•	Offered to make another appointment when a patient cancelled an appointment.
		•	If a patient declined to make another appointment after canceling, documented in the patient's medical record and deleted the appointment in a computer schedule.
		•	If a patient wanted to reschedule, found a new appointment time.
		•	Entered the patient's name and contact information in the new appointment time. In a computer schedule, changed the date and time using the original appointment or copied the original appointment.
		•	Repeated the new date and time to the patient if using the telephone or filled out an appointment card for a patient in the office.
		•	If the patient missed an appointment without canceling, draw a line through the appointment in ink on the daily schedule and labeled the appointment "No-Show."
		•	Telephoned any patients who missed appointments without canceling if office policy.
		Ⓐ	Displayed sensitivity when managing appointments.

Trial 1	Trial 2	Point Value	Performance Standards
		●	Documented the missed appointment in the medical record with any information available.
		∗	Completed the procedure within 10 minutes.
			TOTALS

Chart	
Date	

Evaluation of Student Performance

EVALUATION CRITERIA			COMMENTS
Symbol	Category	Point Value	
∗	Critical Step	16 points	
●	Essential Step	6 points	
Ⓐ	Affective Competency	6 points	
▷	Theory Question	2 points	
Score calculation: 100 points − ___ points missed ___ Score Satisfactory score: 85 or above			

2008 CAAHEP Competencies Achieved
Psychomotor (Skills) ☑ V. 1. Manage appointment schedule, using established priorities. ***Affective (Behavior)*** ☑ V. 2. Implement time management principles to maintain effective office function.

2015 CAAHEP Competencies Achieved
Psychomotor (Skills) ☑ VI. 1. Manage appointment schedule, using established priorities. ***Affective (Behavior)*** ☑ VI. 1. Display sensitivity when managing appointments.

ABHES Competencies Achieved
☑ 7.b. Utilize Electronic Medical Records (EMR) and Practice Management Systems ☑ 8 d. Apply scheduling principles

EVALUATION OF COMPETENCY

Procedure 42-4: Scheduling Inpatient or Outpatient Diagnostic Tests or Procedures

Name: ______________________ Date: ______________

Evaluated by: ______________________ Score: ______________

Performance Objective

Outcome:	Schedule an inpatient or outpatient diagnostic test or procedure.
Conditions:	Given the following: patient medical record and insurance information, name of test or procedure to be scheduled, telephone, and telephone number of facility and department to schedule the test or procedure.
Standards:	Time: 10 minutes. Student completed procedure in ________ minutes. Accuracy: Satisfactory score on the Performance Evaluation Checklist.

Performance Evaluation Checklist

Trial 1	Trial 2	Point Value	Performance Standards
		•	Assembled necessary information about the patient.
		•	Determined the facility and department to call for scheduling using the medical record or a diagnostic test or procedure requisition.
		•	Determined the time frame for scheduling from the physician order.
		•	Asked the patient about preferred days and times for scheduling.
		•	Obtained preauthorization from the patient's insurance if necessary.
		•	Placed a telephone call to the department where the test or procedure would be scheduled and identified the test to be scheduled.
		•	Provided the patient's name and demographic information as needed.
		•	Provided patient insurance information and preauthorization number as needed.
		•	Set up a specific day and time for the procedure.
		•	Informed the patient of the date and time for the test or procedure.
		•	Provided verbal and written instructions about preparation for the test or procedure.
		Ⓐ	Displayed sensitivity to patient preferences when making an appointment for a procedure.
		•	Sent an electronic or paper requisition to the facility or gave a paper requisition to the patient to take to the test.
		•	Documented the scheduled diagnostic test or procedure in the patient's medical record.

Trial 1	Trial 2	Point Value	Performance Standards
		●	Included patient instructions in the documentation.
		✶	Completed the procedure within 10 minutes.
			TOTALS

CHART	
Date	

Evaluation of Student Performance

EVALUATION CRITERIA			COMMENTS
Symbol	**Category**	**Point Value**	
✶	Critical Step	16 points	
●	Essential Step	6 points	
Ⓐ	Affective Competency	6 points	
▷	Theory Question	2 points	
Score calculation: 100 points − ___ points missed ___ Score Satisfactory score: 85 or above			

2008 CAAHEP Competency Achieved
Psychomotor (Skills) ☑ V. 2. Schedule patient admissions and/or procedures.

2015 CAAHEP Competencies Achieved
Psychomotor (Skills) ☑ VI. 2. Schedule a patient procedure. ***Affective (Behavior)*** ☑ VI. 1. Display sensitivity when managing appointments.

ABHES Competencies Achieved
☑ 8.d.1. Schedule of in- and out-patient procedures

EVALUATION OF COMPETENCY

Procedure 42-5: Scheduling Inpatient or Outpatient Admissions

Name: ______________________ Date: ______________

Evaluated by: ______________________ Score: ______________

Performance Objective

Outcome:	Schedule an inpatient or outpatient admission for a patient
Conditions:	Given the following: patient's medical record and insurance information, reason for admission, telephone, and telephone number of the facility and admitting department.
Standards:	Time: 10 minutes. Student completed procedure in __________ minutes.
	Accuracy: Satisfactory score on the Performance Evaluation Checklist.

Performance Evaluation Checklist

Trial 1	Trial 2	Point Value	Performance Standards
		●	Assembled patient demographic and insurance information.
		●	Determined the reason for the outpatient or inpatient admission.
		●	Determined the time frame for the admission from the physician's orders.
		●	Discussed preferred days and times with the patient.
		●	Obtained preauthorization from the patient's insurance company.
		●	Called the admissions department to schedule the admission.
		●	Provided the patient's name and demographic information as needed.
		●	Provided patient insurance information and preauthorization number.
		●	Provided the patient diagnosis or reason for the admission.
		●	Set up a specific day and time for the admission.
		●	Provided admitting orders as needed and faxed to the admitting department or nursing floor.
		●	If patient was to be admitted directly from the office, arranged transport, obtained consent forms, and prepared a patient transfer form.
		●	If the patient was to be admitted at a future date, informed the patient of the date and time, and provided written instructions for any preoperative needs or procedure.
		●	Documented the admission and instructions given to the patient in the patient's medical record.

Trial 1	Trial 2	Point Value	Performance Standards
		●	For a direct admission from the office, identified any documents sent with the patient.
		*	Completed the procedure within 10 minutes.
			TOTALS

CHART	
Date	

EVALUATION CRITERIA			COMMENTS
Symbol	**Category**	**Point Value**	
*	Critical Step	16 points	
●	Essential Step	6 points	
Ⓐ	Affective Competency	6 points	
▷	Theory Question	2 points	

Score calculation: 100 points
− ____ points missed
____ Score

Satisfactory score: 85 or above

2008 CAAHEP Competency Achieved
Psychomotor (Skills)   ☑ V. 2. Schedule patient admissions and/or procedures.

2015 CAAHEP Competency Achieved
Psychomotor (Skills)   ☑ VI. 2. Schedule a patient procedure.

ABHES Competencies Achieved
☑ 8.d.2. Apply scheduling principles: Admission or hospital procedures

43 Medical Records Management

CHAPTER ASSIGNMENTS

✓ After Completing	Date Due	Study Guide Pages	STUDY GUIDE ASSIGNMENTS (CTA = Critical Thinking Activity)	Possible Points	Points You Earned
		1205	Pretest	10	
		1206	Term Key Term Assessment	13	
		1206-1209	Evaluation of Learning questions	29	
		1209	CTA A: Filing Units: Alphabetic	10	
		1210	CTA B: Alphabetic Filing	8	
		1210	CTA C: Filing Units: Terminal Digit	8	
		1210	CTA D: Numeric Filing	8	
		1211	CTA E: Filing Reports and Correspondence	8	
			Evolve Site: Filing Medical Records Using the Alphabetic Filing System (Record points earned)		
			Evolve Site: Filing Medical Records Using the Terminal Digit Filing System (Record points earned)		
			Evolve Site: Guided Practice: Adding Supplementary Items to Established Patient File	10	
			Evolve Site: Apply Your Knowledge questions	10	
			Evolve Site: Video Evaluations	27	
		1205	Posttest	10	
			ASSIGNMENTS ADDITIONAL		
			TOTAL POINTS		

Notes

✓ When Assigned By Your Instructor	Study Guide Pages	Practices Required	LABORATORY ASSIGNMENTS (Procedure Number and Name)	Score*
	1213	2	**Practice for Competency 43-1:** Preparing a Medical Record Textbook reference: pp. 1102-1103	
	1215-1217		**Evaluation of Competency** 43-1: Preparing a Medical Record	*
	1213	3	**Practice for Competency** 43-2: Filing Patient Records: Alphabetic Textbook reference: p. 1107	
	1219-1220		**Evaluation of Competency** 43-2: Filing Patient Records: Alphabetic	*
	1213	3	**Practice for Competency** 43-3: Filing Patient Records—Numeric Textbook reference: p. 1108	
	1221-1222		**Evaluation of Competency** 43-3: Filing Patient Records—Numeric	*
	1213	3	**Practice for Competency** 43-4: Filing Reports Textbook reference: p. 1110	
	1223-1224		**Evaluation of Competency** 43-4: Filing Reports	*
			ADDITIONAL ASSIGNMENTS	

Notes

Name ______________________________ Date ______________

PRETEST

True or False

_______ 1. The patient owns the original medical record.

_______ 2. The main way to enter information into an electronic health record (EHR) is to use a scanner.

_______ 3. Medical record files or filing rooms should always be locked when the office is closed.

_______ 4. Color-coded labels are used for alphabetic filing of paper medical records but not for numeric file systems.

_______ 5. Outguides are placed where a paper medical record has been removed from the filing shelves.

_______ 6. If a numeric medical record system is used for filing, the filing system is indirect.

_______ 7. In an alphabetic filing system, prefixes such as van, von, and de are the third filing unit.

_______ 8. The medical record of a married woman is filed under her last name and her husband's first name.

_______ 9. In a terminal digit numeric filing system, the last group of two digits is the first filing unit.

_______ 10. The length of time that medical records must be retained can vary depending on the age of the patient.

POSTTEST

True or False

_______ 1. The patient controls the information in the medical record and access to it.

_______ 2. An EHR system is less expensive to initiate than a paper record system.

_______ 3. If shelving units are used to store paper medical records, folders with side tabs should be used.

_______ 4. Use of a current year label helps identify inactive paper medical records.

_______ 5. An outguide is placed in the individual medical record when removing papers to file new reports.

_______ 6. In an alphabetic medical record filing system for paper medical records, the patient's surname is the first filing unit.

_______ 7. If a business name includes an acronym, it is filed as if it were spelled out in full.

_______ 8. Hyphenated names are indexed as one filing unit in an alphabetic filing system.

_______ 9. A numeric terminal digit filing system is commonly used in hospitals and large clinics.

_______ 10. Medical records for minors can be destroyed 7 years after the record becomes inactive.

KEY TERM ASSESSMENT

Directions: Match each key term with its definition.

_______ 1. Acronym
_______ 2. Active record
_______ 3. Cross-index
_______ 4. Electronic signature
_______ 5. Filing system
_______ 6. Inactive record
_______ 7. Indexing units
_______ 8. Medical record management
_______ 9. Outguide
_______ 10. Sorter
_______ 11. Surname
_______ 12. Tab
_______ 13. Terminal digit filing

A. A device that facilitates putting papers or records in alphabetic or numeric order
B. To file under one unit and use a guide or card filed under another unit that refers to the primary filing location
C. Pieces of information used to identify a correct filing location
D. The way in which records are arranged such as alphabetically or numerically
E. A cardboard or plastic card to insert in a file when a medical record is removed
F. A word formed from the first letters in a name
G. An electronic sound, symbol, or process added to an electronic record that indicates intent to sign
H. The medical record of a patient who has not been seen within the past 2 to 3 years, or some other time frame specified by a given medical office
I. A projection of a folder that extends beyond the top or side of the folder
J. Activities related to the creation, management, use, and disposition of patient medical records
K. The medical record of a patient who has been seen within a time frame specified by the office (usually 2 to 3 years)
L. Last name or family name of an individual
M. Record-keeping method in which the last digits are used as the first filing unit

EVALUATION OF LEARNING

Directions: Fill in each blank with the correct answer.

1. Discuss the ownership of a paper medical record.

____

____

2. What happens to the old paper medical record after transition to an electronic health record (EHR) system?

____

____

3. What equipment and supplies are used for creation and storage of paper medical records?

____

____

4. What is the advantage of using color-coded labels on medical record file folders?

____

____

5. List seven common categories for chart dividers.

____

____

6. How is an outguide used when filing medical records?

____

____

7. What is the most common method used to organize a new paper medical record for a patient?

____

____

8. What is the difference between a direct filing system and an indirect filing system?

____

____

9. What is the first indexing unit if an alphabetic filing system is used?

____

10. How are names with prefixes filed if an alphabetic filing system is used?

____

11. How are hyphenated names filed if an alphabetic filing system is used?

____

12. What is the second filing unit if the patient's name is Mary Johnson White?

____

13. How is the medical record of a married woman filed if an alphabetic filing system is used?

____

14. What are two advantages of a numeric filing system for paper medical records?

____

____

15. Compare and contrast a terminal digit filing system with a consecutive filing system.

____

____

16. What are four types of documents that might be filed using a subject filing system?

____

17. Identify two ways that documents might be arranged within a subject category.

____

18. Describe the form and function of a tickler file.

____

____

19. What are three factors that influence the decision to choose an alphabetic or chronological filing system for patient records?

____

____

20. What is the process for removing a record from the file?

____

____

21. Before returning medical records to the files, what are the three things the medical assistant should do to condition the records?

____

____

22. How are reports and letters filed into existing medical records?

____

____

____

23. What are three measures to prevent misplaced records?

____

____

____

24. How is an electronic medical record updated?

____

____

____

25. What conditions should be present in the storage area for active or inactive medical records?

____

____

____

26. How are medical records selected to be moved to the location of inactive records?

____

____

27. How long should the medical records of minors be retained? Why?

____

____

____

28. How long should the records of adult patients be retained? Why?

____

____

29. How should computerized records be stored?

____

____

CRITICAL THINKING ACTIVITIES

A. Filing Units: Alphabetic

Identify the filing units in the following list of names:

Name	Unit 1	Unit 2	Unit 3	Unit 4
Diane Riel				
George A. Ricker, Jr.				
Marie A. von Hayden				
Mrs. Carolyn Richenburg				
Robert T. Van Wilder				
Maria Rivera Santos				
G. A. Rickers				
James D. Smith-Richards				
The Blackburn Daily Times				
Uptown Management Corp.				

B. Alphabetic Filing

Arrange the names in the column on the left in correct filing order in the spaces on the right.

Diane Riel	1.
George A. Ricker, Jr.	2.
Marie A. von Hayden	3.
Mrs. Carolyn Richenburg	4.
Robert T. Van Wilder	5.
Maria Rivera Santos	6.
G. A. Rickers	7.
James D. Smith-Richards	8.

C. Filing Units: Terminal Digit

Identify the filing units in the following numbers assuming that a terminal digit system is used with two digits in each group.

Number	Unit 1	Unit 2	Unit 3
01-23-52			
22-19-08			
62-43-33			
00-82-99			
15-66-18			
21-19-44			
66-01-11			
21-18-08			

D. Numeric Filing

Arrange the following numbers in the column on the left in correct filing order in the spaces on the right assuming that a terminal digit filing system is used.

01-23-52	1.
22-19-08	2.
62-43-33	3.
00-82-99	4.
15-66-18	5.
21-19-44	6.
66-01-11	7.
21-18-08	8.

E. Filing Reports and Correspondence

Indicate which section of the paper medical record for each of the following reports would be filed in by writing the name of the report in the correct section of the table below.

1. Report of shoulder x-ray
2. Report of complete blood count
3. Report of laparoscopic cholecystectomy
4. Discharge summary from hospitalization
5. History and physical examination report
6. Progress note dictated at the most recent patient visit
7. Letter from consulting physician regarding a consultation visit by the patient
8. Report of MRI scan of left knee

Section of Medical Record	Reports to Be Filed in this Section
Progress notes	
History and physical examination	
Laboratory reports	
Diagnostic testing	
Hospital reports	
Immunizations/medications	
Correspondence	

Notes

PRACTICE FOR COMPETENCY

Procedure 43-1: Preparing a Medical Record. Prepare a medical record.

Procedure 43-2: Filing Patient Records—Alphabetic. File medical records using the alphabetic system.

Procedure 43-3: Filing Medical Records—Numeric. File medical records using the terminal digit system.

Procedure 43-4: Filing Reports. File reports and correspondence in medical records.

Notes

EVALUATION OF COMPETENCY

Procedure 43-1: Preparing a Medical Record

Name: ______________________ Date: ______________________

Evaluated by: ______________________ Score: ______________________

Performance Objective

Outcome:	Prepare a medical record for a new patient.
Conditions:	Given the following: new patient information form, Notice of Privacy Practices and acknowledgment form, file folder, metal fasteners, name labels, alphabetic labels, miscellaneous chart labels, chart dividers, preprinted forms, and a two-hole punch.
Standards:	Time: 10 minutes. Student completed procedure in __________ minutes.
	Accuracy: Satisfactory score on the Performance Evaluation Checklist.

Performance Evaluation Checklist

Trial 1	Trial 2	Point Value	Performance Standards
		●	Greeted the patient and introduced yourself.
		●	Identified the patient and verified that the patient was a new patient.
		●	Asked the patient to complete a patient registration form, read an NPP, and sign an acknowledgment form.
		▷	Explained why the patient was being given an NPP and being asked to sign an acknowledgement form.
		●	Checked the registration form for accuracy and legibility.
		●	Photocopied the patient's insurance card.
		▷	Stated the purpose of copying the card.
		●	Entered the data on the completed registration form into the computer.
		●	Assembled supplies needed to prepare the medical record.
			Typed the patient's full name on the name label
		●	The patient's name was in transposed order.
		●	The name was typed using correct spacing.
		●	The patient's name was spelled correctly.
		●	Attached two color-coded labels to the side tab that corresponded to the first two letters of the patient's last name.
		●	Attached the labels using the indentations on the tab.
		●	Attached the name label immediately above the alphabetical label.
		●	Attached additional labels to the folder as required.

Trial 1	Trial 2	Point Value	Performance Standards
		●	Inserted chart dividers onto the metal fasteners.
		●	Placed the original registration form in front of the medical record.
		●	Placed the signed NPP acknowledgment form in the record.
		●	Placed the photocopy of the insurance card (copy) in the appropriate section of the record.
		●	Labeled preprinted forms with required information.
		▷	Stated examples of preprinted forms included in the medical record.
		●	Punched holes into the forms if required.
		●	Inserted each form under its proper chart divider.
		●	Checked the medical record to make sure it was prepared properly.
		Ⓐ	Maintained the privacy and integrity of the medical record.
		✶	Completed the procedure within 10 minutes.
			TOTALS

Evaluation of Student Performance

EVALUATION CRITERIA			COMMENTS
Symbol	**Category**	**Point Value**	
✶	Critical Step	16 points	
●	Essential Step	6 points	
Ⓐ	Affective Competency	6 points	
▷	Theory Question	2 points	
Score calculation: 100 points – ___ points missed ___ Score Satisfactory score: 85 or above			

2008 CAAHEP Competencies Achieved
Psychomotor (Skills) ☑ V. 3. Organize a patient's medical record. ☑ V. 6. Use office hardware and software to maintain office systems. ☑ V. 8. Maintain organization by filing. ☑ IX. 3. Apply HIPAA rules in regard to privacy/release of information. ☑ IX. 8. Apply local, state, and federal health care legislation and regulation appropriate to the medical assisting practice setting. ***Affective (Behavior)*** ☑ IX. 3. Recognize the importance of local, state, and federal legislation and regulations in the practice setting.

2015 CAAHEP Competencies Achieved
Psychomotor (Skills) ☑ VI. 3. Create a patient medical record. ☑ VI. 4. Organize a patient's medical record. ☑ X.2.a. Apply HIPAA rules in regard to privacy. ***Affective (Behavior)*** ☑ X.2. Protect the integrity of the medical record

ABHES Competencies Achieved
☑ 4. c. Follow established policies when initiating or terminating medical treatment. ☑ 4. f. Comply with federal, state, and local health laws and regulations as they relate to healthcare settings.. ☑ 7.b. Utilize electronic medical records (EMR) and practice management sytems. ☑ 8. a. Gather and process documents.

Notes

EVALUATION OF COMPETENCY

Procedure 43-2: Filing Patient Records: Alphabetic

Name: ______________________ Date: ______________

Evaluated by: ______________________ Score: ______________

Performance Objective

Outcome:	File patient records using an alphabetic filing system.
Conditions:	Given the following: patient records with patient names, alphabetic sorter, file cabinet or shelves, outguides, and index cards.
Standards:	Time: 10 minutes. Student completed procedure in ________ minutes.
	Accuracy: Satisfactory score on the Performance Evaluation Checklist.

Performance Evaluation Checklist

Trial 1	Trial 2	Point Value	Performance Standards
		•	Gathered the records and removed any elastic bands or paper clips.
		•	Secured any loose sheets of paper.
		•	Sorted the records alphabetically by last name.
		*	Found the correct location in the file for each record.
		•	Slid the record in front of the outguide and removed the outguide from the shelf or drawer.
		•	Stored the outguide with other unused outguides.
		•	Removed any index card from the outguide and discarded or stored according to office policy.
		•	Filed each record until all records were filed.
		*	Maintained the privacy of all medical records.
		*	Completed the procedure within 10 minutes.
			TOTALS

Evaluation of Student Performance

EVALUATION CRITERIA			COMMENTS
Symbol	**Category**	**Point Value**	
∗	Critical Step	16 points	
●	Essential Step	6 points	
Ⓐ	Affective Competency	6 points	
▷	Theory Question	2 points	
Score calculation: 100 points − ___ points missed ___Score Satisfactory score: 85 or above			

2008 CAAHEP Competencies Achieved
Psychomotor (Skills) ☑ V. 5. File patient medical records. ☑ V. 8. Maintain organization by filing.

2015 CAAHEP Competencies Achieved
Psychomotor (Skills) ☑ VI. 4. Organize a patient's medical record. ☑ X.2.a. Apply HIPAA rules in regard to privacy.

ABHES Competencies Achieved
☑ 8. a. Gather and process documents.

EVALUATION OF COMPETENCY

Procedure 43-3: Filing Patient Records: Numeric

Name: ______________________ Date: ______________

Evaluated by: ______________________ Score: ______________

Performance Objective

Outcome:	File patient records using a terminal digit filing system.
Conditions:	Given the following: Patient records with terminal digit labels, file cabinet or shelves, numeric sorter, outguides, and index cards.
Standards:	Time: 10 minutes. Student completed procedure in __________ minutes.
	Accuracy: Satisfactory score on the Performance Evaluation Checklist

Performance Evaluation Checklist

Trial 1	Trial 2	Point Value	Performance Standards
		●	Gathered the records and removed any elastic bands or paper clips.
		●	Secured any loose sheets of paper.
		●	Sorted the records according to the terminal digit indexing units.
		*	Found the correct location in the file for each record based on the final group of numbers.
		*	Refined search based on the middle group of numbers and then the first group of numbers.
		●	Slid the record in front of the outguide and removed the outguide from the shelf or drawer.
		●	Stored the outguide with other unused outguides.
		●	Removed any index card from the outguide and discarded or stored according to office policy.
		●	Filed each record until all records were filed.
		*	Maintained the privacy of all medical records.
		*	Completed the procedure within 10 minutes.
			TOTALS

Evaluation of Student Performance

EVALUATION CRITERIA			COMMENTS
Symbol	**Category**	**Point Value**	
∗	Critical Step	16 points	
●	Essential Step	6 points	
Ⓐ	Affective Competency	6 points	
▷	Theory Question	2 points	
Score calculation: 100 points – ___ points missed ___Score Satisfactory score: 85 or above			

2008 CAAHEP Competencies Achieved
Psychomotor (Skills) ☑ V. 4. File medical records. ☑ V. 8. Maintain organization by filing.

2015 CAAHEP Competencies Achieved
Psychomotor (Skills) ☑ VI. 5. File patient medical records. ☑ X.2.a. Apply HIPAA rules in regard to privacy.

ABHES Competencies Achieved
☑ 8. a. Gather and process documents.

EVALUATION OF COMPETENCY

Procedure 43-4: Filing Reports

Name: ______________________ Date: ______________

Evaluated by: ______________________ Score: ______________

Performance Objective

Outcome:	File reports, correspondence, and other material in a paper patient record.
Conditions:	Given the following: Medical records, assorted reports, letters or other material to be filed, hole punch, tape, stapler, and sorter.
Standards:	Time: 10 minutes. Student completed procedure in ________ minutes.
	Accuracy: Satisfactory score on the Performance Evaluation Checklist.

Performance Evaluation Checklist

Trial 1	Trial 2	Point Value	Performance Standards
		●	Assembled materials to be filed and necessary supplies.
		●	Removed paper clips, pins, or other extraneous materials from records or materials to be filed.
		●	Mended any tears with tape.
		●	Stapled related pages together.
		●	Punched holes as needed.
		●	Verified that each report was initialed by the physician.
		●	Set aside any report without initials to be returned for physician review.
		●	Sorted reports alphabetically or numerically depending on the office filing system.
		●	Assembled all reports for a particular patient.
		●	Located the patient's medical record.
		*	Inserted the reports into the medical record in the correct location in reverse chronological order.
		●	Inserted dividers into the medical record if necessary.
		●	Put the record back together as needed.
		●	Replaced the record in the file.
		●	Repeated until all the reports for all patients were filed.
		●	If the record could not be located in the file, placed the report back in sorter or in the pocket of the outguide according to office policy.

Trial 1	Trial 2	Point Value	Performance Standards
		Ⓐ	Maintained the privacy and integrity of each medical record.
		✶	Completed the procedure within 10 minutes.
			TOTALS

Evaluation of Student Performance

EVALUATION CRITERIA			COMMENTS
Symbol	**Category**	**Point Value**	
✶	Critical Step	16 points	
●	Essential Step	6 points	
Ⓐ	Affective Competency	6 points	
▷	Theory Question	2 points	
Score calculation: 100 points − ___ points missed ___ Score Satisfactory score: 85 or above			

2008 CAAHEP Competencies Achieved

Psychomotor (Skills)

☑ V. 3. Organize a patient's medical record.
☑ V. 8. Maintain organization by filing.

2015 CAAHEP Competencies Achieved

Psychomotor (Skills)

☑ VI. 4. Organize a patient's medical record.
☑ X.2.a. Apply HIPAA rules in regard to privacy.

Affective (Behavior)

☑ X.2. Protect the integrity of the medical record.

ABHES Competencies Achieved

☑ 8. a. Gather and process documents.

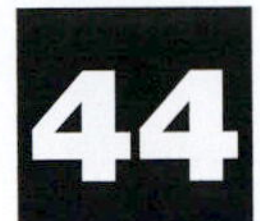

44 Written Communications

CHAPTER ASSIGNMENTS

✓ After Completing	Date Due	Study Guide Pages	STUDY GUIDE ASSIGNMENTS (CTA = Critical Thinking Activities)	Possible Points	Points You Earned
		1229	Pretest	10	
		1230	Term Key Term Assessment	17	
		1230-1232	Evaluation of Learning questions	24	
		1232-1233	CTA A: Parts of a Letter	6	
		1233	CTA B: Letter Styles	6	
		1233	CTA C: Parts of Speech	19	
		1234	CTA D: Proofreading	10	
			Evolve Site: Quiz Show—Spelling (Record points earned)		
			Evolve Site: Comma Exercise (Record points earned)		
			Evolve Site: Hyphen Exercise (Record points earned)		
			Evolve Site: Guided Practice: Proofreading Written Correspondence	10	
			Evolve Site: Apply Your Knowledge questions	10	
			Evolve Site: Video Evaluation	8	
		1229	Posttest	10	
			ADDITIONAL ASSIGNMENTS		
			TOTAL POINTS		

Notes

✓ When Assigned By Your Instructor	Study Guide Pages	Practices Required	LABORATORY ASSIGNMENTS (Procedure Number and Name)	Score*
	1235	2	**Practice for Competency** 44-1: Composing a Business Letter Textbook reference: pp. 1121-1122	
	1239-1241		**Evaluation of Competency** 44-1: Composing a Business Letter	*
	1235-1238	3	**Practice for Competency** 44-2: Sending a Fax Textbook reference: pp. 1127-1128	
	1243-1244		**Evaluation of Competency** 44-2: Sending a Fax	*
			ADDITIONAL ASSIGNMENTS	

Notes

Name ________________________________ Date ______________

PRETEST

True or False

_______ 1. Business letters are more formal than personal correspondence in form and content.

_______ 2. The body of a business letter is double spaced.

_______ 3. The name of the individual sending a business letter should always be keyed so that it appears in print below the handwritten signature.

_______ 4. If an additional form or printed material is included with a letter, this should be indicated in an end notation.

_______ 5. In the semiblock letter style, all lines of the letter are left justified.

_______ 6. An adverb modifies a verb, adjective, or other adverb.

_______ 7. Sentence fragments and comma splices are errors that should always be corrected in a business letter.

_______ 8. A comma should be used to separate two sentences that are not joined by a conjunction or separated by a period.

_______ 9. The common headings for a memo (memorandum) are: TO, FROM, SUBJECT, and DATE.

_______ 10. Because e-mail and fax transmissions are considered secure, they are good ways to transmit confidential information about patients.

POSTTEST

True or False

_______ 1. All business letters sent from the medical office are dictated by the physician and prepared by office staff.

_______ 2. There should be exactly two blank lines between the date line and the inside address of a business letter.

_______ 3. The standard closing of a business letter is "Sincerely yours."

_______ 4. If a letter has been dictated by the physician and prepared by the medical assistant (MA), a reference line should be included below the typed signature.

_______ 5. In the modified block letter style, the date line, complimentary close, and printed signature may be lined up at the center of the letter.

_______ 6. A conjunction joins words, phrases, or clauses in a sentence.

_______ 7. When two sentences are connected without punctuation, it is called a comma splice.

_______ 8. A comma should be used to set off information that could be omitted from a sentence without changing the meaning.

_______ 9. A memo (memorandum) may be used to inform office staff about the time and place of a staff meeting.

_______ 10. Many office photocopy machines will collate and staple documents, as well as copy on both sides of a piece of paper.

KEY TERM ASSESSMENT

Directions: Match each key term with its definition.

_______ 1. Collate
_______ 2. Complimentary closing
_______ 3. Duplex
_______ 4. Email
_______ 5. Fax
_______ 6. Full block style
_______ 7. Grammar
_______ 8. Left justified
_______ 9. Letterhead
_______ 10. Memo (memorandum)
_______ 11. Modified block style
_______ 12. Proofread
_______ 13. Right-justified
_______ 14. Salutation
_______ 15. Semiblock style
_______ 16. Simplified letter style
_______ 17. Template

A. A format for business letters where the date line, complimentary close, and printed signature line are aligned at the center and all other parts of the letter are left justified
B. A letter format in which all elements are left justified, the greeting is replaced by a subject line in all capital letters, and the complimentary close and typed signature are replaced by a typed signature in all capital letters
C. A form of communication within a company that is usually short and limited to one subject
D. A letter format where all parts of the letter begin at the left margin
E. To assemble the pages of a document in numerical order
F. To identify and correct errors in a document
G. A standard form to which additional information can be added as needed
H. A letter format similar to modified block style, but all paragraphs are indented
I. Type that is aligned with the right margin of a document
J. Written communication sent from one computer to another using telecommunication
K. A sheet of stationery preprinted with information about a business, including name, address, telephone number, and other information.
L. The study of accepted rules used to create meaning in a language
M. To produce double-sided copies by storing images from both sides of the original in the memory of a photocopier
N. Lines of type that begin at the left margin of a document
O. Transmission of scanned, printed material by telephone
P. The greeting that begins a letter
Q. Words used as a polite ending to a letter before the writer's signature

EVALUATION OF LEARNING

Directions: Fill in each blank with the correct answer.

1. What is letterhead stationery?

____

____

2. What is included in the heading of a letter?

____

3. Where is the inside address located on a letter?

____

4. What is the correct salutation for a business letter to William Masterson, MD, including punctuation?

____

5. What spacing is used in the body of a letter?

____

6. Give examples of at least two acceptable complimentary closings for a business letter.

____

7. How many lines below the complimentary closing should the typed signature be placed? Why?

____

8. What are three examples of end notations for a letter?

____

9. Compare and contrast full block letter style with modified block letter style.

____

____

10. What is the advantage of using the simplified letter style?

____

11. Identify the eight parts of speech.

____

12. What type of sentence is composed of one independent clause?

____

13. What is a compound sentence?

____

14. What is a complex sentence?

____

15. What is a sentence fragment?

____

16. When does a comma splice occur?

____

17. Identify at least six occasions when a comma should be used.

____

____

____

____

18. When does the spell check feature of a word processing program fail to find errors?

____

19. What is the format of a memo (memorandum)?

____

____

20. Give three examples of individuals that a MA might communicate with via e-mail.

____

____

21. Compare the tone of an e-mail with that of a business letter.

____

22. What is secure messaging within the EHR and when is it useful?

____

____

23. What features on a photocopier are helpful when photocopying a multiple-page document?

____

____

24. What information should be included on the cover sheet for fax transmissions from a medical office?

____

____

CRITICAL THINKING ACTIVITIES

A. Parts of a Letter

Refer to the letter in Chapter 44, Figure 44-2. Identify the following parts of that letter.

1. Inside address: _______________

____

____

2. Salutation: _______________

____

____

3. First three words of the body of the letter: _______________

____

____

4. Complimentary close: _______________

____

____

5. Printed signature: ____

____

____

6. End notation(s): ____

____

____

B. Letter Styles

Name the letter style(s) to which each of the following apply:

1. Date line is left justified: ____

2. Instead of a salutation, a reference line is included in all caps: ______________________

3. The body of the letter is single spaced with two spaces between paragraphs: ______________

____

4. Paragraphs are indented: ____

5. The complimentary close is right justified or at the center: ______________________

6. The inside address is left justified: ____

C. Parts of Speech

Enter each word in the following sentence into the table below under the heading of the correct part of speech.
My name is Christine Walters, and I have worked continuously at a nephrology practice for the past 3 years.

Noun(s)	Pronoun(s)	Verb(s)	Adjective(s)	Adverb(s) Article(s)	Preposition(s)	Conjunction(s)

D. Proofreading

Proofread the passage on the left. In the lines on the right, correct each mistake, including spelling, punctuation, and grammar. If no correction of the italicized word or words is required, write "none."

1. Patient instructed in *perfromance* of range of	1.
2. motion activities, especially for the *weak, right*	2.
3. *lower, extremity.* He was instructed to use both	3.
4. hands *to assisting* in extension of the knee and	4.
5. ankle, flexion of the toes, as well *as invershun*	5.
6. and eversion of the foot. The *pateint* was able	6.
7. to demonstrate all exercises, *included those*	7.
8. done *as assistave* exercises. The patient could	8.
9. *verbalized* understanding of the need to keep all	9.
10. joints *mobile.*	10.

PRACTICE FOR COMPETENCY

Procedure 44-1: Composing a Business Letter. Practice preparing business letters and preparing envelopes using the following two letters. Assume you are using letterhead stationery. Your position: MA.

Letter 1:
Content: You received an invoice (bill) from Physicians' Medical Supply Company, 22 Birkwood Street, Western, XY 44770. It includes a charge for three boxes of extra small gloves, but you only received two boxes. The purchase order number was 12345. You need the extra box of gloves.
Format: Full block using letterhead stationery. Use 1-inch margins. Be sure the letter has at least two paragraphs and that the body of the letter is centered on the page. Prepare an envelope to accompany the letter.

Letter 2:
Content: Dr. Warner asks you to contact the following patient and ask her to schedule a physical examination. The patient's name and address are Lucille Freeman, 22 White Circle, Western, XY 44770. When you check the patient's medical record, you notice that the patient has not been seen for 2 years. Dr. Warner prefers to perform an annual physical examination.
Format: Simplified style using letterhead stationery. Prepare an envelope.

Procedure 44-2: Sending a Fax. Practice the procedure to send a fax using the following cover sheets.

Composing a Letter in SimChart® for the Medical Office Using a Letter Template
Using the Simulation Playground, select the **Correspondence** icon on the **Front Office** tab and select **Missed Appointment** under **Letters** on the **Info Panel**. Click on the **Patient Search** button and locate Monique Jones (DOB 6/23/1985). After selecting Ms. Jones, note that today's date and her information comes up in the date line, inside address lines and salutation line of the letter template. Enter the information to inform the patient that she missed an appointment with Dr. Martin this morning. Click the **Save to Patient Record** Button. To print the letter, click on the **Find Patient** icon and select Monique Jones. View her record on the **Clinical Care** tab. Select the letter you composed and saved under **Correspondence** and click the **Print** button.

WESTERN MEDICAL CENTER
109 RIVER STREET
WESTERN, XY 44770

PHONE: (490) 555-6464
FAX: (490) 668-1414

To:	From:
Fax:	Pages:
Phone:	Date:
Re:	CC:

☐ URGENT ☐ FOR REVIEW ☐ PLEASE COMMENT ☐ PLEASE REPLY ☐ PLEASE RECYCLE

CONFIDENTIALITY STATEMENT:
The documents accompanying this transmission may contain confidential information that is protected under the Privacy Act of 1974. It is being faxed to you after appropriate patient authorization or under circumstances that do not require patient authorization. This information is intended only for the use of the intended recipient(s). The authorized recipient(s) of this information is/are prohibited from disclosing this information to any other party unless permitted to do so by law or regulation.

If the reader of this mess is not the intended recipient(s) or the employee or agent responsible for delivering the attached information to the intended recipient(s), please note that any dissemination, distribution, or copying of this information is strictly prohibited. **Anyone who receives this information in error should notify the sender immediately and arrange for the return or destruction of the transmitted information.**

MESSAGE:

WESTERN MEDICAL CENTER
109 RIVER STREET
WESTERN, XY 44770

PHONE: (490) 555-6464
FAX: (490) 668-1414

To:

From:

Fax:

Pages:

Phone:

Date:

Re:

CC:

☐ URGENT ☐ FOR REVIEW ☐ PLEASE COMMENT ☐ PLEASE REPLY ☐ PLEASE RECYCLE

CONFIDENTIALITY STATEMENT:
The documents accompanying this transmission may contain confidential information that is protected under the Privacy Act of 1974. It is being faxed to you after appropriate patient authorization or under circumstances that do not require patient authorization. This information is intended only for the use of the intended recipient(s). The authorized recipient(s) of this information is/are prohibited from disclosing this information to any other party unless permitted to do so by law or regulation.

If the reader of this mess is not the intended recipient(s) or the employee or agent responsible for delivering the attached information to the intended recipient(s), please note that any dissemination, distribution, or copying of this information is strictly prohibited. **Anyone who receives this information in error should notify the sender immediately and arrange for the return or destruction of the transmitted information.**

MESSAGE:

WESTERN MEDICAL CENTER
109 RIVER STREET
WESTERN, XY 44770

PHONE: (490) 555-6464
FAX: (490) 668-1414

To:	From:
Fax:	Pages:
Phone:	Date:
Re:	CC:

☐ URGENT ☐ FOR REVIEW ☐ PLEASE COMMENT ☐ PLEASE REPLY ☐ PLEASE RECYCLE

CONFIDENTIALITY STATEMENT:
The documents accompanying this transmission may contain confidential information that is protected under the Privacy Act of 1974. It is being faxed to you after appropriate patient authorization or under circumstances that do not require patient authorization. This information is intended only for the use of the intended recipient(s). The authorized recipient(s) of this information is/are prohibited from disclosing this information to any other party unless permitted to do so by law or regulation.

If the reader of this mess is not the intended recipient(s) or the employee or agent responsible for delivering the attached information to the intended recipient(s), please note that any dissemination, distribution, or copying of this information is strictly prohibited. **Anyone who receives this information in error should notify the sender immediately and arrange for the return or destruction of the transmitted information.**

MESSAGE:

EVALUATION OF COMPETENCY

Procedure 44-1: Composing a Business Letter

Name: ______________________ Date: ______________

Evaluated by: ______________________ Score: ______________

Performance Objective

Outcome:	Compose and key a business letter.
Conditions:	Given the following: letterhead stationery, blank stationery, and typewriter or computer and printer.
Standards:	Time: 10 minutes. Student completed procedure in _______ minutes.
	Accuracy: Satisfactory score on the Performance Evaluation Checklist.

Performance Evaluation Checklist

Trial 1	Trial 2	Point Value	Performance Standards
		•	Assembled materials.
		•	Determined the address of the recipient.
		•	Set up the letter according to selected format.
		•	Listed and organized essential content for the letter.
		•	Inserted the date on the second or third line below the letterhead.
		•	Placed the inside address 4 to 10 lines below the date at the left margin (to center the body of the letter on the page).
		•	Placed the salutation two lines below the inside address followed by a colon.
		•	Placed a subject line two lines below the salutation, if desired.
		•	Began the body of the letter two lines below the subject line (or salutation if no subject line was used).
		•	Single-spaced the letter with double spacing between paragraphs.
		•	Began paragraphs at the left margin or indented according to the letter style being used.
		•	Summarized the contents or most important ideas in the final paragraph of the letter.
		•	Placed the complimentary close two spaces below the final paragraph of the letter followed by a comma.
		•	Placed the typed signature four lines below the complimentary close with a title on the line below if appropriate.

Trial 1	Trial 2	Point Value	Performance Standards
		●	Added reference line, enclosure notation, and/or distribution notation as needed below the typed signature.
		●	Began a second page 1 inch from the top including the name of the recipient, the date, and the page number in the top left corner.
		●	Included at least two lines of the body of the letter on the second page, if one was used.
		*	Made sure that there were no errors in the letter using the computer and manual proofreading.
		●	Printed the letter.
		●	Signed the letter or obtained the appropriate signature.
		●	Made one copy of the letter for the file and additional copies for any individuals identified in the distribution notation.
		●	Prepared an envelope (Procedure 43-3: Preparing Envelopes for Mailing).
		●	Inserted the letter in the envelope and placed in the designated area to be mailed.
		●	Filed the copy of the letter according to office policy.
		*	Completed the procedure within 10 minutes.
			TOTALS

Evaluation of Student Performance

EVALUATION CRITERIA			COMMENTS
Symbol	Category	Point Value	
*	Critical Step	16 points	
●	Essential Step	6 points	
Ⓐ	Affective Competency	6 points	
▷	Theory Question	2 points	
Score calculation: 100 points – ___ points missed ___ Score Satisfactory score: 85 or above			

2008 CAAHEP Competency Achieved
Psychomotor (Skills) ☑ IV. 10. Compose professional/business letters.

2015 CAAHEP Competencies Achieved
Psychomotor (Skills) ☑ V. 8. Compose professional correspondence utilizing electronic technology.

ABHES Competencies Achieved
☑ 7.a. Perform basic keyboarding skills ☑ 8.a. Gather and process documents

Notes

EVALUATION OF COMPETENCY

Procedure 44-2: Sending a Fax

Name: ______________________ Date: ______________

Evaluated by: ______________________ Score: ______________

Performance Objective

Outcome:	Send a fax.
Conditions:	Given the following: fax machine, cover sheet, pen, and document to be faxed.
Standards:	Time: 5 minutes. Student completed procedure in ________ minutes.
	Accuracy: Satisfactory score on the Performance Evaluation Checklist.

Performance Evaluation Checklist

Trial 1	Trial 2	Point Value	Performance Standards
		●	Prepared the cover sheet including name, address, and fax and telephone number of the recipient, telephone number of the sender, and number of pages (including cover sheet).
		●	Placed any message to the sender at the bottom of the cover sheet.
		●	Organized all pages of the fax with the cover sheet first.
		●	Placed pages in the fax machine, face up or face down as required by the machine.
		●	Entered the fax number, including extra digits if required.
		●	Verified that the fax number was correct as it appeared in the window.
		●	Pressed the correct button to send the fax.
		●	Returned to remove the fax and verify that it had been sent.
		●	Filed the original document appropriately.
		*	Completed the procedure within 5 minutes.
			TOTALS

Evaluation of Student Performance

EVALUATION CRITERIA			COMMENTS
Symbol	Category	Point Value	
∗	Critical Step	16 points	
●	Essential Step	6 points	
Ⓐ	Affective Competency	6 points	
▷	Theory Question	2 points	
Score calculation: 100 points − ___ points missed ___ Score Satisfactory score: 85 or above			

2008 CAAHEP Competency Achieved
Psychomotor (Skills) ☑ IX. 3. Apply HIPAA rules in regard to privacy/release of information.

2015 CAAHEP Competencies Achieved
Psychomotor (Skills) ☑ X. 2. Apply HIPAA rules in regard to a. privacy or b. release of information.

ABHES Competencies Achieved
☑ 8.a. Gather and process documents

45 Mail

CHAPTER ASSIGNMENTS

✓ After Completing	Date Due	Study Guide Pages	STUDY GUIDE ASSIGNMENTS (CTA = Critical Thinking Activity)	Possible Points	Points You Earned
		1249	Pretest	10	
		1250	Term Key Term Assessment	7	
		1250-1252	Evaluation of Learning questions	30	
		1252-1253	CTA A: Classifications of Mail	6	
		1253	CTA B: Insurance and Delivery Confirmation Services	6	
		1253	CTA C: Determining Postage	8	
			Evolve Site: Apply Your Knowledge questions	10	
			Evolve Site: Video Evaluations	10	
		1249	Posttest	10	
			ADDITIONAL ASSIGNMENTS		
			TOTAL POINTS		

Notes

✓ When Assigned By Your Instructor	Study Guide Pages	Practices Required	LABORATORY ASSIGNMENTS (Procedure Number and Name)	Score*
	1255	3	**Practice for Competency** 45-1: Processing Incoming Mail Textbook reference: pp. 1137-1138	
	1257-1258		**Evaluation of Competency** 45-1: Processing Incoming Mail	*
	1255	3	**Practice for Competency** 45-2: Looking Up a ZIP Code Textbook reference: p. 1141	
	1259-1260		**Evaluation of Competency** 45-2: Looking Up a ZIP Code	*
	1255	3	**Practice for Competency** 45-3: Preparing Envelopes for Mailing Textbook reference: p. 1144	
	1261-1262		**Evaluation of Competency** 45-3: Preparing Envelopes for Mailing	*
			ADDITIONAL ASSIGNMENTS	

Notes

Name ____ Date ____________________

PRETEST

True or False

_______ 1. The ZIP + 4 gives more specific information about the destination of a letter than the 5-digit ZIP code.

_______ 2. The delivery time for Priority Mail is approximately the same as for First-Class Mail.

_______ 3. Standard Post is used by the medical office to mail packages.

_______ 4. The post office has machines that can read barcodes but not printed addresses.

_______ 5. The attention line of the address is placed directly below the recipient line.

_______ 6. The barcode free area of an envelope is at the lower right side of the envelope.

_______ 7. The address must be printed directly on an envelope.

_______ 8. A letter should be folded first in half and then in thirds to place in a number $6\frac{3}{4}$ envelope.

_______ 9. The medical office may purchase a postage meter for more efficient processing of the mail.

_______ 10. The same postage is required for a large envelope as a standard business envelope of the same weight.

POSTTEST

True or False

_______ 1. A postal barcode is often added to first-class letters by the post office to identify the letter's destination.

_______ 2. The fastest way to send an item through the USPS is Priority Mail Express.

_______ 3. A Return Receipt is usually combined with Certified Mail for proof of both mailing and receipt.

_______ 4. If the medical assistant (MA) opens mail for a physician, each item should be stamped with the date.

_______ 5. The attention line of the address should be placed below and to the left of the city, state, and ZIP line.

_______ 6. The address of an envelope should be printed or hand-printed using plain block letters.

_______ 7. A letter is folded exactly the same way to place in a window envelope as in a number $6\frac{3}{4}$ envelope.

_______ 8. Postage can be purchased for a postage meter by telephone, through the Internet, or from the post office.

_______ 9. Stamps can be printed in the office using an online postage service.

_______ 10. Postage meters only print postage on tapes that are applied to letters (i.e. they do not print postage directly on envelopes).

KEY TERM ASSESSMENT

Directions: Match each key term with its definition.

_______ 1. Annotate
_______ 2. Barcode clear zone
_______ 3. Metered mail
_______ 4. Postage meter
_______ 5. Postal barcode
_______ 6. ZIP code
_______ 7. ZIP + 4 code

A. The area on the lower right-hand corner of a card or letter, which is left clear for the postal barcode to be printed
B. A more detailed mailing code consisting of the original 5-digit ZIP code followed by a hyphen and four additional digits
C. A 5-digit code that identifies the post office to which a given piece of mail is to be delivered
D. Mail for which the postage has been applied using a postage meter
E. To underline or highlight important words and phrases in correspondence
F. A machine that automatically stamps a piece of mail with the correct postage
G. A series of vertical bars of two lengths, which represent the delivery address of a piece of mail that facilitates automated sorting of mail

EVALUATION OF LEARNING

Directions: Fill in each blank with the correct answer.

1. What is a ZIP + 4 code, and how is it different from a 5-digit ZIP code?

____

2. How does the USPS use barcodes?

____

____

3. Describe each of the following classifications of mail:

Priority Mail Express: ____

First-Class Mail: ____

Priority Mail: ____

Standard Post: ____

Media Mail: ____

4. What is Certified Mail?

____

5. Why does the medical office usually use Return Receipt instead of Signature Confirmation to obtain a record of the individual who signed for receipt of a mailed item?

____

____

6. When is a Certificate of Mailing obtained?

____

7. What service limits delivery of an item of mail specifically to the addressee?

8. What services are included when an item of mail is sent Registered Mail?

9. What service should be purchased for an item of value sent through the mail?

10. What are the advantages of using a private delivery service instead of the USPS to deliver packages?

11. What are general guidelines for sorting mail in the medical office?

12. If the MA opens mail for the physician, what should he or she do as soon as each item is opened?

13. How should letters regarding patients be arranged for the physician?

14. Why do some physicians ask the MA to annotate their correspondence?

15. How should the physician's mail be handled when he or she is on vacation?

16. What happens to a piece of mail that has a printed address after it has been mailed?

17. Name three pieces of automated equipment used by the USPS.

18. If an organization line is used in an address, where does the USPS recommend that it be placed?

19. What should be included in the bottom line of a delivery address?

20. What is the recommendation regarding punctuation in the address of an envelope?

21. Where should instructions such as Personal or Confidential be placed on an envelope?

____

22. Where should instructions for special services such as Certified or Registered be placed on an envelope?

____

23. What is the barcode clear zone, and where is it located on an envelope?

____

24. How does the MA prepare an envelope with the address directly on the envelope?

____

____

25. How does the MA prepare envelopes for a mailing of more than 30 envelopes?

____

____

26. Describe how to fold a letter for a standard #10 business envelope and for a window envelope.

____

____

27. Describe three ways to add postage to envelopes.

____

____

28. What are six safety measures to keep in mind when using a postage meter?

____

____

____

29. How can the MA obtain additional postage for a postage meter?

____

30. What services are offered by online postage services?

____

____

CRITICAL THINKING ACTIVITIES

A. Classifications of Mail

Identify the classification of mail you would use to mail each of the following items using the USPS.

1. Patient bill: _______________
2. Order form for office supplies: _______________
3. Package containing two books (needs to arrive in 2 to 3 days): _______________

4. Package containing two books (no rush): ____________________

5. Specimen for testing (weighs 9 oz): ____________________

6. Package of office supplies weighing 16 lb: ____________________

B. Insurance and Delivery Confirmation Services

For each of the following items identify whether the item should be insured, if Delivery Confirmation should be obtained, and/or if a Return Receipt should be obtained.

1. X-ray of the hip mailed to another physician: ____________________

2. Item of jewelry worth $12.00: ____________________

3. Item of jewelry worth $650.00: ____________________

4. Letter informing a patient that a physician is retiring: ____________________

5. Letter informing a patient that he or she must find a new physician for failing to keep appointments: ____________________

____

6. Official letter that must be received by a specific deadline: ____________________

C. Determining Postage

For each of the following, determine the correct postage (post office price) using the USPS website (www.usps.com).

First Class (rates as of 4/20/2012):

1. Letter in a #10 envelope weighing 2 oz from ZIP code 19101 to 60606: ____________________

2. Letter in a square envelope weighing 1 oz from ZIP code 19101 to 60606: ____________________

Priority Mail (from post office):

3. Package weighing 4 lb 6 oz from ZIP code 19101 to 60606: ____________________

4. Envelope weighing 14 oz from ZIP code 19101 to 60606: ____________________

Priority Mail Express (from post office):

5. Letter weighing 2 oz (small flat rate envelope) from ZIP code 02114 to 90806: ____________________

6. Letter weighing 2 oz (ordinary envelope) from ZIP code 02114 to 60606: ____________________

Standard Post and/or Media Mail:

7. Package of 3 boxes of gloves weighing 3 lb 2 oz from ZIP code 19101 to 60606: ____________________

8. Package of books weighing 4 lb 8 oz from ZIP code 02114 to 90806: ____________________

Notes

PRACTICE FOR COMPETENCY

Procedure 45-1: Processing Incoming Mail. Process incoming mail.

Procedure 45-2: Looking Up a ZIP Code. Look up ZIP codes for the following addresses to prepare envelopes or mailing labels for Procedure 45-3 using the USPS website (www.usps.com).

Centers for Disease Control and Prevention
1600 Clifton Road
Atlanta, GA [ZIP + 4]

National Institutes of Health
9000 Rockville Pike
Bethesda, MD [ZIP + 4]

Centers for Medicare and Medicaid Services
7500 Security Boulevard
Baltimore, MD [ZIP + 4]

U.S. Department of Health and Human Services
200 Independence Avenue, S.W.
Washington, DC [ZIP + 4]

Procedure 45-3: Preparing Envelopes for Mailing. Prepare envelopes of various sizes for mailing, weigh, and look up correct postage form your location using the USPS website. Be sure to include ZIP + 4 from Procedure 45-2.

Notes

EVALUATION OF COMPETENCY

Procedure 45-1: Processing Incoming Mail

Name: ______________________ Date: ______________

Evaluated by: ______________________ Score: ______________

Performance Objective

Outcome:	Process incoming mail.
Conditions:	Given the following: letter opener, date stamp, stamp pad, paper clips, stapler, pen or highlighter, and transparent tape.
Standards:	Time: 10 minutes. Student completed procedure in ________ minutes.
	Accuracy: Satisfactory score on the Performance Evaluation Checklist.

Performance Evaluation Checklist

Trial 1	Trial 2	Point Value	Performance Standards
		●	Assembled supplies in a work area large enough to make several piles.
		●	Arranged all envelopes so they faced in the same direction.
		●	Placed any envelopes marked "personal" or "confidential" to the side.
		●	Tapped the lower edge of the first envelope on the desk so contents fell to the bottom.
		●	Used a letter opener to open the envelope along the top edge, and removed the contents of the envelope.
		●	Checked to make sure the envelope was empty.
		●	Unfolded and flattened contents of the envelope.
		●	Stamped the date on the first page, preferably in the upper right corner.
		●	Checked to be sure the letter contained an inside address.
		●	Discarded the envelope if the letter contained an inside address; if not, stapled the envelope to the letter.
		●	Fastened enclosures to the letter with a paper clip.
		●	Wrote "no" beside an enclosure notation if any enclosures were missing.
		●	Mended any tears with tape.
		●	Used a highlighter or pen to annotate important points if directed to by the physician.
		●	Attached a sticky note indicating action that should be taken in response to the correspondence as needed.
		●	Opened additional envelopes in the same way until all mail was opened.

Trial 1	Trial 2	Point Value	Performance Standards
		●	Separated mail into piles of urgent mail, letters, or reports containing patient information or results, medical journals, advertising, and other categories as needed.
		●	Arranged letters and reports containing patient information in alphabetical order.
		●	Found and used a paper clip to attach the appropriate paper medical record to each letter or report containing medical information.
		●	Arranged the mail for each recipient from most important on top to least important on the bottom.
		●	Distributed each stack of mail to the appropriate individual.
		▷	Explained why efficient mail sorting helps maintain office effectiveness.
		✶	Completed the procedure within 10 minutes.
			TOTALS

Evaluation of Student Performance

EVALUATION CRITERIA			COMMENTS
Symbol	**Category**	**Point Value**	
✶	Critical Step	16 points	
●	Essential Step	6 points	
Ⓐ	Affective Competency	6 points	
▷	Theory Question	2 points	
Score calculation: 100 points − ___ points missed ___ Score Satisfactory score: 85 or above			

2008 CAAHEP Competency Achieved
Psychomotor ☑ IV.10. Compose professional business letters.

2015 CAAHEP Competency Achieved
Psychomotor ☑ V.8. Compose professional correspondence utilizing electronic technology.

ABHES Competencies Achieved
☑ 8. a. Gather and process documents

EVALUATION OF COMPETENCY

Procedure 45-2: Looking Up a ZIP Code

Name: ______________________________ Date: ______________

Evaluated by: ______________________________ Score: ______________

Performance Objective

Outcome:	Find the correct ZIP + 4 code for a given address.
Conditions:	Given the following: computer with Internet access, pen and pencil, address with incorrect and/or missing ZIP code.
Standards:	Time: 3 minutes. Student completed procedure in ________ minutes.
	Accuracy: Satisfactory score on the Performance Evaluation Checklist

Performance Evaluation Checklist

Trial 1	Trial 2	Point Value	Performance Standards
		●	Opened the computer's web browser and entered the web address for the United States Postal Service.
		●	From the USPS home page, selected "Find a ZIP code."
		●	On the "Search by Address" tab, entered the complete delivery address.
		✶	Copied the correct ZIP + 4 code on a piece of paper or used the computer copy function to copy and past into a computer file.
		✶	Completed the procedure within 3 minutes.
			TOTALS

Evaluation of Student Performance

EVALUATION CRITERIA			COMMENTS
Symbol	**Category**	**Point Value**	
✶	Critical Step	16 points	
●	Essential Step	6 points	
Ⓐ	Affective Competency	6 points	
▷	Theory Question	2 points	
Score calculation: 100 points − ____ points missed ____ Score Satisfactory score: 85 or above			

2008 CAAHEP Competency Achieved
Psychomotor ☑ IV.10. Compose professional business letters.

2015 CAAHEP Competency Achieved
Psychomotor ☑ V.8. Compose professional correspondence utilizing electronic technology.

ABHES Competencies Achieved
☑ 8. a. Gather and process documents.

EVALUATION OF COMPETENCY

Procedure 45-3: Preparing Envelopes for Mailing

Name: ______________________ Date: ______________________

Evaluated by: ______________________ Score: ______________________

Performance Objective

Outcome:	Prepare envelopes for mailing.
Conditions:	Given the following: envelope, other items to be mailed, pen, typewriter, computer and printer, postal scale, postage meter (optional), and/or stamps.
Standards:	Time: 3 minutes. Student completed procedure in __________ minutes.
	Accuracy: Satisfactory score on the Performance Evaluation Checklist.

Performance Evaluation Checklist

Trial 1	Trial 2	Point Value	Performance Standards
		•	Determined the exact address to be used for the envelope.
		•	Selected an envelope of the appropriate size.
		•	Decided on a means to address the envelope (e.g., typewriter, envelope wizard, label template, label program).
		*	Keyed or typed the address correctly according to USPS guidelines including the ZIP + 4 code.
		•	If using an envelope without letterhead, keyed the return address in the upper left corner of the envelope.
		•	Added any special notations such as "personal" or "confidential" below the return address in the upper left corner of the envelope.
		•	Added any mailing instructions on the right side of the envelope below the postage area.
		•	Folded and placed the letter or item to be mailed in the envelope and sealed it.
		•	Weighed the piece of mail if it contained more than two sheets of paper or if the envelope was larger than 6 1/8″ × 11½″.
		•	Calculated and applied the correct amount of postage.
		•	If a postage meter was used, processed all envelopes to be mailed that day.
		•	Sorted envelopes and other items to be mailed according to size.
		•	Separated any items with special mailing instructions to be taken to the post office.
		•	Placed items with postage in a mailbox or requested a pickup from the postal service.

Trial 1	Trial 2	Point Value	Performance Standards
		●	Set special items aside to be taken to the post office.
		✶	Completed the procedure within 10 minutes.
			TOTALS

Evaluation of Student Performance

EVALUATION CRITERIA			COMMENTS
Symbol	Category	Point Value	
✶	Critical Step	16 points	
●	Essential Step	6 points	
Ⓐ	Affective Competency	6 points	
▷	Theory Question	2 points	
Score calculation: 100 points – ____ points missed ____Score Satisfactory score: 85 or above			

2008 CAAHEP Competency Achieved
Psychomotor ☑ IV.10. Compose professional business letters.

2015 CAAHEP Competency Achieved
Psychomotor ☑ V.8. Compose professional correspondence utilizing electronic technology.

ABHES Competencies Achieved
☑ 8. a. Gather and process documents.

46 Managing Practice Finances

CHAPTER ASSIGNMENTS

✓ After Completing	Date Due	Study Guide Pages	STUDY GUIDE ASSIGNMENTS (CTA = Critical Thinking Activity)	Possible Points	Points You Earned
		1267	Pretest	10	
		1268	Term Key Term Assessment	24	
		1268-1271	Evaluation of Learning questions	29	
		1271	CTA A: The Charge Slip	8	
		1272	CTA B: Posting Transactions	8	
		1272	CTA C: Writing Checks	6	
		1272	CTA D: Endorsing Checks	6	
			Evolve Site: Guided Practice: Preparing a Bank Deposit	10	
			Evolve Site: Guided Practice: Writing Checks in Payment of Bills	10	
			Evolve Site: Apply Your Knowledge questions	10	
			Evolve Site: Video Evaluations	15	
		1267	Posttest	10	
			ADDITIONAL ASSIGNMENTS		
			TOTAL POINTS		

Notes

✓ When Assigned By Your Instructor	Study Guide Pages	Practices Required	LABORATORY ASSIGNMENTS (Procedure Number and Name)	Score*
	1273-1278	3	**Practice for Competency** 46-1: Completing a Patient Charge Slip Textbook reference: pp. 1152-1155	
	1287-1288		**Evaluation of Competency** 46-1: Completing a Patient Charge Slip	*
	1273-1278	3	**Practice for Competency** 46-2: Posting Charges Textbook reference: p. 1155	
	1289-1290		**Evaluation of Competency** 46-2: Posting Charges	*
	1273-1281	3	**Practice for Competency** 46-3: Posting Payments and/or Adjustments Textbook reference: pp. 1156-1157	
	1291-1292		**Evaluation of Competency** 46-3: Posting Payments and/or Adjustments	*
	1273-1283	3	**Practice for Competency** 46-4: Writing a Check Textbook reference: pp. 1163-1164	
	1293-1294		**Evaluation of Competency** 46-4: Writing a Check	*
	1273-1285	1	**Practice for Competency** 46-5: Preparing a Bank Deposit Textbook reference: p. 1165	
	1295-1296		**Evaluation of Competency** 46-5: Preparing a Bank Deposit	*
			ADDITIONAL ASSIGNMENTS	

Notes

Name ____________________ Date ____________

PRETEST

True or False

_______ 1. In the cash basis of accounting, income is entered when an item is sold or a service is provided.

_______ 2. Money owed to the medical practice by patients makes up the accounts receivable.

_______ 3. Practice management billing programs are usually based on the traditional pegboard system of bookkeeping.

_______ 4. A superbill contains a list of procedures commonly performed in the medical office.

_______ 5. An adjustment always reduces the balance of a patient's account.

_______ 6. If a computer billing program is used, the office will not create a manual day sheet.

_______ 7. A money market account usually has features of both a savings account and a checking account.

_______ 8. Each bank in the United States has a unique identification number.

_______ 9. Business accounting programs can often create and print checks.

_______ 10. To replenish the petty cash fund, the medical assistant can use any cash payment by a patient.

POSTTEST

True or False

_______ 1. If income is entered when an item is sold, the accrual basis of accounting is being used.

_______ 2. Each patient account is one of the accounts payable.

_______ 3. A daily journal is a chronological record of charges and payments for each day.

_______ 4. A superbill is an itemized charge slip.

_______ 5. The patient ledger shows only the charges and payments for a patient on a specific day.

_______ 6. All transactions posted to the computer are reflected in the day sheet of the day they were posted.

_______ 7. To receive interest on a checking account, it is usually necessary to maintain a minimum balance.

_______ 8. The MICR line is printed in magnetic ink across the bottom of a check.

_______ 9. If the medical assistant makes a mistake on a check, the check should be shredded or destroyed.

_______ 10. Every time money is taken from petty cash, a receipt should be completed.

KEY TERM ASSESSMENT

Directions: Match each key term with its definition.

_______ 1. ABA routing number
_______ 2. Accounting
_______ 3. Accounts payable
_______ 4. Accounts receivable
_______ 5. Accrual basis of accounting
_______ 6. Adjustment
_______ 7. Assets
_______ 8. Bookkeeping
_______ 9. Cash basis of accounting
_______ 10. Cashier's check
_______ 11. Certified check
_______ 12. Charge slip
_______ 13. Credit
_______ 14. Day sheet
_______ 15. Debit
_______ 16. Disbursements
_______ 17. Fee schedule
_______ 18. Ledger
_______ 19. Liabilities
_______ 20. MICR line
_______ 21. Payee
_______ 22. Petty cash
_______ 23. Reconciling
_______ 24. Superbill

A. Accounting method where income is entered when payment is received
B. A posting that is subtracted from an account balance
C. Accounting method where income is entered at the time of sale
D. An itemized charge slip usually also containing diagnosis codes and procedure codes
E. A form used to keep track of charges and payments at the time of a patient visit
F. A nine-digit number that identifies an individual bank
G. In accounting, the amount owed by a business to creditors
H. A check on an individual account that a bank assumes responsibility for
I. The person to whom a check is made out
J. A line of numbers across the bottom of a check that are read by a magnetic character reader
K. A cash account kept in a business office to pay for incidentals
L. A change to a patient account that is neither a charge nor a payment
M. List of charges for specific procedures that may be performed in a medical office
N. In accounting, a combination of property owned and money owed to a business
O. The outstanding bills of a business such as a medical office
P. Money paid out
Q. A posting that is added to an account balance
R. Making sure that two financial records agree
S. Systematic recording and reporting of financial transactions
T. A book, card, or computer account used to record financial transactions
U. The process of posting charges and payments and balancing financial records
V. The chronological record of daily transactions
W. Total amount owed to a business for goods and services
X. A check drawn on a bank instead of an individual account

EVALUATION OF LEARNING

Directions: Fill in each blank with the correct answer.

1. What is the difference between the cash basis and the accrual basis of accounting?

____

____

2. What generates income in the medical office?

____

____

3. What are three types of financial records used in a bookkeeping system?

____

____

4. If patient charges are recorded using a computer billing program, where must the data about the charge be entered? Why is it sufficient to enter the data once?

____

____

5. Why does a charge slip (superbill) usually contain diagnosis and procedure codes?

____

____

6. How does the medical assistant (MA) know what to charge a patient for a specific procedure?

____

____

7. If the office typically charges $65.00 to perform an electrocardiogram, is this the amount paid by all patients? Why or why not?

____

____

8. How is information arranged in the patient account ledger?

____

9. What are four ways that payments are made to a patient account?

____

____

10. What is the difference between a credit adjustment and a debit adjustment? Give one example of each.

____

____

11. When an insurance company pays an amount that is lower than the usual charge, how is the patient's balance due returned to zero?

____

____

12. What information is recorded on a day sheet?

____

13. What does it mean to "close the day," and why is this important for accurate financial record-keeping?

____

____

14. Describe three types of bank accounts.

____

____

____

15. Describe the services and function of a checking account.

____

16. What is the advantage of maintaining a savings account or money market account compared with a checking account?

____

____

17. Differentiate between a cashier's check and a certified check. Which is used more often?

____

____

18. What is the MICR (magnetic ink character recognition) line on a check, and what information does it contain?

____

____

19. Identify three ways that checks can be generated or bills can be paid, and describe how information is recorded.

____

____

____

____

20. What should the MA do if he or she writes a check incorrectly?

____

____

21. What are common precautions for accepting checks in the medical office?

____

____

____

22. If a medical office accepts credit or debit cards, what policies should be in place?

____

____

23. How is the cash drawer balanced at the end of the day?

____

____

24. What is necessary before a check can be cashed or deposited? How is this handled in a medical office?

____

____

25. What is the difference between a special endorsement and a restricted endorsement?

____

____

26. Identify five reasons why the monthly bank statement may not agree with the medical office's calculation of the bank balance in a checking account.

____

____

____

27. What steps must be taken to reconcile a bank account?

____

____

____

28. What financial accounts does a medical office usually have, and what do those accounts include?

____

____

29. How is a petty cash fund (account) managed?

____

____

____

CRITICAL THINKING ACTIVITIES

A. The Charge Slip

Refer to the completed charge slip in your textbook (Figure 46-2), and identify the following information.

1. The name of the insured person: _______________
2. The patient's insurance ID number: _______________
3. The charge for the patient's office visit: _______________
4. The patient's telephone number: _______________
5. The name of the diagnostic test performed: _______________
6. The balance owed by the patient: _______________
7. The patient's birth date: _______________
8. The patient's physician: _______________

B. Posting Transactions

Identify whether each of the following transactions would be posted as a charge, a payment, or an adjustment in the computer billing program or on a pegboard day sheet.

1. Office visit: ___
2. Check from insurance company: ___
3. Tetanus injection: ___
4. Dipstick urinalysis: ___
5. Insurance excluded amount: ___
6. Professional courtesy discount: ___
7. Spirometry test: ___
8. Patient check: ___

C. Writing Checks

Demonstrate how to write the following amounts in words on a check.

1. $76.42 ___ DOLLARS
2. $189.28 ___ DOLLARS
3. $1,020.00 ___ DOLLARS
4. $6.40 ___ DOLLARS
5. $16.04 ___ DOLLARS
6. $382.00 ___ DOLLARS

D. Endorsing Checks

Identify if each of the following is a blank endorsement, restrictive endorsement, or special endorsement.

1. *Maria S. Sanchez* ___
2. Pay to the order of: Robert A. Wilson
   Maria S. Sanchez ___
3. Robert A. Wilson
   Acct. # 12345-67890 ___
4. For deposit only
   Robert A. Wilson ___
5. Pay to the order of: Diane M. Casey
   Frederick Underwood ___
6. For deposit Acct. # 3456-78901
   Edward B. Young ___

PRACTICE FOR COMPETENCY

Use the following information to practice Procedures 46-1 through 46-3. Use today's date for all work.

FEE SCHEDULE				
Office Visit, New Patient			**Office Visit, Established Patient**	
			99211 Nurse/Minimal OV	$ 24.00
99201	Problem Focused OV*	$ 31.00	99212 Problem Focused OV	$ 32.00
99202	Exp** Problem Focused OV	$ 50.00	99213 Exp Problem Focused OV	$ 40.00
OFFICE PROCEDURES				
36415	Venipuncture Collection	$ 12.00	93000 ECG*** w/interpretation	$ 89.00
81002	Urinalysis w/o micro, non-automated	$ 22.00	94010 Spirometry	$ 78.00
87880	Strep test (rapid)	$ 21.00	94640 Nebulizer Treatment	$ 49.22

*OV—office visit
**Exp—Expanded
***ECG—electrocardiogram

PATIENT INFORMATION

Ken Thomas 398 Larkin Avenue Anytown, AL 12345 (123) 784-1118 DOB: 10/25/1961 Diagnosis: Hypertension Procedures: Problem-focused office visit Previous Balance: $45.00 Payment: $10.00 by patient check on bank #242-XX/110	Account Number: 72605 Established Patient of Jean Burke, NP Name of Insured: self Insurance Plan: Blue Cross Blue Shield Insurance ID: 783-21-2215 Group # 55124T

Tai Yan Martin Way Apt. 241 Anytown, AL 12345 (123) 963-3691 DOB: 4/7/1956 Diagnosis: Streptococcal sore throat Procedures: Problem-focused office visit, Strep test (rapid) Previous Balance: -0- Payment: $10.00 by check on bank # 02-XX/502 Cash Discount: - $10.00 (professional courtesy adjustment)	Account Number: 72087 New Patient of Jean Burke, NP Name of Insured: Tai Yan Insurance Plan: Blue Cross Blue Shield Insurance ID: 666-59-8431 Group: 3547BY

Anna Richardson 11 Pruitt Lane Anytown, AL 12345 (123) 122-3987 DOB: 02/14/1978 Diagnoses: Chest pain; Hypertension Procedures: Expanded problem-focused office visit, ECG Previous Balance: $15.00	Account Number: 35418 Established Patient of Dr. Martin Name of Insured: self Insurance Plan: MetLife Insurance ID:347-46-9514 Group: 95364R

Monique Jones 1875 Wellington Springs Court Anytown, AL 12345 (123) 588-9994 DOB: 6/23/1985 Previous Balance: $39.00 Insurance Payment for Visit 9/02/XX: $26.00 by check on bank #602-XX/110 Insurance Excluded Amount: $13.00	Account Number: 89643 Established Patient of Dr. Martin Name of Insured: Monique Jones Insurance Plan: Blue Cross Blue Shield Insurance ID: 278-23-2324 Group: 7851J

Procedure 46-1: Completing a Patient Charge Slip. Fill out charge slips for Ken Thomas, Tai Yan, and Anna Richardson using today's date and time. The forms are located on the next pages.

Create superbills for Ken Thomas, Tai Yan, and Anna Richardson using SimChart® for the Medical Office. In the Simulation Playground, select **Superbill** from the **Coding and Billing** Info Panel, and enter the information as requested. Save each page before progressing to the next page.

Procedure 46-2: Posting Charges. Post charges for Ken Thomas, Tai Yan, and Anna Richardson for the information above. Use a separate transaction entry form for each patient. For code, use the CPT code.

Transaction Entry

Date	Pt #	Patient Name	Provider	Code	Description	Amount

Transaction Entry

Date	Pt #	Patient Name	Provider	Code	Description	Amount

Transaction Entry

Date	Pt #	Patient Name	Provider	Code	Description	Amount

Walden-Martin Family Medical Clinic
1234 Anystreet
Anytown, AL 12345
123-123-1234

James Martin, MD	NPI # 23456781XX
Julie Walden, MD	NPI # 34567891XX
Jean Burke, NP	Tax ID 52-XX63777

Patient Name and Address	Birthdate	Subscriber Name	Provider Name	Today's Date
	Account #	Insurance Company	Insurance Phone #	Time
Telephone No.		Insurance ID #	Group/Plan #	Sex
				Male ☐ Female ☐

√	DESCRIPTION	CPT	FEE	√	DESCRIPTION	CPT	FEE	√	DESCRIPTION	CPT	FEE
	OFFICE VISIT				**IMMUNIZATIONS**				**PROCEDURES**		
	NEW PATIENT				Imm. admin, one	90471			EKG w/interpretation	93000	
	Problem Focused	99201			Imm. admin, each add'l	90472			Spirometry	94010	
	Exp. Prob. Focused	99202			Influenza < 3	90657			Inhalation treatment	94640	
	Detailed	99203			Influenza 3 and >	90658			Remove skin tag <15	11200	
	Comp/Mod MDM	99204			Medicare code	G0008			Cerumen removal	69210	
	Comp./High MDM	99205			Varicella	90716			Wart destruction < 14	17110	
	ESTABLISHED PATIENT				DTaP	90700			I & D abscess	10060	
	Minimal/Nurse Visit	99211			Td adult	90718					
	Problem Focused	99212			Rubella	90706					
	Exp. Problem Focused	99213			MMR	90707			**OTHER**		
	Detailed	99214			Hep B Child	90744					
	Comprehensive	99215			Hep B Adult	90746					
	Post-op Exam	99024			IPV	90713					
	WELL VISIT				**WELL VISIT**				**LABORATORY**		
	NEW PATIENT				ESTABLISHED PATIENT				Blood collection Vein	36415	
	Infant–1 year	99381			Infant–1 year	99391			Venipuncture, Medicare	G0001	
	1 yr–4 yr	99382			1 yr–4 yr	99392			Finger stick, glucose	82948	
	5 yr – 11 yr	99383			5 yr –11 yr	99393			Hemoccult, guaiac	82270	
	12 yr–17 yr	99384			12 yr–17 yr	99394			Strep, rapid	87880	
	18 yr –39 yr	99385			18 yr –39 yr	99395			UA, dipstick (manual)	81000	
	40 yr –64 yr	99386			40 yr –64 yr	99396			UA, automated	81003	
	65 yr and over	99387			65 yr and over	99397			Urine pregnancy	81025	

DIAGNOSTIC CODES (ICD-10-CM)

☐ R10.9 Abdominal Pain	☐ E11.9 Diabetes II–Non Ins	☐ H66.9_ Otitis Media	☐ Z23 Immunization Encounter
☐ E63.4 AllergicReaction	☐ K57.92 Diverticulitis	☐ J02.9 Pharyngitis	☐ Z00.12_ Well Child Check
☐ D64.9 Anemia	☐ K57.90 Diverticulosis	☐ M06.9 Rheumatoid Arthritis	☐ Z00.0_ Well Adult
☐ D51.0 Anemia, Pernicious	☐ R60.9 Edema	☐ R06.02 Short of Breath	☐ ________
☐ I12.9 Angina Pectoris	☐ R51 Headache	☐ J32.9 Sinusitis	☐ ________
☐ I49.9 Arrhythmia, Cardiac	☐ R31.9 Hematuria	☐ L19.8 Skin Tag(s)	☐ ________
☐ I70.0 Atherosclerosis, Aorta	☐ B00.9 Herpes Zoster	☐ J02.0 Streptococcal Sore Throat	☐ ________
☐ J45.909 Asthma	☐ I10 Hypertension	☐ N39.0 Urinary Tract Infection	☐ ________
☐ M54.9 Back Pain	☐ E03.9 Hypothyroidism	**RETURN APPOINTMENT**	**BALANCE DUE**
☐ J20._ Bronchitis, Acute	☐ H61.2_ Impacted Cerumen	________ Days	Total Charge $
☐ J42 Bronchitis, Chronic	☐ J10.1 Influenza	________ Weeks	Amount Paid $
☐ R07.9 Chest Pain	☐ K58.9 Irritable Bowel Syndrome	________ Months	Previous Bal $
☐ J44.9 COPD	☐ M19.0 Osteoarthritis	________ PRN	Adjustment $
☐ E10.0 Diabetes I–Ins. Dep	☐ M19.0 Osteoarthritis		Balance Due $

Notes

Walden-Martin Family Medical Clinic
1234 Anystreet
Anytown, AL 12345
123-123-1234

James Martin, MD — NPI # 23456781XX
Julie Walden, MD — NPI # 34567891XX
Jean Burke, NP — Tax ID 52-XX63777

Patient Name and Address	Birthdate	Subscriber Name	Provider Name	Today's Date
	Account #	Insurance Company	Insurance Phone #	Time
Telephone No.		Insurance ID #	Group/Plan #	Sex
				Male ☐ Female ☐

√	DESCRIPTION	CPT	FEE	√	DESCRIPTION	CPT	FEE	√	DESCRIPTION	CPT	FEE
	OFFICE VISIT				**IMMUNIZATIONS**				**PROCEDURES**		
	NEW PATIENT				Imm. admin, one	90471			EKG w/interpretation	93000	
	Problem Focused	99201			Imm. admin, each add'l	90472			Spirometry	94010	
	Exp. Prob. Focused	99202			Influenza < 3	90657			Inhalation treatment	94640	
	Detailed	99203			Influenza 3 and >	90658			Remove skin tag <15	11200	
	Comp/Mod MDM	99204			Medicare code	G0008			Cerumen removal	69210	
	Comp./High MDM	99205			Varicella	90716			Wart destruction < 14	17110	
	ESTABLISHED PATIENT				DTaP	90700			I & D abscess	10060	
	Minimal/Nurse Visit	99211			Td adult	90718					
	Problem Focused	99212			Rubella	90706					
	Exp. Problem Focused	99213			MMR	90707			**OTHER**		
	Detailed	99214			Hep B Child	90744					
	Comprehensive	99215			Hep B Adult	90746					
	Post-op Exam	99024			IPV	90713					
	WELL VISIT				**WELL VISIT**				**LABORATORY**		
	NEW PATIENT				ESTABLISHED PATIENT				Blood collection Vein	36415	
	Infant–1 year	99381			Infant–1 year	99391			Venipuncture, Medicare	G0001	
	1 yr–4 yr	99382			1 yr–4 yr	99392			Finger stick, glucose	82948	
	5 yr – 11 yr	99383			5 yr –11 yr	99393			Hemoccult, guaiac	82270	
	12 yr–17 yr	99384			12 yr–17 yr	99394			Strep, rapid	87880	
	18 yr –39 yr	99385			18 yr –39 yr	99395			UA, dipstick (manual)	81000	
	40 yr –64 yr	99386			40 yr –64 yr	99396			UA, automated	81003	
	65 yr and over	99387			65 yr and over	99397			Urine pregnancy	81025	

DIAGNOSTIC CODES (ICD-10-CM)

☐ R10.9 Abdominal Pain	☐ E11.9 Diabetes II–Non Ins	☐ H66.9_ Otitis Media	☐ Z23 Immunization Encounter
☐ E63.4 AllergicReaction	☐ K57.92 Diverticulitis	☐ J02.9 Pharyngitis	☐ Z00.12_ Well Child Check
☐ D64.9 Anemia	☐ K57.90 Diverticulosis	☐ M06.9 Rheumatoid Arthritis	☐ Z00.0_ Well Adult
☐ D51.0 Anemia, Pernicious	☐ R60.9 Edema	☐ R06.02 Short of Breath	☐ ________
☐ I12.9 Angina Pectoris	☐ R51 Headache	☐ J32.9 Sinusitis	☐ ________
☐ I49.9 Arrhythmia, Cardiac	☐ R31.9 Hematuria	☐ L19.8 Skin Tag(s)	☐ ________
☐ I70.0 Atherosclerosis, Aorta	☐ B00.9 Herpes Zoster	☐ J02.0 Streptococcal Sore Throat	☐ ________
☐ J45.909 Asthma	☐ I10 Hypertension	☐ N39.0 Urinary Tract Infection	☐ ________
☐ M54.9 Back Pain	☐ E03.9 Hypothyroidism	**RETURN APPOINTMENT**	**BALANCE DUE**
☐ J20._ Bronchitis, Acute	☐ H61.2_ Impacted Cerumen	______ Days	Total Charge $
☐ J42 Bronchitis, Chronic	☐ J10.1 Influenza	______ Weeks	Amount Paid $
☐ R07.9 Chest Pain	☐ K58.9 Irritable Bowel Syndrome	______ Months	Previous Bal $
☐ J44.9 COPD	☐ M19.0 Osteoarthritis	______ PRN	Adjustment $
☐ E10.0 Diabetes I–Ins. Dep	☐ M19.0 Osteoarthritis		Balance Due $

Notes

Walden-Martin Family Medical Clinic
1234 Anystreet
Anytown, AL 12345
123-123-1234

James Martin, MD
Julie Walden, MD
Jean Burke, NP

NPI # 23456781XX
NPI # 34567891XX
Tax ID 52-XX63777

Patient Name and Address	Birthdate	Subscriber Name	Provider Name	Today's Date
	Account #	Insurance Company	Insurance Phone #	Time
Telephone No.		Insurance ID #	Group/Plan #	Sex
				Male ☐ Female ☐

√	DESCRIPTION	CPT	FEE	√	DESCRIPTION	CPT	FEE	√	DESCRIPTION	CPT	FEE
	OFFICE VISIT				**IMMUNIZATIONS**				**PROCEDURES**		
	NEW PATIENT				Imm. admin, one	90471			EKG w/interpretation	93000	
	Problem Focused	99201			Imm. admin, each add'l	90472			Spirometry	94010	
	Exp. Prob. Focused	99202			Influenza < 3	90657			Inhalation treatment	94640	
	Detailed	99203			Influenza 3 and >	90658			Remove skin tag <15	11200	
	Comp/Mod MDM	99204			Medicare code	G0008			Cerumen removal	69210	
	Comp./High MDM	99205			Varicella	90716			Wart destruction < 14	17110	
	ESTABLISHED PATIENT				DTaP	90700			I & D abscess	10060	
	Minimal/Nurse Visit	99211			Td adult	90718					
	Problem Focused	99212			Rubella	90706					
	Exp. Problem Focused	99213			MMR	90707			**OTHER**		
	Detailed	99214			Hep B Child	90744					
	Comprehensive	99215			Hep B Adult	90746					
	Post-op Exam	99024			IPV	90713					
	WELL VISIT				**WELL VISIT**				**LABORATORY**		
	NEW PATIENT				ESTABLISHED PATIENT				Blood collection Vein	36415	
	Infant–1 year	99381			Infant–1 year	99391			Venipuncture, Medicare	G0001	
	1 yr–4 yr	99382			1 yr–4 yr	99392			Finger stick, glucose	82948	
	5 yr – 11 yr	99383			5 yr –11 yr	99393			Hemoccult, guaiac	82270	
	12 yr–17 yr	99384			12 yr–17 yr	99394			Strep, rapid	87880	
	18 yr –39 yr	99385			18 yr –39 yr	99395			UA, dipstick (manual)	81000	
	40 yr –64 yr	99386			40 yr –64 yr	99396			UA, automated	81003	
	65 yr and over	99387			65 yr and over	99397			Urine pregnancy	81025	

DIAGNOSTIC CODES (ICD-10-CM)

☐ R10.9 Abdominal Pain	☐ E11.9 Diabetes II–Non Ins	☐ H66.9_ Otitis Media	☐ Z23 Immunization Encounter
☐ E63.4 AllergicReaction	☐ K57.92 Diverticulitis	☐ J02.9 Pharyngitis	☐ Z00.12_ Well Child Check
☐ D64.9 Anemia	☐ K57.90 Diverticulosis	☐ M06.9 Rheumatoid Arthritis	☐ Z00.0_ Well Adult
☐ D51.0 Anemia, Pernicious	☐ R60.9 Edema	☐ R06.02 Short of Breath	☐ ____________
☐ I12.9 Angina Pectoris	☐ R51 Headache	☐ J32.9 Sinusitis	☐ ____________
☐ I49.9 Arrhythmia, Cardiac	☐ R31.9 Hematuria	☐ L19.8 Skin Tag(s)	☐ ____________
☐ I70.0 Atherosclerosis, Aorta	☐ B00.9 Herpes Zoster	☐ J02.0 Streptococcal Sore Throat	☐ ____________
☐ J45.909 Asthma	☐ I10 Hypertension	☐ N39.0 Urinary Tract Infection	☐ ____________
☐ M54.9 Back Pain	☐ E03.9 Hypothyroidism	**RETURN APPOINTMENT**	**BALANCE DUE**
☐ J20._ Bronchitis, Acute	☐ H61.2_ Impacted Cerumen		Total Charge $
☐ J42 Bronchitis, Chronic	☐ J10.1 Influenza	_______ Days	Amount Paid $
☐ R07.9 Chest Pain	☐ K58.9 Irritable Bowel Syndrome	_______ Weeks	Previous Bal $
☐ J44.9 COPD	☐ M19.0 Osteoarthritis	_______ Months	Adjustment $
☐ E10.0 Diabetes I–Ins. Dep	☐ M19.0 Osteoarthritis	_______ PRN	Balance Due $

Notes

Procedure 46-3: Posting Payments and/or Adjustments. Post payment (CHECK) for Ken Thomas. Post payment (CHECK) and credit adjustment (CRADJ) for Tai Yan. Post insurance payment (INSPAY) and insurance adjustment (INSADJ) for Monique Jones. Use a separate transaction entry form for each patient. The codes are given in parentheses.

Transaction Entry

Date	Pt #	Patient Name	Provider	Code	Description	Amount

Transaction Entry

Date	Pt #	Patient Name	Provider	Code	Description	Amount

Transaction Entry

Date	Pt #	Patient Name	Provider	Code	Description	Amount

Post charge(s), payment (if any) and adjustment (if any) for Ken Thomas, Tai Yan, and Anna Richardson using SimChart® for the Medical Office. In the Simulation Playground, select **Ledger** from the **Coding and Billing** Info Panel, and enter the information as requested. Add rows as needed. Save when all charges, payments and adjustments have been added

Procedure 46-4: Writing a Check. Write checks to pay the following bills beginning with check number 1837 found on p. 1283 Use today's date. The beginning balance brought forward is $4,482.21. Complete each check stub.

a. Write a check for $822.00 to Mitchell Associates for rent.
b. Write a check for $329.62 to ABC Pharmacy for medical supplies.
c. Write a check for $219.64 to Holt Office Supply for office supplies.

Procedure 46-5: Preparing a Bank Deposit. Prepare a bank deposit slip for the checks received from June Simmons, Robert Underwood, and Standard Health HMO (for Marie Richards). Use today's date. Place the practice name (Western Medical Center) on the deposit slip found on p. 1285.

Notes

1837

DATE

TO

FOR

BALANCE BROUGHT FORWARD		
DEPOSITS		
BALANCE		
AMT THIS CK		
BALANCE CARRIED FORWARD		

1837

BLACKBURN PRIMARY CARE ASSOCIATES, PC
1990 Turquiose Drive
Blackburn, WI 54937
608-459-8857

94-72/1224

DATE

PAY TO THE ORDER OF $

DOLLARS

DERBYSHIRE SAVINGS
Member FDIC
P.O. BOX 8923
Blackburn, WI 54937

FOR

⑈055003⑈ 446782011⑈ 678800470

SAMPLE

1838

DATE

TO

FOR

BALANCE BROUGHT FORWARD		
DEPOSITS		
BALANCE		
AMT THIS CK		
BALANCE CARRIED FORWARD		

1838

BLACKBURN PRIMARY CARE ASSOCIATES, PC
1990 Turquiose Drive
Blackburn, WI 54937
608-459-8857

94-72/1224

DATE

PAY TO THE ORDER OF $

DOLLARS

DERBYSHIRE SAVINGS
Member FDIC
P.O. BOX 8923
Blackburn, WI 54937

FOR

⑈055003⑈ 446782011⑈ 678800470

SAMPLE

1839

DATE

TO

FOR

BALANCE BROUGHT FORWARD		
DEPOSITS		
BALANCE		
AMT THIS CK		
BALANCE CARRIED FORWARD		

1839

BLACKBURN PRIMARY CARE ASSOCIATES, PC
1990 Turquiose Drive
Blackburn, WI 54937
608-459-8857

94-72/1224

DATE

PAY TO THE ORDER OF $

DOLLARS

DERBYSHIRE SAVINGS
Member FDIC
P.O. BOX 8923
Blackburn, WI 54937

FOR

⑈055003⑈ 446782011⑈ 678800470

SAMPLE

Notes

DEPOSIT TICKET

BANK OF OHIO
223 MAIN STREET
WESTERN, OH 44770

DATE:______________________

	DOLLARS	CENTS
CURRENCY		
COIN		
CHECKS (LIST SEPARATELY)		
1		
2		
3		
4		
5		
6		
7		
8		
9		
10		
11		
12		
13		
14		
15		
16		
17		
18		
19		
20		
TOTAL FROM ATTACHED LIST:		
TOTAL		

:50 2000001:: 0073872061"

Total Deposit [ ] Total Items [ ]

Notes

EVALUATION OF COMPETENCY

Procedure 46-1: Completing a Patient Charge Slip

Name: ______________________ Date: ______________

Evaluated by: ______________________ Score: ______________

Performance Objective

Outcome:	Complete a patient charge slip.
Conditions:	Given the following: blank charge slip, patient information form or computer data, daily patient schedule, calculator, and fee schedule.
Standards:	Time: 10 minutes. Student completed procedure in __________ minutes.
	Accuracy: Satisfactory score on the Performance Evaluation Checklist.

Performance Evaluation Checklist

Trial 1	Trial 2	Point Value	Performance Standards
		•	Completed the top part of a patient charge slip manually, using a computer, or by printing a label from the computer.
		•	Verified that the patient's name, date of birth, insurance, insurance group and ID numbers, and name of the subscriber have been entered or have printed correctly.
		•	Entered the patient's previous balance on the bottom of the charge slip.
		•	Used the fee schedule to fill in the fee in the box beside the code and name of each procedure performed during the office visit.
		•	Completed the bottom of the charge slip by entering the total charges, payments, and any adjustments.
		•	Totaled the new balance at the bottom of the charge slip correctly.
		•	Completed any other information requested on the charge slip including diagnosis.
		*	Completed the entire charge slip accurately.
		*	Completed the procedure within 10 minutes.
			TOTALS
			Superbill in SimChart® for the Medical Office
		•	Selected a patient, created an encounter, and selected **Superbill** on the **Coding and Billing** tab.
		•	Documented copayment amount and amount paid.
		•	Calculated and entered total charges.
		•	Calculated and entered amount due.

Trial 1	Trial 2	Point Value	Performance Standards
		●	Entered diagnosis code(s), and selected ICD-9 or ICD-10.
		●	Entered CPT codes and fee for all services received.
		●	Selected New or Est appropriately and entered correct rank of diagnosis for each CPT code.
		●	Saved each page before progressing to a new page.
		●	Entered all required information and submitted the superbill.
		✶	Completed the entire charge slip accurately.
		✶	Completed the procedure within 10 minutes.
			TOTALS

Evaluation of Student Performance

EVALUATION CRITERIA			COMMENTS
Symbol	Category	Point Value	
✶	Critical Step	16 points	
●	Essential Step	6 points	
Ⓐ	Affective Competency	6 points	
▷	Theory Question	2 points	
Score calculation: 100 points − ___ points missed ___ Score Satisfactory score: 85 or above			

2008 CAAHEP Competency Achieved
Psychomotor (Skills) ☑ VI. 2.b. Perform billing procedures.

2015 CAAHEP Competencies Achieved
Psychomotor (Skills) ☑ VII.1.a. Perform accounts receivable procedures to patient accounts including posting charges. ☑ VII. 4. Inform a patient of financial obligations for services rendered.

ABHES Competencies Achieved
☑ 8.b. Perform billing and collection procedures: 1. Accounts payable and accounts receivable.

EVALUATION OF COMPETENCY

Procedure 46-2: Posting Charges

Name: ______________________________ Date: ______________

Evaluated by: ______________________________ Score: ______________

Performance Objective

Outcome:	Post charges to the patient account.
Conditions:	Given the following: patient charge slip, patient ledger card or computer account, fee schedule, and pen and/or computer.
Standards:	Time: 5 minutes. Student completed procedure in __________ minutes.
	Accuracy: Satisfactory score on the Performance Evaluation Checklist.

Performance Evaluation Checklist

Trial 1	Trial 2	Point Value	Performance Standards
		●	Posted total charges in the column labeled "charges" of a manual ledger card or the first charge on the first line of a transaction entry screen in a computer program or ledger in SimChart® for the Medical Office.
		●	If using a computer system, posted each additional charge on a new line.
		●	If using a manual system, entered the total charge in the balance column. If using a computer system, saved work after all charges were posted.
		✶	Entered the charges and calculated the new balance accurately.
		✶	Completed the procedure within 5 minutes.
			TOTALS

Evaluation of Student Performance

EVALUATION CRITERIA			COMMENTS
Symbol	**Category**	**Point Value**	
✶	Critical Step	16 points	
●	Essential Step	6 points	
Ⓐ	Affective Competency	6 points	
▷	Theory Question	2 points	
Score calculation: 100 points – ____ points missed ____ Score Satisfactory score: 85 or above			

2008 CAAHEP Competency Achieved
Psychomotor (Skills) ☑ VI. 2.b. Perform billing procedures

2015 CAAHEP Competency Achieved
☑ VII.1.a. Perform accounts receivable procedures to patient accounts including posting charges.

ABHES Competencies Achieved
☑ 8.b. Perform billing and collection procedures: 1. Accounts payable and accounts receivable.

EVALUATION OF COMPETENCY

Procedure 46-3: Posting Payments and/or Adjustments

Name: ______________________________ Date: ____________________

Evaluated by: ______________________________ Score: ____________________

Performance Objective

Outcome:	Post payments and/or adjustments.
Conditions:	Given the following: Patient ledger card or computer account, cash or check from the patient or check from the insurance carrier, calculator, stamp with a restrictive endorsement, stamp pad, and pen.
Standards:	Time: 5 minutes. Student completed procedure in __________ minutes.
	Accuracy: Satisfactory score on the Performance Evaluation Checklist.

Performance Evaluation Checklist

Trial 1	Trial 2	Point Value	Performance Standards
		•	Located the patient account in the computer or selected the patient ledger card.
		•	Posted a payment from a completed patient charge slip to the patient account accurately using the same line or screen as the charges for that day.
		•	Included the check number in a manual system or used the correct code for a patient payment in a computer system.
		•	Posted an insurance payment under the date the payment was received.
		•	Used a new line for an insurance payment in a manual system or on a patient ledger in SimChart® for the Medical Office.
		•	Used the correct code or designation for an insurance payment.
		•	Entered the amount excluded by the insurance carrier as a negative adjustment in the adjustment column of a manual system and using the code for insurance write off in a computer system.
		•	Calculated or verified the patient balance and saved work in a computer system.
		*	Posted payment and any adjustment accurately, and calculated correct new patient balance.
		•	Endorsed a check using a stamp with the restrictive endorsement "For deposit only" and the number of the checking account.
		•	Placed a processed check or cash in the designated drawer or money box.
		*	Completed the procedure within 5 minutes.
			TOTALS

Evaluation of Student Performance

EVALUATION CRITERIA			COMMENTS
Symbol	**Category**	**Point Value**	
∗	Critical Step	16 points	
●	Essential Step	6 points	
Ⓐ	Affective Competency	6 points	
▷	Theory Question	2 points	
Score calculation: 100 points − ___ points missed ___ Score Satisfactory score: 85 or above			

2008 CAAHEP Competencies Achieved
Psychomotor (Skills) ☑ VI. 2.b. Perform billing procedures ☑ VI. 2. d. Post adjustments

2015 CAAHEP Competency Achieved
Psychomotor (Skills) ☑ VII. 1. Perform accounts receivable procedures to patient accounts including posting: b. payments, c. adjustments.

ABHES Competencies Achieved
☑ 8.b. Perform billing and collection procedures 1. Accounts payable and accounts receivable. 2. Post adjustments

EVALUATION OF COMPETENCY

Procedure 46-4: Writing a Check

Name: ______________________ Date: ______________

Evaluated by: ______________________ Score: ______________

Performance Objective

Outcome:	Write a check, and record and calculate new account balance.
Conditions:	Given the following: checks, check register or check stubs, bill to be paid, and pen.
Standards:	Time: 5 minutes. Student completed procedure in ______ minutes.
	Accuracy: Satisfactory score on the Performance Evaluation Checklist.

Performance Evaluation Checklist

Trial 1	Trial 2	Point Value	Performance Standards
		●	Selected a bill to be paid.
		●	Using a pen, wrote the date on the date line.
		●	Wrote the name of the payee on the correct line.
		●	Wrote the amount of the check in numbers in the box next to the dollar sign.
		●	Used a decimal between the number of dollars and the number of cents.
		●	Wrote the amount of the check in words on the line below the name of the payee correctly.
		●	Expressed the number of cents as a fraction over 100.
		●	Drew a line from the end of the fraction to the word "dollars."
		●	Wrote the invoice number, account number, and/or purpose of the check on the memo line.
		●	Completed the checkbook stub or register including the date, check number, payee, amount of the check, and reason for the check.
		●	Added any deposits since the previous check and entered the new balance.
		●	Subtracted the amount of the check from the previous balance and entered the balance carried forward.
		●	Drew a single line through a minor mistake, corrected the error, and initialed the correction.
		*	Wrote the check for the correct amount using the correct format with minor corrections as necessary.
		●	Wrote "void" across the any check with a major mistake and entered "void" on the check stub or in the check register.
		●	Placed a voided check in the folder with accounts payable records.

Trial 1	Trial 2	Point Value	Performance Standards
		●	Prepared an envelope to mail the payment (or used the envelope -supplied by the vendor).
		●	Clipped the prepared check to the envelope with the payment slip and placed in the designated place for review and signature by the physician authorized to sign office checks.
		∗	Completed the procedure within 5 minutes.
			TOTALS

Evaluation of Student Performance

EVALUATION CRITERIA			COMMENTS
Symbol	Category	Point Value	
∗	Critical Step	16 points	
●	Essential Step	6 points	
Ⓐ	Affective Competency	6 points	
▷	Theory Question	2 points	
Score calculation: 100 points – ___ points missed ___ Score Satisfactory score: 85 or above			

ABHES Competencies Achieved
☑ 8.b. Perform billing and collection procedures: 1. Accounts payable and accounts receivable

EVALUATION OF COMPETENCY

Procedure 46-5: Preparing a Bank Deposit

Name: ______________________________ Date: ____________________

Evaluated by: ______________________________ Score: ____________________

Performance Objective

Outcome:	Prepare a bank deposit.
Conditions:	Given the following: account deposit slip, deposit itemization record from a day sheet (optional), cash and checks received as payments, calculator, and bank deposit envelope or bag.
Standards:	Time: 10 minutes. Student completed procedure in __________ minutes.
	Accuracy: Satisfactory score on the Performance Evaluation Checklist.

Performance Evaluation Checklist

Trial 1	Trial 2	Point Value	Performance Standards
		•	Obtained an account deposit slip and placed a date on it. If using the deposit itemization from a day sheet, wrote the name of the medical practice and the account number.
		•	Counted any currency and coins, and entered the totals on the correct line of the deposit slip.
		•	Stamped each check with a restrictive endorsement (if not already done).
		•	Wrote the amount of each check on a separate line of the bank deposit detail.
		•	Used the numerator of the fractional ABA number, check number or name on the checking account to identify each check on the itemization.
		•	Totaled all checks and entered the total correctly.
		*	Totaled the cash and check amounts and entered as the total amount of the bank deposit.
		•	Made a copy of the deposit slip and deposit itemization.
		•	Placed the cash, checks, deposit slip, and deposit itemization (if separate) in a bank envelope or bank deposit bag.
		•	Recorded the amount of the deposit in the check register or on the check stub nearest to the date of deposit.
		•	Recorded the amount of the deposit in the accounts payable record according to office policy.
		•	Filed the copy of the bank deposit and bank deposit itemization as well as the bank deposit receipt after making the deposit.
		*	Completed the procedure within 10 minutes.
			TOTALS

Evaluation of Student Performance

EVALUATION CRITERIA			COMMENTS
Symbol	Category	Point Value	
∗	Critical Step	16 points	
●	Essential Step	6 points	
Ⓐ	Affective Competency	6 points	
▷	Theory Question	2 points	
Score calculation: 100 points − ___ points missed ___ Score Satisfactory score: 85 or above			

2008 CAAHEP Competency Achieved
Psychomotor (Skills) ☑ VI. 1. Prepare a bank deposit.

2015 CAAHEP Competency Achieved
Psychomotor (Skills) ☑ VII. 2. Prepare a bank deposit

ABHES Competencies Achieved
☑ 8. b. Perform billing and collection procedures: 1. Accounts payable and accounts receivable.

47 Medical Coding

CHAPTER ASSIGNMENTS

✓ After Completing	Date Due	Study Guide Pages	STUDY GUIDE ASSIGNMENTS (CTA = Critical Thinking Activity)	Possible Points	Points You Earned
		1301	Pretest	10	
		1302	Term Key Term Assessment	14	
		1302-1306	Evaluation of Learning questions	35	
		1306	CTA A: Evaluation and Management Codes	10	
		1307-1308	CTA B: CPT Codes	40	
		1308-1309	CTA C: HCPCS Codes	10	
		1309-1310	CTA D: Diagnosis Codes	100	
		1311	CTA E: Code Format	8	
			Evolve Site: Guided Practice: Assigning CPT Codes	10	
			Evolve Site: Apply Your Knowledge questions	10	
		1301	Posttest	10	
			ADDITIONAL ASSIGNMENTS		
			TOTAL POINTS		

Notes

✓ When Assigned By Your Instructor	Study Guide Pages	Practices Required	LABORATORY ASSIGNMENTS (Procedure Number and Name)	Score*
	1313	3	**Practice for Competency** 47-1: Performing CPT Coding Textbook reference: pp. 1175-1177	
	1315-1316		**Evaluation of Competency** 47-1: Performing CPT Coding	*
	1313	3	**Practice for Competency** 47-2: Performing HCPCS Coding Textbook reference: p. 1178	
	1317-1318		**Evaluation of Competency** 47-2: Performing CPT Coding	*
	1313	3	**Practice for Competency** 47-3: Performing ICD Coding Textbook reference: pp. 1185-1187	
	1319-1320		**Evaluation of Competency** 47-3: Performing ICD Coding	*
			ADDITIONAL ASSIGNMENTS	

Notes

Name ________________________________ Date ______________

PRETEST

True or False

_______ 1. The radiology section of the current procedural terminology (CPT) coding manual is the largest and has the most codes.

_______ 2. CPT codes for surgical procedures automatically include all services related to the surgery.

_______ 3. There are different codes for office visits for new patients and established patients.

_______ 4. The type of physical examination is a major factor in determining the correct code for the office visit.

_______ 5. Medical decision making is not taken into account when selecting a CPT code for an office visit.

_______ 6. If an injection is given to a patient with Medicare, a Healthcare Common Procedure Coding System (HCPCS) Level II code is required for the medication.

_______ 7. International Classification of Disease, 9th edition (ICD-9-CM) codes and ICD-10-CM codes both end with an alphabetic character.

_______ 8. ICD-9-CM codes for patients who are having physical examinations begin with the letter V.

_______ 9. Coding books or online codes in the medical office must be updated every 2 to 3 years.

_______ 10. If a diagnosis or "impression" includes the words "rule out," it should not receive an ICD code.

POSTTEST

True or False

_______ 1. The CPT manual is arranged according to body system.

_______ 2. CPT codes consist of five digits and may also include a two-digit modifier.

_______ 3. In addition to office visits, CPT codes are used for physician visits to patients in nursing homes.

_______ 4. A problem-focused patient history includes information about the patient's family history.

_______ 5. The CPT code should always be chosen from the alphabetic index.

_______ 6. HCPCS Level II codes are arranged alphabetically by letter, then numerically.

_______ 7. Sometimes two or more codes are required to accurately reflect a patient's diagnosis.

_______ 8. ICD-9-CM codes may contain up to seven alphanumeric characters.

_______ 9. The ICD code should always be selected from the tabular list, not the alphabetic index.

_______ 10. All ICD-10-CM codes have at least two digits after the decimal point.

KEY TERM ASSESSMENT

Directions: Match each key term with its definition.

_______ 1. Established patient
_______ 2. Inpatient
_______ 3. Medical necessity
_______ 4. Modifier
_______ 5. Morphology
_______ 6. NEC
_______ 7. Neoplasm
_______ 8. New patient
_______ 9. NOS
_______ 10. Outpatient
_______ 11. Panel
_______ 12. Sequela
_______ 13. Surgical package
_______ 14. Upcoding

A. A diagnosis code that is not otherwise specified
B. For billing purposes, a patient who has not received services during the past 3 years from any physician in a medical practice
C. Surgical services covered by a single procedure code that includes a preoperative visit, postoperative care, and local anesthesia
D. A patient who has been formally admitted to a health care facility
E. An addition to a CPT code that indicates unusual circumstances related to the procedure
F. A group of diagnostic tests done in one machine at the same time
G. The study of structure and form.
H. A patient who has been receiving services from the same medical practice on a regular basis
I. Any condition that results from a disease, injury, or treatment for a disease or injury
J. A patient who has not been admitted to a health care facility
K. Using a code to obtain a higher level of reimbursement than is justified by medical procedures performed.
L. A diagnosis code that is not elsewhere classified
M. Abnormal growth or tumor
N. Health care that is reasonable and necessary for a patient based on evidence-based clinical standards of care.

EVALUATION OF LEARNING

Directions: Fill in each blank with the correct answer.

1. What are three reasons for the development of procedure codes?

____

____

2. How and when were the CPT and HCPCS coding systems developed?

____

____

3. What are level I HCPCS codes? Level II codes?

____

4. What are the six sections of the CPT manual?

____

____

5. What are Category II codes? Category III codes?

____

____

6. What is a modifier and how is it used?

7. What are several pieces of information that may be significant when looking up a procedure in the index?

8. What types of services are covered in the Evaluation and Management section of the CPT manual?

9. Identify seven factors that affect the level of service when identifying evaluation and management (E/M) codes.

10. What factors must be considered when determining a code in the E/M section of the CPT manual?

11. Differentiate between a problem-focused medical history and a detailed history.

12. Differentiate between an expanded problem-focused physical examination and a comprehensive examination.

13. What factors influence the level of medical decision making?

14. How are anesthesia services reimbursed?

15. What is a physical status modifier, and how are physical status modifiers used in relation to anesthesia services?

16. What services are included in a code for surgical services (surgical package)?

17. What are the four subsections of the Radiology section of the CPT manual?

____

____

18. When coding for a cardiac panel, can the coder use a separate code for each test in the panel if all tests were done? Why or why not?

____

____

19. How does the medical office code for a blood test for a cardiac panel if the specimen was drawn in the office by the medical assistant (MA) and sent out to the hospital laboratory for testing?

____

20. What types of procedures are included in the Medicine section of the CPT manual?

____

____

21. Describe HCPCS Level II codes.

____

____

22. Give several examples of services that require HCPCS codes.

____

____

23. Describe the process for looking up HCPCS codes.

____

____

24. Describe the history of the International Classification of Disease coding system.

____

____

____

25. What are several new features of ICD-10-CM codes compared with ICD-9-CM codes?

____

____

26. What is contained in the two parts of the ICD-10-CM manual?

____

____

27. What is the format of an ICD-9-CM code? An ICD-10-CM code?

____

____

____

____

____

28. Describe the steps to look up a diagnosis code properly.

____

____

____

____

29. What are "Z" codes, and when are they used?

____

____

____

30. What are external cause codes and when are they used?

____

____

____

31. What is the difference between "Excludes 1" and "Excludes 2" when found under an ICD-10-CM category code?

____

____

____

32. If a patient has two related conditions, which is coded first?

____

33. What is a sequela, and how does it affect the ICD-10-CM code?

____

____

34. How does Medicare use medical necessity related to diagnosis and procedure coding?

____

____

34. What are National Coverage Determinations (NCDs)?

____

35. Differentiate between upcoding and downcoding? Why might each occur?

____

____

CRITICAL THINKING ACTIVITIES

A. Evaluation and Management Codes

Select the best code for the E/M service for each of the following:

1. New patient is seen in the office for gradual onset of joint pain (polyarthralgia) and reddened areas on her face with a complete history and review of systems, and a comprehensive examination of the patient's musculoskeletal, cardiovascular, and integumentary systems. ______________________

2. Follow-up visit in the office for a patient with asthma requiring minor adjustment of medication. ____________

3. Office visit for an established patient with arteriosclerotic heart disease who is now complaining of increasing frequency of chest tightness during and after exercise. The cardiovascular history was reviewed and the cardiovascular system was examined with referral to a cardiologist. ______________________

4. An established patient is seen in the office for the second in a series of three hepatitis B injections given by the nurse. ______________________

5. A 30-year-old woman is seen for an initial consultation because of a large and uncomfortable bunion on her right foot. The orthopedic surgeon performs a problem-focused history and problem-focused physical examination.

   ____

6. A new patient is seen in the office for a sore throat with fever. ______________________

7. A patient is seen in a nursing home for an initial evaluation. Although elderly, the patient does not have significant health problems, so the history and physical examination are detailed. ______________________

8. An infant is seen for routine 4-month preventative care, including a routine examination and immunizations. The child has been a patient since birth. ______________________

9. The physician examines an established patient in the emergency room after a fall from a bicycle where the child hit and bruised her head but did not lose consciousness. ______________________

10. A young man who complains of pain in the right hand, which may be due to carpal tunnel syndrome is seen for an initial office consultation by an orthopedic surgeon. The history and physical examination are expanded problem-focused. ______________________

B. CPT Codes

Identify the most specific CPT code for the following services.

Anesthesia Section

1. Anesthesia for burr holes for intracranial procedure ______________________
2. Anesthesia for total knee arthroplasty ______________________
3. Anesthesia for amniocentesis ______________________
4. Anesthesia for thoracoplasty ______________________
5. Qualifying circumstances modifier for anesthesia complicated by emergency conditions ______________________

Surgery Section

1. The patient has closed treatment of a fracture of the clavicle with manipulation. ______________________
2. A 6-year-old boy has a tonsillectomy and adenoidectomy. ______________________
3. A patient has a biopsy of the cornea. ______________________
4. A female patient has a plastic repair of an urethrocele. ______________________
5. The patient has a wart frozen with liquid nitrogen. ______________________
6. The patient has a reconstruction of a dislocating patella. ______________________
7. The patient has a laparoscopic cholecystectomy. ______________________
8. The patient has a thoracoplasty with closure of a bronchopleural fistula. ______________________
9. The patient has a diagnostic amniocentesis. ______________________
10. The patient has a partial cystectomy (simple). ______________________

Radiology Section

1. The patient receives a chest x-ray, two views (AP and lateral). ______________________
2. A patient has thyroid imaging done in nuclear medicine. ______________________
3. The patient has a complete x-ray examination of both hips (two views). ______________________
4. A patient has an ultrasound of the thyroid gland (neck). ______________________
5. The patient has retrograde urography with a KUB. ______________________

Pathology and Laboratory

1. The MA performs a dipstick urinalysis and reads the test manually. ______________________
2. The patient receives a urine culture and colony count. ______________________
3. A spun microhematocrit is performed on blood from a capillary puncture. ______________________

4. The MA performs a rapid strep test (Streptococcus, group A by immunoassay with direct optical observation).
____

5. The patient has a comprehensive metabolic panel blood test. _______________

6. The patient has blood drawn to test for copper. _______________

7. A patient has a prothrombin time (blood test). _______________

8. The patient has a blood test for rubella antibodies. _______________

9. The patient has one blood test that includes cholesterol, lipoprotein, and triglycerides (lipid panel).
____

10. The patient has a blood test for total serum cholesterol. _______________

Medicine Section

1. A patient receives a 12-lead electrocardiogram (ECG) with interpretation. _______________

2. The patient receives an intramuscular injection of antibiotic. _______________

3. The patient receives an inhalation (nebulizer) treatment in the office. _______________

4. The patient has an audiometry screening test, pure tone, air only. _______________

5. The patient has allergy testing by intradermal tests, and the physician interprets and makes a report.
____

6. A new patient receives an ophthalmological examination and evaluation with initiation of diagnostic and treatment program, intermediate. _______________

7. A patient receives an osteopathic manipulative treatment, two body regions. _______________

8. A patient receives in intravenous infusion for hydration, 47 minutes. _______________

9. A patient is given a cholinesterase inhibitor challenge test for myasthenia gravis.
____

10. A patient is given 24-hour electrocardiographic monitoring (Holter monitor) including recording, scanning analysis, and physician review and interpretation. _______________

C. HCPCS Codes

Identify the specific HCPCS codes for the following services:

1. The patient receives a pair of wooden underarm crutches: _______________

2. Injection of ceftazidine 350 mg: _______________

3. The patient receives an electric heat pad, moist: _______________

4. Cervical traction equipment for over the door: _______________

5. Injection, lincomycin HCl 250 mg: ______________________

6. Transcutaneous electrical joint stimulation device system: ______________________

7. Tubular dressing, 1 yard: ______________________

8. Infusion, albumin (human) 5%, 250 mL: ______________________

9. Knee orthosis with joints, prefabricated including fitting and adjustment: ______________________

10. Dynamic adjustable ankle extension/flexion device: ______________________

D. Diagnosis Codes

Identify diagnosis codes for the following diagnoses:

		ICD-9-CM	ICD-10-CM
1.	Portal cirrhosis		
2.	Hiatal (diaphragmatic) hernia		
3.	Malignant tumor of the urinary system (primary)		
4.	Candidal vaginitis		
5.	Calcific tendinitis, left ankle and foot		
6.	Primary thrombocytopenia		
7.	Carpal tunnel syndrome (right side)		
8.	Breast, fibrocystic disease		
9.	Congestive heart failure		
10.	Hypercholesterolemia		
11.	Peripheral polyneuropathy		
12.	Seborrheic dermatitis		
13.	Sports physical examination		
14.	Closed fracture of the right scapula (initial encounter)		
15.	Idiopathic gout of the right great toe		
16.	Foreign body in the eye (external)		
17.	Routine child health examination without abnormal findings		
18.	Osteoporosis (postmenopausal)		
19.	Hypertrophic subaortic stenosis		
20.	Benign neoplasm of right female breast		
21.	Measles without complications		
22.	Supervision of normal first pregnancy		
23.	Congenital talipes equinovarus (clubfoot)		

		ICD-9-CM	ICD-10-CM
24.	Weight loss, cause unknown		
25.	Juvenile rheumatoid arthritis, acute (systemic onset, multiple sites)		
26.	Acute otitis media, both ears		
27.	Atrial paroxysmal tachycardia		
28.	Initial encounter for scalp laceration		
29.	Preterm labor without delivery, third trimester		
30.	Chondromalacia of the left patella		
31.	Type 1 diabetes mellitus with diabetic polyneuropathy		
32.	Type 2 diabetes mellitus (without complications)		
33.	Diabetes insipidus		
34.	Ganglion, right hand		
35.	Enlarged prostate		
36.	Routine gynecologic examination (normal findings)		
37.	Conjunctivitis, both eyes (acute)		
38.	Psoriasis		
39.	Iron deficiency anemia		
40.	Unstable angina		
41.	Left inguinal hernia without obstruction or gangrene		
42.	*Salmonella* enteritis		
43.	Encounter for initial prescription of contraceptive pills		
44.	High-risk pregnancy, first trimester		
45.	Ingrowing nail		
46.	Hives		
47.	Gastroesophageal reflux disease (GERD)		
48.	Auditory hallucination		
49.	Head lice		
50.	Mitral valve prolapse		

E. Code Format

Choose the letter of the type of code for which each of the following descriptions is true. (Each answer may be used more than once.)

a. ICD-10-CM codes
b. CPT codes
c. HCPCS codes

________ 1. Consists only of five numbers without a decimal

________ 2. Used to code the patient's diagnosis

________ 3. Contains two levels of codes

________ 4. A two-digit modifier added to the code gives more information

________ 5. Consists of three to seven alphanumeric characters

________ 6. Contains codes describing evaluation and management

________ 7. Used to bill Medicare for supplies, materials, and injections

________ 8. More specific codes can have more characters than less specific codes

Notes

PRACTICE FOR COMPETENCY

Procedure 47-1: Performing CPT Coding. Look up CPT codes for the following:

1. Patient seen in a nursing home by the office physician for subsequent nursing facility care, problem-focused interval; history, problem-focused examination, and straightforward medical decision making:

   ____

2. Urine pregnancy test by visual color comparison method: ______________________________
3. Spinal chiropractic manipulative treatment—one region: ______________________________
4. Role-play a tactful discussion with a provider who has checked the box to bill for a urine pregnancy test for a 24-year-old male.

Procedure 47-2: Performing HCPCS Coding. Look up HCPCS codes for the following:

1. Injection: ceftriaxone sodium 250 mg: ______________________________
2. One foot arch support, removable, premolded, longitudinal: ______________________________
3. Injection: vitamin B_{12} cyanocobalamin 500 mcg: ______________________________

Procedure 47-3: Performing ICD-10-CM Coding. Look up ICD-10-CM codes for the following diagnoses:

	ICD-9-CM	ICD-10-CM
1. Pernicious anemia:	____________	____________
2. Hematuria:	____________	____________
3. Lumbar intervertebral disc disorder:	____________	____________

4. Role-play a tactful discussion with a provider who has checked the box to bill for a pregnancy test for the patient with a diagnosis of pernicious anemia.

Notes

EVALUATION OF COMPETENCY

Procedure 47-1: Performing CPT Coding

Name: ______________________ Date: ______________________

Evaluated by: ______________________ Score: ______________________

Performance Objective

Outcome:	Perform CPT coding for procedures
Conditions:	Given the following: charge slip or procedure to look up code for, medical record, index card with a diagnosis for which the procedure is not medically necessary, and CPT manual.
Standards:	Time: 10 minutes. Student completed procedure in ________ minutes.
	Accuracy: Satisfactory score on the Performance Evaluation Checklist.

Performance Evaluation Checklist

Trial 1	Trial 2	Point Value	Performance Standards
		•	Found name of procedure to look up from charge slip or other document.
		•	Determined any necessary additional information from the patient's medical record.
		•	For evaluation and management services, identified if the patient is a new patient or an established patient.
		•	For evaluation and management services, identified the location where the patient was seen.
		•	Located the name of the procedure in the index.
		•	From the information in the index, located the correct range of codes in the list of codes.
		▷	Stated the reason for coding from the list of codes instead of the index.
		✶	Selected the correct code from the list of codes
		•	If the service was unusual, decided if a modifier was needed.
		✶	Selected the correct modifier, if one was needed
		•	Verified that the procedure code has a reasonable correlation with the diagnosis code.
		Ⓐ	Demonstrated tact when participating in role play to discuss the lack of correlation between diagnosis and procedure code.
		•	Entered the correct code on the charge slip, on any other document, and in the computer as needed.
		✶	Completed the procedure within 10 minutes.
			TOTALS

Evaluation of Student Performance

EVALUATION CRITERIA			COMMENTS
Symbol	Category	Point Value	
∗	Critical Step	16 points	
●	Essential Step	6 points	
Ⓐ	Affective Competency	6 points	
▷	Theory Question	2 points	
Score calculation: 100 points − ____ points missed ____ Score Satisfactory score: 85 or above			

2008 CAAHEP Competency Achieved
Psychomotor (Skills) ☑ VIII. 1. Perform procedural coding

2015 CAAHEP Competencies Achieved
Psychomotor (Skills) ☑ IX.1. Perform procedural coding ☑ IX.3. Utilize medical necessity guidelines ***Affective (Behavior)*** ☑ IX.1. Utilize tactful communication skills with medical providers to ensure accurate code selection.

ABHES Competencies Achieved
☑ 8. c. Process insurance claims: 3. Perform diagnostic and procedural coding.

EVALUATION OF COMPETENCY

Procedure 47-2: Performing HCPCS Coding

Name: ______________________ Date: ______________________

Evaluated by: ______________________ Score: ______________________

Performance Objective

Outcome:	Perform HCPCS coding for services or equipment
Conditions:	Given the following: charge slip or procedure to look up code for, medical record, and HCPCS manual.
Standards:	Time: 10 minutes. Student completed procedure in ________ minutes.
	Accuracy: Satisfactory score on the performance Evaluation Checklist

Performance Evaluation Checklist

Trial 1	Trial 2	Point Value	Performance Standards
		●	Found name of service or item to look up from charge slip or other document.
		●	Determined any necessary additional information from the patient's medical record.
		●	Located the name of the service or item in the index. Found name of medication in the Table of Drugs.
		●	From the information in the index, located the correct code or range of codes in the list of codes.
		▷	Stated the reason for coding from the list of codes instead of the index.
		*	Selected the correct code from the list of codes
		●	Validated that the code was appropriate for the patient's insurance.
		●	Entered the correct code on the charge slip, on any other document, and in the computer as needed.
		*	Completed the procedure within 10 minutes.
			TOTALS

EVALUATION CRITERIA			COMMENTS
Symbol	**Category**	**Point Value**	
∗	Critical Step	16 points	
●	Essential Step	6 points	
Ⓐ	Affective Competency	6 points	
▷	Theory Question	2 points	
Score calculation: 100 points − ___ points missed ___ Score Satisfactory score: 85 or above			

2008 CAAHEP Competency Achieved
Psychomotor (Skills) ☑ VIII. 1. Perform procedural coding.

2015 CAAHEP Competency Achieved
Psychomotor (Skills) ☑ IX.1. Perform procedural coding

ABHES Competencies Achieved
☑ 8. c. Process insurance claims: 3. Perform diagnostic and procedural coding.

EVALUATION OF COMPETENCY

Procedure 47-3: Performing ICD Coding

Name: ______________________________ Date: ____________________

Evaluated by: ______________________________ Score: ____________________

Performance Objective

Outcome:	Perform ICD coding for a patient's diagnosis
Conditions:	Given the following: charge slip or diagnosis to look up code for, medical record, index card with a procedure that the diagnosis does not reasonably support, and an ICD-9-CM or ICD-10-CM manual.
Standards:	Time: 5 minutes. Student completed procedure in ________ minutes.
	Accuracy: Satisfactory score on the Performance Evaluation Checklist.

Performance Evaluation Checklist

Trial 1	Trial 2	Point Value	Performance Standards
		●	Found diagnosis to look up from charge slip or other document.
		●	Determined any necessary additional information from the patient's medical record.
		●	Decided on the key word or phrase to look for in the alphabetic index.
		●	Looked under as many terms as necessary to locate the diagnosis in the alphabetic index.
		●	From the information in the index, located the correct range of codes to look under in the tabular list.
		▷	Stated the reason for coding from the tabular list instead of the index.
		●	Checked all potential codes against the diagnosis to identify the most specific code.
		●	If there was a list of possible fifth (ICD-9-CM) or seven (ICD-10-CM) characters, selected the most specific letter to use as a final character
		✶	Selected the correct code from the list of codes.
		●	Verified that the diagnosis code has a reasonable correlation with the procedure listed on an index card.
		Ⓐ	Demonstrated tact when participating in role play to discuss the lack of correlation between diagnosis and procedure code.
		●	Entered the correct code on the charge slip, on any other document, and in the computer as needed.
		✶	Completed the procedure within 5 minutes.
			TOTALS

EVALUATION CRITERIA			COMMENTS
Symbol	Category	Point Value	
∗	Critical Step	16 points	
●	Essential Step	6 points	
Ⓐ	Affective Competency	6 points	
▷	Theory Question	2 points	
Score calculation: 100 points – ___ points missed ___ Score Satisfactory score: 85 or above			

2008 CAAHEP Competency Achieved
Psychomotor (Skills) ☑ VIII. 2.Perform diagnostic coding.

2015 CAAHEP Competencies Achieved
Psychomotor (Skills) ☑ IX.2. Perform diagnostic coding ☑ IX.3. Utilize medical necessity guidelines ***Affective (Behavior)*** ☑ IX.1. Utilize tactful communication skills with medical providers to ensure accurate code selection.

ABHES Competencies Achieved
☑ 8. c. Process insurance claims: 3. Perform diagnostic and procedural coding.

48 Medical Insurance

CHAPTER ASSIGNMENTS

✓ After Completing	Date Due	Study Guide Pages	STUDY GUIDE ASSIGNMENTS (CTA = Critical Thinking Activity)	Possible Points	Points You Earned
		1325	Pretest	10	
		1326 1327	Term Key Term Assessment: A. General Insurance Terms B. Insurance Plans and Methods of Reimbursement	27 11	
		1327-1331	Evaluation of Learning questions	35	
		1331-1332	CTA A: Primary and Secondary Insurance	10	
		1332	CTA B: Managed Care Plans	5	
		1332	CTA C: The Insurance Claim Form	10	
			Evolve Site: Guided Practice: Obtaining a Managed Care Referral	10	
			Evolve Site: Apply Your Knowledge questions	10	
		1325	Posttest	10	
			ADDITIONAL ASSIGNMENTS		
			TOTAL POINTS		

Notes

✓ When Assigned By Your Instructor	Study Guide Pages	Practices Required	LABORATORY ASSIGNMENTS (Procedure Number and Name)	Score*
	1333-1334	3	**Practice for Competency** 48-1: Interpreting Information on an Insurance Card Textbook reference: p. 1200	
	1341-1342		**Evaluation of Competency** 48-1: Interpreting Information on an Insurance Card	*
	1333-1334	3	**Practice for Competency** 48-2: Verifying Insurance Eligibility and Benefits Textbook reference: p. 1201	
	1343-1344		**Evaluation of Competency** 48-2: Verifying Insurance Eligibility and Benefits	*
	1333-1335	3	**Practice for Competency** 48-3: Obtaining Insurance Preauthorization (Precertification) Textbook reference: pp. 1201-1202	
	1345-1346		**Evaluation of Competency** 48-3: Obtaining Insurance Preauthorization (Precertification)	*
	1335-1339	3	**Practice for Competency** 48-4: Completing and Reviewing an Insurance Claim Form Textbook reference: pp. 1205-1209	
	1347-1349		**Evaluation of Competency** 48-4: Completing and Reviewing an Insurance Claim Form	*
	1336	3	**Practice for Competency** 48-5: Communicating Effectively Related to Insurance and/or Managed Care Textbook reference: p. 1213	
	1351-1352		**Evaluation of Competency** 48-5: Communicating Effectively Related to Insurance and/or Managed Care	*
			ADDITIONAL ASSIGNMENTS	

Notes

Name ____ Date ____________________

PRETEST

True or False

_______ 1. Capitation is a term meaning that the insurance carrier pays a specific amount for each service.

_______ 2. If an individual obtains health insurance through employment, it is usually through a group plan.

_______ 3. If a patient's insurance is a Staff Model HMO, the patient must usually pay an annual deductible.

_______ 4. If a patient is covered by more than one health insurance plan, the primary insurance must be billed first.

_______ 5. If a patient is covered by more than one health insurance policy, insurance may pay more than 100% of charges.

_______ 6. Usually the medical office accepts assignment of benefits.

_______ 7. A patient covered by traditional indemnity insurance always requires a written referral to see a specialist.

_______ 8. Precertification by the insurance carrier is usually required if a patient will be scheduled for surgery.

_______ 9. Patients with Medicare Part B must pay an annual deductible before any other services are covered.

_______ 10. A patient's usual health insurance plan will deny any claim for a work-related injury.

POSTTEST

True or False

_______ 1. Health insurance for the spouses and dependents of active military personnel is called TRICARE.

_______ 2. The age for eligibility for Medicare is 65.

_______ 3. The amount of money that is paid to an insurance carrier for insurance coverage is called a benefit.

_______ 4. If a child is covered by insurance plans through both parents, the birthday rule establishes the primary insurance.

_______ 5. Medicare supplemental insurance is always the primary insurance.

_______ 6. If a physician participates in the Medicare plan, he or she must accept assignment of benefits.

_______ 7. In an HMO, the primary care provider controls a patient's access to specialty services and specialists.

_______ 8. PPOs cover in-network and out-of-network services.

_______ 9. Both Medicare and Medicaid usually have different names in different states.

_______ 10. A separate medical record should be established for a patient being seen for a work-related injury.

Term KEY TERM ASSESSMENT

A. General Insurance Terms

Directions: Match each insurance term with its definition.

_______ 1. Advanced Beneficiary Notice of Noncoverage (ABN)
_______ 2. Assignment of benefits
_______ 3. Beneficiary
_______ 4. Birthday rule
_______ 5. Carrier
_______ 6. Coinsurance
_______ 7. Coordination of benefits
_______ 8. Copayment
_______ 9. Deductible
_______ 10. Eligibility
_______ 11. Participating provider (PAR)
_______ 12. Explanation of benefits (EOB)/remittance advice
_______ 13. Fee-for-service
_______ 14. Formulary
_______ 15. Guarantor
_______ 16. Indemnity
_______ 17. Insured
_______ 18. Medicare Administrative Contractor (MAC)
_______ 19. Preauthorization/precertification
_______ 20. Premium
_______ 21. Primary care provider
_______ 22. Primary insurance
_______ 23. Referral
_______ 24. Reimbursement
_______ 25. Secondary insurance
_______ 26. Signature on file (SOF)
_______ 27. Utilization review

A. Rules followed by insurance companies so that no claim is reimbursed at more than 100% of the charges
B. An obligation to provide compensation for loss or damage
C. Physician who has a contractual agreement with a third party payor
D. The insurance carrier that must be billed first
E. Insurance that an individual has in addition to primary insurance
F. A statement issued by the insurance carrier explaining reimbursement or denial of a claim
G. A person who can receive benefits under an insurance plan
H. A person with financial responsibility for a bill
I. Written notification that a patient must pay for a covered service if denied by Medicare
J. Reviewing proposed or current care to determine medical necessity
K. A fixed amount of money that the patient must pay for any health care service
L. The signature of the patient is maintained by the medical office to authorize submission of insurance claims
M. Verification from an insurance carrier that a procedure or diagnostic test will be covered
N. Authorization for insurance reimbursement to be made to the provider of health service
O. The physician chosen by a patient to provide general medical care and also authorize additional medical services
P. An amount of money that an insured person must pay annually before health services are covered
Q. A percentage of the payment for health services that the patient is responsible for
R. Enrollment status related to a health insurance plan
S. The rule that determines which insurance is primary for the children of two parents who have a family health plan
T. An insurance carrier's official list of covered medications
U. The person named on an insurance certificate
V. The amount paid for a procedure by insurance
W. An amount of money paid in a given period to purchase health insurance
X. An insurance company
Y. Insurance reimbursement that is based on the services provided and the amount charged
Z. A multi-state independent agency that administers Medicare claims
AA. Directing a patient to a specialist physician or therapy

B. Insurance Plans and Methods of Reimbursement

Directions: Match each insurance plan or reimbursement method with its description.

_______ 1. Capitation

_______ 2. CHAMPVA

_______ 3. Diagnosis-related groups

_______ 4. Group plan

_______ 5. Managed care

_______ 6. Medicaid

_______ 7. Medicare

_______ 8. Resource-based relative value scale (RBRVS)

_______ 9. TRICARE

_______ 10. Usual, customary, and reasonable (UCR)

_______ 11. Workers' compensation

A. A movement to reduce health care costs while providing quality care

B. Covers lost wages and health care costs of workers injured on the job or who suffer from work-related illnesses

C. Establishes the fee schedule for Medicare Part B based on the service provided and the geographic location of the provider

D. The government insurance program for low-income individuals and families

E. A fixed amount is paid to the provider per member for a specific time period

F. Provides medical care to spouses and dependents of individuals on active duty in the military

G. Provides insurance coverage for the elderly, permanently disabled, and individuals with end-stage kidney disease

H. Covers dependents of military personnel with service-connected disabilities

I. Insurance payment based on a physician's usual charge and the customary charge of other physicians in the same area

J. A system to determine Medicare reimbursement for a hospital stay based on the patient's diagnosis

K. One insurance policy that covers a group of people

EVALUATION OF LEARNING

Directions: Fill in each blank with the correct answer.

1. Briefly describe the history of health insurance in the United States.

____

____

____

____

2. Identify three ways for individuals and families to obtain health insurance coverage.

____

____

3. What is the tax advantage to obtaining health insurance through the employer?

____

____

4. What types of payments must the insured person make for health care?

____

____

5. If both parents have health insurance through their employers, what determines which parent's insurance is primary for their children? Is it the same if the parents are divorced?

____

____

____

6. What is a participating provider (PAR)? A nonparticipating provider (nonPAR)?

____

____

____

7. What are two ways that fee-for-service insurance plans determine the amount they will pay for services?

____

____

8. What is meant by managed care?

____

____

9. What is the function of the primary care provider in a managed care plan?

____

____

10. What is the cost to patients if they seek services outside a managed care plan?

____

____

11. Describe each of the following managed care plans:

    a. Staff model HMO: ____

    ____

    b. Network model HMO: ____

    ____

    c. Preferred provider organization (PPO): ____

    ____

    d. Exclusive provider organization (EPO): ____

    ____

    e. Independent practice association (IPA): ____

    ____

    f. Point-of-service (POS) plan: ____

    ____

12. Identify three differences between Medicare Part A and Medicare Part B.

____

____

13. What are Medicare Part B payments based on, and how is the allowable charge calculated?

____

____

14. What part of the bill for services is the patient covered by Medicare Part B responsible for if the physician -participates in the Medicare program? If the physician does not participate?

____

____

15. If a patient is covered by Medicaid insurance, what portion of the bill is the patient responsible for?

____

16. What additional services are covered by Medicaid that other health insurance is usually not responsible for?

____

____

17. Why do some physicians refuse to accept Medicaid patients?

____

____

18. What organization oversees the Children's Health Insurance Program?

____

____

19. Describe who receives benefits under the government TRICARE plan, and describe the three levels of service briefly.

____

____

20. What group of people is covered by CHAMPVA?

____

____

21. Describe who purchases workers' compensation insurance and when claims must be filed to this program.

____

____

____

22. Why is a separate medical record established for a patient who is being treated for a work-related injury or illness?

____

23. What is the difference between verifying eligibility status and verifying insurance benefits?

24. What is the process of preauthorization/precertification?

25. What is a referral and how are referrals used in managed care?

26. How is the term "formulary" used by managed care organizations?

27. What is the CMS-1500 claim form?

28. Identify the three boxes on the CMS-1500 form that require signatures, who must sign, and what each signature authorizes. What can replace the signature for each for most insurance carriers?

29. What are the recommendations for completing insurance forms to facilitate optical scanning?

30. Identify three advantages of submitting insurance claims electronically.

31. What is the purpose of an insurance claims register?

32. What information is contained on a remittance advice (RA) or explanation of benefits (EOB) form?

33. How should the medical assistant (MA) handle an insurance claim that was denied?

____

____

34. What type of communication skills should the medical assistant use when communicating with third party representatives and/or patients related to managed care and/or insurance?

____

____

35. What is the major difference between Medicare fraud and abuse?

____

____

CRITICAL THINKING ACTIVITIES

A. Primary and Secondary Insurance

In the Swann family, the mother has insurance from her own employment (individual plan) and the father has insurance from his employment (family plan). The mother's birthday is January 31, and her husband's birthday is May 10. Whose insurance is the primary insurance and whose is the secondary insurance (if any) for each of the following family members?

1. mother primary insurance: ______________________

   secondary insurance: ______________________

2. father primary insurance: ______________________

   secondary insurance: ______________________

3. son primary insurance: ______________________

   secondary insurance: ______________________

4. daughter primary insurance: ______________________

   secondary insurance: ______________________

In the McGrath family, the mother has insurance from her own employment (family plan) and the father has insurance from his employment (family plan). The mother's birthday is January 31, and her husband's birthday is May 10. Whose insurance is the primary insurance and whose is the secondary insurance (if any) for each of the following family members?

5. mother primary insurance: ______________________

   secondary insurance: ______________________

6. father primary insurance: ______________________

   secondary insurance: ______________________

7. son primary insurance: ______________________

   secondary insurance: ______________________

8. daughter primary insurance: ______________________

   secondary insurance: ______________________

Eleanor Whitby is 68, and her husband Jeremy Whitby is 69. Eleanor is a retired office worker with Medicare (Part A and Part B) and an individual Medigap insurance policy through her previous employment. Jeremy is covered by Medicare Part A because he is older than 65, but he is still employed full time and has health insurance from his employer (individual policy). Which is the primary and which is the secondary insurance (if any) for each for medical office charges?

9. Eleanor primary insurance: ____________________

secondary insurance: ____________________

10. Jeremy primary insurance: ____________________

secondary insurance: ____________________

B. Managed Care Plans

For each of the following types of managed care plans, choose the letter that describes access to out-of-network services for a subscriber (member).

a. Plan does not pay for out-of-network services (except for emergencies)

b. Out-of-network services are available at a higher cost

1. Staff model HMO: ____________________
2. Network model HMO: ____________________
3. Preferred provider organization (PPO): ____________________
4. Exclusive provider organization (EPO): ____________________
5. Point-of-service (POS) plan: ____________________

C. The Insurance Claim Form

Looking at the CMS-1500 health insurance claim form in Figure 48-3, identify which box should be used for each of the following pieces of information.

1. The patient's address: ____________________
2. The name of the insured: ____________________
3. If an outside laboratory was used: ____________________
4. If the physician accepts assignment of benefits: ____________________
5. The CPT code pointer of the first procedure: ____________________
6. The patient's birth date: ____________________
7. If there is another insurance plan: ____________________
8. The NPI number of the referring physician: ____________________
9. The balance owed by the patient: ____________________
10. The federal tax ID number: ____________________

PRACTICE FOR COMPETENCY

Procedure 48-1: Interpreting Information on an Insurance Card

Obtain copies of at least three medical insurance cards including a Medicare card. You may use Figure 48-1 and 48-2 from your textbook. The third card may be your own insurance card or a card provided by your instructor.

1. Examine each card carefully and make a list of information found on the front of each card and the back of each card.
2. Write several questions that a patient might ask that could be answered with information found on the cards.
3. With a classmate, practice asking and answering questions about insurance plans to prepare for role play.

Procedure 48-2: Verifying Insurance Eligibility and Benefits

Role-play situations with a classmate where you telephone to verify a patient's insurance. Assemble information before the role play. Assume the part of both the medical assistant and the insurance representative.

Describe to a classmate the process to verify eligibility and benefits using an insurance carrier website.

Procedure 48-3: Obtaining Insurance Preauthorization/Precertification

Role play the following situation first as a medical assistant and then as a third party representative/patient. One student should call for preauthorization/precertification, and the other student should represent ABC Insurance Company. At the final step, one student should role play the medical assistant and the other student should be the patient.

The patient, Linda Fuhr, is a female, DOB: 2/24/1957, who was initially seen at Fresno Medical Center for a urinary tract infection. On further examination, the patient was found to have an elevated bilirubin and a history of alcoholism with suspected alcoholic cirrhosis of the liver. Use the sample insurance card on the following page. The ordering physician's name is Goeff Lohman, Fresno Medical Center, telephone number (555) 452-1100, NPI 34567890XX. The patient's diagnoses are (1) jaundice, (2) alcohol dependence, uncomplicated. Look up any procedure codes and diagnosis codes before making the telephone call. Fresno Medical Center is located at 2000 Ocean Drive, Fresno, CA 93765. Memorial Hospital is located at 6200 Appleton Way, Fresno, CA 93765. If you have access to SimChart® for the Medical Office, it may be helpful to print and fill out a Prior Authorization Request form from the Forms Repository

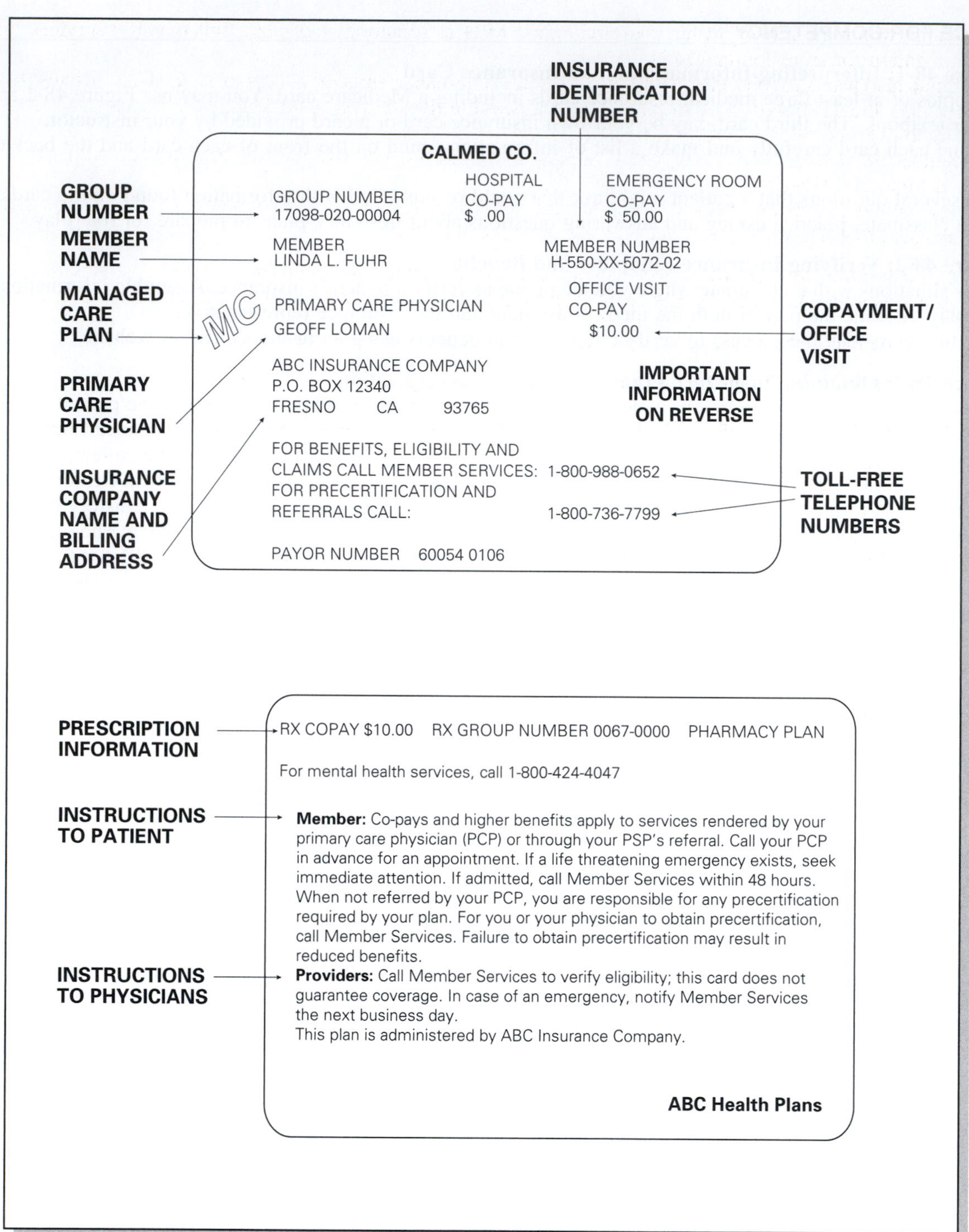
INSURANCE
IDENTIFICATION
NUMBER
CALMED CO.
GROUP
NUMBER
GROUP NUMBER
17098-020-00004
HOSPITAL
CO-PAY
$ .00
EMERGENCY ROOM
CO-PAY
$ 50.00
MEMBER
NAME
MEMBER
LINDA L. FUHR
MEMBER NUMBER
H-550-XX-5072-02
MANAGED
CARE
PLAN
MC
PRIMARY CARE PHYSICIAN
GEOFF LOMAN
OFFICE VISIT
CO-PAY
$10.00
COPAYMENT/
OFFICE
VISIT
PRIMARY
CARE
PHYSICIAN
ABC INSURANCE COMPANY
P.O. BOX 12340
FRESNO CA 93765
IMPORTANT
INFORMATION
ON REVERSE
INSURANCE
COMPANY
NAME AND
BILLING
ADDRESS
FOR BENEFITS, ELIGIBILITY AND
CLAIMS CALL MEMBER SERVICES: 1-800-988-0652
FOR PRECERTIFICATION AND
REFERRALS CALL: 1-800-736-7799
TOLL-FREE
TELEPHONE
NUMBERS
PAYOR NUMBER 60054 0106
PRESCRIPTION
INFORMATION
RX COPAY $10.00 RX GROUP NUMBER 0067-0000 PHARMACY PLAN
For mental health services, call 1-800-424-4047
INSTRUCTIONS
TO PATIENT
Member: Co-pays and higher benefits apply to services rendered by your primary care physician (PCP) or through your PSP's referral. Call your PCP in advance for an appointment. If a life threatening emergency exists, seek immediate attention. If admitted, call Member Services within 48 hours. When not referred by your PCP, you are responsible for any precertification required by your plan. For you or your physician to obtain precertification, call Member Services. Failure to obtain precertification may result in reduced benefits.
INSTRUCTIONS
TO PHYSICIANS
Providers: Call Member Services to verify eligibility; this card does not guarantee coverage. In case of an emergency, notify Member Services the next business day.
This plan is administered by ABC Insurance Company.
ABC Health Plans

(Modified from Fordney*: Insurance handbook for the medical office*, ed 13, St. Louis, 2014, Saunders.)

1. Dr. Lohman wants the patient to have an abdominal MRI at Memorial Hospital. Call member services to obtain preauthorization for an abdominal MRI.
2. Dr. Lohman also wants to refer the patient to Dr. Lionel Whitman, a surgeon at Fresno Medical Associates (telephone number (555) 452-1280, NPI # 67890123XX) for a possible liver biopsy. Call Member Services at ABC Insurance Company to obtain a referral for the patient.
3. Call Member Services at ABC Insurance Company to obtain preauthorization for Dr. Whitman to perform a liver biopsy at Memorial Hospital.
4. Role play calling the patient and informing her that she can schedule an appointment with Dr. Whitman, and you will make sure that his office receives a copy of the referral form.

Questions to ask when MA is calling for insurance preauthorization or referral: (Answer telephone as "Member Services, ABC Insurance Company"). Record your answers for each telephone call on a separate piece of paper.

1. What is the patient's name? ____________________
2. What is the patient's birth date? ____________________
3. What is the patient's insurance member number? Group number? ____________________
4. Physician's name and telephone number: ____________________
5. Physician's office name? ____________________
6. Physician's NPI number? ____________________
7. Facility that will perform a diagnostic test or surgery? ____________________
8. Facility address and phone number where diagnostic test or surgery will be performed?

   ____
9. Physician to whom the patient is being referred? ____________________
10. NPI number of physician to whom patient is referred? ____________________
11. Patient diagnosis (diagnoses) and diagnosis code(s)? Please specify if it is an ICD-9 or ICD-10 code.

   ____

   A. ____________________

   B. ____________________
12. Procedure(s) and procedure code(s)? ____________________

   A. ____________________

When answering the telephone as an ABC representative, after taking the information, tell the caller that it will take 24 to 48 hours to process the request.

Procedure 48-4: Completing/Reviewing the CMS-1500 Insurance Claim Form. Using the patient information and charge slips from Chapter 44 (Practice for Competency, Procedure 44-1), complete insurance claim forms for Ken Thomas and Tai Yan. Look up codes as needed.
Use the following address as needed:

BLUE CROSS BLUE SHIELD
1500 SUMMIT AVE
ANYTOWN, AL 12345

For Medicare:
NATIONAL HERITAGE INSURANCE CO
276 PINE STREET
WESTERN RIDGE XY 44779

In addition, complete an insurance claim form for the following:

Monique Jones	Patient number: 89643
1875 Wellington Springs Court	Established patient of Dr. Martin
Anytown, AL 12345	Name of insured: Monique Jones
(123) 588-9994	Insurance plan: Blue Cross Blue Shield
DOB: 6/23/1985	

10/18/XX	Expanded problem focused OV (99212)	$32.00
	Venipuncture collection (36415)	$10.00
Diagnoses:	Inflammatory polyarthropathy	
	Discoid lupus erythematosus	

Enter the information to complete insurance claims in SimChart® for the Medical Office using the Simulation Playground. It may be necessary to create an encounter and superbill, if you have not already done so, before you can create a claim. Print each claim and review it for accuracy.

Procedure 48-5 Communicating Effectively Related to Insurance and/or Managed Care
Role play three situations (as a medical assistant talking to a third party representative, a physician, and a patient) to practice professional and tactful communication related to third party requirements.

HEALTH INSURANCE CLAIM FORM

APPROVED BY NATIONAL UNIFORM CLAIM COMMITTEE (NUCC) 02/12

PICA　　　　　　　　　　　　　　　　　　　　　　　　　　PICA

CARRIER

1. MEDICARE (Medicare#) MEDICAID (Medicaid#) TRICARE (ID#DoD#) CHAMPVA (Member ID#) GROUP HEALTH PLAN (ID#) FECA BLK LUNG (ID#) OTHER (ID#)

1a. INSURED'S I.D. NUMBER (For Program in Item 1)

2. PATIENT'S NAME (Last Name, First Name, Middle Initial)

3. PATIENT'S BIRTH DATE MM DD YY SEX M F

4. INSURED'S NAME (Last Name, First Name, Middle Initial)

5. PATIENT'S ADDRESS (No., Street)

6. PATIENT RELATIONSHIP TO INSURED Self Spouse Child Other

7. INSURED'S ADDRESS (No., Street)

CITY STATE

8. RESERVED FOR NUCC USE

CITY STATE

ZIP CODE TELEPHONE (Include Area Code) ( )

ZIP CODE TELEPHONE (Include Area Code) ( )

9. OTHER INSURED'S NAME (Last Name, First Name, Middle Initial)

10. IS PATIENT'S CONDITION RELATED TO:

11. INSURED'S POLICY GROUP OR FECA NUMBER

a. OTHER INSURED'S POLICY OR GROUP NUMBER

a. EMPLOYMENT? (Current or Previous) YES NO

a. INSURED'S DATE OF BIRTH MM DD YY SEX M F

b. RESERVED FOR NUCC USE

b. AUTO ACCIDENT? YES NO PLACE (State)

b. OTHER CLAIM ID (Designated by NUCC)

c. RESERVED FOR NUCC USE

c. OTHER ACCIDENT? YES NO

c. INSURANCE PLAN NAME OR PROGRAM NAME

d. INSURANCE PLAN NAME OR PROGRAM NAME

10d. CLAIM CODES (Designated by NUCC)

d. IS THERE ANOTHER HEALTH BENEFIT PLAN? YES NO *If yes*, complete items 9, 9a, and 9d.

READ BACK OF FORM BEFORE COMPLETING & SIGNING THIS FORM.

12. PATIENT'S OR AUTHORIZED PERSON'S SIGNATURE I authorize the release of any medical or other information necessary to process this claim. I also request payment of government benefits either to myself or to the party who accepts assignment below.

SIGNED ______ DATE ______

13. INSURED'S OR AUTHORIZED PERSON'S SIGNATURE I authorize payment of medical benefits to the undersigned physician or supplier for services described below.

SIGNED ______

PATIENT AND INSURED INFORMATION

14. DATE OF CURRENT ILLNESS, INJURY, or PREGNANCY(LMP) MM DD YY QUAL.

15. OTHER DATE QUAL. MM DD YY

16. DATES PATIENT UNABLE TO WORK IN CURRENT OCCUPATION FROM MM DD YY TO MM DD YY

17. NAME OF REFERRING PROVIDER OR OTHER SOURCE

17a. 17b. NPI

18. HOSPITALIZATION DATES RELATED TO CURRENT SERVICES FROM MM DD YY TO MM DD YY

19. ADDITIONAL CLAIM INFORMATION (Designated by NUCC)

20. OUTSIDE LAB? YES NO $ CHARGES

21. DIAGNOSIS OR NATURE OF ILLNESS OR INJURY Relate A-L to service line below (24E) ICD Ind.

A. B. C. D.
E. F. G. H.
I. J. K. L.

22. RESUBMISSION CODE ORIGINAL REF. NO.

23. PRIOR AUTHORIZATION NUMBER

24. A. DATE(S) OF SERVICE From MM DD YY To MM DD YY	B. PLACE OF SERVICE	C. EMG	D. PROCEDURES, SERVICES, OR SUPPLIES (Explain Unusual Circumstances) CPT/HCPCS MODIFIER	E. DIAGNOSIS POINTER	F. $ CHARGES	G. DAYS OR UNITS	H. EPSDT Family Plan	I. ID. QUAL.	J. RENDERING PROVIDER ID. #
1								NPI	
2								NPI	
3								NPI	
4								NPI	
5								NPI	
6								NPI	

PHYSICIAN OR SUPPLIER INFORMATION

25. FEDERAL TAX I.D. NUMBER SSN EIN

26. PATIENT'S ACCOUNT NO.

27. ACCEPT ASSIGNMENT? (For govt. claims, see back) YES NO

28. TOTAL CHARGE $

29. AMOUNT PAID $

30. Rsvd for NUCC Use $

31. SIGNATURE OF PHYSICIAN OR SUPPLIER INCLUDING DEGREES OR CREDENTIALS (I certify that the statements on the reverse apply to this bill and are made a part thereof.)

SIGNED DATE

32. SERVICE FACILITY LOCATION INFORMATION

a. NPI b.

33. BILLING PROVIDER INFO & PH # ( )

a. NPI b.

NUCC Instruction Manual available at: www.nucc.org　　*PLEASE PRINT OR TYPE*　　APPROVED OMB-098-1197 FORM 1500 (02-12) PENDING

HEALTH INSURANCE CLAIM FORM

APPROVED BY NATIONAL UNIFORM CLAIM COMMITTEE (NUCC) 02/12

PICA | PICA

CARRIER

1. MEDICARE (Medicare#) | MEDICAID (Medicaid#) | TRICARE (ID#DoD#) | CHAMPVA (Member ID#) | GROUP HEALTH PLAN (ID#) | FECA BLK LUNG (ID#) | OTHER (ID#)

1a. INSURED'S I.D. NUMBER (For Program in Item 1)

2. PATIENT'S NAME (Last Name, First Name, Middle Initial)

3. PATIENT'S BIRTH DATE MM | DD | YY — SEX M ☐ F ☐

4. INSURED'S NAME (Last Name, First Name, Middle Initial)

5. PATIENT'S ADDRESS (No., Street)

6. PATIENT RELATIONSHIP TO INSURED — Self ☐ Spouse ☐ Child ☐ Other ☐

7. INSURED'S ADDRESS (No., Street)

CITY | STATE

8. RESERVED FOR NUCC USE

CITY | STATE

ZIP CODE | TELEPHONE (Include Area Code) ( )

ZIP CODE | TELEPHONE (Include Area Code) ( )

9. OTHER INSURED'S NAME (Last Name, First Name, Middle Initial)

10. IS PATIENT'S CONDITION RELATED TO:

11. INSURED'S POLICY GROUP OR FECA NUMBER

a. OTHER INSURED'S POLICY OR GROUP NUMBER

a. EMPLOYMENT? (Current or Previous) ☐ YES ☐ NO

a. INSURED'S DATE OF BIRTH MM | DD | YY — SEX M ☐ F ☐

b. RESERVED FOR NUCC USE

b. AUTO ACCIDENT? ☐ YES ☐ NO — PLACE (State)

b. OTHER CLAIM ID (Designated by NUCC)

c. RESERVED FOR NUCC USE

c. OTHER ACCIDENT? ☐ YES ☐ NO

c. INSURANCE PLAN NAME OR PROGRAM NAME

d. INSURANCE PLAN NAME OR PROGRAM NAME

10d. CLAIM CODES (Designated by NUCC)

d. IS THERE ANOTHER HEALTH BENEFIT PLAN? ☐ YES ☐ NO ***If yes***, complete items 9, 9a, and 9d.

READ BACK OF FORM BEFORE COMPLETING & SIGNING THIS FORM.

12. PATIENT'S OR AUTHORIZED PERSON'S SIGNATURE I authorize the release of any medical or other information necessary to process this claim. I also request payment of government benefits either to myself or to the party who accepts assignment below.

SIGNED ____________ DATE ____________

13. INSURED'S OR AUTHORIZED PERSON'S SIGNATURE I authorize payment of medical benefits to the undersigned physician or supplier for services described below.

SIGNED ____________

PATIENT AND INSURED INFORMATION

14. DATE OF CURRENT ILLNESS, INJURY, or PREGNANCY(LMP) MM | DD | YY QUAL.

15. OTHER DATE QUAL. MM | DD | YY

16. DATES PATIENT UNABLE TO WORK IN CURRENT OCCUPATION FROM MM | DD | YY TO MM | DD | YY

17. NAME OF REFERRING PROVIDER OR OTHER SOURCE

17a. | 17b. NPI

18. HOSPITALIZATION DATES RELATED TO CURRENT SERVICES FROM MM | DD | YY TO MM | DD | YY

19. ADDITIONAL CLAIM INFORMATION (Designated by NUCC)

20. OUTSIDE LAB? ☐ YES ☐ NO — $ CHARGES

21. DIAGNOSIS OR NATURE OF ILLNESS OR INJURY Relate A-L to service line below (24E) ICD Ind.

A. ____ B. ____ C. ____ D. ____
E. ____ F. ____ G. ____ H. ____
I. ____ J. ____ K. ____ L. ____

22. RESUBMISSION CODE | ORIGINAL REF. NO.

23. PRIOR AUTHORIZATION NUMBER

	24. A. DATE(S) OF SERVICE From MM DD YY	To MM DD YY	B. PLACE OF SERVICE	C. EMG	D. PROCEDURES, SERVICES, OR SUPPLIES (Explain Unusual Circumstances) CPT/HCPCS	MODIFIER	E. DIAGNOSIS POINTER	F. $ CHARGES	G. DAYS OR UNITS	H. EPSDT Family Plan	I. ID. QUAL.	J. RENDERING PROVIDER ID. #
1											NPI	
2											NPI	
3											NPI	
4											NPI	
5											NPI	
6											NPI	

PHYSICIAN OR SUPPLIER INFORMATION

25. FEDERAL TAX I.D. NUMBER SSN EIN

26. PATIENT'S ACCOUNT NO.

27. ACCEPT ASSIGNMENT? (For govt. claims, see back) ☐ YES ☐ NO

28. TOTAL CHARGE $

29. AMOUNT PAID $

30. Rsvd for NUCC Use $

31. SIGNATURE OF PHYSICIAN OR SUPPLIER INCLUDING DEGREES OR CREDENTIALS (I certify that the statements on the reverse apply to this bill and are made a part thereof.)

SIGNED DATE

32. SERVICE FACILITY LOCATION INFORMATION

a. NPI b.

33. BILLING PROVIDER INFO & PH # ( )

a. NPI b.

NUCC Instruction Manual available at: www.nucc.org *PLEASE PRINT OR TYPE* APPROVED OMB-098-1197 FORM 1500 (02-12) PENDING

HEALTH INSURANCE CLAIM FORM

APPROVED BY NATIONAL UNIFORM CLAIM COMMITTEE (NUCC) 02/12

PICA | PICA | CARRIER

1. MEDICARE (Medicare#) | MEDICAID (Medicaid#) | TRICARE (ID#DoD#) | CHAMPVA (Member ID#) | GROUP HEALTH PLAN (ID#) | FECA BLK LUNG (ID#) | OTHER (ID#)

1a. INSURED'S I.D. NUMBER (For Program in Item 1)

2. PATIENT'S NAME (Last Name, First Name, Middle Initial)

3. PATIENT'S BIRTH DATE MM DD YY SEX M F

4. INSURED'S NAME (Last Name, First Name, Middle Initial)

5. PATIENT'S ADDRESS (No., Street)

6. PATIENT RELATIONSHIP TO INSURED Self Spouse Child Other

7. INSURED'S ADDRESS (No., Street)

CITY | STATE

8. RESERVED FOR NUCC USE

CITY | STATE

ZIP CODE | TELEPHONE (Include Area Code) ( )

ZIP CODE | TELEPHONE (Include Area Code) ( )

9. OTHER INSURED'S NAME (Last Name, First Name, Middle Initial)

10. IS PATIENT'S CONDITION RELATED TO:

11. INSURED'S POLICY GROUP OR FECA NUMBER

a. OTHER INSURED'S POLICY OR GROUP NUMBER

a. EMPLOYMENT? (Current or Previous) YES NO

a. INSURED'S DATE OF BIRTH MM DD YY SEX M F

b. RESERVED FOR NUCC USE

b. AUTO ACCIDENT? PLACE (State) YES NO

b. OTHER CLAIM ID (Designated by NUCC)

c. RESERVED FOR NUCC USE

c. OTHER ACCIDENT? YES NO

c. INSURANCE PLAN NAME OR PROGRAM NAME

d. INSURANCE PLAN NAME OR PROGRAM NAME

10d. CLAIM CODES (Designated by NUCC)

d. IS THERE ANOTHER HEALTH BENEFIT PLAN? YES NO *If yes*, complete items 9, 9a, and 9d.

READ BACK OF FORM BEFORE COMPLETING & SIGNING THIS FORM.

12. PATIENT'S OR AUTHORIZED PERSON'S SIGNATURE I authorize the release of any medical or other information necessary to process this claim. I also request payment of government benefits either to myself or to the party who accepts assignment below.

SIGNED ______ DATE ______

13. INSURED'S OR AUTHORIZED PERSON'S SIGNATURE I authorize payment of medical benefits to the undersigned physician or supplier for services described below.

SIGNED ______

PATIENT AND INSURED INFORMATION

14. DATE OF CURRENT ILLNESS, INJURY, or PREGNANCY(LMP) MM DD YY QUAL.

15. OTHER DATE QUAL. MM DD YY

16. DATES PATIENT UNABLE TO WORK IN CURRENT OCCUPATION FROM MM DD YY TO MM DD YY

17. NAME OF REFERRING PROVIDER OR OTHER SOURCE

17a. | 17b. NPI

18. HOSPITALIZATION DATES RELATED TO CURRENT SERVICES FROM MM DD YY TO MM DD YY

19. ADDITIONAL CLAIM INFORMATION (Designated by NUCC)

20. OUTSIDE LAB? YES NO $ CHARGES

21. DIAGNOSIS OR NATURE OF ILLNESS OR INJURY Relate A-L to service line below (24E) ICD Ind.

A. ___ B. ___ C. ___ D. ___

E. ___ F. ___ G. ___ H. ___

I. ___ J. ___ K. ___ L. ___

22. RESUBMISSION CODE | ORIGINAL REF. NO.

23. PRIOR AUTHORIZATION NUMBER

24. A. DATE(S) OF SERVICE From MM DD YY To MM DD YY	B. PLACE OF SERVICE	C. EMG	D. PROCEDURES, SERVICES, OR SUPPLIES (Explain Unusual Circumstances) CPT/HCPCS MODIFIER	E. DIAGNOSIS POINTER	F. $ CHARGES	G. DAYS OR UNITS	H. EPSDT Family Plan	I. ID. QUAL.	J. RENDERING PROVIDER ID. #
1								NPI	
2								NPI	
3								NPI	
4								NPI	
5								NPI	
6								NPI	

25. FEDERAL TAX I.D. NUMBER SSN EIN

26. PATIENT'S ACCOUNT NO.

27. ACCEPT ASSIGNMENT? (For govt. claims, see back) YES NO

28. TOTAL CHARGE $

29. AMOUNT PAID $

30. Rsvd for NUCC Use $

31. SIGNATURE OF PHYSICIAN OR SUPPLIER INCLUDING DEGREES OR CREDENTIALS (I certify that the statements on the reverse apply to this bill and are made a part thereof.)

SIGNED DATE

32. SERVICE FACILITY LOCATION INFORMATION

a. NPI b.

33. BILLING PROVIDER INFO & PH # ( )

a. NPI b.

PHYSICIAN OR SUPPLIER INFORMATION

NUCC Instruction Manual available at: www.nucc.org *PLEASE PRINT OR TYPE* APPROVED OMB-098-1197 FORM 1500 (02-12) PENDING

Notes

EVALUATION OF COMPETENCY

Procedure 48-1 Interpreting Information on an Insurance Card

Name: ______________________ Date: ______________

Evaluated by: ______________________ Score: ______________

Performance Objective

Outcome:	Interpret information on an insurance card.
Conditions:	Given the following: sample insurance cards.
Standards:	Written list of information and paper. Time for role play: 20 minutes. Student completed procedure in __________ minutes. Accuracy: Satisfactory score on the Performance Evaluation Checklist.

Performance Evaluation Checklist

Trial 1	Trial 2	Point Value	Performance Standards
		●	Used at least three insurance cards to make a list of information found on the front of insurance cards and on the back of insurance cards.
		●	Wrote a short paper analyzing one sample insurance card
		●	Included insurance carrier name and contact information, subscriber name and identifying information, patient payment responsibility for various services (if present), and the type of insurance plan in the short paper.
		●	Participated in role play situation playing the part of the medical assistant to answer specific questions about the insurance plan related to a specific insurance card.
		●	Participated in role play situation playing the part of a patient asking questions about amount of co-pay, referral process, patient responsibility in a life-threatening emergency related to a specific insurance card.
		Ⓐ	Displayed sensitivity when communicating with the simulated patient about insurance plan requirements.
		*	Handed in the list of information and short paper analyzing an insurance card to instructor.
		*	Completed the role play part of the procedure within 20 minutes.
			TOTALS

Evaluation of Student Performance

EVALUATION CRITERIA			COMMENTS
Symbol	**Category**	**Point Value**	
∗	Critical Step	16 points	
●	Essential Step	6 points	
Ⓐ	Affective Competency	6 points	
▷	Theory Question	2 points	
Score calculation: 100 points − ___ points missed ___ Score Satisfactory score: 85 or above			

2008 CAAHEP Competencies Achieved
Psychomotor (Skills) ☑ VII.2. Apply third party guidelines. ***Affective (Behavior)*** ☑ VII.3. Communicate in language the patient can understand regarding managed care and insurance plans.

2015 CAAHEP Competencies Achieved
Psychomotor (Skills) ☑ VIII.1. Interpret information on an insurance card ***Affective (Behavior)*** ☑ VIII.3. Show sensitivity when communicating with patients regarding third party requirements.

ABHES Competencies Achieved
☑ 8. c. Process insurance claims: 1. Differentiate between procedures of private, federal, and state payers.

EVALUATION OF COMPETENCY

Procedure 48-2 Verifying Insurance Eligibility and Benefits

Name: ______________________________ Date: ______________

Evaluated by: ______________________________ Score: ______________

Performance Objective

Outcome:	Verify insurance or managed care eligibility
Conditions:	Given the following: patient insurance information, telephone, computer, pen and paper.
Standards:	Time: 20 minutes. Student completed procedure in ________ minutes.
	Accuracy: Satisfactory score on the Performance Evaluation Checklist.

Performance Evaluation Checklist

Trial 1	Trial 2	Point Value	Performance Standards
		●	Assembled information about patient insurance plan including name of carrier, telephone number or web address, patient name, patient date of birth, subscriber number, and group number.
		●	If using the telephone called and asked a third party representative to verify that the patient was eligible for benefits.
		●	Recorded effective date and termination date (if any) of eligibility.
		●	Requested information about the patient's deductible, copayment and/or coinsurance.
		●	Determined if the proposed service was covered and if preauthorization or precertification would be required.
		▷	Described situations when preauthorization or precertification is usually necessary.
		●	If using a plan website, logged in and found the patient using name, date of birth and/or subscriber number.
		●	Verified that the correct patient was found on a website and viewed eligibility information.
		●	Noted eligibility information on an office form or in the patient's medical record according to office policy.
		●	Attached electronic verification of eligibility to the patient's EHR or printed and filed in a paper-based medical record.
		Ⓐ	Interacted tactfully with third party representatives.
		✶	Completed the procedure within 20 minutes.
			TOTALS

Evaluation of Student Performance

EVALUATION CRITERIA			COMMENTS
Symbol	Category	Point Value	
∗	Critical Step	16 points	
●	Essential Step	6 points	
Ⓐ	Affective Competency	6 points	
▷	Theory Question	2 points	
Score calculation: 100 points − ___ points missed ___ Score Satisfactory score: 85 or above			

2008 CAAHEP Competencies Achieved
Psychomotor (Skills) ☑ VII.2. Verify eligibility for managed care services. ***Affective (Behavior)*** ☑ VII.1. Demonstrate assertive communication with managed care and/or insurance providers

2015 CAAHEP Competencies Achieved
Psychomotor (Skills) ☑ VIII.2. Verify eligibility for services including documentation ***Affective (Behavior)*** ☑ VIII.1. Interact professionally with third party representatives.

ABHES Competencies Achieved
☑ 8. c. Process insurance claims: 1. Differentiate between procedures of private, federal, and state payors

EVALUATION OF COMPETENCY

Procedure 48-3: Obtaining Insurance Preauthorization

Name: ______________________ Date: ______________

Evaluated by: ______________________ Score: ______________

Performance Objective

Outcome:	Obtain insurance preauthorization (precertification).
Conditions:	Given the following: patient medical record, patient insurance information, physician's directions about the service to be provided, computer or paper preauthorization (precertification) request form, pen, telephone
Standards:	Time: 20 minutes. Student completed procedure in ________ minutes. Accuracy: Satisfactory score on the Performance Evaluation Checklist

Performance Evaluation Checklist

Trial 1	Trial 2	Point Value	Performance Standards
		●	Assembled information to request preauthorization (precertification) • Patient demographic information • Patient insurance information • Information about service to be provided including diagnosis code(s) and procedure code(s) • Forms as needed • Pen, computer • Telephone (optional)
		●	Assembled additional information including physician's NPI number.
		●	If additional information was needed, obtained from the medical record or physician (or other provider).
		●	Completed preauthorization or precertification form, or called the patient's insurance carrier and provided all information requested.
		●	Requested preauthorization or precertification by completing an online form, a paper form, or by telephone and supplied all necessary information.
		●	If using the telephone, completed the request form manually before placing the call.
		▷	Described times when precertification or preauthorization would be required.
		●	Submitted from electronically or by mail as appropriate.
		●	Informed the patient that he or she could not obtain service until the preauthorization/precertification was approved by the insurance carrier.
		●	When approval was received, notified the patient, instructed the patient to schedule the service, and sent a copy as needed to any other physician or provider of service.
		●	Filed a copy of the approval form in the patient's medical record.

Trial 1	Trial 2	Point Value	Performance Standards
		Ⓐ	Demonstrated tactful behavior when requesting additional information from a provider.
		Ⓐ	Demonstrated professional interaction with a third party representative.
		Ⓐ	Showed sensitivity when communicating with a patient related to preauthorization or precertification.
		∗	Completed the procedure within 20 minutes.
			TOTALS

Evaluation of Student Performance

EVALUATION CRITERIA			COMMENTS
Symbol	**Category**	**Point Value**	
∗	Critical Step	16 points	
●	Essential Step	6 points	
Ⓐ	Affective Competency	6 points	
▷	Theory Question	2 points	
Score calculation: 100 points − ___ points missed ___ Score Satisfactory score: 85 or above			

2008 CAAHEP Competencies Achieved

Psychomotor (Skills)

☑ VII.4. Obtain precertification, including documentation.
☑ VII.5. Obtain preauthorization, including documentation.

Affective (Behavior)

☑ VII.1. Demonstrate assertive communication with managed care and/or insurance providers.

2015 CAAHEP Competencies Achieved

Psychomotor (Skills)

☑ VIII.3. Obtain precertification or preauthorization including documentation.

Affective (Behavior)

☑ VIII.1. Interact professionally with third party representatives.
☑ VIII.2. Display tactful behavior when communicating with medical providers regarding third party requirements
☑ VIII.3. Show sensitivity when communicating with patients regarding third party requirements.

ABHES Competencies Achieved

☑ 8. c. Process insurance claims: 2. Differentiate managed care: i.e. HMO, PPO, IPA including referrals and pre-certification.

EVALUATION OF COMPETENCY

Procedure 48-4: Completing and Reviewing an Insurance Claim Form

Name: ______________________ Date: ______________

Evaluated by: ______________________ Score: ______________

Performance Objective

Outcome:	Complete (or review) an insurance claim form.
Conditions:	Given the following: patient information form or computer screen, patient account or ledger, photocopy of patient's insurance card, insurance claim form, computer with medical billing program or SimChart® for the Medical Office, printer, and pen.
Standards:	Time: 15 minutes. Student completed procedure in ________ minutes.
	Accuracy: Satisfactory score on the Performance Evaluation Checklist.

Performance Evaluation Checklist

Trial 1	Trial 2	Point Value	Performance Standards
		●	Assembled information and supplies.
		●	If creating a paper claim, used capital letters without commas, dollar signs, or other punctuation unless specifically instructed.
		●	In the carrier section entered the name and address of the insurance carrier using correct address format.
		●	Entered the type of insurance.
		●	Entered the ID number and group number of the insured individual as shown on photocopy of the insurance card.
		●	Entered patient information accurately.
		●	Identified the patient's relationship to the insured.
		●	If the insured was not the patient, entered the required information about the insured.
		●	Entered the patient's marital status and employment status.
		●	Entered complete information about any secondary insurance as needed.
		●	Entered information related to the cause of the patient's condition(s).
		●	Identified if the patient did or did not have other insurance.
		●	Validated the patient signature on the form to allow insurance billing and assignment of benefits.
		●	Entered Signature on File (SOF) in boxes authorizing permission.
		▷	Explained how to obtain signatures if they were not on file.
		*	Completed the patient and insured information section accurately and completely.

Trial 1	Trial 2	Point Value	Performance Standards
		•	Entered any special information required by a specific insurance carrier as needed.
		•	Entered the name and identifying number of the referring physician, if any.
		•	Entered dates of hospitalization if services were provided in the hospital.
		•	Checked the correct box to identify if outside laboratory services were provided.
		•	Entered the ICD indicator to identify which version of ICD codes was being reported.
		•	Entered up to twelve ICD codes.
		•	Entered reference numbers for a Medicaid resubmission, referral, preauthorization, and/or precertification.
		•	Entered information about the first procedure including date(s) of service, place of service, CPT or HCPCS Level II code and modifiers, letter to point to the appropriate diagnosis, charges, number of units, and the NPI number or other ID number.
		•	Entered complete information about each additional procedure.
		•	Entered the tax identification number and checked if the Social Security number or employer identification number was used.
		•	Entered the patient account number, if any.
		•	Checked the correct box to indicate acceptance of assignment of benefits.
		•	Entered the total charges, total amount paid, and total balance due.
		•	Entered SOF or the physician's legal signature including credentials and date.
		•	Entered the name, address, and telephone number of the billing facility, and the name of the facility where services were provided, if different.
		•	Entered the NPI number or other ID number for the billing facility and facility where services were provided, if different.
		•	Made a copy of a paper claim and filed in an insurance claims file.
		•	Reviewed the claim for accuracy before submission.
		*	Completed the physician or supplier section accurately and completely.
			Completing the insurance claim in SimChart® for the Medical Office
		•	Selected **Claim** for the correct patient after the superbill and ledger were created and verified the auto-populated details.
		•	Validated that the HIPAA form and date were on file for the patient on the **Encounter Notes** tab and saved.
		•	Completed all information on the **Charge Capture** screen and saved.
		•	Printed the claim and manually double checked to be sure all information was correct.
		•	Submitted the claim after entering the date of service and saving.

Trial 1	Trial 2	Point Value	Performance Standards
		✶	The information on the claim form was complete and correct.
		✶	Completed the procedure within 15 minutes.
			TOTALS

Evaluation of Student Performance

EVALUATION CRITERIA			COMMENTS
Symbol	**Category**	**Point Value**	
✶	Critical Step	16 points	
●	Essential Step	6 points	
Ⓐ	Affective Competency	6 points	
▷	Theory Question	2 points	
Score calculation: 100 points – ____ points missed ____ Score Satisfactory score: 85 or above			

2008 CAAHEP Competencies Achieved
Psychomotor (Skills) ☑ VII. 3. Complete insurance claim forms. *Affective (Behavior)* ☑ VIII.1. Work with physician to achieve the maximum reimbursement.

2015 CAAHEP Competency Achieved
Psychomotor (Skills) ☑ VIII.4. Complete an insurance claim form.

ABHES Competencies Achieved
☑ 8. c. Process insurance claims

Notes

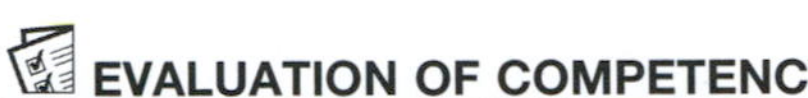

EVALUATION OF COMPETENCY

Procedure 48-5 Communicating Effectively Related to Insurance and/or Managed Care

Name: ______________________________ Date: ____________________

Evaluated by: ______________________________ Score: ____________________

Performance Objective

Outcomes:	1. Interact professionally with third party representatives 2. Display tactful behavior when communicating with medical providers related to insurance or managed care. 3. Show sensitivity when communicating with patients regarding third party requirements.
Conditions:	Given the following: Pen, paper, computer with printer.
Standards:	Written paper. Time for role play: 30 minutes. Student completed procedure in __________ minutes. Accuracy: Satisfactory score on the Performance Evaluation Checklist.

Performance Evaluation Checklist

Trial 1	Trial 2	Point Value	Performance Standards
		●	Reviewed principles of effective communication in textbook.
		●	Worked with at least two other students to create three role play situations: A. Medical assistant and managed care provider representative related to denied insurance claim; B. Medical assistant and physician related to denied request for a diagnostic test; C. Medical assistant and patient related to denied insurance claim.
		●	Reviewed all situations and gave constructive feedback to other students.
		●	Participated in role play as a medical assistant for each situation demonstrating professional communication with a third party representative, tact with a physician, and sensitivity with a patient.
		●	Wrote a short summary of the role play experience using a computer related to the situation created and explained effective communication techniques used.
		●	Printed paper and handed in to instructor.
		Ⓐ	Interacted professionally in role play with third party representative.
		Ⓐ	Displayed tactful behavior in role play with physician.
		Ⓐ	Demonstrated sensitivity in role play when explaining insurance denial to a patient.
		✶	Completed the role play part of the procedure within 30 minutes.
			TOTALS

Evaluation of Student Performance

EVALUATION CRITERIA			COMMENTS
Symbol	Category	Point Value	
∗	Critical Step	16 points	
●	Essential Step	6 points	
Ⓐ	Affective Competency	6 points	
▷	Theory Question	2 points	
Score calculation: 100 points − ___ points missed ___ Score Satisfactory score: 85 or above			

2008 CAAHEP Competency Achieved
Affective (Behavior) ☑ VII.1. Demonstrate assertive communication with managed care and/or insurance providers. ☑ VII.2. Demonstrate sensitivity in communicating with both providers and patients. ☑ VII.3. Communicate in language the patient can understand regarding managed care and insurance plans.

2015 CAAHEP Competencies Achieved
Affective (Behavior) ☑ VIII.1. Interact professionally with third party representatives. ☑ VIII.2. Display tactful behavior when communicating with medical providers regarding third party requirements ☑ VIII.3. Show sensitivity when communicating with patients regarding third party requirements.

ABHES Competencies Achieved
☑ 5.c. Intervene on behalf of the patient regarding issues/concerns that may arise, i.e. insurance policy information, medical bills, physician/provider orders, etc.

Billing and Collections

CHAPTER ASSIGNMENTS

✓ After Completing	Date Due	Study Guide Pages	STUDY GUIDE ASSIGNMENTS (CTA = Critical Thinking Activity)	Possible Points	Points You Earned
		1357	Pretest	10	
		1358	Term Key Term Assessment	10	
		1358-1360	Evaluation of Learning questions	23	
		1361	CTA A: Cycle Billing	10	
		1361	CTA B: Adjustments	8	
		1362	CTA C: Aging Accounts	8	
			Evolve Site: Apply Your Knowledge questions	10	
			Evolve Site: Video Evaluation	5	
		1357	Posttest	10	
			ADDITIONAL ASSIGNMENTS		
			TOTAL POINTS		

Notes

✓ When Assigned By Your Instructor	Study Guide Pages	Practices Required	LABORATORY ASSIGNMENTS (Procedure Number and Name)	Score*
	1363	3	**Practice for Competency** 49-1: Processing Patient Statements Textbook reference: p. 1220	
	1367-1368		**Evaluation of Competency** 49-1: Processing Patient Statements	*
	1363	1	**Practice for Competency** 49-2: Posting an NSF Check Textbook reference: pp. 1221-1222	
	1369-1370		**Evaluation of Competency** 49-2: Posting an NSF Check	*
	1363-1364	1	**Practice for Competency** 49-3: Processing a Credit Balance and Refund Textbook reference: pp. 1222-1223	
	1371-1372		**Evaluation of Competency** 49-3: Processing a Credit Balance and Refund	*
	1365-1366	1	**Practice for Competency** 49-4: Creating an Accounts Receivable Aging Record Textbook reference: p. 1225	
	1373-1374		**Evaluation of Competency** 49-4: Creating an Accounts Receivable Aging Record	*
	1366	1	**Practice for Competency** 49-5: Writing a Collection Letter Textbook reference: p. 1231	
	1375-1376		**Evaluation of Competency** 49-5: Writing a Collection Letter	*
			ADDITIONAL ASSIGNMENTS	

Notes

Name ________________________________ Date ______________

PRETEST

True or False

_______ 1. The first bill is usually sent to the patient the day after a patient visit.

_______ 2. Almost all medical offices do monthly billing from the office.

_______ 3. Credit agreements with patients must be in writing even if the patient is not charged interest.

_______ 4. A check written on an account that does not have sufficient funds is called an overdraft.

_______ 5. When a check is reported lost, the bank should be notified to stop payment on the check.

_______ 6. If a patient overpays his or her account, the office usually issues a refund to the patient.

_______ 7. The medical assistant must create an accounts receivable aging report manually at least once a month.

_______ 8. Overdue accounts older than 120 days are definitely subject to collection activity.

_______ 9. The first time a claim message is used on a patient's bill is when the bill is older than 120 days.

_______ 10. It is illegal to call a patient at his or her place of employment about an overdue bill.

POSTTEST

True or False

_______ 1. Medical offices usually send a bill to patients to collect copayments.

_______ 2. The billing cycle is a term used to describe how long it takes to prepare bills for mailing.

_______ 3. Sending some patient bills every week is usually more efficient than sending all bills at the end of the month.

_______ 4. The bank only charges a fee to the account a nonsufficient funds (NSF) check is written on.

_______ 5. When a check is returned by the bank for not sufficient funds (NSF check), the amount of the check is added to the patient's account balance.

_______ 6. If a patient has a credit balance, it means that the office owes the patient money.

_______ 7. Accounts are first considered overdue at 90 days after the date billed.

_______ 8. The medical office can sue patients for overdue accounts in small claims court.

_______ 9. The best time to call a patient about an overdue bill is after 9:00 PM.

_______ 10. A written truth in lending statement is required if the medical office makes an agreement for monthly payments.

KEY TERM ASSESSMENT

Directions: Match each key term with its definition.

_______ 1. Account aging

_______ 2. Balance due

_______ 3. Bankruptcy

_______ 4. Claim message

_______ 5. Credit balance

_______ 6. Collection agency

_______ 7. Overdraft

_______ 8. Patient statement

_______ 9. Skip

_______ 10. Truth in lending

A. Money owed by the medical office to a patient, usually due to an overpayment

B. A check (or draft) that exceeds the amount of funds in a bank account

C. Total amount owed

D. A firm that is in the business of collecting overdue accounts

E. The process of finding out how long specific account balances have been outstanding

F. Legal requirement to provide written terms of a loan in language that can be easily understood

G. The legal process by which the debts of an individual or business are resolved if they cannot be paid

H. Messages encouraging payment of a bill, usually attached to or printed on the monthly statement

I. Account for which no billing information is available

J. A bill sent to a patient that contains charges, payments and adjustments

EVALUATION OF LEARNING

Directions: Fill in each blank with the correct answer.

1. What is the advantage to the office of a weekly billing cycle?

____

____

2. If the medical office bills every week, how are patient accounts usually divided?

____

____

3. What are two ways that bills can be produced?

____

____

4. Give examples of two special situations that may affect billing.

____

____

5. What is overdraft protection?

____

____

6. When should the medical office stop payment on a check?

____

____

7. How should the medical assistant (MA) handle a check that is returned for insufficient funds?

8. When does a credit balance occur in a patient account, and how is a credit balance handled?

9. When is a patient account considered overdue?

10. What are the usual categories of overdue accounts when an accounts receivable aging record is created?

11. What is the usual progression in collection activity when a patient's account is overdue?

12. Why is it recommended to place a telephone call regarding an overdue account in addition to placing claim messages on the bill?

13. When does the office need to have a written credit arrangement with a patient?

14. What does a truth in lending statement include, and when should it be sent to a patient?

15. Identify three methods to try to trace a patient whose bill is returned with the notation "address unknown."

16. If the three methods identified in the previous question fail to locate a "skip," what should the medical office do to try to collect a bill?

17. What is the process for sending a patient account to a collection agency?

18. How should a collection agency payment be entered on the patient's ledger card and on the day sheet?

19. What is small claims court, and how might it be used by the medical office?

20. If a patient has died, how and when should the bill for services rendered before death be sent?

21. If the bill of a deceased individual is not paid promptly, how should the MA follow up?

22. What is the status of outstanding medical bills if a person declares bankruptcy under Chapter 7? Under Chapter 13?

23. Describe briefly how each of the following laws affects credit and collection activities in the medical office:
    a. Equal Credit Opportunity Act:
    b. Fair Debt Collection Practices Act:
    c. Federal Truth in Lending Act:
    d. Fair Credit Reporting Act:
    e. Bankruptcy Abuse and Consumer Protection Act of 2005:

CRITICAL THINKING ACTIVITIES

A. Cycle Billing

Assume that a billing cycle is used in which patients with a last name beginning with the letters A-E are billed the first week of the month; the second week, F-L; the third week, M-S; and the fourth week, T-Z. Identify which week each of the following patients would be billed.

1. John T. Sanders ____________________
2. Eileen McDonald ____________________
3. Winston A. Robertson ____________________
4. Tracy Marie Jordan ____________________
5. Julian W. Allen ____________________
6. Edward Elliot Hubbard ____________________
7. Joanne Mason-Taylor ____________________
8. Diane von Bohlen ____________________
9. Carolyn Ann Oppenheimer ____________________
10. Douglas P. Benson ____________________

B. Adjustments

For each of the following situations identify whether the MA will post the transaction to the patient account as a negative adjustment (reduces the patient balance), a payment, or a positive adjustment (increases the patient balance).

1. Patient pays $50.00 by check, which is an overpayment of $25.00:

2. Patient's check for $25.00 is returned by the bank marked "Not sufficient funds:"

3. A collection agency payment is received, and the patient balance is zero:

4. A check from an insurance company is received for a patient account:

5. A patient pays a copayment of $10.00 at the time of the visit:

6. A patient is given a discount of $15.00 for paying the bill in cash:

7. A check is issued as a refund for a patient overpayment:

8. The insurance company identifies $12.00 of the patient charge as an excluded amount:

C. Aging Accounts

Assume that accounts are aged from the date of billing. If you are aging accounts on 10/30/XX, select the letter of the correct length of time that each of the following accounts has been outstanding.

a. Current (0 to 30 days)
b. 31 to 60 days
c. 61 to 90 days
d. 91 to 120 days
e. Older than 120 days

_______ 1. Service provided on 7/4/XX, billed on 8/1/XX

_______ 2. Service provided on 9/22/XX, billed on 10/3/XX

_______ 3. Service provided on 8/13/XX, billed on 8/22/XX

_______ 4. Service provided on 4/18/XX, billed on 4/25/XX

_______ 5. Service provided on 5/13/XX, billed on 6/6/XX

_______ 6. Service provided on 6/19/XX, billed on 7/12/XX

_______ 7. Service provided on 6/25/XX, billed on 7/18/XX

_______ 8. Service provided on 7/18/XX, billed on 8/15/XX

PRACTICE FOR COMPETENCY

Procedure 49-1: Processing Patient Statements. Using practice management software or SimChart® for the Medical Office, practice printing selected patient bills and placing them in window envelopes.

Create a manual statement for Darla Sissle with a due date of 9/26/XX using the format and information from Figure 49-1 in your textbook. Add a payment from the patient of $20.00 on 8/15/XX.

Procedure 49-2: Posting an NSF Check. The bank has returned Tai Yan's check No. 938 for $10.00 marked NSF (not sufficient funds). Your bank charges $15.00 for each returned check. Using today's date, enter the returned check as a positive adjustment as well as the bank fee on the patient ledger below. Use parentheses around each positive adjustment in the ADJMT column, and add the amount to the running balance in the BALANCE column. (Parentheses are used for positive adjustments and negative numbers in manual accounting.) Then post the adjustments in SimChart® for the Medical Office. Post each adjustment on a separate line.

Date	Professional Service	Fee	Payment	Adjustment	New Balance
X/XX/XX	87880, 99201	$53.00	$10.00	$0.00	$32.00

Procedure 49-3: Processing a Credit Balance and Refund. You receive check No. 332 in the amount of $50.00 on 6/15/XX from James Winston for payment of charges for an office visit 3 weeks before. Mr. Winston did not realize that his insurance deductible was already paid. Enter the payment on the patient ledger below. Remember to post negative amounts in parentheses.

Prepare a refund for James Winston to bring the balance of his account to zero. Post the refund on the line below the payment as a negative adjustment. Write a check to James Winston for the refund amount using the first check form below. Leave the signature line blank, because you are not authorized to sign checks. The old balance of the checking account is $4,166.82. Complete the check stub. Prepare a letter to James Winston informing him that you are enclosing a check for the amount of his overpayment. His address is James Winston, 25 Magnolia Lane, Western, XY 44970. Inform him that he can call you at extension 24 if he has any questions. Assume that you will print the letter on office letterhead, and sign the letter using your own name and the title Medical Assistant on the next line. This means that a reference line is not necessary. Specify the check on the enclosure line. (Enc: Check #1837)

Date	Professional Service	Fee	Payment	Adjustment	New Balance
6/1/20XX	99397	$120.00	$10.00	$0.00	$110.00
6/15/20XX	Ins payment	$0.00	$85.00	$25.00	$0.00

1837

DATE ____

TO ____

FOR ____

BALANCE BROUGHT FORWARD		
DEPOSITS		
BALANCE		
AMT THIS CK		
BALANCE CARRIED FORWARD		

BLACKBURN PRIMARY CARE ASSOCIATES, PC
1990 Turquiose Drive
Blackburn, WI 54937
608-459-8857

1837

94-72/1224

DATE ____

PAY TO THE ORDER OF ____ $ ____

____ DOLLARS

DERBYSHIRE SAVINGS
Member FDIC
P.O. BOX 8923
Blackburn, WI 54937

FOR ____

⑈055003⑈ 446782011⑈ 678800470

SAMPLE

1838

DATE ____

TO ____

FOR ____

BALANCE BROUGHT FORWARD		
DEPOSITS		
BALANCE		
AMT THIS CK		
BALANCE CARRIED FORWARD		

BLACKBURN PRIMARY CARE ASSOCIATES, PC
1990 Turquiose Drive
Blackburn, WI 54937
608-459-8857

1838

94-72/1224

DATE ____

PAY TO THE ORDER OF ____ $ ____

____ DOLLARS

DERBYSHIRE SAVINGS
Member FDIC
P.O. BOX 8923
Blackburn, WI 54937

FOR ____

⑈055003⑈ 446782011⑈ 678800470

SAMPLE

1839

DATE ____

TO ____

FOR ____

BALANCE BROUGHT FORWARD		
DEPOSITS		
BALANCE		
AMT THIS CK		
BALANCE CARRIED FORWARD		

BLACKBURN PRIMARY CARE ASSOCIATES, PC
1990 Turquiose Drive
Blackburn, WI 54937
608-459-8857

1839

94-72/1224

DATE ____

PAY TO THE ORDER OF ____ $ ____

____ DOLLARS

DERBYSHIRE SAVINGS
Member FDIC
P.O. BOX 8923
Blackburn, WI 54937

FOR ____

⑈055003⑈ 446782011⑈ 678800470

SAMPLE

Procedure 49-4: Creating an Accounts Receivable Aging Record. Create a patient aging report based on information from the accounts of the following patients. Assume that you are creating the report on 11/30. Bills were sent on the first day of the month after an insurance payment was received: 8/1, 9/1, 10/1, or 11/1. Beside each account on the report, mark the action that should be taken according to Procedure 49-4.

Daryl P. Sanders
24 Lakeview Drive
Western, XY 44970

Date	Professional Service	Fee	Payment	Adjustment	New Balance
6/4/XX	99202, cash payment	55.00	20.00		35.00
6/28/XX	Ins. ck #219		20.00		15.00

Lloyd Hanson
10 High Street
Western, XY 44970

Date	Professional Service	Fee	Payment	Adjustment	New Balance
7/15/XX	99204, 93000, ck #664	150.00	15.00		135.00
7/28/XX	Ins ck #604 (for 6/15)		128.00	7.00	0.00
8/25/XX	99212	48.00	15.00		33.00

Maria Rivera Santos
160 Underwood Street
Western, XY 44970

Date	Professional Service	Fee	Payment	Adjustment	New Balance
9/28/XX	99204, ck #259	135.00	27.00		108.00

Thomas Maxwell
1100 Main Street
Western, XY 44970

Date	Professional Service	Fee	Payment	Adjustment	New Balance
9/1/XX	99213, 81002, 98000, ck #22	122.00	50.00		72.00
10/12/XX	99212, ck #602	48.00	15.00		105.00
10/15/XX	Ins ck #2298 (for 9/1)		56.00	16.00	33.00

Account Aging Report

Patient Name	Last Payment	Current 0 - 30	Past 31 - 60	Past 61 - 90	Past 91 - 120	Past 121+	Total Balance

Procedure 49-5: Writing a Collection Letter. Write a collection letter to each individual on the aging report above if you marked the account: "Payment is now overdue." Instruct the recipient to pay the bill or contact the office to make other arrangements. Use the date of 11/30/XX and assume that the letters will be printed on office letterhead. Sign any letter using your own name and use the title, Medical Assistant, on the next line.

EVALUATION OF COMPETENCY

Procedure 49-1: Processing Patient Statements

Name: ______________________________ Date: ____________________

Evaluated by: ______________________________ Score: ____________________

Performance Objective

Outcome:	Process patient statements.
Conditions:	Given the following: computer, patient accounts, paper or statement forms, window envelopes with two windows, word processing program (optional) and postage.
Standards:	Time: 15 minutes. Student completed procedure in __________ minutes.
	Accuracy: Satisfactory score on the Performance Evaluation Checklist.

Performance Evaluation Checklist

Trial 1	Trial 2	Point Value	Performance Standards
		•	Located patient accounts with outstanding balances after insurance payments in the computer database.
		•	Selected accounts to be billed.
		•	Printed patient statements using paper forms or forms generated by the computer program and/or created one or more patient bills manually using a word processing program.
		•	Verified that statements printed correctly.
		•	Folded statements so that the practice and patient name and address would be facing outward.
		•	Inserted statements in window envelopes.
		•	Verified that name, address and return address were visible through the windows.
		•	Placed postage on envelopes and set aside for mailing.
			Preparing a Patient Statement Using SimChart® for the Medical Office
		•	Selected **Patient Statement** from the **Form Repository** and selected the correct patient.
		•	Verified that the information that has populated the top part of the Patient Statement form is correct.
		•	Entered all charges and payments since the last visit correctly.
		•	Saved the statement to the patient record.
		•	Opened the patient record, opened the saved statement and printed the statement.

Trial 1	Trial 2	Point Value	Performance Standards
		*	Prepared statement(s) correctly for mailing.
		*	Completed the procedure within 15 minutes.
			TOTALS

Evaluation of Student Performance

EVALUATION CRITERIA			COMMENTS
Symbol	**Category**	**Point Value**	
*	Critical Step	16 points	
●	Essential Step	6 points	
Ⓐ	Affective Competency	6 points	
▷	Theory Question	2 points	
Score calculation: 100 points − ___ points missed ___ Score Satisfactory score: 85 or above			

2008 CAAHEP Competencies Achieved
Psychomotor (Skills) ☑ VI. 2.b. Perform billing procedures. ☑ VI. 3. Utilize computerized office billing systems.

2015 CAAHEP Competency Achieved
Psychomotor (Skills) ☑ VII.4. Inform a patient of financial obligations for services rendered

ABHES Competencies Achieved
☑ 7. b. Utilize Electronic Medical Records (EMR) and Practice Management Systems. ☑ 8. b. Perform billing and collection procedures: 1. Accounts payable and accounts receivable.

EVALUATION OF COMPETENCY

Procedure 49-2: Posting an NSF Check

Name: ______________________ Date: ______________

Evaluated by: ______________________ Score: ______________

Performance Objective

Outcome:	Post a check returned for not sufficient funds (NSF).
Conditions:	Given the following: computer, patient accounts, returned check, patient ledger, billing software, pen, and calculator.
Standards:	Time: 20 minutes. Student completed procedure in ________ minutes.
	Accuracy: Satisfactory score on the Performance Evaluation Checklist.

Performance Evaluation Checklist

Trial 1	Trial 2	Point Value	Performance Standards
		●	Selected the correct computer screen for entering a transaction and selected the correct patient ledger.
		●	Created a new transaction for the patient in the computer account, and posted the returned check using the code(s) for NSF check and bank fee (for returned check).
		●	Wrote "NSF check" and "returned check fee" in the professional service column of the ledger.
		●	Entered zero in the other fields as needed and verified that the new balance is increased by the amount of the returned check and bank fee.
		▷	Explained the difference between a negative adjustment and a positive adjustment.
			Posting an NSF check on a Day Sheet in SimChart® for the Medical Office
		●	Selected **Day Sheet** from the **Coding and Billing** Info Panel.
		●	Entered "NSF check and fee" in the **SERVICE** field.
		●	Entered the total of the returned check and bank fee in the **ADJMT** field.
		●	Found the patient's old balance from their ledger and entered in the **OLD BALANCE** field.
		●	Added the total of the bank fee and returned check and placed in the **NEW BALANCE** field.
		●	Entered zeros in the other columns.
		●	When totaling the adjustment column of the day sheet, subtracted the adjustment from the total of other adjustments.
		●	Notified the patient by telephone or letter that the check was returned and a fee was charged. Enclosed an updated statement with a letter.

Trial 1	Trial 2	Point Value	Performance Standards
		●	Spoke to the patient professionally, or used a professional tone in the letter.
		Ⓐ	Displayed sensitivity to the patient's feelings when informing the patient of payment conditions such as a bank check or money order.
		✶	Completed the procedure within 20 minutes.
			TOTALS

Evaluation of Student Performance

EVALUATION CRITERIA			COMMENTS
Symbol	**Category**	**Point Value**	
✶	Critical Step	16 points	
●	Essential Step	6 points	
Ⓐ	Affective Competency	6 points	
▷	Theory Question	2 points	
Score calculation: 100 points – ____ points missed ____ Score Satisfactory score: 85 or above			

2008 CAAHEP Competencies Achieved

Psychomotor (Skills)

☑ VI.2.g. Post nonsufficient fund (NSF) check.

Affective (Behavior)

☑ VI.1. Demonstrate sensitivity and professionalism when handling accounts receivable activities with clients.

2015 CAAHEP Competencies Achieved

Psychomotor (Skills)

☑ VII.1. c. Perform accounts receivable procedures to patient accounts including posting: adjustments.
☑ VII.4. Inform a patient of financial obligations for services rendered.

Affective (Behavior)

☑ VII.1. Demonstrate professionalism when discussing patient billing record.
☑ VII.2. Display sensitivity when requesting payment for services rendered.

ABHES Competencies Achieved

☑ 7. b. Utilize Electronic Medical Records (EMR) and Practice Management Systems.
☑ 8. b. Perform billing and collection procedures: 3. Payment procedures: i.e. credit balance, non-sufficient funds, refunds.

EVALUATION OF COMPETENCY

Procedure 49-3: Processing a Credit Balance and a Refund

Name: ______________________ Date: ______________

Evaluated by: ______________________ Score: ______________

Performance Objective

Outcome:	Process a credit balance and issue a refund.
Conditions:	Given the following: computer, patient accounts, payment check(s), computer billing program, pen, and calculator.
Standards:	Time: 20 minutes. Student completed procedure in ________ minutes.
	Accuracy: Satisfactory score on the Performance Evaluation Checklist.

Performance Evaluation Checklist

Trial 1	Trial 2	Point Value	Performance Standards
		●	Located the ledger or account of the correct patient after receiving payment.
		●	Created a new line or transaction for the patient in the computer account, and posted the overpayment using the correct code (patient check or insurance check) linked to the charges being paid.
		●	Noted that the balance due is a negative number.
		▷	Explained the meaning of a negative number as a balance in the accounts receivable.
		●	Calculated the amount to be refunded and the recipient of the refund.
		●	Added a new row and entered "Refund to [patient or insurance] as the professional service.
		●	Entered the amount of the refund in the adjustment field as a positive number. Entered the correct code in a practice management program.
		●	Verified that the account balance was zero.
		●	Wrote a check for the refund amount to the correct recipient using correct check format leaving the signature line blank.
		●	Completed the check stub or check register in the checkbook correctly.
		Ⓐ	Wrote a professional letter to the recipient including the reason for the refund and signed it.
		●	Prepared an envelope and left letter, check and envelope in the correct place to obtain an authorized signature on the check.
		*	Completed the procedure within 20 minutes.
			TOTALS

Evaluation of Student Performance

EVALUATION CRITERIA			COMMENTS
Symbol	**Category**	**Point Value**	
∗	Critical Step	16 points	
●	Essential Step	6 points	
Ⓐ	Affective Competency	6 points	
▷	Theory Question	2 points	
Score calculation: 100 points – ___ points missed ___ Score Satisfactory score: 85 or above			

2008 CAAHEP Competencies Achieved
Psychomotor (Skills) ☑ VI.2.e. Process a credit balance. ☑ VI.2.f. Process refunds. ***Affective (Behavior)*** ☑ VI.1. Demonstrate sensitivity and professionalism in handling accounts receivable activities with clients.

2015 CAAHEP Competencies Achieved
Psychomotor (Skills) ☑ VII.1. c. Perform accounts receivable procedures to patient accounts including posting: adjustments. ***Affective (Behavior)*** ☑ VIII.2. Demonstrate professionalism when discussing patient billing record.

ABHES Competencies Achieved
☑ 7. b. Utilize Electronic Medical Records (EMR) and Practice Management Systems. ☑ 8. b. Perform billing and collection procedures: 3. Payment procedures: i.e. credit balance, non-sufficient funds, refunds.

EVALUATION OF COMPETENCY

Procedure 49-4: Creating an Accounts Receivable Aging Record

Name: ______________________________ Date: ____________________

Evaluated by: ______________________________ Score: ____________________

Performance Objective

Outcome:	Create and examine an accounts receivable aging record.
Conditions:	Given the following: computer with medical billing software, patient accounts, accounts receivable aging record analysis form (optional), and pen.
Standards:	Time: 20 minutes. Student completed procedure in ________ minutes.
	Accuracy: Satisfactory score on the Performance Evaluation Checklist.

Performance Evaluation Checklist

Trial 1	Trial 2	Point Value	Performance Standards
		•	Used the reports function of the computer billing program to print an aging report for patients and insurance companies, or created the report manually from individual patient ledgers.
		•	Reviewed the accounts on the report and marked the appropriate action for each account according to office policy.
		•	Marked all accounts less than 31 days old: "No action needed."
		•	Marked accounts with unpaid insurance claims older than 31 days: "Follow up with insurance."
		•	Marked accounts 31 to 60 days old with paid insurance claims according to office policy (e.g., "Payment is now due").
		•	Marked accounts 61 to 90 days old with paid insurance claims according to office policy (e.g., "Payment of this bill is now overdue. Please pay the balance or contact the office.").
		•	Marked accounts 91 to 120 days old with paid insurance claims according to office policy (e.g., "Telephone patient").
		•	Participated in role play as a medical assistant simulating a collection telephone call for a patient with a balance that is over 91 days old.
		Ⓐ	Demonstrated professionalism in in discussing the patient's billing record.
		Ⓐ	Displayed sensitivity when requesting payment for overdue amounts.
		•	Reviewed previous collection attempts for accounts over 120 days.
		•	Set aside accounts over 120 days to write collection letters (Procedure 49-5).
		•	Recorded all action taken beside each account on the report.
		•	Documented any telephone calls and/or collection letter in the progress notes of the patient's medical record.

Trial 1	Trial 2	Point Value	Performance Standards
		*	Analyzed outstanding accounts accurately, and indicated appropriate follow-up.
		*	Completed the procedure within 20 minutes.
			TOTALS

Chart	
Date	

Evaluation of Student Performance

EVALUATION CRITERIA			COMMENTS
Symbol	**Category**	**Point Value**	
*	Critical Step	16 points	
●	Essential Step	6 points	
Ⓐ	Affective Competency	6 points	
▷	Theory Question	2 points	
Score calculation: 100 points – ___ points missed ___ Score Satisfactory score: 85 or above			

2008 CAAHEP Competency Achieved
Psychomotor (Skills) ☑ VI.2.c. Perform collection procedures.

2015 CAAHEP Competencies Achieved
Psychomotor (Skills) ☑ VII.4. Inform a patient of financial obligations for services rendered. ***Affective (Behavior)*** ☑ VII.1. Demonstrate professionalism when discussing patient billing record. ☑ VII.2. Display sensitivity when requesting payment for services rendered.

ABHES Competencies Achieved
☑ 8. b. Perform billing and collection procedures.

EVALUATION OF COMPETENCY

Procedure 49-5: Writing a Collection Letter

Name: ______________________________ Date: ________________

Evaluated by: ______________________________ Score: ________________

Performance Objective

Outcome:	Write a collection letter.
Conditions:	Given the following: accounts receivable aging report, computer, patient accounts, letterhead stationery, envelope, and printer.
Standards:	Time: 10 minutes. Student completed procedure in __________ minutes.
	Accuracy: Satisfactory score on the Performance Evaluation Checklist

Performance Evaluation Checklist

Trial 1	Trial 2	Point Value	Performance Standards
		●	Determined which accounts were over 120 days old from an accounts receivable aging report.
		●	Reviewed accounts over 120 days to be sure that there are no extenuating circumstances for which the patient might be given more time to pay.
		●	Set up a letter for an account over 120 days using the format preferred by the office. If using SimChart® for the Medical Office, selected **Collection Letter** from the **Correspondence** Info Panel.
		●	Identified the patient's address by selecting the correct patient in the computer billing program or SimChart® for the Medical Office.
		●	Included the outstanding balance, the date charges were incurred, the service provided, and date by which payment is expected in the letter.
		●	Entered the provider name and medical assistant signature in the letter.
		●	Printed the letter and saved the letter to the patient record.
		●	Prepared an envelope.
		●	If office policy, copied the letter and filed in a collection follow-up file.
		●	Placed the letter in the envelope and mailed the letter.
		*	Created an error-free letter and envelope.
		*	Completed the procedure within 10 minutes.
			TOTALS

Evaluation of Student Performance

EVALUATION CRITERIA			COMMENTS
Symbol	Category	Point Value	
✶	Critical Step	16 points	
●	Essential Step	6 points	
Ⓐ	Affective Competency	6 points	
▷	Theory Question	2 points	
Score calculation: 100 points – ____ points missed ____ Score Satisfactory score: 85 or above			

2008 CAAHEP Competencies Achieved
Psychomotor (Skills) ☑ IV.10. Compose professional/business letters. ☑ VI.2.c. Perform collection procedures. ☑ IX.8. Apply local, state, and federal health care legislation and regulation appropriate to the medical office setting. ***Affective (Behavior)*** ☑ VII.1. Demonstrate sensitivity and professionalism when handling accounts receivable activities with patients. ☑ IX.3. Recognize the importance of local, state, and federal legislation and regulations in the practice setting.

2015 CAAHEP Competencies Achieved
Psychomotor (Skills) ☑ V.8. Compose professional correspondence using electronic technology. ☑ VII.4. Inform a patient of financial obligations for services rendered.

ABHES Competencies Achieved
☑ 7. a. Perform basic keyboarding skills. ☑ 8. b. Perform billing and collection procedures.

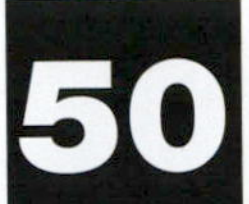

The Medical Assistant as Office Manager

CHAPTER ASSIGNMENTS

✓ After Completing	Date Due	Study Guide Pages	STUDY GUIDE ASSIGNMENTS (CTA = Critical Thinking Activity)	Possible Points	Points You Earned
		1381	Pretest	10	
		1382	Key Term Assessment	19	
		1382-1386	Evaluation of Learning questions	34	
		1386	CTA A: Equipment Inventory List	10	
		1386	CTA B: Supply Inventory List	10	
		1386-1387	CTA C: Community Resources	5	
		1387	CTA D: Incident Report	7	
			Evolve Site: Apply Your Knowledge questions	10	
			Evolve Site: Video Evaluations	12	
		1381	Posttest	10	
			ADDITIONAL ASSIGNMENTS		
			TOTAL POINTS		

Notes

✓ When Assigned By Your Instructor	Study Guide Pages	Practices Required	LABORATORY ASSIGNMENTS (Procedure Number and Name)	Score*
	1389	3	**Practice for Competency** 50-1: Creating an Environmental Checklist and Performing a Safety Inspection Textbook Reference: pp. 1239-1240	
	1393-1395		**Evaluation of Competency** 50-1: Creating an Environmental Checklist and Performing a Safety Inspection	*
	1390	3	**Practice for Competency** 50-2: Complying with Safety Signs, Symbols, and Labels Textbook Reference: p. 1240	
	1397-1398		**Evaluation of Competency** 50-2: Complying with Safety Signs, Symbols, and Labels	*
	1390	2	**Practice for Competency** 50-3: Performing Routine Maintenance of Equipment Textbook reference: p. 1242	
	1399-1400		**Evaluation of Competency** 50-3: Performing Routine Maintenance of Equipment	*
	1391	1	**Practice for Competency** 50-4: Taking a Supply or Equipment Inventory Textbook reference: p. 1245	
	1401-1402		**Evaluation of Competency** 50-4: Taking a Supply or Equipment Inventory	*
	1391	3	**Practice for Competency** 50-5: Locating and Facilitating Referrals to Community Resources Textbook reference: pp. 1249-1250	
	1403-1404		**Evaluation of Competency** 50-5: Locating and Facilitating Referrals to Community Resources	*

✓ When Assigned By Your Instructor	Study Guide Pages	Practices Required	LABORATORY ASSIGNMENTS (Procedure Number and Name)	Score*
	1391	1	**Practice for Competency** 50-6: Completing an Incident Report Textbook reference: p. 1252	
	1405-1406		**Evaluation of Competency** 50-6: Completing an Incident Report	*
			ADDITIONAL ASSIGNMENTS	

Name ______________________________ Date ______________

PRETEST

True or False

_______ 1. Stationery, envelopes, and billing forms should be located in the administrative area of the medical office.

_______ 2. Old telephone logs should be shredded if they are discarded.

_______ 3. Rigid biohazard waste containers are usually stored under the sink in an examination room.

_______ 4. The waiting room often has a sign requesting that patients pay copayments at the time of the visit.

_______ 5. Falls are a common cause of workplace injury.

_______ 6. Treatment rooms or special procedure rooms are usually kept a little warmer than examination rooms.

_______ 7. The medical assistant (MA) is usually responsible for changing the plastic liners in biohazard waste containers.

_______ 8. The doors to the laboratory and medical records storage for paper medical records may have additional locks.

_______ 9. Areas where x-ray is used should be marked with signs.

_______ 10. An equipment inventory includes the date of purchase, cost, and serial number of each piece of equipment.

POSTTEST

True or False

_______ 1. Business operations may be performed at the front desk or separate area of the medical office.

_______ 2. Each examination room should have a sink and wall-mounted paper towel dispenser.

_______ 3. Biohazard waste containers with a plastic liner only need to be covered at night.

_______ 4. The medical office may have a display rack with informational brochures in the waiting room.

_______ 5. Tripping or slipping without falling may still cause workplace injuries.

_______ 6. A good temperature for the office waiting room is 70°F to 72°F.

_______ 7. All cleaning is done at night in the medical office by an outside cleaning company.

_______ 8. Controlled substances should always be stored in an area with two locks and two separate keys.

_______ 9. Exit signs should be yellow with black lettering.

_______ 10. A supply inventory is used to keep records for tax purposes.

KEY TERM ASSESSMENT

Directions: Match each key term with its definition.

_______ 1. Back order
_______ 2. Depreciation
_______ 3. Gross pay
_______ 4. Inventory
_______ 5. Invoice
_______ 6. Minutes
_______ 7. Net pay
_______ 8. *Per diem*
_______ 9. Policy
_______ 10. Procedure
_______ 11. Purchase order (PO) number
_______ 12. Reorder point
_______ 13. Risk management
_______ 14. Salary
_______ 15. Service contract
_______ 16. Social Security tax (FICA)
_______ 17. Vendor
_______ 18. Warranty
_______ 19. W-4 form

A. A written record of the proceedings of a meeting
B. The form used to claim allowances for federal income tax reporting
C. The total amount earned in a time period by an employee before any deductions
D. A guiding principle for the management of a medical office or business
E. A tax collected from employees to fund the Social Security program
F. A fixed amount of wages that does not depend on the number of hours worked
G. A detailed list of items in stock or in possession of an individual or business
H. A promise by the manufacturer to repair or replace defective parts in an item during a specific time period
I. A term used for items ordered that cannot be shipped immediately, usually because they are out of stock
J. A number on a supply inventory that indicates when a specific item should be reordered
K. A list of the steps to handle a certain situation or perform a certain task
L. The actual amount of money paid directly to an employee after taxes and other deductions
M. An agreement that provides for service for a piece of equipment after the warranty expires
N. An itemized bill for items that have not been prepaid
O. Employees who are scheduled by the day according to office needs
P. Accounting methods to record the loss of value of a property or piece of equipment over time
Q. The process of assessing risk and putting policies and procedures in place to minimize it
R. A company from whom supplies or equipment is purchased
S. A number assigned by a business to authorize and keep track of an order

EVALUATION OF LEARNING

Directions: Fill in each blank with the correct answer.

1. Write a general statement identifying the type of equipment and supplies needed in the administrative area of the medical office.

   a. Equipment: ____

   ____

   b. Supplies: ____

   ____

2. Write a general statement identifying the type of equipment and supplies needed for examination rooms and treatment rooms.

   a. Equipment: ____

   ____

b. Supplies: ______________________________

____

3. What are four common signs that might be found in a medical office waiting room?

____

____

4. What are areas within the medical office that can often be locked separately and are often kept locked at night?

____

____

5. List five activities that are considered part of routine maintenance.

____

____

____

6. Identify two important components for controlling the air in the medical office.

____

____

7. What parts of the medical office are MAs usually responsible for cleaning and/or tidying?

____

____

____

8. What are five general guidelines recommended by the Occupational Safety and Health Administration (OSHA) to maintain workplace safety?

____

____

____

9. What should be included in a safety plan for a medical office?

____

____

____

10. What are five examples of signs that should be present in the medical office?

____

____

____

11. What are two common symbols that may appear on safety signs or labels without text?

12. Identify two reasons why it is important to maintain an accurate inventory of equipment.

13. Describe how service contracts work. When do they go into effect?

14. What are some helpful things to do when a new piece of equipment is placed into service?

15. Name five types of information that should be included on a supply inventory list.

16. What is the reorder point on a supply inventory list? How is it used?

17. What is the MA's responsibility for restocking administrative and clinical areas?

18. Why is a tracking number or purchase order number useful when ordering supplies?

19. Identify three steps the MA should take when supplies are delivered.

20. How can staff meetings help create an environment for teamwork?

21. Describe two methods to prepare meeting participants, keep a meeting running smoothly, and keep track of decisions made during the meeting.

22. What paperwork is required for a new employee?

23. What are five things that must be documented in an employee's payroll record?

24. Identify three types of deductions that the employer must withhold from an employee paycheck.

25. What is unemployment tax, and how is it paid?

26. When preparing payroll checks for employees, what five items of information must be recorded in the payroll record for each employee?

27. What is the MA's responsibility in relation to the physician and office schedule?

28. Differentiate between a policy and a procedure.

29. Identify three reasons why it is valuable for organizations to have procedure manuals available.

30. Identify eight types of community resources to which patients might be referred for information or services.

31. Give four examples of damage or injury that should be covered by the medical office's general property and/or liability insurance.

____

____

32. What kind of protection is provided by professional liability insurance?

____

____

33. List four types of compliance reporting that might be required for a medical office.

____

____

34. Describe when incident reports are completed and how they fit into the risk management plan of an organization.

____

____

CRITICAL THINKING ACTIVITIES

A. Equipment Inventory List

Create an inventory list of equipment in the clinical laboratory of your medical assisting program. Include the name of each piece of equipment, a description, and a serial number or school ID number. Set up your list with columns for at least three dates to check off items when you take inventory.

B. Supply Inventory List

Working with at least one classmate, set up a supply inventory list for at least 15 supply items that might be used during the physical examination. The categories should include the following: item name, quantity in stock, reorder point, and quantity to reorder. For this assignment, a supply meets one or more of the following conditions:

- It is consumed in use.
- It is expendable, and if it is damaged, it will be replaced rather than repaired.
- It costs less than $250.00.

Assume that your office wants to keep a 3-month supply of each item on hand. Assume that 100 patients are seen in the office each day, 5 days a week. Assume that there will be a 2-week delay between the time the order is placed and the time the order is received.

C. Community Resources

Describe the types of community services that might be appropriate for each of the following patients:

1. Patient discharged from the hospital after hip replacement surgery.

____

2. Elderly patient who lives alone with limited mobility and no family members living in the community.

____

3. Male patient (65 years old) diagnosed with inoperable lung cancer with planned radiation treatments. Wife does not drive.

____

____

4. Family with a 6-year-old child who sustains an injury resulting in permanent paralysis from the waist down.

5. Elderly couple with the wife diagnosed with Alzheimer disease and who cannot be left alone. Husband still drives. Daughter lives in the community.

D. Incident Report

You are working in a medical office, and a patient falls while a medical assistant is helping the patient to step up to the examination table. The physician is called, assists the patient to get up, and finds a large bruise on the right hip but no other apparent injury. The physician orders an x-ray of the right hip, and instructs the patient to telephone if any problems arise later. The physician documents the examination and findings in the patient's medical record. It is office policy to fill out an incident report for any fall that occurs in the office. Make a list of all information that you would have to include on the incident report.

Notes

PRACTICE FOR COMPETENCY

Procedure 50-1: Creating an Environmental Checklist and Performing a Safety Inspection. Expand the following checklist adhering to the guidelines outlined in Procedure 50-1. Make three copies of your revised checklist. Use it to inspect at least two rooms in your own home, and use it to inspect a medical office environment. After completing the inspections, write down any problems that could not be fixed during the inspection. Discuss with your classmates the difference between safety hazards in the home and safety hazards in the medical office.

Safety Inspection Checklist

Date: ____________ Person Making Inspection: ______________________________

Label as C if there are no problems; label as NC if a problem is found.

	C or NC	Problem/Action Taken
General Visual Inspection		
Walkways		
Electrical Cords and Plugs		
Storage Areas		
Lighting		
Safety Signs, Symbols, and Labels		
Storage and Labeling of Chemicals/Biohazards		

Plan to Correct Items that Could not be Corrected During Inspection:

1.

2.

3.

4.

5.

Procedure 50-2: Complying with Safety Signs, Symbols, and Labels. Make a table with three columns. In the first column, list common safety signs, symbols, and labels that are found in the medical office and their appearance. In the second column, describe the appropriate location for the sign, symbol or label. In the third column, describe actions that the medical assistant should take to comply with the sign, symbol, or label and to make sure that patients are not placed at risk. Role play instructing a coworker or patient about the meaning of at least three signs or symbols.

Procedure 50-3 Performing Routine Maintenance of Equipment. Perform routine maintenance of both administrative and clinical equipment such as the autoclave, electrocardiograph, photocopier, and/or fax machine. Complete an equipment maintenance log for each item.

Equipment Maintenance Log			
Equipment Description:			
Serial Number:	**Model Number:**		
			Initials
Date:	**Action Taken/Comments:**		

Equipment Maintenance Log			
Equipment Description:			
Serial Number:	**Model Number:**		
			Initials
Date:	**Action Taken/Comments:**		

Procedure 50-4: Taking a Supply or Equipment Inventory. Take a supply and equipment inventory using the lists you prepared for Critical Thinking Activities B and C. Prepare a list of supplies to be ordered.

Procedure 50-5: Locating and Facilitating Referrals to Community Resources. Make a list of community resources to which patients may be referred including visiting nurse services, homemaker services, meal delivery, senior services, etc. Role play facilitating referrals for three of the situations described in Critical Thinking Activity D.

Procedure 50-6: Completing an Incident Report. Use the following information to complete an incident report. Role play the situation with a classmate, and take turns playing the patient. An elderly lady falls while you are helping her to step up to the examination table landing on her right side. The physician is called, assists the injured patient to get up, and finds a large tender area on the right hip but no other apparent injury. An x-ray is done in the office which is normal. The physician instructs the patient to telephone if any problems arise later and documents the examination and findings in the injury log. It is office policy to fill out an incident report for any fall that occurs in the office and the physician asks you (MA) to fill out the incident report.

WALDEN-MARTIN
FAMILY MEDICAL CLINIC
1234 ANYSTREET ANYTOWN, ANYSTATE 1234
PHONE 123-123-1234 FAX 123-123-5678

Incident Report

Date: ____________ Time: ____________

Incident type: ☐ Staff ☐ Patient ☐ Visitor ☐ Equipment/property

Witness: ☐ Staff ☐ Patient ☐ Visitor

Department: ____________ Exact location: ____________

Medical team: ____________

Patient reason for visit: ____________ Medication incident: ☐ Yes ☐ No

Incident description: [ ] Immediate actions and outcomes: [ ]

Contributing factors: [ ] Prevention: [ ]

Next of kin/guardian notified/patient? ☐ Yes ☐ No ☐ N/A Medical staff notified? ☐ Yes ☐ No ☐ N/A

Reported by: ____________ Position: ____________

Contact phone number: ____________

Other persons involved: ____________ Position: ____________

Contact phone number: ____________

Medical report (Document patient's assessment and list investigations and treatments):

____

Provider: ____________ Designation: ____________

Provider signature: ____________ Date/time: ____________

Notes

EVALUATION OF COMPETENCY

Procedure 50-1: Creating an Environmental Checklist and Performing a Safety Inspection

Name: ______________________ Date: ______________

Evaluated by: ______________________ Score: ______________

Performance Objective

Outcome:	1. Create an environmental checklist and perform a safety inspection.
Conditions:	Given the following: area to be inspected, pen and paper (or computer and word processing file) to create an environmental checklist
Standards:	Time: 1 hour. Student completed procedure in __________ minutes. Accuracy: Satisfactory score on the Performance Evaluation Checklist.

Performance Evaluation Checklist

Trial 1	Trial 2	Point Value	Performance Standards
		●	Using the form below, added specific items to inspect to create a checklist of hazards to be inspected for including: clear walkways and tripping hazards; electrical hazards; proper storage of boxes; adequate lighting; dry floors; and proper labels and storage of biohazards, medications and chemicals.
		●	Made a general inspection to be sure that all floors were dry and all furniture and fixtures in good repair. Then filled out the appropriate parts of the checklist.
		●	Made a detailed inspection as required for each section on the checklist and filled out the checklist. Included a check for appropriate safety signs, symbols, and/or labels.
		●	Noted any problems and either fixed the problem or removed a potential hazard. Recorded any action performed and/or needed action on the checklist.
		●	Checked for walkways that were wide enough for usual traffic without anything to obstruct the walkway or cause a tripping hazard.
		●	Checked all electrical cords and plugs to ensure that there was no fraying or malfunction.
		●	Checked all storage areas for clear tops of cabinets and proper storage of supplies without potential to fall.
		●	Made sure all light bulbs worked. Either changed burned out bulbs or made a note to have them changed.
		●	Noted any areas with inadequate lighting.
		●	Made sure that all biohazards, chemicals or other potentially hazardous materials were labeled correctly and stored in secure areas away from patients.
		*	Filled out the checklist completely.
		●	After filling out the checklist, made a written plan to respond to any areas that could not be corrected during the inspection.
		*	Completed the procedure within 1 hour.
			TOTALS

Safety Inspection Checklist		
Date: ___________ Person Making Inspection: ___________		
Label as C if there are no problems; label as NC if a problem is found.		
	C or NC	**Problem/Action Taken**
General Visual Inspection		
Walkways		
Electrical Cords and Plugs		
Storage Areas		
Lighting		
Safety Signs, Symbols, and Labels		
Storage and Labeling of Chemicals/Biohazards		
Plan to Correct Items that Could not be Corrected During Inspection:		
1.		
2.		
3.		
4.		
5.		

Evaluation of Student Performance

EVALUATION CRITERIA			COMMENTS
Symbol	Category	Point Value	
✶	Critical Step	16 points	
●	Essential Step	6 points	
Ⓐ	Affective Competency	6 points	
▷	Theory Question	2 points	
Score calculation:	100 points – ____ points missed ____ Score		
Satisfactory score: 85 or above			

2008 CAAHEP Competencies Achieved
Psychomotor (Skills) ☑ XI.2. Evaluate the work environment to identify safe vs. unsafe working conditions ☑ XI.3. Develop a personal (patient and employee) safety plan. ☑ XI.4. Develop an environmental safety plan.

2015 CAAHEP Competency Achieved
Psychomotor (Skills) ☑ XII.5. Evaluate the work environment to identify unsafe working conditions

Notes

EVALUATION OF COMPETENCY

Procedure 50-2: Complying with Safety Signs, Symbols, and Labels

Name: ______________________ Date: ______________

Evaluated by: ______________________ Score: ______________

Performance Objective

Outcome:	Comply with safety signs, symbols, and labels
Conditions:	Given the following: safety signs (or pictures of safety signs), biohazard trash container with lid, paper medical record with allergy label, computer with printer (color if possible).
Standards:	Printed signs and written description of role play. Time for role play: 20 minutes. Student completed procedure in _____ minutes. Accuracy: Satisfactory score on the Performance Evaluation Checklist.

Performance Evaluation Checklist

Trial 1	Trial 2	Point Value	Performance Standards
		•	Used computer to locate and print examples of safety signs and symbols including a sign for authorized personnel only, a sign indicating radiation with a radiation symbol, and a sign for an eyewash station and/or shower.
		•	Wrote on the back of the sign where such a sign should be located in the medical office.
		•	Participated in a role play situation as a medical assistant to instruct a patient who was preparing to enter a room with a sign for authorized personnel only.
		•	Participated in a role play situation as a medical assistant to instruct a patient what an eyewash station is used for.
		•	Participated in a role play situation to instruct a patient who was about to discard a used tissue in a biohazard waste container.
		•	Participated in a role play situation to question a patient about possible pregnancy before allowing entry to a room marked with a radiation symbol.
		•	Wrote a short description of the role play identifying appropriate actions of the medical assistant.
		•	Handed in the signs and written description to the instructor
		*	Completed the role play part of the procedure within 20 minutes.
			TOTALS

Evaluation of Student Performance

EVALUATION CRITERIA			COMMENTS
Symbol	**Category**	**Point Value**	
✱	Critical Step	16 points	
●	Essential Step	6 points	
Ⓐ	Affective Competency	6 points	
▷	Theory Question	2 points	
Score calculation: 100 points – ____ points missed ____ Score Satisfactory score: 85 or above			

2008 CAAHEP Competency Achieved
Psychomotor (Skills) ☑ XI.1. Comply with safety signs, symbols, and labels

2015 CAAHEP Competency Achieved
Psychomotor (Skills) ☑ XII.1. Comply with: a. safety signs, b. symbols, c. labels.

EVALUATION OF COMPETENCY

Procedure 50-3: Performing Routine Maintenance of Equipment

Name: ______________________________ Date: ______________

Evaluated by: ______________________________ Score: ______________

Performance Objective

Outcome:	Perform equipment maintenance and document on equipment maintenance log.
Conditions:	Given the following: piece of equipment to be maintained, cloth for dusting, maintenance log sheet, and supplies necessary for the piece or equipment (such as paper, batteries, toner, fluids, etc).
Standards:	Time: 10 minutes. Student completed procedure in __________ minutes.
	Accuracy: Satisfactory score on the Performance Evaluation Checklist.

Performance Evaluation Checklist

Trial 1	Trial 2	Point Value	Performance Standards
		●	Located the piece of equipment to be maintained.
		●	Checked all electrical cords to be sure there is no fraying or malfunction.
		●	Checked the piece of equipment for cracks, dents, or other damage, obvious impairment or malfunction.
		●	Checked any keyboard or keypad for cracks, faded numbers, or other impairment.
		▷	Explained what to do if the piece of equipment was damaged.
		●	Dusted or cleaned the outside or case of the piece of equipment according to manufacturer's directions.
		●	Checked leads and other wires, or other tubing.
		●	Checked or changed batteries, fluid, toner, or other essential components.
		●	Scheduled any required maintenance if appropriate.
		*	Filled out the equipment maintenance log correctly.
		*	Completed the procedure within 10 minutes.
			TOTALS

Equipment Maintenance Log			
Equipment Description:			
Serial Number:	**Model Number:**		
			Initials
Date:	**Action Taken/Comments:**		

Evaluation of Student Performance

EVALUATION CRITERIA			COMMENTS
Symbol	**Category**	**Point Value**	
✶	Critical Step	16 points	
●	Essential Step	6 points	
Ⓐ	Affective Competency	6 points	
▷	Theory Question	2 points	
Score calculation: 100 points − ___ points missed ___ Score Satisfactory score: 85 or above			

2008 CAAHEP Competencies Achieved
Psychomotor (Skills) ☑ V.9. Perform routine maintenance of office equipment with documentation. ☑ XI.2. Evaluate the work environment to identify safe vs. unsafe working conditions.

2015 CAAHEP Competency Achieved
Psychomotor (Skills) ☑ VI.8. Perform routine maintenance of administrative or clinical equipment. ☑ XII.5. Evaluate the work environment to identify unsafe working conditions.

ABHES Competencies Achieved
☑ 8. e. 1. Perform routine maintenance of administrative equipment.

EVALUATION OF COMPETENCY

Procedure 50-4: Taking a Supply Inventory

Name: ______________________ Date: ______________

Evaluated by: ______________________ Score: ______________

Performance Objective

Outcome:	Take a supply and equipment inventory.
Conditions:	Given the following: inventory list, notebook or cards, items to inventory, and pen.
Standards:	Time: 15 minutes. Student completed procedure in __________ minutes.
	Accuracy: Satisfactory score on the Performance Evaluation Checklist.

Performance Evaluation Checklist

Trial 1	Trial 2	Point Value	Performance Standards
		•	Obtained list of items in inventory, inventory notebook, or box of inventory cards.
		•	Checked each item in the inventory record against items present in the area being inventoried.
		•	Validated serial numbers or equipment and checked the expiration date of supplies.
		•	Discarded any expired supplies and did not include in the inventory count.
		•	Documented any missing piece of equipment after making an effort to locate.
		•	Documented any item that needed repair.
		•	Flagged any supplies close to or below the reorder point as needing to be reordered.
		•	Checked that information on the inventory card or list was correct and complete.
		•	Made sure that the storage space was tidy and arranged so that items with the oldest expiration date were at the front of the storage area.
		•	Placed inventory cards, list, or book in the proper location for follow-up.
		*	Completed the procedure within 15 minutes.
			TOTALS

Evaluation of Student Performance

EVALUATION CRITERIA			COMMENTS
Symbol	**Category**	**Point Value**	
∗	Critical Step	16 points	
●	Essential Step	6 points	
Ⓐ	Affective Competency	6 points	
▷	Theory Question	2 points	
Score calculation: 100 points – ___ points missed ___ Score Satisfactory score: 85 or above			

2008 CAAHEP Competency Achieved
Psychomotor (Skills) ☑ V.10. Perform an office inventory.

2015 CAAHEP Competency Achieved
Psychomotor (Skills) ☑ VI.9. Perform an inventory with documentation

ABHES Competencies Achieved
☑ 8. e. Maintain inventory equipment and supplies.

EVALUATION OF COMPETENCY

Procedure 50-5: Locating and Facilitating Referrals to Community Resources

Name: ______________________ Date: ______________

Evaluated by: ______________________ Score: ______________

Performance Objective

Outcome:	1. Develop a current list of community resources. 2. Facilitate referrals to community resources.
Conditions:	Given the following: local telephone book, office list of community resources, computer and printer, local hospital newsletter(s), library access, local newspapers, pen, and notepad.
Standards:	Time: 45 minutes. Student completed procedure in ________ minutes. Accuracy: Satisfactory score on the Performance Evaluation Checklist.

Performance Evaluation Checklist

Trial 1	Trial 2	Point Value	Performance Standards
		●	Researched local sources to identify community agencies.
		●	As resources were identified, created a list.
		●	Included pertinent information such as name, services available, address, telephone number, web address, contact information, and other useful information.
		●	Included resources for organizations/support groups that can assist patients and family members of patients experiencing terminal illness.
		●	Included resources for complementary and alternative medicine practices (CAM).
		●	Transferred handwritten list to a computer document.
		●	Grouped resources by category and alphabetized within each group.
		●	Obtained physician approval of finished list.
		●	Updated the list when information changed, new resources were identified.
		●	Used a list of community resources for patients to make recommendations to patients and families.
		●	Wrote a two-page report identifying the specific steps a medical assistant should take to facilitate referrals for a patient who needs a handicap placard for their automobile and a patient not taking their prescribed brand name medication because they cannot afford it.
		●	Handed list of resources and two-page report in to instructor.
		*	Completed the procedure within 30 minutes.
			TOTALS

Evaluation of Student Performance

EVALUATION CRITERIA			COMMENTS
Symbol	**Category**	**Point Value**	
∗	Critical Step	16 points	
●	Essential Step	6 points	
Ⓐ	Affective Competency	6 points	
▷	Theory Question	2 points	
Score calculation: 100 points − ___ points missed ___Score Satisfactory score: 85 or above			

2008 CAAHEP Competency Achieved
Psychomotor (Skills) ☑ IV.12. Develop and maintain a current list of community resources related to patients' healthcare needs.

2015 CAAHEP Competency Achieved
Psychomotor (Skills) ☑ V.9. Develop a current list of community resources related to patients' healthcare needs. ☑ V.10. Facilitate referrals to community resources in the role of a patient navigator.

ABHES Competencies Achieved
☑ 5. b. 3. List organizations/support groups that can assist patients and family members of patients experiencing terminal illness. ☑ 9.i. Identify community resources and complementary and alternative medicine practices (CAM).

EVALUATION OF COMPETENCY

Procedure 50-6: Completing an Incident Report

Name: ______________________ Date: ______________

Evaluated by: ______________________ Score: ______________

Performance Objective

Outcome:	Complete an incident report.
Conditions:	Given the following: incident report form (such as Incident Report Form from SimChart® for the Medical Office or OSHA form 301), computer (if SimChart is used), pen, notes from witnesses to the incident
Standards:	Time: 20 minutes. Student completed procedure in ________ minutes.
	Accuracy: Satisfactory score on the Performance Evaluation Checklist.

Performance Evaluation Checklist

Trial 1	Trial 2	Point Value	Performance Standards
		•	Interviewed all individuals involved in the incident and all witnesses and make notes as needed to complete the written incident report.
		•	Obtained an incident report form and fill in information about the person (or persons) who are the main subject of the incident including name, date of birth, and address.
		•	If using SimChart® for the Medical Office, opened an Incident Report form on the Office section of the Form Repository and entered the information required.
		•	Completed any information about health care provided, including the names and identifying formation for physicians or health care professionals who provided treatment.
		•	Included pertinent information to describe the incident in detail including time, location (address, building, room number), what happened, and any injury or illness that resulted from the incident.
		•	Included the name and contact information of the individual to whom the incident was reported.
		•	Reviewed the report with the subject of the incident if possible before signing the report and obtaining the signature of the subject on a paper report if possible. Also obtained a supervisor's signature on a paper report.
		•	If creating a computer report, saved the report when it was complete.
		*	Completed the procedure within 20 minutes.
			TOTALS

Evaluation of Student Performance

EVALUATION CRITERIA			COMMENTS
Symbol	**Category**	**Point Value**	
∗	Critical Step	16 points	
●	Essential Step	6 points	
Ⓐ	Affective Competency	6 points	
▷	Theory Question	2 points	
Score calculation: 100 points – ___ points missed ___ Score Satisfactory score: 85 or above			

2008 CAAHEP Competency Achieved
Psychomotor (Skills) ☑ IX.6. Complete an incident report.

2015 CAAHEP Competency Achieved
Psychomotor (Skills) ☑ X.7. Complete an incident report related to an error in patient care.

ABHES Competencies Achieved
☑ 4. e. Perform risk management procedures.

51 Obtaining Employment

CHAPTER ASSIGNMENTS

✓ After Completing	Date Due	Study Guide Pages	STUDY GUIDE ASSIGNMENTS (CTA = Critical Thinking Activity)	Possible Points	Points You Earned
		1409	Pretest	10	
		1409	Term Key Term Assessment	5	
		1410-1412	Evaluation of Learning questions	24	
		1412-1416	CTA A: Preparing a Résumé	15	
		1416-1417	CTA B: Preparing a Cover Letter	10	
		1417	CTA C: References	10	
		1418	CTA D: Interview Questions	10	
			Evolve Site: Apply Your Knowledge questions	10	
		1409	Posttest	10	
			ADDITIONAL ASSIGNMENTS		
			TOTAL POINTS		

Notes

Name ________________________________ Date ______________

PRETEST

True or False

_______ 1. Networking to find employment means applying for jobs using the Internet.

_______ 2. It is recommended to limit a résumé to one page.

_______ 3. Hobbies and other personal information are included in the last section of a résumé.

_______ 4. A functional résumé is recommended when an individual wants to change to a different type of work.

_______ 5. Begin a résumé with your name, address, telephone number, and e-mail address.

_______ 6. The medical assisting externship and volunteer work should not be included under Work Experience.

_______ 7. When describing job duties, use all past tense or all participle forms of verbs.

_______ 8. It is assumed that a medical assistant (MA) has a valid CPR (cardiopulmonary resuscitation) certification, and it is not necessary to put this information on the résumé.

_______ 9. The MA should always ask permission before using a supervisor's name as a reference.

_______ 10. The MA may ask about a salary range during the interview.

POSTTEST

True or False

_______ 1. Using several methods to identify potential employers is an important step to find a job.

_______ 2. If a résumé is submitted to an employer, it is not necessary to complete a job application.

_______ 3. A résumé that categorizes experience according to skills is called a chronological résumé.

_______ 4. When including information about education, it should be listed with the most recent first.

_______ 5. The high school and date diploma was received should always be included on a résumé.

_______ 6. It is important not to leave gaps of time unaccounted for on a chronological résumé.

_______ 7. Job duties may be summarized in bullet form on a résumé.

_______ 8. The names and addresses of three personal references should be listed on the résumé.

_______ 9. Résumés can be sent through the mail, attached to e-mail, by fax, or attached to an online application.

_______ 10. The interviewer should not ask about marital status or number of children during a job interview.

Term KEY TERM ASSESSMENT

Directions: Match each key term with its definition.

_______ 1. Burnout

_______ 2. Continuing education unit (CEU)

_______ 3. Cover letter

_______ 4. Networking

_______ 5. Résumé

A. A summary of information about a person that describes education, work experience, and other information

B. A letter sent with one or more documents (such as a résumé) to provide an explanation

C. Contacting acquaintances and their contacts who may know of potential jobs

D. Disillusionment with work and physical or emotional exhaustion

E. A standard measure of qualified instruction or contact hours as defined by a specific profession

EVALUATION OF LEARNING

Directions: Fill in each blank with the correct answer.

1. What are the two parts of successful job hunting?

____

____

2. What are three questions the MA might ask himself or herself when setting goals for job hunting?

____

____

____

3. Identify three resources to identify potential employers other than newspaper or Internet advertisements.

____

____

____

4. Describe what a résumé is and identify its function.

____

____

____

5. Should an MA include personal information on a résumé? Why or why not?

____

____

6. Describe three styles of résumés.

____

____

____

7. What information should be included on a résumé?

____

____

8. What specific information should be included in the education section of a résumé?

____

____

____

9. Discuss two ways that previous experience can be presented, and give the advantages and disadvantages of each.

10. In a previous job at a supermarket, the MA often helped put price tags on new items and arrange them in the store. Describe this using the past tense as she might include it on a résumé.

11. In a previous job at a retail store, the MA worked at the cash register. Describe this using the participle form of the verb as it would appear in a bulleted list.

12. What are three types of information that might be included in the "Special Skills" section of a résumé?

13. How should the MA prepare a list of references?

14. What format should be used for the final version of a résumé?

15. What is the purpose of a cover letter when sending out résumés?

16. What are the advantages and disadvantages of faxing a résumé?

17. In addition to a résumé, what information should the MA bring when applying for a job?

18. Identify six specific ways that the MA can make a favorable impression during a job interview.

19. What kinds of questions might an MA ask during a job interview?

____

____

20. What kind of follow-up is appropriate after a job interview?

____

____

21. After obtaining employment, how can the MA keep his or her administrative and clinical skills current?

____

____

22. Identify three specific actions an MA can take to avoid or respond to job burnout.

____

____

23. Identify four benefits for members of a national professional organization.

____

____

24. Identify four routes that an MA may take to advance his or her career.

____

____

CRITICAL THINKING ACTIVITIES

A. Preparing a Résumé

Complete the following information as a basis for preparing your résumé. Then create a professional résumé.

1. Identify the kind of job(s) you are looking for:

   First choice

   Second choice

2. Summarize your education beginning with your most recent:

   Name of school ______________________________

   City ______________________ State ______________________

   Dates attended: ______/______/______ to ______/______/______

   Degree: ______________________ Date: ______/______/______

Major (or courses completed if you did not graduate):

Awards, GPA (if higher than 3.0), Dean's list (dates):

Previous education (beyond high school)

Name of school ______________________________

City ______________________________ State ______________

Dates attended: ______/______/______ to ______/______/______

Degree: ______________ Date: ______/______/______

Major (or courses completed if you did not graduate):

____

____

Awards, GPA (if higher than 3.0), Dean's list (dates):

____

Provide information for other educational experience.

____

____

Other relevant training and dates of completion such as first-aid training, CPR training, and computer training.

Other skills including foreign languages spoken and skills you have learned but never practiced in an externship or work setting.

3. Summarize your experience in the health care field beginning with your most recent. Include your medical assisting externship.

   Name of organization or physician: ______________________________

   City ______________________________ State ______________

   Dates of experience: ______/______/______ to ______/______/______

   Type of experience or job title: ______________________________

   Indicate if the following apply: Externship/Practicum ________ Volunteer ________ Part-time ________

   Summer ________

Identify your duties and responsibilities, one per line. Use a consistent form (e.g., "prepared patients for examinations," "responsible for preparing patients for examinations").

____

____

____

____

Identify any special accomplishments, promotions, or other positive outcomes from this position.

____

____

Next most recent health-related experience:

Name of organization or physician: ____________________

City ____________________ State ____________________

Dates of experience: ______/______/______ to ______/______/______

Type of experience or job title: ____________________

Indicate if the following apply: Externship/Practicum ______ Volunteer ______ Part-time ______

Summer ______

Identify your duties and responsibilities, one per line. Use a consistent form (e.g., "prepared patients for examinations," or "responsible for preparing patients for examinations").

____

____

____

____

Identify any special accomplishments, promotions, or other positive outcomes from this position.

____

____

Next most recent health-related experience:

Name of organization or physician: ____________________

City ____________________ State ____________________

Dates of experience: ______/______/______ to ______/______/______

Type of experience or job title: ____________________

Indicate if the following apply: Externship/Practicum ______ Volunteer ______ Part-time ______

Summer ______

Identify your duties and responsibilities, one per line. Use a consistent form (e.g., "prepared patients for examinations," or "responsible for preparing patients for examinations").

____

____

____

____

Identify any special accomplishments, promotions, or other positive outcomes from this position.

____

____

Provide information for other experience in the health care field.

____

____

4. Identify work experience that is not related to health care. Include all full-time jobs, but if you have not been employed consistently, include part-time and/or summer employment, volunteer experience, or time spent as a homemaker.

   Employer (or organization): ______________________________

   City ______________________________ State ______________

   Dates of experience: ______/______/______ to ______/______/______

   Type of experience or job title: ______________________________

   Indicate if the following apply: Externship/Practicum ________ Volunteer ________ Part-time ________

   Summer ________

   Identify your duties and responsibilities, one per line. Use a consistent form (e.g., "prepared patients for examinations," or "responsible for preparing patients for examinations").

   ____

   ____

   ____

   ____

   Identify any special accomplishments, promotions, or other positive outcomes from this position.

   ____

   ____

   Provide information for other work experience.

   ____

   ____

   Next most recent experience:

   Employer (or organization): ______________________________

   City ______________________________ State ______________

   Dates of experience: ______/______/______ to ______/______/______

   Type of experience or job title: ______________________________

   Indicate if the following apply: Externship/Practicum ________ Volunteer ________ Part-time ________

   Summer ________

Identify your duties and responsibilities, one per line. Use a consistent form (e.g., "prepared patients for examinations," or "responsible for preparing patients for examinations").

____

____

____

____

Identify any special accomplishments, promotions, or other positive outcomes from this position.

____

____

Provide information for other work experience.

____

____

Next most recent experience:

Employer (or organization): ______________________________

City ______________________________ State ______________________________

Dates of experience: ______/______/______ to ______/______/______

Type of experience or job title: ______________________________

Indicate if the following apply: Externship/Practicum ________ Volunteer ________ Part-time ________

Summer ________

Identify your duties and responsibilities, one per line. Use a consistent form (e.g., "prepared patients for -examinations," or "responsible for preparing patients for examinations").

____

____

____

____

Identify any special accomplishments, promotions, or other positive outcomes from this position.

____

____

Provide information for other work experience.

____

____

B. Preparing a Cover Letter

Complete the following information to help you prepare a cover letter to accompany your résumé when you look for a job.

1. Describe in one sentence the reason that you are currently seeking a job.

____

____

2. Describe the type of position you seek (job title, full-time, and/or part-time) and when you will be available to begin working.

____

____

3. Describe your personal qualifications in a few sentences focusing on your strengths as a person, as well as your skills.

____

____

C. References

Complete the following information to help you prepare a list of at least three references. If possible, include a -supervisor from employment and/or externship and an instructor or coach from your educational program. Indicate if you have already obtained permission from the person to use him or her as a reference.

Name: ____________________ Permission Requested: ____________________

This person's relationship to you: ____________________

Contact information:

Employer: ____________________ Job Title: ____________________

Address: ____________________

Telephone Number: ____________________

Name: ____________________ Permission Requested: ____________________

This person's relationship to you: ____________________

Contact information:

Employer: ____________________ Job Title: ____________________

Address: ____________________

____

Telephone Number: ____________________

Name: ____________________ Permission Requested: ____________________

This person's relationship to you:

Contact information:

Employer: ____________________ Job Title: ____________________

Address: ____________________

Telephone Number: ____________________

Provide information for two other references.

____

____

D. Interview Questions

Prepare a personalized and thoughtful response to each of the following questions you might be asked during a job interview.

1. Where do you see yourself in 5 years?

____

____

____

2. Describe a difficult situation you have had at work and how you handled it.

____

____

____

3. What could you contribute to our office?

____

____

____

4. What are some of your weaknesses or areas you need to work on?

____

____

____

5. What would your medical assisting instructor say about you if I were to call her for a reference?

____

____

____